MODERN PERSPECTIVES IN PSYCHIATRY
Edited by John G. Howells

1

MODERN PERSPECTIVES
IN
CHILD PSYCHIATRY

MODERN PERSPECTIVES
IN
CHILD PSYCHIATRY

Edited by

JOHN G. HOWELLS
M.D., D.P.M.

Consultant Psychiatrist, Department of Family Psychiatry,
Ipswich and East Suffolk Hospital

INTRODUCTION TO THE AMERICAN EDITION
by
E. JAMES ANTHONY
M.D.

BRUNNER/MAZEL *Publishers* · New York

CONTENTS

★   ★   ★

PART ONE

SCIENTIFIC BASIS OF CHILD PSYCHIATRY

THE MAKING OF A DISCIPLINE

E. James Anthony
B.SC., M.D., D.P.M., F.A.P.A.

Blanche F. Ittleson Professor of Child Psychiatry,
Washington University School of Medicine, St. Louis
President, International Association of Child Psychiatry
and Allied Professions

The Clinician's Dilemma

Every psychiatric clinician worth his salt operates with a double set of aspirations that combine to make his life more dissonant than would seem necessary. One part of him would want to use himself as a sensitive clinical instrument functioning through a conglomerate of hunches, intuitions, preconcepts, subjective impressions and what D. H. Lawrence would refer to as 'belly feelings.' By means of such experiential 'frames' he develops the inward conviction of being in touch with the richer, more relevant and universal aspects of reality as pertaining to his patients. The other side to him, perhaps a relic of his earlier premedical and medical training, hankers after the testable, the measurable and the scientifically objective. However, in pursuing such canons, he may find himself reducing the total picture of reality to a more atomistic and statistically manageable form but at the same time losing in meaningfulness and validity.

Gill has aphoristically termed this "the dilemma between the significant and the exact," and every textbook that aims at being compendious tries to solve the problem by including a selection of both 'soft' and 'hard' facts, hoping thereby to satisfy both sets of needs. The present book is no exception to this general tendency and its editor acknowledges succinctly in his preface the unevenness prevalent in the field of psychiatry and the existence of untested speculations alongside systematic investigation and experiment. It would be too much to expect, even in a British textbook, even in a predominantly Maudsley one, that all speculation would be rigorously eradicated and that skepticism would reign supreme. The book, in fact, sets out commendably to reflect the state of the art, which is relatively muddled; and no attempt is made at an editorial level to resolve this confusion or speciously inject order or clarity or connection when this is contrary to the nature of things. The contributors were invited to be selective, not exhaustive in their reviews; but since they range, on a semantic differential, over extremes of tough- and tender-mindedness, hardness and softness, objectivity and subjectivity, and quantitativeness and qualitativeness, every degree of scientific tightness and looseness is present. On the whole, however, there is much less fiction present than there would be in a comparable American book, and far less dependence on mythology. Psychoanalysis is not regarded as providing a scientific basis to child psychiatry and receives not even a mention in the index—all of which would be inconceivable in a multi-authored volume generated in this country.

This will prove its main value in the United States: to present not so much a modern as a different perspective, and many American clinicians will profitably undergo a corrective cognitive experience to counterbalance their own staple viewpoint. To what extent will it help to resolve the clinician's dilemma? Hardly, if at all, since the significant and the exact are as much at odds here as in any local production. Loevinger has maintained that no one-sided resolution of this issue should be sought, since "the function of the researcher is to look for what is objective, behavioristic, and quantifiable without losing the sense of the problem." On the other hand, she felt that "the function of the clinician is to preserve the depth and complexity of the problem without putting it beyond the reach of objective and quantifiable realization." She added the humorous comment that "in the battle of the sexes, so in the clinical research dialogue, if either side wins, the cause is lost." Eysenck and Winnicott may make strange bedfellows and it may seem premature to put them together under the same bedclothes, but unless tentative efforts are made in this direction the clinician will try to resolve his dilemma by evading the issue. Here again this book scores on the side of scientific virtue, but not overwhelmingly, since one psychoanalyst does not make a Freudian millennium, especially when the factor analyst is dominantly represented.

Judging from the balance preserved in these pages, it would seem that the clinician in child psychiatry is fated for a good many years to live with these apparently incompatible scientific urges. He may perhaps even thrive clinically (albeit confusedly) on such a regime! More books with this amount of objectivity and empiricism will gradually make inroads on his subjectivity and propel him in the direction of greater exactitude and measurement; which brings me to consider the general state of the science (or art) of child psychiatry today.

The Problem of Science versus Art

If one were to be so bold as to equate the objective, testable and measurable with the scientific and the subjective, intuitive and qualitative with the artistic, then one might depict child psychiatry at its present stage as an art struggling to become a science, a metamorphosis to be desired, expected and encouraged, but for optimal functioning never to be completed if a clinical orientation is to be preserved. The scientific approach in its purest form could wither many a patient (or is this the clinician's bias?) unseasoned with those ineluctable attributes of empathy, sympathy and sensitivity. The right proportion for the mixture is a matter for the individual clinician and is largely self-selective. There are those who veer toward the art form, using their personalities and perceptiveness as instruments of therapy, and there are those who rely almost exclusively on external measures that can be carefully dosed. The particular proclivity is presumably determined by unknown psychodevelopmental forces.

The present status of child psychiatry also poses a developmental problem. Its precocious growth has precluded a solid scientific underpinning, so that it has become a discipline or developed the semblance of a discipline without undergoing a basic disciplinary training. Without the help of systematic research, its superstructure of ideas, culled from every conceivable source—from psychoanalysis to sociology—is in grave danger of subsiding. There is ample evidence, less apparent in this sensible book, of what Popper referred to as pseudoscientific tendencies, meaning the accumulation of beliefs and dogmatically held preconceptions that are mostly irrefutable, untestable, unrepeatable, but omnisciently interpretative.

A less critical assessment would be inclined to regard child psychiatry as a pre-science, occupied, as an appropriate reflection of its developmental stage, with relevance rather than rigor and with the assembling of broad-ranging observations rather than of conclusive evidence. The established sciences have all undergone such prescientific historical eras during which myth and magic have been ascendant, so it should not be surprising that newcomers repeat the same course. Perhaps it is asking too much of a young discipline, so strongly oriented toward treatment and amelioration, to exercise scientific rigor in its infancy. The psychiatry of adults is in much the same predicament, since not only are its origins immersed in witchcraft but its modern practice is no less infiltrated with magic. In fact, there is much to suggest that both psychiatries, of the child and the adult, are (citing Popper again) historical sciences whose fundamental activity is not in testing universal hypotheses and predicting specific events but in exploring the past and establishing continuities by means of meaningful connections (Jaspers' *Verständliche Zusammenhange*).

Whether it is at all possible to go beyond a pseudoscience, or pre-science or historical science, in dealing with such complex phenomena as human attitudes and behavior is a moot point. One can sharpen one's Occam razor and shave off redundant entities for the sake of reducing the diverse elements of psychopathological life to manipulable proportions, but often only at the expense of validity. One may need to recognize that there are unascertainable complexities that simply cannot be reduced without serious loss of meaning. It is again to the credit of this book that complexity is, for the most part, given its due, and attempts to attenuate it are confined to the chapters on learning theory, and expectably so. The S-R proponents have always been notoriously intolerant of labyrinthine complications and entanglements.

The capacity to live tolerantly with redundancy, ambiguity and incompatibility is not regarded here as a scientific virtue but as an inevitable, and perhaps necessary, phase of development. Its presence must remain a matter of concern to all workers in the field until manifestly shown to be unneeded. The tough-minded have raised objections that, generally speaking, prescientific techniques and attitudes do little more than foster a prescientific body of theory and delay the development of a genuine science. They have expressed alarm that uncontrolled and untested hypotheses will overwhelm the field and leave it a victim to idiosyncratic and whimsical ideas that do nothing but mischief. Speculators should be confined to their armchairs and relinquish the field to experimentalists. Bearing in mind Kurt Lewin's remark that there is nothing more practical than a good theory, how is it possible to discipline theorists to stay within the ambience of facts? This would be tantamount to smothering the infant science in its cradle. Ideas vary greatly in their usefulness and relevance; how can one recognize the good from the bad, the serious from the trivial, the productive from the worthless? Preceptors from the past have offered sage advice that is difficult to follow. Pasteur, for example, cautions the student while studying, observing and experimenting not to remain content with "the surface of things," but offers no suggestions as to how to recognize ideas in depth. Poincaré observes that ideas can be stratified hierarchically and that the worker should learn to eschew unproductive and to cultivate productive ones; but he fails to reveal how one can distinguish those of high yield. Polanyi's point of view is perhaps the most acceptable both from the aspect of generating new ideas and keeping the flow under control. According to him, any scientific field is exposed to the operations of "artificial selection" whereby the population of ideas at any particular time is kept within bounds by the formation of "minute inquisitions" conducted by the established roster of specialists. Although the inquisition insures that no unfounded propositions are let through, it unfortunately does not allow for the fact that well-founded propositions may also be kept out because they are disturbing to prevailing ideas or because they do not point in the direction to which scientific enthusiasm at that time happens to be channeled.

At the present time, it is obvious from this well-documented book that the 'inquisition' in child psychiatry is less critical than one might wish, but this again may be a reflection of the stage of a discipline-in-the-making. We need a large population of ideas if we are ever to learn how to ask the right questions to be tested. In place of a rigorous inquisition, the false elements can be gradually eliminated by a haphazard system of intuitions, guesswork, collective experience, past results, etc.; wobbly, but not unworkable. We can see all these at work in these various chapters. There is no concluding inquisition by the editor, but the reader is left to make his own 'artificial selection' from the population of ideas, which indicates succinctly the state of the art (or science). This inquisition of one is perhaps not the best way with which to govern a science but it is the best of all possible methods now.

Culture and Cognitive Style

A blind reading of papers from cross-cultural sources will convince anyone that cultures have cognitive styles and that irrespective of agreements or disagreements authors from the same scientific culture sound alike. Even such antithetical characters as Eysenck and Winnicott exude something peculiarly British and, although divided by theory, method and personality, are patently 'birds of a feather.' All the contributors exhibit this indefinable quality that cannot be quite explained in psycholinguistic or cognitive terms. An analysis of sentiment might bring one nearest to this shared generality. On completing one's reading of the book, even though many of the chapters are *réchauffés*, one is left with the impression of honesty, reliability, down-to-earth matter-of-factness, practicality, skepticism (in its best sense), modest understatement and helpfulness. One feels that most of these authors are doing their best to (using a current piece of jargon) 'tell it like it is' without coating the pill or gilding the gingerbread. They are never (or hardly ever) verbose or literary. The sparse style carries its own special conviction.

A second process of conditioning reinforces the first. People prefer to read authors with a similar cognitive style, and it is for this reason that science, as Rousseau reminded us, does not travel. Bibliographies are revealing in this respect. American writers for the most part quote American sources and the British tend to stick to their erstwhile empire. Some might find this insular but a majority should find it refreshing to be introduced to a different frame of reference with a different point of view set in a different style. How dull foreign travel would be if everyone spoke the same language! It is for this purpose that one hopes that many

American workers in the children's field will read this other account of their discipline.

Who Is a Child Psychiatrist?

Child psychiatry incorporates a host of professionals such as child psychiatrists, psychologists, social workers, psychotherapists, specialists in mental deficiency, special educators, speech therapists, child care workers and so on. This book is generally aimed at the child psychiatrist, which allows it to remain at a good scientific level. The basic model in the clinical section is a medical one and this enhances the unity of approach. An American textbook, lacking this basis in neuropsychiatry, would be more conflicted around this point and therefore more disparate in its presentation. For the general practitioner, not overly concerned with the dynamic trimmings, the British approach could be of more practical value since it presents the bread-and-butter of clinical work with much less recourse to interpretation and much greater emphasis on organization.

The British child psychiatrist is only now beginning to obtain a professional identity stemming from specialized training. There are as yet no divisions of child psychiatry in medical schools headed by professors of child psychiatry nor any endowed chairs of child psychiatry. The Americans are therefore ahead in terms of professional recognition, but they would still be most unlikely to produce a textbook of child psychiatry with a first half devoted to a scientific basis dealing with research methodology, ethology, genetics, Piagetian theory, learning theory and sections on perceiving, thinking, remembering, and imagining, and a second half to the clinical applications of these. Which leads us to wonder what is wrong with American child psychiatry and why is it that the British with a still poorly organized field of child psychiatry can bring out a book with at least some pretentions to being truly scientific.

This is not to say that this book is entirely successful in what it sets out to do. It is a sad commentary on child psychiatry that no child psychiatrist was found competent enough to contribute to the scientific basis of the book and bears out the miserable fact that child psychiatrists, apart from a few, are not researchers although passionate consumers of other people's research.

The book also fails to accomplish the mysterious leap from basic research and theory to clinical application that would have made the entire project a resounding success. The reason for this lies once again in the stage of the art (or the stage of the science). The art has mostly gone its own intuitive way because the scientific basis has been lacking. Now that a scientific basis has been provided, the gap between the basic scientist and clinician still remains to be bridged but it may take some time before the latter will avail himself of the new props provided. The basic science will need to be integrated into the training programs in child psychiatry before the gap can be closed. This will mean the creation of a new breed of child psychiatrists whose understanding of fundamental theory and research will not only equal their grasp of clinical practice but will in a real way contribute to it. The attempt made in this book to bring the science and art together, although tenuous at its best, is a genuine pioneering effort and needs to be brought to the notice of all practitioners in this field.

We have to remember that this accomplishment owes little to the academic organization of the field. Until recently in Britain the child psychiatrist could be anyone who had worked in a child guidance clinic or mental deficiency colony. Winnicott was of the opinion that any pediatrician who had been analyzed could function as a child psychiatrist, and Lewis, on the other hand, felt that any general psychiatrist could function as a child psychiatrist when confronted by a disturbed child. The Americans over the past two decades have insisted that only those who have received two years of supervised training at approved training centers are eligible to sit for the specialized examination in child psychiatry.

None of this will ensure the emergence of an authentic scientific discipline of child psychiatry. Only basic research in this field carried out by child psychiatrists familiar with the clinical problems of the field, only the systematic application of this basic research to the clinical case, and only a specialized training that teaches both the basic science as well as its application to clinical child psychiatry will ensure not only the survival of child psychiatry as a discipline but its continued growth as an applied science.

Having considered the book in general in relation to child psychiatry as an academic discipline in a state of rapid evolution, I want now to consider certain aspects of the book that have unusual interest to the field or are more than straightforward reviews.

N=1 and the Plausibility of Dr. Winnicott

Dr. Winnicott has spent most of his productive working life on the thin edge of probability and his dynamic 'brinkmanship' has brought many a tough-minded, hard-nosed, both-feet-on-the-ground organicist to his first exhilarating experience of the 'psychobiologically improbable.' He is as much a phenomenon on the British scene as Eysenck and has roused as much love and hate. It is well-nigh impossible for him to be unoriginal and, like Picasso, his bizarre 'squiggles' have opened up new worlds of psychological exploration. The magnificent thing about the 'squiggle' test, that makes it unlike any other, is that it is carried out in a mutual interchange with the patient. Its purpose is to reach rapidly into the interior of the patient and extract the essentials dealing with current problems in the outside world. Its method is to juxtapose the interacting 'selves' of tester and testee so that the two can procreate a deeper image ostensibly emerging from within one of them, preferably the patient. It is a most imaginative use of outer resources and is as good an externalizing method as the administrator makes it. It works for Winnicott but whether it would work for others is more than doubtful. As with some of Picasso's less earth-bound flights, it is not easy to evaluate the essential seriousness of the 'squiggle.'

For example, it is difficult to believe that with the help of eleven 'squiggles' highly significant and relevant data could be obtained on mother-fixation, early separation experience, the symptomatic consequence of a 'weaning gap,' the genesis of depression, the suppression of fantasy and the direction of sublimation; but, as James Whistler once retorted when challenged about the length of time it took to throw paint on a canvas, a lifetime of experience is represented in the interpretation offered. I would therefore be ready to accept Winnicott's translation of 'squiggle' language, although I would balk at believing that a defense mechanism such as splitting could be made to disappear as the result of three sessions. Defenses are not built in a day, nor do they succumb in an hour.

It is surprising how frequently Winnicott gets to the heart of the matter, and a good example of this is his comparison of child analysis and child psychiatry in their interminable and terminable perspectives. The analyst's motto is "how much may I be allowed to do in this case?" and the child psychiatrist's motto: "how little need I do?" My colleagues will not like this at all although most child guidance clinics in the United States are overburdened with cases, and community psychiatry with its emphasis on brief measures is an outcome of this situation. This is therefore not an example of psychoanalytic arrogance but a clear view of conditions, making full use of the 'facilitating environment,' an accurate history and the child's ability to take advantage of the professional helper to arrive at his 'areas of distress' where his incapacitating defenses were first organized. According to Winnicott, the child psychiatrist's job is to "help those who are doing the mental nursing to understand the value of what is being done."

Now what about the problem of N=1? Winnicott is aware of this when he remarks in a footnote that "naturally no one case can cover the vast range of child psychiatry" and promises a future book of many such cases. Nevertheless, the problem remains since the case of Mark is used prototypically. Now there is no doubt that Freud succeeded in making a number of valid generalizations on the basis of exceedingly minute samples but in the hands of lesser people this could and has proved disastrous. It is an axiom of modern empirical science that generalization across cases requires a sampling of many since the single-case method provides no indication as to whether a particular relationship applies to 'all others, many others, a few others or no others.' In technical language, there are zero degrees of freedom with regard to individual differences even though each observation may be founded on hundreds of degrees of freedom with respect to samples of the individual's behavior entering into the correlation between dependent and independent variables. This means, as Janis has emphasized, that the single-case commentator cannot be sure that his findings can be generalized to any broad class of individuals.

However, an N of 1 has been successfully employed by others besides Freud and one can cite in this context the classic work of Ebbinghaus on memory which was carried out on only one subject, namely himself. More recently, Dukes has discussed five conditions that would scientifically warrant the use of $N = 1$, and in one of these—problem-centered research—it can be extremely helpful in clarifying questions, defining variables and indicating approaches, which is somewhat descriptive of what Winnicott is attempting to accomplish with his squiggles. He himself would undoubtedly eschew this research jacket into which I have tried to fit him.

Sense and Nonsense, Fact and Fiction in Eysenckian Psychology

Gwynne Jones, a student of Eysenck's offers a fairly sound introduction to research methodology which should be made required reading for every resident in child psychiatry on this side of the ocean. So often residents leave their training centers as accomplished therapists but with little or no knowledge of how to carry out or assess research and with little or no enthusiasm for investigation. If this should continue, child psychiatry will gradually die as a scientific discipline. Child psychiatrists must learn to acquire reliable knowledge for themselves and not be so dependent on other disciplines. They have established a scientific symbiosis with psychologists, who supposedly provide them with a scientific basis which they can then supposedly apply to the treatment of patients. This is in theory. In practice, the child psychiatrist either altogether does without basic science, which he may see as too academically remote, or resorts surreptitiously or openly to the theory provided by psychoanalysis. The eclectic child psychiatrist borrows mostly from the clinical practice of neighboring disciplines—psychiatry, neurology and pediatrics—and rarely from different basic sciences. Much of this is exemplified in this present book, in which there should surely be an intermediate section demonstrating how the findings of basic science can be applied in practice to the clinical field. This missing section is a key enterprise for some future compendium.

Eysenckian psychology is not scientifically impressed by the clinician, particularly the dynamic psychotherapist, and there is sense to what Gwynne Jones says when he stigmatizes the tendency of clinicians "to develop an attitude of mind in which scepticism gives way to belief, humility to confidence, curiosity to dogmatism and respect for a theory is dependent more on its intellectual and emotional appeal, and the authority of its proposer than on its empirical validation." He is also right in pointing out that these tendencies are most evident in child psychiatry and I would agree with him that a major reason for this is that tenderminded humanitarians are especially attracted to work with children. In any meeting of child psychiatrists, 'bleeding hearts' are very much in evidence, so that a concentration of effort goes toward helping their patients with well-established methods rather than finding out new etiological facts about them.

Jones rightly dismisses the operability of the unhealthy symbiosis (verging on parasitism) between psychologist and psychiatrist and concludes that it is "better by far for each to carry out independent research, the psychologist employing the concepts of experimental psychology and making his own relevant observations, and the clinician employing the concepts of psychopathology and carrying out his own experiments." That is, if he can, but who is going to show him how, and is he likely to want to learn? This chapter should prove encouraging to him, especially if he can find reassurance in the remark that "the prime requirement for effective research is a certain attitude of mind, not methodological sophistication."

It is at this point that I would have parted company with Jones and constructed the rest of the chapter differently. For example, when discussing the tactics of science, he is likely to befuddle the timid reader that I have in mind by his exposition of the five classical methods of experimentation described by Mill over a hundred years ago. I would have introduced him gently to research design, research methods and elementary statistical analyses by means of real examples, step-by-step, rather in the way of the logical progression by which a case study is built up. What the average clinician needs is a good research cook book with all the ingredients nicely provided and with a nice end-product to whet his appetite and keep him interested. While I therefore applaud this first effort in child psychiatry to introduce the clinician to research, I think the future compendiums should bear in mind the way in which a clinician functions and build on that. It makes no sense to mention random sampling, tests of significance or null hypothesis in a few sentences when the clinical reader remains vague as to exactly what dependent and independent variables are.

The application of learning theory to child psychiatry is written with all of Eysenck's habitual skill and verve, so that one begins to feel that there must be *something* to this controversial factor analysis, especially when everything turns out so neatly and one feels with Pippa that God's in His heaven and all's right with the world. The chaotic lumber room of the average clinician's mind might feel that it seems too good to be true, but every resident should be exposed to the sharpness of thinking achieved by learning theorists. I would make it required reading for the new clinician to peruse the passage at the beginning of the section on personality, starting with: "Suppose we were to take a very large random group of children coming to a child guidance clinic; and suppose that we note down for each child the presence or absence of a large number of different items of behavior," and through the next six pages in order to obtain a brand new perspective on psychopathology. The plausibility of Dr. Winnicott to which we succumbed earlier is nothing compared with the plausibility of Dr. Eysenck, although the former is a divergent and the latter a convergent type of thinker. When Eysenck links his model to that of Galen, I become ready to allow that in spite of his basic lack of experience with emotionally disturbed children there must be something to his schema if Galen, separated by over a thousand years, arrived at similar conclusions. The introverted child who is neurotic has personality problems, conditions more rapidly and can be treated successfully by deconditioning; the extroverted child who is neurotic has conduct problems, conditions with difficulty and can be treated (less successfully) by socialization through conditioning and perhaps stimulant drugs. What more can one need?

Since learning theory is slowly penetrating some of the clinics in this country, this lucid account might help to pave the way for a good study by a conventionally trained research child psychiatrist whose positive findings might well start a new era in clinic practice. It should not be done by an Eysenckian psychologist because no one will accept the results in the guidance world, just as no psychotherapist has stopped practicing because Eysenck has demonstrated that his treatment is no better than no treatment.

What's Right with Child Psychiatry?

Having discussed so much that is deficient in the training and practice of the child psychiatrist, one must, for the sake of justice, add that this book generates a great deal of pleasure by its nice layout, the absence of gross overlapping of content and the final feeling it gives the reader that he has covered the known field such as it is. In this respect, the book does the field a good service in that it conveys an impression of systematized knowledge that is to some extent illusional. The average child psychiatrist has much less in his head than is in this book, especially in the portion contained in the basic science section. He will, therefore, feel more of a child psychiatrist having read this book than before, and it should make him aware that he has a discipline in which common sense, intuition and research have combined to produce an interesting and intriguing body of knowledge of which he should not feel altogether ashamed (British understatement!).

One gets a view of the child psychiatrist in relation to his basic science 'host,' the psychologist, and to the ethologist, the geneticist, the Piagetian, the learning theorist, the mental deficiency expert and many others who are out to help him in the way that they know how. The syndromes considered seem randomly selected but they do cover a lot of essential ground between them.

As one puts down the book, some very quotable and pertinent remarks stick in the mind. From the editor: "There is little doubt that we are on the edge of a more questioning attitude towards the scientific basis of psychoanalysis. In some quarters there is a desire to start afresh and to make a new approach based upon systematic research." This has been true for the last few decades in Britain, where psychoanalysis has always had a weak foothold, but it would take the British adventurous spirit 'to start afresh'; the American child psychiatrists are far too organized and stabilized to attempt anything so revolutionary; and why would they want to when, according to their experience, the 'tried and true' works so well.

Dr. Warren reminds us of the sad and surprising fact that after all these years we still lack an adequately controlled long-term follow-up study of children and adolescents with psychiatric disorders. Should this not have first priority in all future research plans in this field? Should not all children's psychiatric centers have built-in follow-up programs of the kind suggested?

Dr. Pinkerton insists that the investigation of psychosomatic disorders demands a "progressive liaison between the disciplines of paediatrics and child psychiatry, so that each reinforces the contribution of the other. In so doing," he says, "we subscribe to the fundamental principle of reintegrating psychological medicine with medicine as a whole. *There can be no finer aim.*" (My italics.) Dr. Pinkerton should speak for us all to pediatricians since he does so persuasively and in a style that would be acceptable to them. I cannot believe that they would reject him as they have rejected many child psychiatrists in this country who have abandoned their stethoscopes and distanced themselves from the medical world. A rapprochement will best be brought about within the marginal areas of brain damage and psychosomatic illness where the use of words as treatment can be made to assume a less prominent role. Furthermore, as the recruitment from pediatrics into child psychiatry increases, as it shows signs of doing, the professional gap should diminish.

Pinkerton alludes to another important disjunctive factor between the two disciplines that can and often does stand in the way of harmonious cooperation in the care of a shared patient. Pediatricians are trained to resolve presenting symptoms by direct treatment as early as possible in the course of a disorder, whereas the child psychiatrist, in contrast, is taught to tolerate the presence of symptoms and direct his attention to the underlying primary factors at the root of the disturbance. Pinkerton says, somewhat easily in my view, that these differing attitudes need not preclude a combined approach to therapy "provided certain safeguards are observed" such as the need to prevent unnecessary physical suffering on the part of the child. I feel that the differences involving time, tolerance and the appreciation of latent psychological forces are more complex and fundamental than he allows and may require repeated and open discussions between the two physicians and even then may foul the collaboration.

The great British empirical tradition comes to the forefront with regard to treatment and particularly in reference to the thorny problem of psychoanalysis. Eysenck espouses conditioning and deconditioning methods because they can be demonstrated to work and Rogers argues cautiously for their use in the future with the added hope that they may help us to increase our knowledge of child development and the development of neurotic illness. "For the time being," he concludes, "we still have to rely on our patiently-acquired empirical skills for much of the treatment of disturbed children." The system of therapy is of less importance to him. It can be couched in Freudian terms "or in those of any other psychological theory to which the therapist is himself an adherent" and the form it assumes will be determined by the child's needs and on the experience and inclinations of the therapist. The most crucial factor is *to make sense of the world* to the child and *to see the world through his eyes*. Without a comprehensive therapeutic system in one's armamentarium this empirical principle is as good as any that I know and should work out reasonably in practice. Group therapy with children is not a major dynamic undertaking in Britain as it is in the United States and Rogers is quite content to have it carried out by occupational therapists. The same is true of family therapy, which is regarded as a mild extension of casework rather than the intensive and technically difficult undertaking into which it has developed in this country. O'Gorman, in his discussion of childhood psychosis, again de-emphasizes the system in favor of ad hoc measures that work. Anyone can achieve success or partial success in the therapy of the psychotic child if he gives over one-fifth of his working day to the child, but this O'Gorman feels is economically impossible. Success is a function of relationship, not of systematic interpretation.

Whither Child Psychiatry?

This book therefore gives an excellent account of British child psychiatry in the latter part of this century. In its empirical philosophy and in its dedication to basic research it has a good deal to teach us in America. Many of the problems with which we are familiar here and which are part of the 'growing pains' (we hope) of a developing discipline receive mention, discussion or emphasis. The conflictual allegiances to medicine and the behavioral sciences seem less disturbing to our British colleagues, but one can sense the pinch every now and then in these pages. These developmental conflicts must then be looked upon as universal, inevitable and perhaps challenging. We must learn not only to live with them but also to thrive on them. We must continue to look to all sources that may help to enrich our theory and practice. I can best sum up my own particular attitude to the past, present and future of child psychiatry by quoting from an address given in the United States by someone, namely myself, who has lived in both worlds (British and American), and to this extent can boast a double perspective:

> In this presentation, I have described the history and progress of the child psychiatrist, who, having duly trained himself as a physician, wandered away into the distant realms occupied by the behavioral scientist—the psychologist, the anthropologist, the sociologist, the educationalist, the psychoanalyst, the philosopher, the social worker, even the economist. Over the past fifty years, he has ranged far and wide, retaining his umbilical tie to the medical world but taking whatever he could from every human experience, even from those whom his medical colleagues might be tempted to describe as charlatans. As Paracelsus said, "The universities do not teach all things, so a doctor must seek out old wives, gypsies, sorcerers, wandering tribes, old robbers and such outlaws and take lessons from them." It is to our great advantage today that William Withering followed this advice with respect to the foxglove. The child psychiatrist has now returned to the schools of medicine and is setting up divisions for this discipline within their walls. He appears ready to settle down and for the next fifty years devote himself to the construction and elaboration of a complex sociopsychobiological system whose concepts can be communicated to colleagues and taught to medical students and whose researches can be replicated around the globe. I am confident that he will not lose his contacts in the outside world and will continue to fraternize with the many friends he has made outside. From time to time, he must refuel by taking stock of the developments in the social sciences and carry them back to the medical and basic sciences. But he must wander, because he is a go-between for the two worlds and

he can serve the useful function of interpreting the one to the other. To quote Paracelsus again (who I am sure would be a psychiatrist if he were alive today), in his defense of his wayfaring: "The wanderings that I have this far accomplished have proved of advantage to me, for the reason that no one's master grows in his own house, nor his teacher behind the stove. Also, all kinds of knowledge are not confined to the fatherland but scattered throughout the whole world. They are not in one man nor in one place. They must be brought together, sought and found where they do exist. Is it not true that knowledge pursues no one but that it must be sought? It is written in the laws that a physician must be a traveler. Not merely to describe countries as to how they wear their trousers, but courageously to attack the problems as to what kind of diseases they possess. The English humors are not the Hungarian, nor the Neapolitan the Prussian; therefore you must go where they are. He who wanders hither and thither gains knowledge of many peoples—experience of all kinds of habits and customs, to see which one would be willing to wear out his shoes and hat. Does not a lover go a long way to see a pretty woman? How much better to pursue a beautiful art!"

In my own professional life, I have tried to practice what Paracelsus preached. I have wandered from one continent to another and have been instructed by the changes—the English humors are certainly not the American ones nor the English language the American language and English habits, apart from tea drinking, are peculiarly difficult to export. I have lived in medical schools most of my life but I have also wandered far and wide among the behavioral sciences. I have wandered between the world of research and of clinical practice. Having surveyed the field, I am deeply aware how much integration in these several fields of knowledge there remains to be accomplished in the next fifty years. Most of all, I have become aware, in wanderings, what an undeserved privilege it is "to pursue a beautiful art."

Center for the Advanced Study
in the Behavioral Sciences
Stanford University
1971

EDITOR'S PREFACE

Growth in psychiatry is necessarily uneven, as advances in the field occur here and there through special circumstances. The present series of 'Modern Perspectives' books aims at bringing the facts from the growing-points in the field of psychiatry to the clinician at as early a stage as possible. A complete coverage of psychiatry is therefore not attempted.

Child Psychiatry was selected for the first book in the series because this field has developed rapidly in recent years. That emotional illness can occur in children is now well recognised. Treatment at an early age not only brings relief to the child, but goes a long way towards guaranteeing emotional health in the adult. Furthermore the understanding of childhood psychopathology is relevant to the treatment of adult emotional illness.

In the past progress in Child Psychiatry has been handicapped by a superfluity of untested speculations. But systematic investigation and experiment are rapidly moving into Child Psychiatry and this is reflected in the first half of the book, which is devoted to the Scientific Basis of Child Psychiatry. The second half of the book covers clinical subjects in which recent developments are evident.

Each chapter is written by an acknowledged expert in that subject, who was entrusted with the task of selecting, appraising and explaining the available knowledge on his subject for the benefit of colleagues who may be less acquainted with it. The book will also be valuable to the psychiatrist in training. Each chapter is not an exhaustive review of the literature on the subject, but contains what the contributor regards as the important material in his field relevant to clinical practice. Thus the bias is clinical rather than academic.

Volumes in the 'Modern Perspectives in Psychiatry Series' are complementary. Readers interested in child psychiatry will wish to know of a companion volume 'Modern Perspectives in International Child Psychiatry', half of which is devoted to psychopathology and the other half to clinical topics. Furthermore, relevant chapters in 'Modern Perspectives in World Psychiatry' include the genetics of schizophrenia, sleeping and dreaming, learning therapy, family psychiatry, and an evaluation of psychoanalysis. These and other volumes are in active preparation at the time of this present reprint.

The Editor wishes to acknowledge his special indebteness to Mrs. Maria-Livia Osborn for her considerable assistance in his editorial work. Much of the preparation of the book is the result of her energetic, painstaking and thoughtful effort. The book has profited greatly from the impeccable literary work of Mr. F. B. Etherington of Oliver and Boyd.

Grateful acknowledgment is also made to the following publishers and editors of journals, and to the authors concerned, for kind permission to reproduce the material mentioned:

The *American Journal of Psychology* (Ch. V, Fig. 4, from an article by L. Ghent in Vol. 69, 1956); the American Orthopsychiatric Association, New York (Ch. V, Fig. 2, from L. Bender's *A Visual Motor Gestalt Test and its Clinical Use*, 1938); *Archives de Psychologie*, Geneva (Ch. V, Fig. 3, from an article by J. Piaget and B. Stettler-von Albertini in Vol. 34, 1934); the *British Medical Journal* (Ch. XIX, Tables I, II, from Dr. D. A. Pond's Goulstonian Lectures, 1961); Butterworth & Co. (Ch. XIX, Table III, from Holzel and Tizard's *Modern Trends in Paediatrics*, 1958); and Cambridge University Press and the Editor of the *British Journal of Psychology* (Ch. V, Fig. 2, from an article by D. E. Berlyne in Vol. 49, 1958).

J. G. H.

PART ONE

SCIENTIFIC BASIS OF
CHILD PSYCHIATRY

I

RESEARCH METHODOLOGY AND

CHILD PSYCHIATRY

H. Gwynne Jones
B.Sc., F.B.Ps.S.

*Senior Lecturer in Psychology, St. George's Hospital Medical School,
University of London*

1

Introduction

Effective clinical practice can only develop in the context of adequate theory concerning pathology. Equally, the adequacy of any scientific theory, although partly determined by its formal characteristics, is dependent upon the quality of the research on which it is based and the quality of the on-going research leading to its progressive modification and refinement. By 'quality' is meant not only the aptness of the design of experiments and the reliability and validity of the observational procedures and measuring techniques, but also the relevance and fruitfulness of the hypotheses tested, and the skill with which separate findings are integrated into a theoretical whole.

The formulation of hypotheses is the core procedure in research and the point at which art and science meet. No experiment can produce findings further-reaching than the implications of the hypotheses placed at risk. A brilliant hypothesis is one which is sufficiently abstract to bring into relation a wide range of apparently isolated facts within the field under study, and has logical implications leading to the formulation of subsidiary hypotheses and the discovery of new facts and relationships. Examples from the physical and biological sciences are well known, but Darwin's hypothesis of 'natural selection' might be mentioned as illustrating an important or even essential factor in the development of fruitful hypotheses. It is unlikely that Darwin could have arrived at his theory concerning the origin of species without being a naturalist who had steeped himself in observations of individual plants and animals over a wide range of species in many parts of the world. To attempt to theorise without adequate observation is to submit oneself to a form of scientific sensory deprivation which impoverishes the scientific intellect.

In the field of psychopathology it is the clinician who is richest in observational experience, and therefore might appear the most likely to make valuable contributions to research. The practitioner's main concern however is, and should be, the immediate welfare of his patients. He cannot withhold treatment when relevant current theories conflict and research findings are ambiguous, but must arbitrarily select working hypotheses and act on them with at least a show of confidence. His main guides in selection can only be common sense, judgement based on experience, and the authoritative statements of those whose professional opinions he has learned to respect. In these circumstances it is not surprising to note a marked tendency for clinicians to develop an attitude of mind in which scepticism gives way to belief, humility to confidence, curiosity to dogmatism, and respect for a theory is dependent more on its intellectual and emotional appeal, and the authority of its proposer, than on its empirical validation. After the completion of this process, and the achievement of seniority, the clinician is likely to make his own authoritative contributions to theory from speculations based on his experience with the claim that they have been verified in clinical practice, although that practice has not followed or may even have violated principles of scientific methodology. This does not imply that speculative generalisations of this nature are necessarily invalid, but merely that they are not necessarily valid and require empirical testing, with the normal scientific precautions against bias and error.

These tendencies are possibly more evident in child psychiatry than in any other branch of medicine. One important factor may be the natural selection by personality type which inevitably occurs during the course of medical training. All clinicians choose the ward and consulting room in preference to the laboratory, but those who enter psychiatry choose to maximise the subjective elements in their assessments and the interpersonal nature of their relationships with patients. Among these, the more tender-minded and humanitarian may be attracted to child psychiatry. Another factor is the lack of knowledge and the uncertainty, even at a taxonomic level, in this field of study.

Lest the last two paragraphs be interpreted as an attack on clinicians made for personal reasons, it may be politic to point out that even 'pure' researchers cannot escape social and psychological influences which tend to pervert their science. Provided it is consistent with known facts, a hypothesis which is falsified by testing is, scientifically speaking, quite as respectable as one which is verified, and by clearing valuable ground may serve a very useful purpose. It is the successful hypotheses, however, which engender a feeling of personal achievement, attract the congratulations of one's colleagues, and lead to professional advancement. The normal processes of social learning therefore foster a tendency for the researcher to become a person who is all too familiar—the 'scientist' who is wedded to a theory, and so neglects to test alternative explanations of his findings and ignores unfavourable evidence. Owing to the ambiguous nature of many psychological data this trend is more evident in psychology than in most other sciences. The dogmatic clinician may well be a successful and valuable therapist, but the dogmatic researcher is a hindrance to the advance of knowledge.

As many clinical and research procedures are mutually incompatible, one possible research strategy is to pair off clinicians and research workers, the former feeding their clinical insights to the latter, who then re-state them in formal terms as hypotheses to be tested in formal experiments. An added attraction of this possibility is that it suggests a fruitful form of collaboration between psychiatrists and psychologists. But in the writer's experience it seldom works in practice. One reason for this failure is that, inevitably, the conceptual systems within which the two members of the team are operating are essentially different, and this leads to a fatal distortion of communication. A second, even more important, reason is that each collaborator loses something vital by his failure to expose himself to the intellectual discipline of the entire research process. The clinician's reflections and speculations are likely to lose their sharpness and rigour from his delegation of the responsibility for testing their validity, and the researcher's experiments, even if methodologically elegant, are likely to be mechanical and sterile when not illuminated by the first-hand observations essential to fruitful research. Better by far for each to carry out independent research, the psychologist employing the concepts of experimental psychology and making his own relevant observations, and the clinician employing the concepts of psychopathology and carrying out his own experiments.

This is not to say that there cannot be fruitful collaboration of this nature in what might be called 'operational research', in which clinical instruments and procedures are submitted to critical examination, modification and re-examination. Experiments concerned with such matters as validating diagnostic procedures or assessing the effects of different forms of therapy would fit into this category.

The purpose of this chapter is to encourage interest in research and to give guidance on matters of methodology. Neither task is at all easy. It requires at least an entire book to deal at all adequately with the problems and methods of science, even without reference to the special problems of research in child psychiatry. Many volumes have been written on the topic, and it must be admitted that they can be very dull and forbidding to the casual reader. Initial interest can be rapidly smothered unless the reader is seeking assistance on a specific problem with which he is grappling. Then the pages spring to life with meaning and relevance. The first step, then, is not to study methodology but to select a problem, a real problem that confronts one daily in the clinic, and to embark on research into it: the rest inevitably follows. The shortcomings of the original crude design and makeshift measures become rapidly evident, and guidance can then be sought for their improvement. The prime requirement for effective research is a certain attitude of mind, not methodological sophistication. Any bias in the experimenter or in the experimental situation must be rigorously excluded or else allowed for, alternative hypotheses to account for the findings must be constantly sought and scrupulously tested, and errors in measurement must be estimated and taken into account when interpreting findings. Above all, prejudice and belief must give way to impartiality and scepticism.

Guidance in the design of experiments and the assessment of data may be obtained from many sources. Two excellent short works by A. E. Maxwell (8, 9), specifically intended for the clinician, may be especially recommended. These might be supplemented by an introductory book on descriptive statistics, e.g. Lindquist (7), and an excellent background account of the logic and methods of science is provided by Cohen and Nagel (3). The remainder of this chapter is devoted to a brief survey of the strategy and tactics of science, and to a consideration of the special problems of research in psychiatry with particular reference to child psychiatry.

2

The Strategy of Science

Science may be defined as organised or systematic knowledge, expressed in terms of general laws concerning events and the relationships between events. These laws facilitate the description of natural phenomena, and enable predictions to be made concerning future events. A highly developed branch of science is characterised by relatively few interrelated general laws or principles from which a great variety of specific propositions may be deduced. A definition of this nature however, while quite apt to science, is not sufficient to exclude other systematic accounts of similar phenomena. By these criteria astrology, for example, would rank as a science. To define science adequately reference must also be made to the method by which knowledge is acquired.

The term 'knowledge' implies a psychological state of belief, and beliefs can be arrived at and maintained in a variety of ways. Cohen and Nagel (3) list four main methods. The *method of tenacity* refers to the stubborn retention of an opinion which has become habitual, in the face of all contradictory evidence. The *method of authority* requires an appeal to some highly respected source, and is characteristic of religious and many political beliefs. Appeal to authority in the form of an expert is inevitable in many situations where an individual lacks the knowledge or skill to arrive at a well-founded opinion of his own, but this does not necessarily imply a belief in the infallibility of the authority. The *method of intuition* is the appeal to self-evident truths such as: 'The shortest distance between two points is a straight line', 'No event can occur without a preceding cause', or 'The Earth is flat.' The *method of reflective inquiry* is the method of science, and aims at independence from subjective bias by examining the relationships between objective data in a logical manner which can be repeated on different occasions and by different individuals. It differs from the other methods in that the beliefs arrived at are tentative, and that the method is flexible, self-correcting and progressive.

Observation and Problem Selection

The starting-point of any scientific inquiry is the recognition of a problem, an area of doubt, so that some informal observation and sifting of the data must occur before research even begins. The selection of the problem area implies the attachment to it of special importance, and therefore indicates that certain preconceptions, the germs of hypotheses, have already formed in the researcher's mind. Such preconceptions are equally evident in the next stage, that of systematic observation in relation to the problem. Observation is never random, attention being directed to those variables which are considered to be relevant to the problem. This selection of variables again indicates the implicit formulation of hypotheses whose nature is partly determined by the observer's knowledge and background. In child psychiatric research, for example, the variables stressed by paediatricians, psychiatrists, psychologists and sociologists may be very different. The majority of scientific observations require the use of special instruments, and the observer has to acquire special skills before he can make use of them and interpret their 'readings'. In the advanced sciences these readings are all measurements of some type, and observation is directed towards the establishment of mathematical relationships between variables.

Closely related to problem selection and observation is the question of classification, which is an important aspect of science. Taxonomic problems loom particularly large in the earlier stages of development of a science. Later, when taxonomic systems are well established, they tend to appear self-evident, but there is no criterion by which one system of classification may be considered more natural than another. The choice between taxonomic systems must be determined by their relative scientific utility. In any classification a trait or group of traits possessed in common is selected to define a class. Thus a porpoise may be classed with the fishes by virtue of its aquatic habitat, external form and method of locomotion, or it may be placed in the mammalian group by virtue of its mammary glands and habit of suckling its young. The latter classification is superior because it leads to more highly organised knowledge of the relationships between animals.

Hypotheses and their Verification

A research project takes a major step forward when the researcher is able, on the basis of his observations and previous knowledge, to suggest a tentative solution of the problem and to state it formally as a hypothesis. A hypothesis differs from a hunch by satisfying certain formal requirements. Primarily it must be verifiable, which means that it can be put to an experimental test. Certain simple hypotheses can be directly tested, but many of the most important scientific hypotheses cannot. These must be so stated that certain logical consequences may be deduced which are themselves testable. For example, Newton's hypothesis of gravitation cannot be directly tested, as no direct observation of the mutual attraction of bodies, proportional to their masses but inversely proportional to the square of their distances, is possible. Implicit in the hypothesis, however, are various empirically testable consequences concerning such superficially different phenomena as the behaviour of tides and the orbits of the planets. The concept of gravitation has the status of a *hypothetical construct* or *intervening variable* in Newton's theory. It is an unobservable which is *operationally defined* by relating it to observables such as those mentioned.

A hypothesis is put forward to account for known facts by describing those facts in an abstract, general and economic fashion. It is essential that logical analysis should be able to show that the relevant facts are described in this way. A hypothesis gains in power, however, when it can be shown to *predict* new facts. Several alternative hypotheses may account equally well for a given set of facts. The choice between them must then rest on the verification of empirical predictions derived from their logical consequences. If two hypotheses do not differ in their logical consequences they only differ in language and, for scientific purposes, are identical unless they can be distinguished in terms of parsimony. A parsimonious hypothesis is one which refers to few systematically interrelated assumptions, and is to be preferred to a hypothesis which, in addition to its main assumptions, includes special *ad hoc* assumptions in order to embrace the full range of relevant facts.

That a hypothesis should be capable of verification implies that it must also be capable of refutation. An excellent illustration is given by Cohen and Nagel. They consider the proposition 'All men are mortal', and point out that, no matter how old an individual man they produce, the proposition cannot be refuted. To become a scientific hypothesis this proposition would need to be modified to a statement such as 'All men die before their two-hundredth birthday'. It is on grounds of lack of refutability and parsimony that many object to psychopathological hypotheses which include the *ad hoc* assumption that, when the behaviour predictable from the main assumptions does not occur, this is due to a 'reaction formation'.

Refutation is of vital importance in science because, although a hypothesis may be verified in a number of particular instances, it can never be confirmed in the sense that it is demonstrated to be true. Each verification increases the confidence with which further predictions can be made, but a scientist can only deal with probabilities, selecting at any one time the hypothesis which is most probable in terms of empirical evidence. A single refutation invalidates a hypothesis in its existing form, although it may survive by the modification of one or more of its assumptions to meet the new facts. Such progressive modification of theory is an essential aspect of science, and, although *ad hoc*, is entirely justified if the new formulation retains its systematic quality and remains as testable as the old.

Consider some hypothesis, *A*, which has the logical implication that event *B* will occur in circumstances *C*. Failure of *B* to occur under conditions *C* is a refutation of *A*, and at the same time makes it logically untenable. When *C* does produce *B*, however, although this is consistent with *A* it may also be consistent with any number of alternative hypotheses, and the possibility that *A* is invalid remains. No finite number of demonstrations of *B* being associated with *C* ensures that this is universally true, any more than finding that every single Irishman one has met has been hot-tempered proves that the same is true of all Irishmen.

A final point about hypothesis selection is that, although the problem being considered may be highly specific, the hypotheses selected for testing should usually be closely related to the main concepts of the general field of study and to current hypotheses in neighbouring problem areas. The aim of any branch of science is to unify knowledge over a broad field, by developing an integrated theory employing a limited number of concepts and systematically interrelated hypotheses in the form of general laws. When, as sometimes happens, a fresh problem forces the development of new concepts and novel hypotheses, this stimulates a re-examination of the entire theoretical structure of the science, and may result in major advances.

3

The Tactics of Science

The discussion so far has been concerned with the broad strategy of science and its logical bases. Equally important are the more detailed tactics employed in specific experiments. These vary according to the nature of the problem and the variables under examination; nevertheless certain general principles may be recognised, and five classical methods of experimentation were described by John Stuart Mill (10) on the basis of earlier suggestions by Francis Bacon. In general, a scientific problem presents itself when unpredictable changes are observed in what is then called the *dependent variable*. Hypotheses are formulated by which these changes are postulated to be associated with or dependent upon changes in one or more *independent variables*. Experiments are carried out to examine and describe the nature of the relationships between the dependent and independent variables, by varying each independent variable systematically and measuring the concomitant changes in the dependent variable. The principle of control requires that all variables other than the independent and dependent variables be held constant: the relationship between the volume and the pressure of a gas, for example, could not be ascertained if the temperature were allowed to vary. Other points for tactical consideration are the method to be adopted to vary the independent variable, the nature of the variations, and the accurate measurement of the concomitant variations of the dependent variable.

Mill's Canons

Mill's experimental canons indicate five basic methods of scientific inquiry:

The Method of Agreement. By this method an invariable antecedent or 'cause' of a phenomenon is sought by examining the antecedents of a plurality of instances of the phenomenon, until a single common antecedent is observed. This is more a principle for systematic observation and hypothesis construction than an experimental method, and fails when the dependent phenomenon, as defined and measured, is a consequence of any one of a number of antecedents. A great many detailed case studies of backward readers or enuretic children, for example, fail to reveal any single circumstance common to all instances. Yet several antecedents which only occur in a proportion of instances have been shown not to be irrelevant to these conditions.

Nevertheless the method of agreement can be useful in eliminating irrelevant circumstances, and is the method underlying the popular medical technique of studying series of patients with a common disorder. If the series is sufficiently large and representative to eliminate chance bias this certainly provides an economical and accurate account of the characteristics of the disorder, but, without the concomitant study of appropriate control groups, the description will include many non-differentiating features.

The Method of Difference. This method introduces the principle of control, instances of both the presence and the absence of the phenomenon under investigation being studied to check on the concomitant presence and absence of the postulated causal antecedents. The strict application of the principle of control is necessary, as the positive and negative instances need to be alike in all other relevant respects. Such a condition is usually impossible to fulfil when only a single pair of instances is studied. Mill was aware of this difficulty and proposed a third method, *the Joint Method of Agreement and Difference*, which is essentially the extension of the method of difference to groups of positive and negative instances.

Frequently, in practice, it is effects rather than causes which are investigated, the positive and negative groups being assembled in terms of the presence or absence of the independent rather than the dependent variable. A psychiatric example would be an investigation of the psychological effects of brain damage, for which a group of brain-damaged patients would be matched, in terms of age, sex, socio-economic status, education and pre-morbid intellectual ability, with a control group of normal subjects, and both groups examined for the postulated effects. Such a study would require additional control groups if the aim was to discover characteristics which differentiated brain-damaged patients from those suffering from other disorders such as psychosis.

The danger with this, as indeed with all, scientific methods is that there is no adequate safeguard against the fallacy of *post hoc, ergo propter hoc*, and no assurance, even when necessary conditions are established, that these are sufficient conditions for the appearance of the phenomenon. Confidence in the findings is vastly increased when one does not need to rely on naturally occurring variations in the independent variable, but can experimentally vary it in a predetermined fashion. This also brings the dependent variable under control and makes possible the practical application of the findings. The distinction between pure and applied science is in many ways artificial, and successful applications may be considered as powerful tests of hypotheses.

The Method of Concomitant Variation. The previous methods are qualitative in nature, requiring the presence or absence of some quality. Difficulties arise when negative instances of a variable cannot be observed. It may then be possible to observe or experimentally induce variations in the magnitude of the variable and look for concomitant variations in related variables. This is the method underlying the establishment of the mathematical laws relating quantitative variables such as volume and pressure in physics, and the less precise reports of *correlations* between variables in psychology and psychiatry. It is a truism to point out that the demonstration of a correlation does not necessarily imply a direct causal relationship, although it supports or may suggest a hypothesis that such a causal relationship exists. Lack of correlation does imply the absence of such a relationship.

When there is a dependent relationship, a correlation cannot indicate its direction. Again this requires the deliberate experimental variation of the postulated independent variable and consequent control of the dependent variable. A demonstrated relationship need not necessarily apply outside the range of variation actually observed.

The Method of Residues. Mill's final method refers to the demonstration of residual systematic variation when known effects are allowed for. A clear example is the discovery of Argon: the expected density of air, calculated from the densities and proportions of its known components, differed from its measured density and indicated the presence of another constituent. In botany, the failure of an appropriate combination of known nutrient substances to support healthy growth led to the discovery of the nutritional importance of trace elements. Less formally, the effects of long-term institutionalisation suggest that the institutional environment lacks certain characteristics of normal social life which are essential to mental health.

Mill proposed these five methods as infallible techniques for the discovery of new knowledge concerning the causes of phenomena. In practice, they cannot even be operated unless preliminary observation and hypothesis construction have suggested the important independent and control variables to be taken into account. Without such selection no experiment would be possible. A discussion of the concept of causality is beyond the scope of this chapter, but the aim of scientific inquiry is the discovery of invariant relationships between variables. In some instances this may be a symmetrical co-relationship, neither variable taking precedence; in others, one (independent) variable precedes the other (dependent) variable in time. Then the former is frequently described as the 'cause' and the latter as the 'effect'.

Other Research Methods

Biological and, in particular, psychological research since the time of Mill have led to the recognition of three other research methods which are important in these sciences:

The Evolutionary or Genetic Method. This method is based on the fact that phenomena may be interrelated by occurring in a developmental sequence, and research is aimed at the discovery of systematic changes in the characteristics of an organism which occur as a function of its age or maturational status, or in which the emergence of a characteristic is dependent on the prior emergence of related characteristics. The genetic method is, of course, particularly relevant to child psychology and psychiatry because of their dependence upon knowledge concerning child development. Piaget's studies of the stages in the development of concepts and conceptual schemata are examples of the application of this method (e.g. 12, 13, 14).

Genetic studies in psychology may be carried out in three ways, each with advantages and disadvantages. The most common method, and the one adopted by Piaget, is *cross-sectional.* Groups of children, each group representing an age level within the span to be covered, are studied simultaneously. The trend of the differences between successive age groups is considered to represent the developmental sequence of the characteristics observed and measured. The main advantage of this technique is that it is economical, allowing conclusions to be drawn about phases in development in a shorter time than that required for the phase to be completed in a developing individual. The main disadvantage is an inevitable violation of the principle of control. Children who were a certain age some years ago cannot be assumed to have been similar in all relevant respects to children of that age now. Social and educational factors, among others, may vary considerably from one period to another. This is well illustrated in another context by studies of the decline of intelligence in the later years of life.

Here cross-sectional studies indicated that such a decline commenced fairly early, even for abilities dependent on previous learning such as vocabulary. More recent studies, however, by use of the *longitudinal method* demonstrate that an individual may continue to extend his vocabulary even into old age. The cross-sectional research had failed to allow for the far more limited educational opportunities of the older subjects.

In the longitudinal method this type of error is avoided, since the same individuals are studied at different ages. This is an example of control by matching, no closer matching of groups being possible than to make different sets of observations of the same subjects on different occasions. The passage of time between the different ages studied cannot be avoided, however, and very little control is possible of the environmental influences to which each individual is subjected between successive assessments. A seven-year-old is potentially many different eight-year-olds, and the particular eight-year-old ultimately studied can only be an imperfect match to himself when younger, and may have undergone certain experiences which directly influence one or more of the variables being investigated. The changes observed cannot then be treated simply as a function of the difference in age. One of the main advantages of the longitudinal method in developmental studies is that it requires the maintenance of close contact with a group of children over a long period, thereby providing an excellent opportunity for the formulation and testing of hypotheses concerning environmental influences affecting development. It is the only satisfactory method when the subsequent courses of development of young children who differ in respect of some non-enduring characteristic are to be compared. For example, if the long-term effects of different responses to toilet training are to be studied, it is important that groups be assembled in the light of careful and systematic first-hand observation of the children's behaviour in the toilet-training situation.

When a longitudinal study is not possible in these circumstances, the experimenter has to resort to the third, the *retrospective*, method of study, reliance being placed on a historical account provided by an unskilled observer in close contact with the child, usually the mother. Such accounts are far from reliable even when restricted to contemporaneous events and behaviour. When retrospective, various additional sources of bias and error make them extremely unreliable. Undoubtedly the main weakness of most research in child psychiatry is that the data are acquired in this way. The retrospective method is most useful when used to supplement cross-sectional studies as a check on environmental factors which might influence the findings.

The Comparative Method. This method is based on reasoning from analogy and the assumption of fundamental similarity in biological processes in different species. In its main form it is the phylogenetic equivalent of the previous, ontogenetic, method. For example, the process of learning shows essential similarities in mammalian and even lower species. Many of the complicating factors in human learning are absent or can be strictly controlled in animal experiments. Thus contemporary learning theory, which is claimed to apply to human beings, is largely based on experiments with the albino rat. Light is considered to be thrown on the manner in which human and rat learning differ by the findings from experiments with chimpanzees and other primates. The comparative method is not however restricted to phylogenetic studies, but may be used in investigations in which the responses of different groups within a species, subnormal and normal children for example, are compared.

Child psychology is linked with the comparative method in two ways. Firstly, in the manner described, developmental studies of lower species are considered to be relevant to theories of child development. Secondly, child studies may be important elements in mixed phylogenetic/ontogenetic investigations. Thus the comparative learning studies already mentioned have been extended with great advantage by carrying out analagous experiments through the series: rats, chimpanzees, pre-verbal children, verbal children and human adults.

The Statistical Method. Statistical procedures have two roles in research: not only do they provide tools for the efficient presentation, description and analysis of data, but also modern statistical science, based on the logic of inductive reasoning, is concerned with the actual design of experiments. It is the latter usage which is implied in the term 'statistical method'; and it is of great importance in psychiatric research whenever, in addition to the independent variable being experimentally manipulated, a host of other variables, many unknown, are related to the dependent variable and, according to the principle of control, need to be held constant. This is impossible in practice, and control has to be exercised statistically.

Statistical arguments are expressed in terms of probabilities and 'chance', and statistical designs ensure that chance is given full scope for its operation. For example, to test a hypothesis that two treatments, *A* and *B*, have differential effects on children of a certain type, it is first necessary to assemble a *sample* from the *population* of children of this type. This sample should be *random*, i.e. each member of the population should have an equal chance of being included in the sample. Then the members of the sample should be randomly assigned to each treatment, and the effects measured. It is then possible to apply a statistical *test of significance* to the difference observed. This is not a direct test of the initial hypothesis, but a test of the *null hypothesis* that the difference is no greater than might occur, through the chance distribution of uncontrolled factors, between any two samples from this population given identical treatments. The test results in a probability statement, and if the probability that the null hypothesis is tenable is slight, it is rejected, and the original hypothesis gains support. The statistical experimental designs most frequently employed in psychiatric research are fully described by Maxwell (8, 9) in the books previously mentioned.

4

Complicating Factors in Psychological Research

The multiplicity of relevant variables has already been mentioned as a complicating factor in psychiatric research. Further complications arise from the fact that these variables frequently interact in a variety of ways. The relationship between any particular pair of independent and dependent variables need not be linear. Scholastic performance, for example, is affected by anxiety, but whereas in the low-anxiety range increased anxiety is associated with higher attainment, this relationship is reversed in the high-anxiety range. Anxiety itself is the product of the interaction of other variables. Special experimental designs and statistical techniques of analysis have been devised to deal with some of these difficulties.

A major source of difficulty in all psychological research is that a human being, unlike an inanimate object, is modified by the very processes of observation and measurement. When an investigation requires repeated assessments, it is essential to include controls for practice effects. Possible placebo effects of various types also need to be taken into consideration. The measurement of psychological variables presents special problems; but these will not be discussed here, as a later chapter is devoted to this topic.

Theoretically many of these problems could be solved by the rigorous application of appropriate complex experimental designs, but a frequent insuperable difficulty, especially in psychopathological research, is that for obvious ethical and practical reasons the variables cannot be experimentally controlled and conclusions have to be drawn from "experiments of nature'. Inevitably, sampling and control is imperfect in these circumstances and the conclusions reached must remain very tentative. Cross-validation, which is always important, is then essential, and should be sought in situations as different as possible from those in which the earlier observations were made. It is often valuable to work out a theoretically adequate experimental design, and then to collect data from naturally occurring events to satisfy the requirements of this design as far as possible. Bowlby's (1) work on the effects of early deprivation is an excellent example of this approach. His early hypotheses have been considerably modified in the light of later work by himself and others (2, 11).

A danger which is frequently difficult to avoid in clinical research is that of criterion contamination, overlap in the assessment of the independent and dependent variables. The scientific weakness of clinical assessment is its global nature and lack of clear specification of the criteria employed. If, for example, it is intended to test the hypothesis that spatial disabilities are characteristic of brain-damaged children by comparing the scores of two groups, brain-damaged and normal, on tests of spatial ability, then it is essential that evidence of spatial disability (from behaviour at interview or informants' accounts) be excluded from the criteria by which children are allocated to the brain-damaged group. Otherwise the findings merely express a tautology, not a relationship between variables. Strauss and Lehtinen's (15) work on brain-injured children is badly marred by this type of contamination.

The special difficulty of child psychology and psychiatry is that the object of study is a developing organism. The actual processes of maturation are studied by the genetic and comparative methods already discussed, but maturational change must also be taken into account, by the operation of experimental control, in the investigation of other processes in children. If for example it is postulated that some environmental influence or pathological process has a harmful effect on the intellectual functioning of a child, this does not necessarily imply that the child's scores on tests of intellectual ability will decline, but that they will not improve at the same rate as those of normal children of the same age and original intellectual status. Much research in child psychology has been concerned with the relative importance of maturation and learning in the acquisition of various skills. Many of the most important experiments in this area derive their value from the high level of control of maturational factors achieved by the use of uniovular twins as matched experimental subjects submitted to different training programmes.

A special feature of maturation, creating major problems for child psychiatry, is the inability of young children to communicate verbally. This prevents the use of the classical methods of adult psychiatry, and has led to the development of play techniques. Responses made in a play situation however, when treated as communications, are altogether more ambiguous than the verbal responses of an adult during an interview. Unfortunately a great deal of child psychiatric research is reported as if no such ambiguity exists, although it is clear that different investigators make very different interpretations of very similar behaviour. Communication is a process worthy of investigation in its own right, and, influenced by developments in information theory, psychologists have paid increasing attention to it in recent years. Investigations into the communicative aspects of play could be of great value to child psychiatry. Meanwhile the conclusions of clinical researchers would be more soundly based if hypotheses deriving from observations of play were tested by varying some aspects of the play experimentally, and making predictions concerning effects observable outside the play situation.

Classification has been mentioned as an essential step in scientific investigation. There is a well-established nosological system in adult psychiatry which, although in many respects inadequate, is clinically useful. Also in the adult field, more experimental approaches to taxonomy, such as that of Eysenck (5), consistently yield quantitative dimensions which can be reliably measured and are relevant to both normal and abnormal psychology. In child psychiatry, however, not only cannot unique pathognomic signs be identified, but classification of disorders in terms of patterns or syndromes is extremely difficult.

Many of the difficulties and complicating factors are demonstrated in a statistical study by Collins *et al.* (4), who examined the correlations between the entries in an 'Item Sheet' routinely completed for all the patients attending a child psychiatric clinic. Children regarded as epileptic, psychotic or very dull were excluded from the sample. The most striking finding was the small amount of correlation in the data, implying that in respect of characteristics of psychiatric interest the children were extremely heterogeneous. The 'factors' emerging from the analysis of the low correlations observed were different for each sex and for different age levels. For example, boys and girls of 8–10 years are each described by three factors. For boys the first factor, labelled 'rebelliousness', refers to disobedience, destructiveness and aggressive behaviour. The second, described as 'rootlessness', refers to lack of a parent or enduring parent substitute or some similar deprivation. The data for girls of the same age also produce a rebelliousness factor, but for them items implying 'rootlessness' are closely associated with this factor, suggesting that a girl of this age who is well established in an enduring family situation is unlikely to rebel, whereas a boy may become aggressive with any type of home background. The second girls' factor is formed by items describing a backward, nervous child who is failing scholastically and socially at school. This factor did not appear in the boys' data. A third, 'anxiety' factor is evident in both boys' and girls' data.

5

Conclusion

A discussion of the difficulties encountered in psychiatric research cannot be concluded without mention of the gap between the complexity and sophistication of many theories widely accepted as valid, and the inadequacy of the empirical data which support them. The failure to submit psychopathological hypotheses to rigorous and repeated empirical validation has had the cumulative effect that many current hypotheses are so formulated that not only is a direct test impossible, but testable consequences cannot be unequivocally deduced from them. They may not be illogical, but they are unscientific by the criteria employed in this chapter. Their intellectual appeal derives from the subjective feeling of 'understanding', and the ability to 'explain' psychological events, once they have occurred, which comes from their use. Their weakness lies in the impossibility of using them to predict future events from knowledge concerning the relevant independent variables.

Owing to the nature and demands of clinical work discussed earlier, it is not surprising that theories of this nature are popular with and even useful to clinicians. They provide a rationale for procedures employed in a situation where action cannot be deferred until more satisfactory procedures are available. Research, however, does not require an elaborate theory, and when a clinician adopts the role of researcher, he should be prepared to limit his theoretical preconceptions to a few relatively simple and clearly testable hypotheses directly relevant to the problem being investigated. Although, even if verified, these may have very limited potentialities for practical application, it is only on the basis of well validated hypotheses of this nature that adequate psychopathological theories can be constructed. A complex theory is, anyway, usually impossible to test *in toto* within the scope of a single investigation, because of the impossibility of systematically varying all the relevant variables in an appropriate manner. Such a theory gains support from the repeated testing of one or more of its consequences, implicit or explicit, in a wide range of experimental investigations.

Research in a clinical setting is complicated by the fact that a clinician is required to deal with a succession of individual cases which cannot, usually, be selected to conform with a prearranged plan of research. One consequence of this is that psychiatric literature abounds with single case studies which, although many may be of didactic value, are mostly of very limited scientific value. Of course, scientific method is entirely applicable to individual cases, and much may be gained by treating the investigation of a single patient as a research problem in miniature (see Jones (6)). A generalisation shown to be valid for one patient often suggests a fruitful hypothesis concerning the disorder from which the patient is suffering, relevant to many patients of the same type.

One way in which a complex theory may be tested is by validating the specific predictions which derive from it concerning a series of individual patients. This type of validation is claimed for most psychopathological theories, but the claim is seldom justified. To test a theory adequately in this way it would be necessary to make formal records of the predictions applicable to each patient, ensuring that the predictions were necessary consequences of the theory, different from those which would be made from rival theories, and of the type which can be unequivocally confirmed or shown to be false. In practice, predictions of this nature are only possible when linked with experimental control of some independent variable. Thus, for example, in child psychopathology acceptable predictions might be of the type: 'If interpretation A is made of the child's play, his play will alter in specified manner X, his behaviour in relation to his mother in specified manner Y, and his responses to test P in specified manner Z.' Provided that such predictions and the tests are reliable in the sense that there is a high level of agreement between different predictors and assessors, the evidence accumulated over a series of cases would be of immense value in assessing the validity of a theory. Even then, however, the statistical analysis of the data would present great difficulties owing to lack of independence between the predictions made about a single individual, and the difficulty of assessing the *a priori* probabilities of many of the predictions.

Many other difficulties of a more specific nature inevitably present themselves in the course of any child psychiatric research, but sufficient have been mentioned in this survey to explain the paucity of well validated findings, and to emphasise the necessity for the researcher to re-examine his procedures constantly, seeking ways to improve his control of relevant variables and eliminate sources of bias in his data. Abstract methodological principles can only indicate the main directions of improvement: the ultimate efficiency of an experimental design depends upon the skill and ingenuity of the experimenter.

REFERENCES

1. BOWLBY, J., 1952. *Maternal Care and Mental Health.* Geneva: World Health Organisation Monographs.
2. BOWLBY, J., AINSWORTH, M., BOSTON, M. and ROSENBLUTH, D., 1956. The effects of mother-child separation: a follow-up study. *Brit. J. Med. Psychol.*, **29**: 211.
3. COHEN, M. R. and NAGEL, E., 1949. *An Introduction to Logic and Scientific Method.* London: Routledge & Kegan Paul.
4. COLLINS, L. F., MAXWELL, A. E. and CAMERON, K., 1962. A factor analysis of some child psychiatric clinic data. *J. Ment. Sci.*, **108**: 274.
5. EYSENCK, H. J., 1952. *The Scientific Study of Personality.* London: Routledge & Kegan Paul.
6. JONES, H. G., 1960. Applied abnormal psychology: the experimental approach. *In* EYSENCK, H. J. (ed.), *Handbook of Abnormal Psychology.* London: Pitman.
7. LINDQUIST, E. F., 1942. *A First Course in Statistics.* Boston: Houghton Mifflin.
8. MAXWELL, A. E., 1958. *Experimental Design in Psychology and the Medical Sciences.* London: Methuen.
9. 1961. *Analysing Qualitative Data.* London: Methuen.
10. MILL, J. S., 1856. *A System of Logic.* London: Longmans.
11. O'CONNOR, N., 1956. The evidence for the permanently disturbing effects of mother-child separation. *Acta Psychol.*, **12**: 174.
12. PIAGET, J., 1928. *Language and Thought of the Child.* London: Routledge & Kegan Paul.
13. 1950. *Judgement and Reasoning in the Child.* New York: Harcourt Brace.
14. 1953. *The Origin of Intelligence in the Child.* London: Routledge & Kegan Paul.
15. STRAUSS, A. A. and LEHTINEN, L. E., 1947. *Psychopathology and Education of the Brain-injured Child.* New York: Grune & Stratton.

II

THE CONTRIBUTION OF ETHOLOGY
TO CHILD PSYCHIATRY

EWAN C. GRANT

B.SC., PH.D.

Research Ethologist, Rubery Hill Hospital, Birmingham

Introduction

In 1872 Darwin (8) published *The Expression of the Emotions in Man and Animals*. Despite this lead there has been no determined attempt to view the behaviour of man from the comparative standpoint, and I think that it is in this field that ethologists can make their greatest contributions. Comparative anatomy and comparative physiology are by now firmly established disciplines, and it is accepted by the great majority of scientists that the human species belongs to the same plane of evolution as the rest of the mammals. In the fields of behaviour and psychology, however, the increase in understanding that is offered by comparative knowledge has been hampered by a persisting feeling that, in this area at least, man is uniquely different. Ethologists have, in the past few decades, built up and justified methods of describing and analysing overt motor behaviour that seem applicable to the complex behaviour of man. An analysis of human behaviour by these methods should have relevance to all forms of psychiatry. Unfortunately it is only in the last few years that ethologists have begun to look at the primates, and extremely few studies have been carried out on the human species. Therefore what I intend to do in this chapter is to give a general outline of the methods of ethology, and then to show how I think they could be applied to the study of human behaviour, and the ways in which this study could be of help to the psychiatrist. Finally I will go over some of the findings and concepts of ethology, and in doing so take a look at some of the behaviour problems of man and child in a new way.

1

Methods of Ethology

Non-social Behaviour

Ethology may be defined as a quantitive study of behaviour, relying for its basic units on simple, described elements of behaviour shown by the particular species that is being studied. Historically it has been developed in the study of the 'instinctive' behaviour of the lower vertebrates and certain invertebrates. Painstaking observation and description of the behaviour and the environment, deliberate or natural reorientation of the environment, followed by redescription of the behaviour, have enabled the stimuli arousing and the stimuli directing and controlling much of the behaviour of these animals, as well as the behaviour itself, to be described with great accuracy. In many cases the rigidity of the response and the particular qualities of the stimuli releasing these responses are very marked.

Social Behaviour

Ethology has made many important contributions in the field of social behaviour, that is, behaviour involving two or more members of the same species, and it is this aspect that is important when discussing its relevance to mental health. Again the original observations were made on the lower vertebrates, Tinbergen's studies on sticklebacks being among the classical early works on social behaviour. In social behaviour the stimuli to which the animal is responding are provided by another animal, and the whole behaviour pattern is of a more dynamic nature than when the stimuli are of an inanimate or at least non-social nature. The practical difficulties that this causes were solved by the extensive use of models and stuffed animals. These could then be placed in appropriate positions and the behaviour of the animals towards them described. This gives the advantage of allowing the stimuli to be directly and precisely controlled, and also allows the responses of a number of individuals to exactly the same situation to be observed. However the use of models has a number of distinct drawbacks, the most important of which is the inability of the performing animal to get its expected response. This becomes more important as the behaviour becomes more variable and less dependent on discrete sign stimuli. In the mammals it is almost impossible to evoke responses to models except in very specific situations.

Units of Behaviour. It is therefore necessary to describe and analyse the behaviour of each of the reacting animals at the same time. The method remains the same, the first essential being a familiarisation with the species in question so that one comes to recognise recurring units of behaviour, which can be described so that they will be recognised by other observers. These units form the elements on which the first analysis is done. The degree to which the behaviour is broken down to form these elements is rather subjectively determined in the initial stages of a study. They are rarely as discrete as a single muscle movement, although this may be necessary for the detailed description of particular aspects of the behaviour, nor are they normally as general as, for example, fighting. They should be fairly clear units, either acts or postures or expressions, which can be

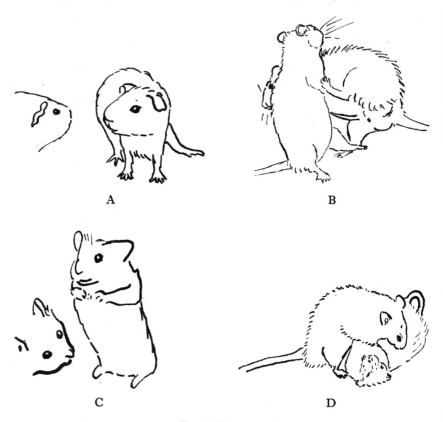

A

B

C

D

FIG. 1. Elements

A: Offensive Sideways Posture, Guinea-pig. B, Left: Defensive Upright Posture Right: Offensive Sideways Posture, Rat. C: Upright Posture, Hamster. D, Top: Aggressive Posture; Bottom, Submissive Posture, Rat.

recognisably described despite probable variations. One should remember that these elements can often be further analysed after the initial study. Fig. 1 shows a few examples of elements that have been used in fairly detailed analyses of these species. By continued observation the situations in which these elements occur and their relation to one another in these situations can be built up. In this way the analysis follows that of other scientific disciplines, that is, breakdown and recognition of constituents followed by a resynthesis of the whole.

Resynthesis. It is this reconstitution that allows the ethologist to describe the behaviour as being controlled by a number of distinct motives. The way in which this is done is by analysing the temporal interrelationships of the elements so that one can see, by their association and sequential arrangement, those elements that combine to form a pattern of behaviour leading to a particular end point. The function of this pattern can be defined both by this end point and by its effect on the responding animal, who will also be displaying a pattern of behaviour that can be defined in the same way. The name given to this pattern, e.g. aggressive drive, is purely descriptive and cannot, at present, be taken to indicate an emotional state equivalent to e.g. anger. However I think most workers would agree that it does indicate some particular central nervous activity. As more comparative evidence becomes available, I think it will become possible to say that this activity is homologous with that of an aggressive man.

Once the behaviour has been described in this way, its development and derivation can be examined by longitudinal studies in the life of the animal and by comparative studies with related species.

Application to Human Behaviour

I am at the present time attempting to use these methods in the study of psychiatric patients, and I have found that when approaching the study of human social behaviour the problem of isolating the elements becomes acute. As a member of the same species one is affected by, and is responding to, the finest grades of expression, and there is a tendency to try to distinguish a very large number of individual elements. In the initial study of the broad outlines of the behaviour, especially behaviour as complex as that of man, the mass of detail that this provides becomes too confusing, and an attempt has to be made to describe larger units within which some variation is included. Having done this, it will be possible to build up sequences of behaviour in the way that it has been done with animals. Fig. 2 is a sequence diagram of a few acts performed by patients in the very circumscribed situation of a first psychiatric interview. This diagram is built up by indicating the most common temporal linkages of the elements by means of arrows. There is, of course, no true analysis here, but it does show some points of interest. The two main acts available to the patient in this situation are either to look at the doctor or to look away from him. These two often simply alternate, although frequently Look At is immediately preceded by Eye Flash, a swift raising of the eyebrows which may be a form of attention-drawing mechanism, as it also frequently immediately precedes speech. However a number of other expressions and gestures are interspersed, and it is interesting to see that those which we might, at the moment, call 'nervous movements' occur while the patient is looking at the doctor and lead to him looking away from the doctor. Those which involve a more extreme form of looking away (cf. 'cut-off' later in this chapter) allow the patient to return his attention to the doctor. Lips In, a tightening of the lips while drawing them between the teeth, which subjectively looks as though it might be interpreted 'I won't say any more', also enables the patient to look back at the doctor. These patterns can also be related to the verbal content of the interview.

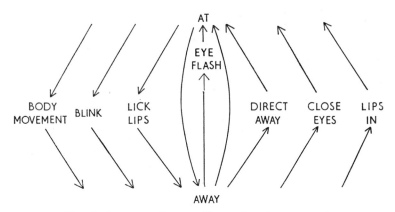

FIG. 2. Sequence diagram (for explanation see text).

Function in Psychiatry. I see the function of the ethologist in modern psychiatry at three levels. There is the help that an observer, who is trained to think of behaviour in quantitative terms, can give in the accurate description of the behaviour displayed by the patients. Secondly there is, what at the moment is only a promise, the possibility that a detailed analysis of human behaviour will provide a biological background of knowledge against which individual problems can be viewed, and which might allow an observer to state the motivation behind particular aspects of behaviour. Finally, with its roots firmly bedded in biology, I believe that the concepts of ethology, and its explanations of behaviour from the points of view of adaptive value and evolutionary origin, can be of value in showing the psychiatrist possible ways in which the behaviour that he sees could have arisen.

2

Aspects of Behaviour

In this part of the chapter I will try to show, using examples from different species of animals, how various kinds of behaviour may have arisen. I will not try in every case to describe an example in human behaviour, since even in the cases that I do mention there is still no experimental evidence that my suggestions are correct. However I hope that at least some of the examples that I describe will remind you of behaviour patterns you have seen, and will give a possible explanation for their occurrence. By demonstrating that some of the disturbed behaviour patterns shown by man have their homologues in the biology of other species and in many cases have an adaptive function, I wish to show that the behaviour itself may not be pathological, but that the pathology lies in the emotional state that fixes this behaviour. Also it may be that this understanding of the possible derivations of these overt behaviour patterns can provide a clue to the causes and definition of the emotional state. This latter must remain tentative until a full analysis of the behaviour of the human species is available.

Flight

I am using the term 'flight' to indicate a tendency to flee. In man and possibly in animals it is associated with the emotion fear.

Reduction of Incoming Stimuli. One function of flight, from the actor's point of view, is to eliminate or to reduce reception of the arousing stimuli. When this elimination is achieved the continuing arousal of the flight motive stops, the motivation dies away and the animal can continue with its normal behaviour. A number of factors might make it difficult or impossible actually to flee; there might be physical limitations, or there might be a strong motive to remain in the same place. In such conditions many animals perform acts or postures which have the effect of reducing the incoming disturbing stimuli; these postures have been called 'cut-off' postures (Chance (6)). The simplest of these postures can be easily derived from intention movements of flight. Thus an animal that is going to flee will first turn away its head, then its forebody. If the movement is stopped at either of these points we have postures in which the animal cannot see the source of the disturbance. This reduces the incoming stimuli and so secondarily reduces the excitement level in the disturbed animal, allowing it to remain where it is. In a number of animals that live in groups, postures that could function in this manner are integrated into the social behaviour, thus allowing submissive animals to stay within the confines of the group in spite of fairly intense flight responses to the dominant animal. Examples of this can be seen in rats, where a number of submissive postures (Fig. 1) involve turning away the head, closing the eyes, drawing back the vibrissae and laying flat the ears, all of which would tend to reduce incoming information.

Cut-off elements that can be seen quite frequently in man are closing the eyes or covering the eyes with the hands. Less obvious examples occur when the person 'refuses' to hear disturbing words. It is interesting to note in this connection that a mechanism has been shown which allows this to be done at a peripheral level. Hernandez-Peon (15) placed a metronome in a room, with a cat which had an electrode attached in its auditory tract. Each time the metronome clicked an impulse was picked up from this electrode. But when a dish of food was shown to the cat, these impulses stopped, indicating that when the attention is elsewhere one may in fact not hear, as well as not pay attention to.

Reduction of Outgoing Stimuli. Another function of flight is to remove the animal from the view of the individual causing the response, i.e. to eliminate the stimuli releasing attack in the other animal. In situations where physical limitations prohibit flight, postures are shown which have a complimentary function to cut-off postures: they reduce outgoing rather than incoming information. In animals these postures are most clearly seen in predator-prey situations. As movement seems to be one of the more essential components releasing attack, stillness is a common feature of these postures and many animals will simply 'freeze' in whatever position they happen to be in. Throughout the mammals the various crouched and hunched postures probably also function in this way. A number of species have morphological developments which, when associated with these postures, form a very effective defence against predators, e.g. the spines of the hedgehog and the scales of the armadillo.

In a number of animals which have been studied, postures of this type appear in social situations when flight responses are prohibited by physical limitations. These postures however appear at higher levels of intensity of motivation than do the cut-off postures. For example in rats, experimental studies have shown that cut-off postures are integrated into the displays that are used during dominance-submission encounters between animals that know each other and between whom the tension is low. Crouching is much more common when strange animals meet and when the intensity level of the encounter is high (Grant (11)). Similarly in macaque monkeys, a crouching posture, which has been described by Chance (5) and Reynolds (21) as having the effect of removing the monkey from the social scene, is only shown by certain animals in periods of extreme stress. Both types of behaviour can of course be shown at the same time, and in many cases this does happen, for example the crouching animal will put its head right down and cover its eyes.

Both types of behaviour are easily seen in man. Simple forms of cut-off such as closing the eyes or turning away the head can be seen during meetings between normal people, and are frequent in psychiatric interviews when matters causing anxiety are raised. In man too a hunched type of posture appears in more intense situations. It can be seen in the normal person when an immediate danger from an unexpected source threatens: the shoulders are raised, the head is lowered and occasionally the arms cover the face; it can be seen in the social situation when a strong fear stimulus is combined with an inability to retreat, e.g. the dependent child confronted with a hostile parent. This type of posture finds its extreme of expression in the withdrawn schizophrenic who has adopted it almost to the exclusion of any other form of expression.

Confusion of Stimuli. Another form of behaviour that is displayed by animals in flight-provoking situations, when for some reason flight is impossible, is the types of display that have been named 'cryptic' or 'Protean' by Chance and Russell (7). This behaviour seems to occur only at very high degrees of intensity, and again it is most common in the predator-prey situations. It takes the form of unexpected and bizarre movements which have the effect of confusing the predator and, by breaking up the normal outline of the animal, again reducing the outgoing information, or rather, in communication language, lowering the signal-noise ratio. A number of highly specialised forms of behaviour can be considered in this category, e.g. the squid ejecting its 'ink' or the lizard that drops its tail off when grabbed by a predator. In mammals there is evidence that certain types of convulsions fulfil this function. It seems possible that the audiogenic seizures of small mammals are aspects of this type of behaviour. Chance (4) has shown (in *Peromyscus maniculatus*, the American deer mouse) that if a possibility of escape is offered, e.g. if a hiding-place is available, the mice will not convulse when exposed to stimuli that could cause them to do so. These responses are not as specific as the term audiogenic implies, because a number of other frightening stimuli can provoke them. It is rare for this behaviour to occur in social situations, but when I have seen it, in a laboratory mouse, it was very effective in stopping the attacks of the aggressive animal. It is interesting to compare this behaviour with the functional epilepsies in man where the attacks are immediately preceded by a frightening situation.

Ambivalence

Situations in which two or more mutually opposing tendencies are simultaneously aroused in the same animal, by the same stimulus or by spacially close stimuli, give rise to ambivalent behaviour. Since ambivalent motivation seems to be the cause of a considerable amount of disturbed behaviour in man, it may be worth while to have a look at the more common of the ways in which ambivalence can be displayed and resolved in other species.

Alternating Expression. The simplest way in which ambivalence can be resolved is by performing the two types of behaviour alternately. Usually when this is done neither pattern is complete, the animal displaying alternating intention movements of each tendency. For example, when a rat is frightened by another and at the same time strongly motivated to approach it, perhaps owing to a sexual attraction, it will move towards it for a short distance and will then move away again over a similar distance, and may go on repeating these movements until the ambivalence is resolved either by one tendency gaining ascendency or by the motivation dying away.

Simultaneous Expression. Both types of behaviour can be displayed at the same time. This may result in part of the body trying to go forward while another part tries to go back, giving rise to long stretched postures, or the animal may make a compromise and position itself on the vector of the two tendencies, so presenting its flank to the stimulus. In animals many of these responses have become stylised and have meaning within the framework of social behaviour. For example, the pivoting dances in the

courtship of certain finches can be analysed as alternating intention movements, the performing male being frightened of his partner as well as
sexually attracted; many species have sideways fighting postures that would
appear to be derived from an ambivalent state between aggression and
flight and that now have a distinct threat meaning to the responding animal.
Morris (19) has used the term 'emancipation' in describing how, in some
species, certain of these elements might have become completely integrated
into, for example, courtship behaviour, and may even be completely
dissociated from their original motivation. However, from the evidence
available, it seems unlikely that this amount of emancipation is present in
mammalian behaviour.

In the primates, including man, where facial gestures are of more
importance, it is easier for the subject to display ambivalent tendencies
simultaneously. There are three major areas of the face which take part
in facial expression, and which may work together or independently.
These are the eyes, the forehead and the mouth. An example can be given
of ambivalence between aggression and fear. The following description is
taken from my own observations, aided by a detailed analysis by Van Hooff
(24) of the facial gestures in monkeys and apes. In man the fully aggressive
face shows the following elements: eyes almost completely open and directed towards the opponent, forehead drawn down and eyebrows drawn
together, lips brought forward and the mouth slightly open. In the frightened face the following elements are shown: eyes closed, scalp drawn back
so that the forehead is smooth, corners of lips drawn right back and lips
parted to show the teeth, which are nearly clenched. In ambivalent states
one or other element can be transposed, e.g. in a frightened subject that is
still showing some assertion the eyes will be open and directed towards the
opponent, in an aggressive subject with a certain amount of fear the corners
of the mouth will be withdrawn. It is difficult to make detailed statements
at present about the function and derivation of these gestures, but very
recently Andrew (2), in a detailed comparative paper on the calls and
expressions of the primates, has put forward some attractive theories. For
example he suggests that the aggressive frown is an exaggerated form of an
intense stare, and he derives the drawing back of the lips from the reflex
gesture that is given in response to an unpleasant taste.

Displacement Activities. In ambivalent situations animals sometimes
perform acts relating to behaviour patterns unconnected with any of the
motives that are being stimulated. These have been called 'displacement
activities' by ethologists. Unfortunately this is different from the way in
which this term has been used by psychoanalysts. The equivalent ethological term to the psychoanalytic 'displacement' is 'redirection' (see
below). Displacement activities are often performed in an abbreviated
form and, subjectively, at a higher energy level than is seen in their normal
occurrence. An example can be taken from the behaviour of rats, where
displacement grooming is common during social fighting. The normal

grooming pattern in these animals follows a fairly stereotyped course. To start with, the head and face are washed, the rat using its forepaws, in strokes which eventually reach from the base of the ears to the tip of the snout. Interspersed with these strokes the animal licks its forepaws. Next the body fur is licked, starting at the forepart of the body and working back to the tail. Finally the animal scratches with its hind legs. In the displaced activity only the forepaw movement is seen, and frequently only one or two quick wipes which may even be disorientated so that they just miss the tip of the snout. In the rat these movements seem to have no signal value, and their function seems to be some release of tension. In birds and fishes, many acts having this derivation have become part of the display and indicate the state of arousal to the other animal; in some cases they have become highly specialised, forming very distinctive signals. In man, many of the 'nervous' movements can be derived in this way, many probably from primitive grooming movements, e.g. passing the hand through the hair or scratching the head or body; with the development of social cultural habits these may be seen as stereotyped picking of fluff from clothes or straightening of ties. An extreme form of displacement has been reported in soldiers in the front line who have fallen asleep during intense conflict. This, of course, also acts as a very effective form of cut-off.

Redirection. As explained above, this term is more or less equivalent to the analysts' 'displacement'. In this case the behaviour patterns of one of the aroused motives are shown, but they are directed on to an irrelevant object. For example, within a social group, an animal that is motivated to attack the dominant animal, but is unable to do so because it is at the same time frightened of it, will redirect its aggression on to a lower ranking member of the group. The object on to which the behaviour is redirected need not be another animal and in many cases is inanimate. Tinbergen (1951) has described a combination of redirection and displacement in the herring gull. In this species pulling up of grass is part of the nest-building behaviour, but when it occurs in territory border disputes as a displacement activity, the grass is snapped at with aggressive head and beak movements. Again examples can be seen in human behaviour: kicking and banging at furniture in the frustrated child, and the aggression released at home by the husband angry at his boss, may be cited as examples. The combination of redirection and displacement can also occasionally be seen: hand movements in the hair may become more and more violent until the person is literally pulling his hair out, or nail biting, which I would also consider as part of the primitive grooming pattern, may become so intense as to cause damage to the quick.

Both displacement and redirection can also be seen when a single strongly motivated tendency is blocked simply by the lack of adequate facilities to release it, rather than because of ambivalence caused by an opposing motivation. This may be an immediate response, as for example when an animal or person gets angry at another who is either not there or

not immediately within reach. The aggression can then be directed on to
any available object, or some tension may be released through displacement activities. On the other hand it may be the result of a build-up of
some tendency over a long period of time spent in an inadequate environment. In this condition very inadequate stimuli can release the motor
patterns of the behaviour. Hediger (14) has described how this can give
rise to some of the typical stereotypes seen in wild animals in the zoo. For
example, in the active hunting animals, where the actual hunting seems to
be under separate motivation from the ingestion of food, stereotyped
ambulatory movements are performed within the confines of the cage. The
increase in homosexual and masturbatory behaviour seen in captive
animals can also be considered as arising in this way. However, in the
mammals at least, it seems to me that boredom itself must be considered
as an important contributory factor in the aetiology of some of these
unadaptive forms of behaviour. For instance it has been shown that the
over-eating of caged rats can be reduced by giving them a simple toy to
play with.

3

The Organisation of Social Behaviour

Territory

An animal in the wild does not wander at random, and the individuals
of many species remain for the greater part of their lives within a fairly
circumscribed area. This area is the home range of the individual concerned. By continuous exploration the individual builds up its knowledge
of this area. Not all parts are equally well known, and the home range of
many animals consists of an interconnecting series of familiar pathways
connecting particular locations, feeding sites, shelters, etc. Within the
home range, although not necessarily topographically central, there is a
home which represents the place of maximum security. The solitary animal
frequently defends a part or all of the home range against members of the
same species, and in social animals the group will defend it against other
groups. This defended area is the territory. The territory may, therefore,
be the same as the home range or may only be the actual home or may be
an area of varying size round the home. In the social animals the individual
may have his own territory within the group territory.

Function of Territory. A number of suggestions have been put forward
as to the function of territory, e.g. distribution of food supply, spacing out
of mates, or an undisturbed area for bringing up the young. Each of these
may be of prime importance in specific cases; whatever the ultimate
function, there is no doubt about the importance to the individual concerned of forming his own territory. Within its own territory the animal
has a very considerable advantage in meetings with other members of its
species. A number of workers have shown how, in border disputes, the

advantage lies first with one animal, then with the other as they move over the border into first one animal's territory, then back into the other's. In those cases where the home range is wider than the territory, the detailed knowledge of the ground is still of advantage to the animal: it can move freely and easily from place to place and in times of danger it can quickly reach a place of refuge. If the topography of this area is disturbed in some way, or if the animal is placed on unknown ground, then its behaviour is considerably altered: its movements are timorous, and in some species a prolonged period of avoidance behaviour ensues.

Marking of Territory. Many species mark their territories, either at the boundaries or, more commonly, at many points both at the boundaries and within the territory. The marking is done in many different ways: the spring song of birds is probably an acoustical marking of territory; optical marking is seen in, for example, the brown bear, which scrapes bark off trees at certain points in its territory. However in the majority of mammals territory marking is olfactory. A number of species have developed special scent glands for this purpose, while many use the normal body products of urine and faeces. This marking is carried out fairly regularly, but any disturbance and particularly an agonistic encounter with a member of its own species will considerably increase the frequency of this behaviour. The main function of this marking is probably to warn off intruders of the same species, but from the performing animal's point of view it seems, in many species, to give a quality of ownership and security. That is to say, if the area is not marked by the individual's own scent, the animal appears much more unsure of itself. A rat that is put into a strange place will urinate at a single point and will use that point as a base for its first tentative explorations, and if it meets another rat it will move back to that point. Ilse (16) has described how the slow loris, a primitive primate, cannot continue with its normal behaviour if its urine markings are washed away, and it will spend a long time re-marking its territory. In a number of animals any new object within the home range is marked in this way. Among social animals this sort of behaviour is associated with dominance, and enurination is part of the behaviour of the dominant animal. Anyone who, like myself, owns a subordinate tom-cat will know of examples of this.

Territorial Behaviour in Man. It would seem that territorial behaviour is still of some importance to man, and the security of a known place becomes very obvious in the mentally ill. However I would like to draw more attention to the personal side of it, the sense of owning and marking as 'mine'. The child who writes his name on his personal belongings is marking territory, and, as in other species, any threat or potential threat to his security will increase this behaviour. This behaviour may be shown in different ways; the child of a friend of mine would place articles of his own clothing at various parts of the house, and the probable explanation of this behaviour occurred when it was seen that he would place them on new things that came into the house and on visitors' bags. In extreme cases it is possible that faeces or urine could be used in the same way. In institutional life, although the place is known, this personal aspect of owning is liable to disappear. This lack still causes quite a lot of distress, despite the fact that a number of authors have already emphasised the importance to the individual of his personal property (e.g. Freeman *et al.* (10)).

Motivation

In animals that normally live solitary lives the usual response towards another member of the same species is either to attack it or to run away from it. As described in the previous section, the particular one of these responses that is shown is very often dependent on whether the animal is on its own territory or not. This behaviour has to be modified in response to members of the opposite sex during the mating season. Even in those species with a clearly marked sexual dimorphism, however, the initial response to a member of the opposite sex is the same as that shown to a member of the same sex, that is, aggression or flight. Much of pairing behaviour has the function of reducing these tendencies and so allowing the pair to come together for mating. This type of behaviour should be distinguished from pre-coitional displays, the main function of which is the simultaneous sexual arousal of each animal, although in this behaviour also both aggressive and flight tendencies can frequently be seen. In the social animals there is usually a tendency for the group to split up during the mating season. This break-up is due to the arousal, at this time, of the aversive tendencies of aggression and flight. Even in those species that come together into colonies for breeding, e.g. the herring gulls and other sea birds, there is a distinct space between pairs, members of which vigorously attack intruders. In this way much of the most distinctive social behaviour shown by the lower vertebrates during the breeding season can be seen to be motivated by a combination of the three distinct and opposing tendencies, mating, aggression and flight (cf Morris (20)). During other seasons the level of social interaction is lower and sexual behaviour seems to disappear.

In mammals there is some evidence that all three tendencies are aroused during all intense social activity. In rats, for example, elements showing sexual arousal can be seen during territorial behaviour between males and during dominance-submission behaviour between males or between females. On the other hand evidence of both aggression and flight can be seen in the pre-coitional behaviour between the sexes. Although there is still little evidence of the type of factors involved, it seems that the balance of these motives in the individual can be disturbed by external factors, resulting in an animal that is biassed towards showing e.g. aggressive behaviour. In extreme cases this results in behaviour so biassed as to be considered abnormal. One factor, that has been shown in a number of species to have a very distinct effect of this sort, is the isolation of a social animal from its fellows. However it cannot be stated exactly whether this bias will be towards flight, aggression or mating in any particular individual. This is presumably dependent on a number of other factors, some of which lie within the past experience of the animal and some in its innate propensities. Although we know little about these factors or about the method by which they affect the behaviour, it looks as though we might have here a phenomenon analogous to the psychopathologies of man, which might well repay further investigation.

Group Structure

Some form of structure is usually evident in the formation of social groups of animals. This structure frequently depends on dominance-submission relationships between the members of the group, so that dominance hierarchies or orders of rank are present. The classic examples of these are the peck orders that occur in flocks of hens, which have been described in detail by Allee (1).

In mammals clearly defined orders of rank are most typically seen in the adult males, the relations of the females and sub-adults to this central hierarchy depending on the particular social organisation of the species. The dominant member of this hierarchy may enjoy priority of access to the food, receptive females, etc. The position of each animal in the order is attained and maintained by combat, which frequently means that the dominant position is held by the largest and strongest member of the group. This is not necessarily so; especially in a newly formed group, a smaller but more active and aggressive member might become dominant. However, there is a positive feedback in the situation, in that the dominant animal, because of the security and advantages of his position, is likely to become the largest and healthiest member of the group, even in situations where abundant food is available for all.

Social Bond. In the face of the aggression present during dominance-submission displays, some strong positive motivation to remain together is required to maintain the cohesion of the group. This is, apparently, a strong attraction towards the dominant animal. A number of authors have commented with surprise upon the strength of this attraction in particular instances, when they have seen an animal that has just been severely beaten crawling back towards its aggressor. A clear example, that will have been seen by many people, is the behaviour of the pet dog that crawls back to its master after being punished for some misdemeanour; although this behaviour is inter-specific the situation is probably the same. Kummer (17) has shown, in baboons, how this behaviour can be derived from that of the infant towards its mother. Among other aspects of the mother figure an important one is its significance as a place of refuge: the infant will flee towards its mother from any frightening stimulus. This aspect of behaviour must be taken into account, together with any positive love approach, when considering ambivalent responses towards hostile parents. As the baboons mature this response is reorientated, firstly towards an older member of its own play or sub-adult group and eventually towards the dominant animal. The response is then displayed even when the dominant animal is itself the frightening stimulus.

Sexual Arousal. The sub-dominant members of these hierarchies are under continuous tension and a part of their attention must be continuously on the dominant member, to whom they must give way either spatially or by appropriate submissive gestures. In some of the monkeys these submissive gestures are derived directly from the sexual behaviour of the female: the submissive animal that has to pass close to the dominant, or suddenly finds himself within the area controlled by the dominant, will 'present', that is, adopt the posture a receptive female adopts when she is ready to be mounted (see e.g. Chance (5)). In groups of laboratory rats, on the other hand, the directing of attention towards the dominant is partly shown by mounting behaviour directed towards him (Grant and Chance (12)). These may be special cases, derived as displacement activities and with no general significance. However it is interesting to consider the possibility of sexual arousal in dominance groups, especially when taken together with the theories of infant sexuality towards the mother and the already considered suggestion that one aspect of the mother figure is transferred to the dominant. The differences in the overt pattern observed in the two animals that I mentioned is probably related to differences in dominance in mating pairs, since in the monkeys the male is the aggressive partner while in the rats the female is the more aggressive.

Imprinting

Imprinting is a translation of the German term *Prägung*, which was used by Lorenz (18) to describe a type of learning that occurs during the 'following' response (an innate tendency to follow moving objects) of the young of nidifugous birds, i.e. birds which are able to walk and leave the nest very shortly after they are hatched, such as ducks and geese. Lorenz originally suggested that it was a unique type of learning in four ways: (1) It is confined to a definite and short period in the life cycle. (2) It is irreversible. (3) It affects responses not yet developed; a bird that is imprinted onto a different species when young may, when adult, react with members of that species as potential mates in preference to its own. (4) It involves learning species characteristics rather than individual characteristics. However later studies have shown that, except perhaps for some rare cases, imprinting is not quite so clearly differentiated as was originally suggested. Only (1) above, and in some cases (3), are now considered essential characteristics of this process. The term is now commonly used to describe any rapid learning which occurs at a definite period of life.

Bird and Chick. The aspects of imprinting to which I wish to draw attention are, firstly, the brief period in the life of the animal during which it may occur, and, secondly, the way in which it leads to a restricting of the stimulus situation which will set off a particular response that was initially given to a wide variety of stimuli. The initial 'following' response of the young nidifugous bird is released by a wide variety of moving objects, e.g. in ducklings Fabricius and Boyd (9) have shown it occurring in response to objects ranging from a moving matchbox to a walking human being. During the performance of this response the bird learns the characteristics of the object it is following, and after this learning, which occurs very quickly, only that object will elicit the behaviour. These birds may subsequently perform towards these objects behaviour normally shown to their parents. Under natural conditions the object concerned is almost always the parent. Comparable learning occurs during the begging response of young nidicolous birds. This behaviour is initially released by a wide variety of stimuli, but is later shown only to the parents. Fear responses are also elicited in these young birds by stimuli having the same characteristics as those releasing the 'following' response. However it appears that the tendency to flee from these stimuli matures rather later than the tendency to follow them. Ambivalence is therefore absent at first, and the imprinting restricts the stimuli releasing the 'following' response so that the animal's tendency to flee from this object, normally the parent, is overcome while still weak. The same development occurs in the nidicolous bird, in which stimuli similar to those which would earlier have released begging responses later cause the bird to crouch down into the nest. Despite this habituation effect of imprinting, there is still probably some ambivalence in the behaviour to the parent once the flight responses are fully developed.

Mother and Child. Evidence of analogous behaviour in mammals is still rather limited, but fairly definite examples have been described in one or two species, and it seems possible that a similar type of learning occurs in the relationship of the human child and its mother. Thus many of the responses appropriate to the mother can be elicited by a wide variety of objects; this is, of course, made use of in artificial feeding, and the smiling response can be elicited in very young babies by quite crude masks, although it later becomes restricted to the parent. Fear of strangers appears at about five to nine months, a little later than the recognition of the mother. Thus the same developmental steps are seen in the human child as have been described in the birds. The experiments of Harlow (13) with infant macaque monkeys make it clear that, in this species at least, the actual response during which the mother figure is learned is not feeding, but probably some form of contact behaviour, e.g. clinging and hugging. Monkeys raised with two forms of surrogate mothers, one of wire and one of rough cloth, would go to the cloth mother when frightened even if it was the wire mother which had 'lactated'. Nor did those animals which only had experience of the wire mother go to her as a place of refuge when frightened.

There is evidence that these various behaviour patterns, feeding, smiling, contact, etc., which help to form the relationship between the child and its mother, have a sensitive period of their own during which learning may occur. This, together with the increase in flight responses, may make it difficult for an adequate relationship to be built up after this period, and these difficulties, as suggested by Bowlby (3), may continue into adult life.

Although ethology is a fairly new discipline it already encompasses a wide variety of information. The topics that I have discussed are necessarily biased by my own interests, but I have at the same time tried to lay emphasis on those points which I believe have relevance to human behaviour and mental health. However the behaviour mechanisms that I have been describing are, to a greater or lesser extent, rigid and stereotyped, and before concluding I must draw attention to the ability, already present in the higher mammals and of great potential in man, to control and direct these tendencies by intelligence. As Russell and Russell (22) have pointed out in their book on human behaviour, the ethological study of these mechanisms may help to provide the knowledge necessary for this intelligent control.

REFERENCES

1. ALLÉE, W. C., 1938. *The Social Life of Animals*. London and Toronto.
2. ANDREW, R. J., 1963. Origin and evolution of the calls and facial expressions of the Primates. *Behaviour*, 20: 1-110.
3. BOWLBY, J., 1952. *Maternal Care and Mental Health*. World Health Organisation Monographs, Series 2.
4. CHANCE, M. R. A., 1954. The suppression of audiogenic hyperexcitement by learning in *Peromyscus maniculatus*. *Brit. J. Anim. Behav.*, 2: 31-35.
5. ——— 1956. Social structure of a colony of *Macaca mulatta*. *Brit. J. Anim. Behav.*, 4: 1-13.
6. ——— 1962. The interpretation of some agonistic postures: the role of cut-off acts and postures. *Symp. Zool. Soc. Lond.*, No. 8: 71-89.
7. CHANCE, M. R. A. and RUSSELL, W. M. S., 1959. Protean displays: a form of allaesthetic behaviour. *Proc. Zool. Soc. Lond.*, 132: 65-70.
8. DARWIN, CH. R., 1872. *The Expression of the Emotions in Man and Animals*. London.
9. FABRICIUS, E. and BOYD, H., 1954. Experiments on the following-reaction of ducklings. *Wildfowl Trust Annual Report* 1952-53: 84-89.
10. FREEMAN, T., CAMERON, J. L. and McGHIE, A., 1958. *Chronic Schizophrenia*. London: Tavistock Publications.
11. GRANT, E. C., 1963. An analysis of the social behaviour of the male laboratory rat. *Behaviour*, 20: 261-281.
12. GRANT, E. C. and CHANCE, M. R. A., 1958. Rank order in caged rats. *Animal Behaviour*, 6: 183-194.
13. HARLOW, H. F., 1959. Affectional responses in the infant monkey. *Science*, 130: 421-423.
14. HEDIGER, N., 1950. *Wild Animals in Captivity*. London.
15. HERNANDEZ-PEON, R., SCHERRER, H. and JOURET, M., 1956. Modification of electric activity in the cochlear nucleus during 'attention' in unanesthetized cats. *Science*, 123: 331-332.

16. ILSE, D. R., 1955. Olfactory marking of territory in two young male loris. *Brit. J. Anim. Behav.*, **3**: 118-120.

17. KUMMER, H., 1957. Soziales Verhalten einer Mantelpaviangruppe. *Beih. Schweiz. Z. Psychol.*

18. LORENZ, K., 1935. Der Kumpan in der Umwelt des Vogels. *J. f. Orn., Leipzig*, **83**: 137-214.

19. MORRIS, D., 1954. The reproductive behaviour of the zebra finch (*Poephila guttata*) with special reference to pseudo-female behaviour and displacement activities. *Behaviour*, **6**: 271-322.

20. ———— 1956. The function and causation of courtship ceremonies. In *L'Instinct dans le Comportement des Animaux et de l'Homme*: 261-286. Paris: Fondation Singer-Polinac.

21. REYNOLDS, V., 1961. Ph.D. Thesis, University of London.

22. RUSSELL, W. M. S. and RUSSELL, C., 1960. *Human Behaviour*. London.

23. TINBERGEN, N., 1951. *The Study of Instinct*. Oxford.

24. VAN HOOFF, J. A. R. A. M., 1962. Facial expressions in higher Primates. *Symp. Zool. Soc. Lond.*, No. 8: 97-125.

III

THE GENETICAL ASPECTS OF

CHILD PSYCHIATRY

VALERIE COWIE

M.D., D.P.M.

Consultant Psychiatrist, the Fountain Hospital Group, Queen Mary's Hospital for Children, Carshalton and St. Ebba's Hospital, Epsom
Assistant Director, Medical Research Council, Psychiatric Genetics Research Unit

1

Introduction

It is most understandable and proper that particular emphasis has been laid on environmental effects in psychiatric disorders of childhood. The ready response of the child to environmental change and the effectiveness of therapeutic manipulation of social and other conditions may, however, distract attention altogether from inborn potentialities. An understanding of constitutional strengths and weaknesses is essential in tackling problems of aetiology. Moreover, by allowing for recognised innate tendencies, treatment itself may be strengthened and made more effective.

Certain fields of child psychiatry have been investigated more thoroughly than others from a genetical point of view. Thus much work has been done on the role of heredity in juvenile delinquency, intelligence and especially mental subnormality. These subjects lend themselves particularly to genetical research, as the case material is usually circumscribed, readily available from fairly static populations and convenient for statistical analysis. On the other hand, though there are some outstanding examples, fewer genetical investigations have been made in the fields of personality differences and neurotic traits in childhood. Even less work has been done on the role of inheritance in childhood psychosis.

This chapter is not intended to be an encyclopaedic review of the literature of genetics in child psychiatry. Instead it will give an account of the different methods of approach to genetical problems in that field, with specific examples. In this way it is hoped to show the scope and the limitations of various existing methods, and to indicate changing trends and future possibilities for increasing our knowledge of the mechanisms of inheritance. Following the discussion of research aspects, there will be a short section on the practical application of genetical information in genetical counselling.

2

Historical Background

As regards background, psychiatric genetics is a special province of the larger field of human genetics. Human genetics began by the recording of pedigrees showing the hereditary transmission of various abnormalities. Systematic studies of this kind were in progress towards the end of the nineteenth century, and they gained new impetus from the rediscovery of the Mendelian laws in 1900. Shortly afterwards, in 1902, the work of Garrod on inborn errors of metabolism introduced biochemical considerations into the study of human genetics. This led in turn to major advances in genetical theory and to the recognition of the relationship between genes and enzymes. The introduction of a biochemical approach has been of great importance in the genetical study of mental disorder. The investigation of such conditions as phenylketonuria, in which inborn metabolic errors are accompanied by mental dysfunction, promises to elucidate other conditions, possibly psychoses, in which chemically mediated and controlled mechanisms may play a part.

Penrose in Britain has done much to establish a scientific basis for genetical research in the field of mental subnormality. He has stressed the need for objective clinical evaluation in terms of actual measurements wherever possible, and the application of biochemical, cytological and other specialised techniques to widen the scope of clinical observation. He himself has set a brilliant example by the imaginative use of statistics to extract the meaning from collected data. Under the influence of Penrose the main growing point of genetical research in the field of child psychiatry has been in relation to mental subnormality.

Against this general background of development in research method, certain special techniques have added their own particular contributions. Twin studies have been especially noteworthy in this respect.

3

Twin Studies

Twin studies are based on the belief that monozygotic twins are identical in their genetical endowment, while dizygotic twins may be expected to be no more alike in this respect than singleton sibs. On this basis it is reckoned that a high concordance for any particular trait between the members of monogzyotic twin pairs indicates a hereditary factor. By the same token, differences between monozygotic twins are taken as evidence in support of environmental effect. The concordance rate between members of twin pairs brought up apart in different environments is considered a particularly sensitive measure of genetical influence.

Twin studies are however of limited value in that, while they may demonstrate the presence of a genetical influence, they do not indicate the mode of hereditary transmission, nor do they provide the kind of information needed for precise genetical calculations such as the estimation of risk figures amongst relatives. Penrose (37) evaluates twin studies as follows:

. . . the most important results of twin studies are those which describe the differences, not similarities, between identical pairs. If we take a pair of monozygotic twins and expose them to any environmental circumstance whatever, they will tend to react in the same manner. They are like two cars, mass produced, from the same factory. Suppose that two such vehicles both break down in the same way after about the same mileage. The first thing we learn is that two cars of the same make have the same defects (which we knew already). We can infer very little about what would happen to cars of different makes in the same circumstances. And this little could be inferred from examining one car instead of a twin pair. Data from twin studies overemphasize the effects of heredity, but they do also remind us that a human being is a physical entity with a chemical constitution ultimately determined genetically.

Despite the limitations of twin study as a technique, there have been some outstanding and classical examples relevant to child psychiatry. These include studies by Rosanoff, Handy and Rosanoff (45) and by Rosanoff, Handy and Plesset (44) in the United States on juvenile delinquents and young children with behaviour disorders who did not appear before the courts; by Kranz (28) in Germany on the institutional re-education of juveniles with personality abnormality; and by Kent (26) in the United States on childhood maladjustment. These studies and others are well reviewed by Shields (49) in the publication of his own work on personality differences and neurotic traits in normal twin schoolchildren, and the Table is abstracted from a tabulation by Shields showing the main results from these twin studies. The high concordance rate, as compared with the discordance rate, between monozygotic pairs with respect to the various traits examined suggests the operation of hereditary factors. The high concordance rates between same-sexed dizygotic twins as compared with those between opposite-sexed dizygotic twins, which shows up well in the figures of Rosanoff and his collaborators, especially with respect to juvenile delinquency, is most probably an environmental effect. Shields (49) investigated personality differences and neurotic traits in normal twin schoolchildren. He found a much closer similarity between monozygotic twins with respect to personality characteristics than between dizygotic twins. The form in which neurotic symptoms were shown seemed to be more closely related to hereditary factors than was the degree of their

PLATE 1

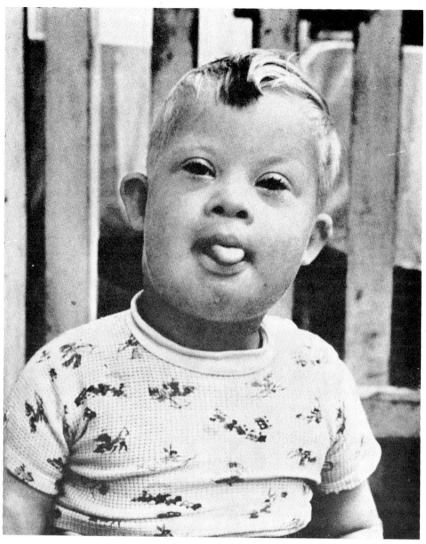

Boy with mongolism. Note the small round head, epicanthic folds, slanting palpebral fissures, broad flat nasal bridge, simple configuration of ears.

(Photograph kindly supplied by Mr. Lepage, Queen Mary's Hospital for Children, Carshalton.)

PLATE 2

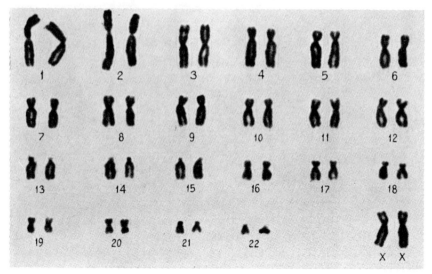

Karyotype of a normal human female cell.

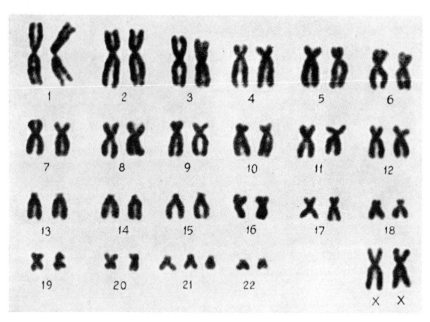

Karyotype of female "standard" mongol cell
(trisomy chromosome No. 21).

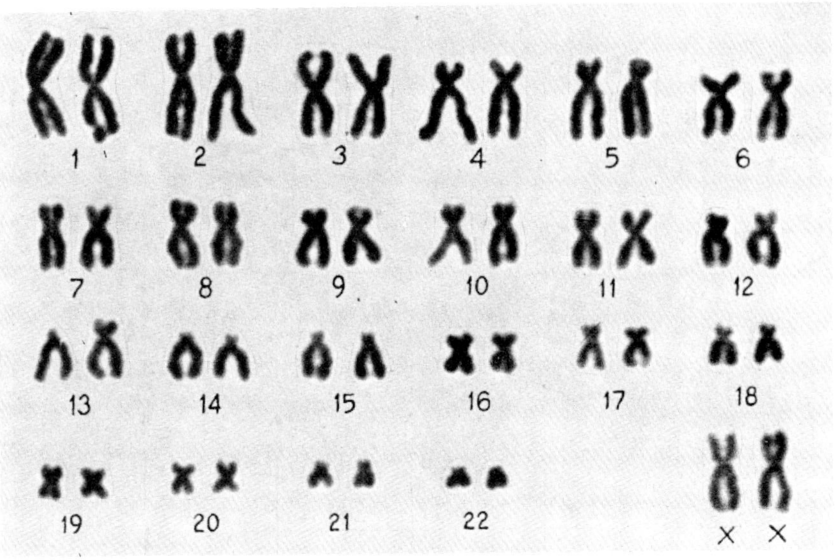

PLATE 3

Karyotype of female "translocation" mongol cell
(translocation 13-15/21).

(Photographs kindly supplied by Dr. J. R. Ellis,
Galton Laboratory, University College, London.)

PLATE 4

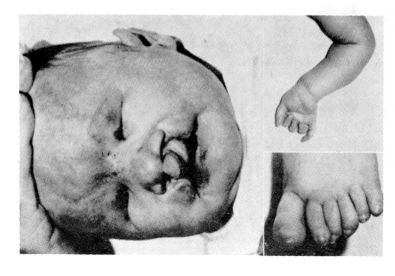

Patient with trisomy 13 15 syndrome. Note especially facial haemangioma, bilateral hare-lip, polydactyly, single palmar crease.

(Photograph kindly supplied by Dr. Klaus Patau, Department of Medical Genetics, University of Wisconsin.)

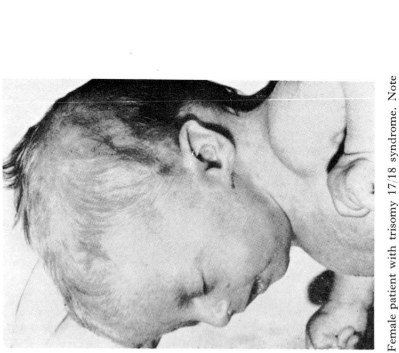

Female patient with trisomy 17/18 syndrome. Note the low-set, malformed ears, micrognathia, small mouth.

(Photograph kindly supplied by Dr. John Edwards, Institute of Child Health, University of Birmingham.)

severity, where the environment appeared to matter more. It was suggested also that genes most often influence neurotic behaviour through their effect on the physical basis of personality; thus disorders such as juvenile delinquency, which are not closely related to personality type, are likely to be determined by heredity to a lesser extent than other disorders, such as psychosomatic disorders, which are so related. Other psychological studies of normal twin schoolchildren have been reviewed very fully by Gedda (17) in Italian, and by Eysenck (14), who together with Prell (Eysenck and Prell (15)) used a battery of personality tests on a series of twin schoolchildren and subjected the results to factor analysis. The high correlation of 0·85 with respect to neuroticism was found between mono-

Non-pyschotic Twin Pairs

(Abstracted from Shields, 1954)

Condition studied	Author (Country)	Year	Uniovular Pairs		Same-sexed Binovular Pairs		Opposite-sexed Binovular Pairs	
			Con-cordant	Dis-cordant	Con-cordant	Dis-cordant	Con-cordant	Dis-cordant
Juvenile Delinquency	Rosanoff et al. (USA)	1934	39	3	20	5	8	32
Behaviour Disorder in Children	,,	,,	41	6	26	34	8	21
Institutional Re-education of Juveniles with Personality Abnormality	Kranz (Germany)	1937	7	4	0	3	2	6
Childhood Mal-adjustment	Kent (USA)	1949	7	0	4	2	2	1

zygotic twins. A lower correlation of 0·22 was found between the dizygotic twins. This suggests very strongly the effect of heredity.

In general these studies provide some evidence to support the view that personality deviation in childhood, whether manifested as juvenile delinquency, non-delinquent behaviour disorder or childhood maladjustment, is to a considerable extent determined by heredity. The conclusion of Eysenck and Prell (15) that the concept of neuroticism derived from factor analysis is not a statistical artefact but a biological unit, and that neurotic predisposition is to a large extent inherited, is of special interest with respect to the work of Slater (50) on the neurotic constitution in adults. Both of these studies support the idea that every individual has inborn potentialities for resistance to or psychological breakdown under stress, and it appears that the neurotic constitution may manifest itself, depending upon the environment, at a very early age.

Turning to childhood psychosis: very little genetical investigation has been made in this field. Kallmann and Roth (25) studied genetic aspects of pre-adolescent schizophrenia, taking a sample of index cases consisting of 52 twins and 50 singletons under the age of 15. A distinct change in the behaviour of a child who previously had seemed to develop normally was taken as a crucial diagnostic feature. Other signs listed by the authors included diminished interest in the environment; blunted or distorted affect; peculiar conduct, especially in motor activity; diffuse anxiety with phobias; bizarre thinking with a tendency towards exaggerated fantasies; and hallucinations. The probands were compared with an adult sample with respect to twin concordance rates and schizophrenia rates for parents and sibs. No significant differences were found between the two samples. This was taken to indicate an early effect in childhood schizophrenia of the same genotype as was assumed to be responsible for the basic symptoms of adult schizophrenia. The observation that the psychoses in the co-twins of early schizophrenia cases occur sometimes before and sometimes after adolescence was taken as further support for this conclusion.

It is not easy to go all the way with Kallmann and Roth in their views. There are obvious difficulties in comparing the psychoses of children and adults, and such comparisons are only doubtfully valid. Furthermore there are reasons for regarding both the schizophrenias of adult life, and the 'schizophrenias' of childhood, as being each of them heterogeneous groups. Genetical studies will no doubt play an important part in the investigation of these heterogeneities. It would be better to pay attention to criteria of a biological kind, such as age of onset, than to ambiguous psychological manifestations when an attempt is made to classify these conditions.

4

Studies of Populations and Special Samples

The study of human genetics has its roots scientifically as well as historically in the study of human families. Although the nineteenth-century fashion of collecting sporadic family material is now long outdated, active work continues along the lines of examining larger communities and samples for familial patterns. The study of population genetics has become a very important branch of human genetics. It is concerned mainly with the statistical treatment of material gathered from defined communities, and the extraction of gene frequencies and of other values which indicate their genetical composition. Especially noteworthy studies in population genetics have been carried out in Scandinavia, where populations fairly circumscribed geographically exist in rural areas and on islands. Moreover careful national records are kept with complete registers of individuals with various notifiable conditions, including congenital defects. This applies particularly to Denmark. The psychiatric aspects of various communities have been thoroughly investigated in Scandinavian population studies.

In recent years outstanding and classical examples include the genetical and neuropsychiatric study of Böök (5) in a North Swedish population; a study of mongolism in Denmark by Øster (33); a methodological, psychiatric and statistical study of a large Swedish rural population by Larsson and Sjögren (30); and an investigation of the epidemiology and genetics of mental deficiency in a South Swedish population by Åkesson (1).

In Britain our facilities do not lend themselves to studies on this scale or of this type. Attempts have been made however, with rewarding results, to study large but less circumscribed populations. Especially noteworthy examples which are of particular relevance to child psychiatry are the surveys carried out under the auspices of the Scottish Council for Research in Education (47), which yielded useful information of genetical significance about the intelligence of Scottish schoolchildren. The work of Douglas (11) and of Douglas and Blomfield (12), for example, on the pre-school child was similarly based on a large population sample, and has provided extremely useful information, with important psychiatric and genetical implications.

Intermediate between the extensive studies of population genetics and the intensive investigation of a specific condition in a selected and circumscribed sample comes work aimed at extracting more general and varied psychiatric information from a given sample. Such work entails the statistical analysis of clinical data. An example is a study of the incidence of neurosis in the children of psychotics (Cowie (9)). This study, which was based on information about the children of hospital patients, set out to find whether there was evidence to disprove the hypothesis based on genetical grounds that there is no increase of neurosis among the children of psychotics. In fact, the findings in this study showed no overall increase in the incidence of neurosis among the children of psychotics. Various interesting effects were noticed, however, suggesting that certain environmental factors associated with parental psychosis may predispose to neurosis in the children. For instance, of the children who showed neurotic signs, a significantly higher proportion had become neurotic within two years following the onset of parental psychosis than at any other period. This was taken to indicate that the onset of psychosis in a parent can constitute an effective stress factor capable of provoking a neurotic reaction in the children, which fits in with general psychiatric observation. Besides such effects, for which there was every reason to suppose an environmental basis, the main findings of this study supported the view that hereditary influences which may play a part in determining psychosis are without any great effect in the determination of neurosis.

The intensive study of circumscribed populations selected with respect to one particular condition has contributed greatly to psychiatric genetics. Works in this category include the study of complex subjects such as juvenile delinquency. They often set out primarily to investigate environmental effects. Outstanding studies of this kind on juvenile delinquency include the work of the Gluecks in the United States (e.g. (18) and (19)). From the careful and detailed observations of these workers, clues emerge as to the interaction of heredity and evironment in the complex aetiology of juvenile delinquency.

Other studies in this class of intensive investigations of particular conditions begin a from specifically clinical and genetical starting-point. Examples of special relevance include the excellent studies of Hallgren in Sweden into the fairly common problems in child psychiatry of specific dyslexia (20) and enuresis (21). With respect to specific dyslexia, Hallgren studied 276 cases, of whom 116 were probands and 160 were secondary cases (sibs and parents of probands). The probands were from the Stockholm Child Guidance Clinic and from a secondary school. He showed that there is a hereditary type of dyslexia in which an autosomal dominant mode of inheritance was almost certainly operative. A calculation of the incidence of specific dyslexia based on a study of consecutive children in a school sample gave an approximate figure as high as 10% for the condition in the general population. Hallgren found no grounds for assuming a direct association between specific dyslexia and left-handedness, though the incidence of left-handedness was higher in the affected children than in their unaffected sibs or in controls. Although the results from Hallgren's selected sample showed no relationship between certain environmental factors, such as broken homes, and specific dyslexia, he pointed out that his series was not a random sample of the normal population. In some of his cases, moreover, there were grounds for assuming that environmental factors had had an adverse effect on the ability to read and write.

In his monograph on enuresis, Hallgren reviews the literature with respect to the familial incidence of the condition. He draws attention to the opinion held by some, including Kanner, that this familial occurrence is not the result of genetical factors but of a 'family tradition' of enuresis. This is, however, not borne out by earlier systematic studies nor by Hallgren's study. Hallgren based his investigation on 229 propositi from the psychiatric departments of two children's hospitals, and on 173 secondary cases from among their relatives. He showed that nocturnal enuresis is aetiologically heterogeneous, there being cases which are primarily genetically determined and others which he terms 'non-genetic'. As regards the mode of inheritance in genetical cases, Hallgren's results indicate either that a single major dominant gene is responsible, the manifestation of which is modified by the action of the external environment and of many genes of small effect (polygenes), or that the condition is determined solely by the interaction of polygenes and the environment. The study underlines the importance of environmental factors, and Hallgren points out that enuresis, at least in its combined nocturnal and diurnal form, can become manifest as a result of unfavourable environmental factors disturbing the emotional security of the child.

I have outlined the findings of these studies to show how, owing to the close interrelationship of both genetical and environmental factors in psychiatric disorders, it is wrong if not impossible to ignore one class of factors while examining the other. Hallgren's investigations are excellent examples of primarily genetical studies which have nevertheless yielded important evidence relating to environmental effects. Without a comprehensive approach such as this, there is a tendency towards biased results which may confuse and delay the answer to aetiological problems.

5
Biochemical Genetics

The older type of family studies, twin studies, population studies and the investigations of selected samples which have just been described are the products chiefly of clinical observation, measurement and statistical analysis. In addition, for many years special techniques have been employed to give particular kinds of information in human genetical studies. Biochemical techniques have been foremost among these, and the study of human biochemical genetics has come to occupy a special place of its own. In Britain one of the leading exponents of human biochemical genetics is Professor Harry Harris, whose textbook on the subject (23) is a valuable and authoritative source of information.

Historically, human biochemical genetics have their roots in the work of Sir Archibald Garrod, who at the beginning of this century introduced the concept of inborn errors of metabolism. His original studies were on conditions such as alkaptonuria, which had little or no psychiatric relevance. Subsequently however many more inborn errors of metabolism have been discovered, which are of special significance to the child psychiatrist since they are associated in greater or lesser degrees with mental defect. The best known amongst these is perhaps phenylketonuria, discovered in 1934 by the Norwegian Fölling. Others in which intellectual impairment is known to occur include galactosaemia, argininosuccinic aciduria, 'maple-syrup urine' disease, the oculocerebrorenal syndrome of Lowe, genetically determined cretinism, citrullinuria and idiopathic hypercalcaemia of infancy.

These genetically determined disorders of metabolism are of special interest in that they pose the question of the relationship between the metabolic error and the mental impairment. We tend to think that there is a direct causal relationship. For instance an amelioration of the mental condition is claimed to follow reduction of the phenylalanine level in the blood in phenylketonuria by means of a special diet. This might suggest that a simple toxic effect on the brain, induced directly by the presence of excessive phenylalanine, had been alleviated. In fact the use of the low phenylalanine diet in phenylketonuria is still empirical, and we do not yet know at all the nature of the connection between the basic metabolic error and the impairment of mental function. The relationship may not be direct. For instance it is not impossible, though not probable on account of dietary and other evidence, that the impairment of mental function on the one hand and the lack of the enzyme phenylalanine hydroxylase on the other may be quite independent of each other as pleiotropic effects of the phenylketonuria gene.

There is good evidence for extending the concept of inborn errors of metabolism to include storage diseases associated with mental subnormality such as the cerebrall ipoidoses and gargoylism, in which large amounts of a mucopolysaccharide are stored. These conditions, which are known to have a hereditary basis, are most probably caused by the genetically determined lack of specific enzymes. In Gaucher's disease, for instance, it has been suggested that a defect in an epimerase enzyme may be responsible for the accumulation of glucose cerebroside (Stein and Gardner (51)).

In those conditions which have been established as inborn errors of metabolism with known specific enzyme defects, and in the storage diseases, biochemical disturbances can be demonstrated clearly. In other clinical conditions with a genetical basis associated with mental subnormality, such as mongolism, biochemical changes of any particular pattern are not at all obvious. However, as in mongolism, there are often widespread changes throughout the whole body, both gross and subtle, and it seems not unreasonable to speculate that these may be biochemically mediated. If this were established, it would extend still further the concept of inborn errors of metabolism. More will be said later in connection with the possibilities for further biochemical investigations along these and other lines in human genetics. Meanwhile another special field of investigation must be introduced, as one which is now leading in human genetics and which holds promise of throwing more light on aetiological problems in psychiatry.

6

Cytogenetics

Until quite recently, our techniques for the visualisation of chromosomes were still so imperfect that up to 1956 we assumed that there were 48 chromosomes in the normal human somatic cell. In the last decade, however, there have been various improvements in the technique of culturing cells from human tissue. Advances have also been made in methods for promoting cell division and arresting it at a phase in which the separate chromosomes are most clearly visible, and in the treatment of cell preparations for photography under the microscope for well-defined pictures of the chromosomes.

In 1956 a paper was published by Tjio and Levan which marked the beginning of a new era in cytology, since when cytogenetics has developed into the main growing point of human genetics. In their classical paper, Tjio and Levan (52) reported for the first time that the human somatic cell has a normal complement of only 46 chromosomes. This was soon verified by other workers using the improved cytological techniques.

The improved techniques of handling cell material have made it possible to get such clear pictures of the chromosomes that one may measure and observe their size, morphology and position of the centromere (the point at which the daughter chromatids are still joined when the dividing chromosome is arrested, for instance under the influence of colchicine). These distinguishing features enable chromosomes to be recognised as members of small groups, and sometimes individually. There have been different systems for classification and nomenclature of the chromosomes, but an international classification was agreed upon at a meeting at Denver, Colorado. This is known as the Denver System (Böök *et al.* (6)), and is now very widely used.

Autosomal Anomalies

Obviously, the next step after the confirmation of the normal human chromosome complement was to look for anomalies of number and form in human chromosomes and to see whether these were associated with clinical effects. It is of special interest to those working in child psychiatry that the first autosomal[1] anomaly associated with a clinical syndrome in man was the triplication or trisomy or chromosome 21 in mongolism. This was discovered by the French workers Lejeune, Gauthier and Turpin (31). Their findings were soon followed by the observation by others of 47 chromosomes in the cells of mongols instead of the usual normal human complement of 46, the extra chromosome in these cases being chromosome No. 21.

The establishment of the genetical basis of mongolism in this way was an important event. For many years it had been suspected that some particular genetical mechanism might be responsible for mongolism, although this view was widely discredited by those who put forward purely environmental hypotheses of various kinds. Some of the early workers believed, for instance, that mongolism was due to the faulty implantation of the ovum in ageing endometrium, because a late maternal age is a common observation in mongolism.

The first observations of trisomy 21 associated with mongolism were followed soon by observations of mongols in whom the cells contained the normal human number of 46 chromosomes and only two chromosomes No. 21, as in normal people (Polani *et al.* (41); Penrose (40a)). One of the 46 chromosomes in the cells of these mongols, however, was abnormal in morphology, and had arisen apparently from chromosomal fusion or translocation between fractured chromosomes 15 and 21. The greater parts of these broken chromosomes had joined to produce the abnormal

---

[1] There are two kinds of chromosomes, the sex chromosomes (*X* and *Y*) and the autosomes. There are 22 pairs of autosomes, and two sex chromosomes, in the normal human somatic cell nucleus.

chromosome. A further abnormality in the cells of these mongols was the absence of one of the pair of No. 15 chromosomes.[1] The extra translocated chromosome and the missing No. 15 therefore brought the total chromosome count to 46. Disregarding the actual number of chromosomes in the cell, however, and thinking in terms of the quantity of genetical material present, mongols with this chromosomal pattern or karyotype carried in their cells approximately the same amount of chromosome material as those trivalent for chromosome 21. Very roughly speaking, they had an extra chromosome 21 joined on to a chromosome 15.

Among the normal relatives of these mongols some, including the mothers, were found to carry the same abnormal fused or translocated chromosome as the mongol, but the total chromosome count in their case was only 45, due to the absence of one of the pair of chromosomes No. 21. Presumably the quantitative balance of chromosomal material was correct in their cells, although the total chromosome number was reduced. The discovery of mongols with chromosomal translocation and having carriers of the same abnormal chromosome among their normal relatives demonstrated a mode of hereditary transmission which, though not very common in mongolism, operates in at least a number of cases.

Trisomy 21 is present in many more mongols than are translocated chromosomes, and the extra chromosome in trisomy arises through a genetical process called non-disjunction. This is failure of separation of chromosomes or of daughter chromatids in cell division, so that one extra chromosome finds its way into a cell. This may occur at one of several stages. It may occur in the parent at gamete formation, or after the zygote destined to become the mongol has been formed by fusion of the parental germ cells. It is supposed that non-disjunction occurs most often in gametogenesis, and the observed maternal age effect would indicate an implication of the ovum rather than of the sperm (Penrose (39)).

Trisomy 21 and one type of chromosomal translocation in mongolism have now been mentioned. There is a third type of chromosomal aberration in mongolism as well. This is translocation or chromosomal fusion between chromosomes of the group containing chromosomes Nos. 21 and 22. Just as in the other translocation type of mongolism, there is a modal number of 46 chromosomes in the cell. One of the group involved, however, is again abnormal in morphology and is abnormally large, so that the mongol is carrying too much genetical material in the cell. Again, normal carriers of the fused chromosome with a reduced total chromosome count are found amongst the normal relatives, though in this type of translocation fathers, and not mothers, have been found to be carriers. Moreover an associated late paternal age effect has been demonstrated in mongolism with this type of translocation (Penrose (40).)

---

[1] This translocation may involve a chromosome 13, 14 or 15, as chromosomes of this group are very alike and difficult to distinguish, but for purposes of this description we will refer to chromosome 15.

Although these chromosomal anomalies have been discovered in association with mongolism, we are still ignorant of the influences by which they make their effects shown in such a widespread manner, affecting probably every tissue of the body and, by no means least, mental function. On the other hand we have various clues as to the kind of influences that might facilitate the chromosomal aberrations responsible. Observations of both maternal and paternal age effects have already been mentioned. It seems that the physique of the mother may be associated with the production of a mongol child at a young maternal age (Coppen and Cowie (8)) and that this in turn may depend upon the endocrinological status of the mother (Rundle, Coppen and Cowie (46)). Clues such as these are worth following to discover the fundamental aetiological factors, which may well be chemical in nature.

To turn from mongolism: two other conditions have been discovered in which repeated observations have been made of a specific autosomal anomaly associated with a characteristic syndrome that includes mental subnormality. These are trisomy for a chromosome of group 13–15, first described by Patau and his co-workers (36), and trisomy for chromosome 17 or 18 (Edwards *et al.* (13)). These trisomies are known by the chromosome group numbers, because it is very difficult to distinguish between chromosomes 13, 14 and 15 by their size and morphology. Similarly it is difficult to distinguish with certainty between chromosome 17 and chromosome 18.

The syndrome associated with trisomy 13–15 consists of multiple deformities including anophthalmia, hare-lip, cleft palate, polydactyly, cardiac defects, capillary haemangiomata, and a cerebral defect which would no doubt lead to severe mental subnormality if the children with this syndrome lived long enough for it to become fully manifest. They die, however, as a rule early in infancy.

The syndrome associated with trisomy 17–18 includes such features as a peculiar facies with low-set ears and a triangular mouth, small chin, cardiac septal defect, many minor physical abnormalities and spasticity. Again there is evidence of retarded mental development, although these children appear unable to survive infancy.

Many sporadic isolated cases have been reported of other autosomal abnormalities with associated physical and mental defects. Mongolism and the trisomies for chromosomes of groups 13–15 and 17–18 are the only clinical syndromes to date which have been established by repeated observation of a number of cases.

Anomalies of the Sex Chromosomes

It will be remembered that the normal human sex chromosome constitutions are *XY* in the male and *XX* in the female. Several clearly defined syndromes associated with anomalies of the sex chromosomes have been recognised and are now well known. The most common of these are the Klinefelter's syndrome, Turner's syndrome and the triplo-X female. In Klinefelter's syndrome the patient is anatomically male with male genitalia, but has the sex chromosome complement XXY. In Turner's syndrome the patient is anatomically female but with a deficiency of ovarian tissue and with various physical signs, and the sex chromosome complement is XO (or in other words, a single X chromosome only). In the triplo-X syndrome the patient is again anatomically female, but has the sex chromosome complement XXX.

From a psychiatric point of view, it is interesting that a higher proportion of patients with these sex chromosome anomalies has been found among populations of the mentally subnormal than could have been expected from figures of incidence in the normal population. A number of surveys have been carried out in schools for the educationally subnormal and in hospitals for the mentally subnormal, with results to bear this out (e.g. Ferguson-Smith (16); Prader *et al.* (42); Hamerton *et al.* (22)). Although there is a tendency towards reduced capacity for intellectual function to be associated with these sex chromosome anomalies, the association is not a constant one. Moreover in contradistinction to the autosomal anomalies, which appear to be strongly associated with severe mental defect, the sex chromosome anomalies appear to be associated with milder degrees of mental retardation.

A tendency for individuals with Klinefelter's syndrome to exhibit schizoid traits as well as to be of subnormal intelligence has been observed by Pasqualini, Vidal and Bur (35). This observation has been made also by Penrose (38), who has noticed a tendency among patients with Klinefelter's syndrome to be truculent, easily offended, suspicious and paranoid. Observation of such traits in patients with Klinefelter's syndrome has not, however, been often reported.

The search for anomalies of the sex chromosomes has been greatly facilitated by two screening techniques which are simpler and much quicker than the culture and observation of chromosomes. These are the examination of cells, usually obtained from a scraping of buccal mucosa, for sex chromatin masses, and the examination of the nuclei of polymorphonuclear leucocytes for the presence of club-shaped projections or 'drumsticks'.

Briefly, with respect to sex chromatin masses, it has been found that in females with a normal sex chromosome complement XX about 50% to 70% of cells have a small intranuclear body close to the nuclear membrane. These intranuclear bodies can be stained clearly. It has been suggested that they are masses of sex chromatin, and that a cell with n times X chromosomes contains $n-1$ of these bodies. Hence a normal female with an XX sex chromosome constitution would be expected to show $2-1$, or one, of these bodies in a number of her cells. A triplo-X female, with three X chromosomes per cell, would show a cellular content of $3-1$, or two, of these bodies. A normal male, on the other hand, would be expected to be deficient in these bodies, as he possesses only one X chromosome. A male with Klinefelter's syndrome however, having the sex chromosome complement XXY, would show $2-1$, or one, sex chromatin body in a proportion of his cells. The sex chromatin bodies and their relationship to the X chromosome was first discovered by Barr and Bertram (3) during experiments with nervous tissue from cats.

The 'drumstick' phenomenon in polymorphonuclear leucocytes was first observed and reported by Davidson and Smith (10). They found a club-shaped projection or 'drumstick' in approximately six out of every 500 polymorph nuclei from females, and none in those from males. This is the basis of a very useful screening test for sex chromosomes anomalies by the examination of blood smears.

Although these tests may be used for preliminary screening for sex chromosome anomalies, the actual culture and examination of chromosomes is lengthy and complicated and requires special skill. It is natural therefore that special populations and abnormal individuals should have been tackled first in the search for chromosomal anomalies. Normal population surveys have still to be done (although newborn babies have been studied) to answer such questions as how compatible sex chromosome anomalies may be with physical and mental normality.

The chromosomes of patients with the main syndromes associated with mental subnormality (besides mongolism) and with psychosis and other psychiatric conditions have been examined, but no characteristic chromosomal anomalies have been found. Special interest has been shown in the chromosomal status of patients with abnormal sexual behaviour. Many years ago the theory had been put forward that male homosexuals are genotypically female (Lang (29)). This was based on the observation of an increased incidence of males among the sibs of homosexuals. The new techniques of chromosome examination however, when applied to series of homosexual patients, have failed to show a conflict between anatomical and chromosomal sex, and provide strong evidence against the theory of Lang (Pare (34); Pritchard (43)). Similarly no incompatibility has been found between somatic and chromosomal sex in the case of transvestites (Barr and Hobbs (4)).

The Limitations of present Cytological Techniques, and possible further Lines of Research

These findings by no means exclude a genetical factor in the aetiology of homosexuality or similar sexual deviations. By the same token, the negative findings in the chromosomal examinations do not rule out hereditary factors in the case of patients with other types of psychiatric disorder, including psychosis. Although there have been great technical improvements recently, our pictures of the chromosomes are still comparatively crude, and show only such changes as differences of number and fairly gross morphology. It is most likely that we are still a long way from being able to detect the subtle differences, probably of a chemical nature, which no doubt lie within the chromosomes and determine the physical and mental constitution of man.

Lines of genetical research may well proceed from this point into the field of molecular biology and again link up with biochemical genetics. The work of Watson, Crick and their colleagues in the Medical Research Council Microbiological Research Unit in Cambridge has laid a foundation for development in this direction. They have worked on the chemical structure of genetical material, and some years ago put forward an ingenious hypothesis for the molecular structure of deoxyribonucleic acid (DNA), of which the chromosomes are supposed to consist (Watson and Crick (53)). They suggested that this molecule is a double helix which can unwind, divide and replicate itself. They have elaborated this hypothesis, and with supportive evidence now postulate a chemical genetical code carried upon this molecule. It is not within the scope of this chapter to discuss these developments, but they are reviewed well and with basic references in a recent annotation of the *Lancet* (Anon. (2)).

One of the most striking facts about observed chromosomal anomalies is their association with mental function. As we have seen, anomalies of both the sex chromosomes and the autosomes are associated with impairment of intellect. They are associated with widespread changes throughout the body, and it would not be surprising if the highly specialised tissue of the central nervous system were particularly susceptible to such far-reaching effects. The solution of the great problem of how these changes are mediated, possibly through altered metabolism, may throw completely new light on our concepts of factors in the aetiology of mental disorder.

7

Genetical Counselling

So far, different fields of genetical research have been considered. Finally, let us turn briefly to the subject of genetical counselling, in which the information gained by research finds practical application to clinical problems. In the field of child psychiatry, genetical counselling is at present confined almost exclusively to problems relating to mental subnormality. Here a good deal is known of the modes of inheritance and of genetical influences operating in different clinical syndromes.

Genetical counselling rests mainly on calculating the risk of various classes of relative being affected similarly to the patient. The Mendelian principles of dominant and recessive modes of genetical transmission play an important part in the calculation of risk figures. It is possible, for example, to advise the parents of a phenylketonuric child that, of children born to them, one out of four is likely to have the phenylketonuria gene in double dose (i.e. to be heterozygote) and to have phenylketonuria. Two out of four are likely to have the phenylketonuria gene in single dose (i.e. to be heterozygotes), but to be clinically free from phenylketonuria. One out of four is likely to be completely free from the phenylketonuria gene, but again to be clinically free from the condition. This advice is based on the knowledge that phenylketonuria is a Mendelian recessive trait, and that the parents therefore each carry the gene in single dose.

It cannot be too strongly emphasised that genetical risk figures are merely expressions of tastistical probability. Although the three genetical types set out above, of children that can be born to parents each carrying the phenylketonuria gene, are theoretically likely to occur in the proportions given, in practice it is possible for them to appear in any proportion. It is possible for example, though not likely, for parents each carrying a single phenylketonuria gene to give birth to a number of children all of whom are phenylketonuric. Alternatively, all the children might be lucky enough to escape completely any inheritance of the gene.

The scope for genetical counselling advice has been extended with the development of techniques for detecting the heterozygote in Mendelian recessive conditions. Until recently the proportion of heterozygous (gene-carrying) sibs of patients homozygous for recessive conditions could be only inferred. One could not tell which possessed the gene and which were free. Now, however, various biochemical methods have been devised to identify individuals as genetical carriers. For example it has been found that, although the heterozygote for the phenylketonuria gene is clinically free from the condition, his response to a phenylalanine tolerance test is moderately abnormal. The response is grossly abnormal in the phenyl-ketonuric homozygote. This effect was first discovered by Hsia and his co-workers (24). Even in the absence of a loading dose of phenylalanine given for the tolerance test, differences in the blood levels of phenylalanine between heterozygotes for phenyolketonuria and homozygous normal subjects have been reported (Knox and Messinger (27)). This makes it possible to detect by chemical means the heterozygous carrier for phenyl-ketonuria. There are situations in which such testing can be of practical value to the individual. For instance, if the sib of a phenylketonuric patient were contemplating marriage, it could be ascertained whether he or she were a carrier of the phenylketonuria gene. If the result of testing were positive, the test could be carried out with the intended spouse. The information obtained would provide a basis for genetical advice about the progeny to be expected from the marriage.

Another class of hereditary conditions where it would be especially helpful in genetical counselling to detect the presence of unexpressed genes are those in which the clinical signs do not become apparent until later in life. Such conditions do not, by definition, come into the realm of child psychiatry. Genetical counselling however is essentially concerned with hereditary problems of the family as a whole, and the problems are frequently concerned with hereditary conditions.

Huntington's chorea, a dominant Mendelian trait, is a classical example of the group of genetical conditions in which the onset of signs is delayed until later life. The mean age of onset for Huntington's chorea is about 35 years. Accordingly the possessor of the gene has often passed on the gene to his or her children before signs of the disease have appeared. So far, no objective or quantifiable test for the early detection of gene carriers in this condition has been devised, though there have been suggestions of non-specific EEG changes which antedate the onset of choreic signs, an increase in psychiatric disturbance of various kinds among those who later develop the disease, and chemical changes which may be associated with the condition, including possible changes in amino-acid metabolism (Seakins and Cowie (48)) and changes in the serum globulin patterns on electrophoresis (McMenemey (32)). Any likely clue is well worth following up, since detection of affected individuals before the reproductive period could to a great extent reduce the incidence of the condition.

Besides biochemical methods, cytogenetical investigations are giving technical information not formerly obtainable in special problems of genetical counselling. The general public are becoming better informed on scientific matters, and it is not uncommon to be asked in a genetical counselling clinic whether the chromosomes are affected. This question is not limited to the lay inquirers. Frequently one's professional colleagues suggest, apparently without any definite clinical grounds for suspicion, that chromosome analysis should be carried out. It should be pointed out that we now have enough evidence to show that, with present techniques, only a limited number of conditions are associated with detectable chromosome changes. Usually they are characterised by quite striking physical changes, including congenital deformities, and by mental subnormality. The occasions on which it would seem profitable to look at the chromosomes are limited, especially as the processes of culture and examination require much time and skill.

There are, however, certain circumstances in which the answer to genetical problems may be greatly modified by information from chromosome analysis. For instance in the case of a young mother, say under 30, who has borne a mongol child, chromosome analysis may show that she is a genetically balanced 15/21 translocation carrier. In that case her chances of bearing further mongols at any age would be likely to be increased. If on the other hand her mongol baby were found to have 21 trisomy, and the mother herself and baby's father had normal karyotypes, we would have no theoretical grounds in cytogenetics for supposing that her chances of bearing further mongols were greater than for mothers in the general population. It has been estimated that for mothers who have borne a mongol under the age of 25 years the risk of bearing a second mongol is something like 50-fold the random risk, whereas there is no increased risk for mothers over the age of 35 (Carter and Evans (7)). It has been suggested, however, that the increased risk for younger mothers is at least partially explained by instances where one or other parent has been found to be a translocation carrier.

As our knowledge of genetical mechanisms advances, there is perhaps an increasing tendency in genetical counselling to present the gloomy picture of a multitude of unlikely dangers. One should remember that the inquirer is often more anxious than the facts warrant, and usually comes expecting to get pessimistic advice. As a rule those who come to the genetical counselling clinic of their own accord are responsible and conscientious people, of the kind who make excellent parents. It is very sad if, on account of unduly pessimistic advice, they should deprive themselves unnecessarily of children. Genetical counselling should never be undertaken in a thoughtless or irresponsible manner. Genetical risks should, of course, be explained, but at the same time reassurance should be given whenever possible, and the advisor should do whatever he can to alleviate the guilt borne by so many parents who feel they have almost wittingly passed on some hereditary condition to their children.

REFERENCES

1. AKESSON, H. O., 1961. *Epidemiology and genetics of mental deficiency in a South Swedish population.* Published from the Institute for Medical Genetics, University of Uppsala.
2. ANON., 1962. The sequence hypothesis. (An annotation). *Lancet,* ii: 81-83.
3. BARR, M. L. and BERTRAM, E. G., (1949). A morphological difference between neurones of the male and female. *Nature,* **163**: 676.
4. BARR, K. L. and HOBBS, G. E., 1954. Chromosomal sex in transvestites. *Lancet,* i: 1109.
5. BÖÖK, J. A., 1953. A genetic and neuropsychiatric investigation of a North Swedish population. *Acta Genet.,* **4**.
6. BÖÖK, J. A., CHU, E. H. Y., FORD, C. E., FRACCARO, M., HARNDEN, D. G., HSU, T. C., HUNGERFORD, D. A., JACOBS, P. A., LEJEUNE, J., LEVAN, A., MAKINO, S., PUCK, T. T., ROBINSON, A., TJIO, J. H., CATCHESIDE, D. G., MULLER, H. J. and STERN C.,, 1960. A proposed standard system of nomenclature of human mitotic chromosomes. *Lancet,* i: 1063.
7. CARTER, C. O. and EVANS, K. A., 1961. Risk of parents who have had one child with Down's syndrome (mongolism) having another child similarly affected. *Lancet,* ii: 785-788.
8. COPPEN, A. and COWIE, V., 1960. Maternal health and mongolism. *Brit. Med. J.,* i: 1843-7.
9. COWIE, V., 1961. The incidence of neurosis in the children of psychotics. *Acta Psychiat. Scandinavica,* **37**: 37-87.
10. DAVIDSON, W. M. and SMITH, D. R., 1954. A morphological sex difference in the polymorphonuclear neutrophil leucocytes. *Brit. Med. J.,* ii: 6.
11. DOUGLAS, J. W. B., 1951. Social class differences in health and survival during the first two years of life: result of a national survey. *Popul. Stud.* **5**: 35.
12. DOUGLAS, J. W. B. and BLOMFIELD, J. M., 1958. *Children Under Five.* London: George Allen and Unwin.
13. EDWARDS, J. H., HARNDEN, D. G., CAMERON, A. H., CROSSE, V. M. and WOLFF, O. H., 1960. A new trisomic syndrome. *Lancet,* i: 787-9.

14. EYSENCK, H. J., 1951. Neuroticism in twins. *Eugen. Rev.*, **43**: 79-82.
15. EYSENCK, H. J. and PRELL, D. B., 1951. The inheritance of neuroticism: an experimental study. *J. Ment. Sci.*, **98**: 441-465.
16. FERGUSON-SMITH, M. A., 1958. Chromatin positive Klinefelter's syndrome (primary micro-orchidism) in a mental deficiency hospital. *Lancet*, i: 928-931.
17. GEDDA, L., 1951. *Studio dei Gemelli*. Rome: Edizione Orizzonte Medico.
18. GLUECK, S. and GLUECK, E., 1950. *Unraveling Juvenile Delinquency*. The Commonwealth Fund, N.Y.
19. 1959. *Predicting Delinquency and Crime*. Cambridge, Mass.: Harvard Univ. Press.
20. HALLGREN, B., 1950. *Specific Dyslexia (Congenital Word-Blindness)*. Copenhagen: Munksgaard.
21. 1957. *Enuresis—a Clinical and Genetical Study*. Copenhagen: Munksgaard.
22. HAMERTON, J. L., JAGIELLO, G. M. and KIRMAN, B. H., 1962. Sex chromosome abnormalities in a population of mentally defective children. *Brit. Med. J.*, i: 220-3.
23. HARRIS, H., 1959. *Human Biochemical Genetics*. Cambridge Univ. Press.
24. HSIA, D. Y-Y., DRISCOLL, K., TROLL, W. and KNOX, W. E., 1956. Heterozygous carriers of phenylketonuria detected by phenylalanine tolerance tests. *Nature*, **178**: 1279-80.
25. KALLMANN, F. J. and ROTH, B., 1956. Genetic aspects of pre-adolescent schizophrenia. *Amer. J. Psychiat.*, **112**: 599-606.
26. KENT, E., 1949. A study of maladjusted twins. *Smith College Studies in Social Work*, **19**, 63-77.
27. KNOX, W. E. and MESSINGER, E. C., 1958. The detection in the heterozygote of the metabolic effect of the recessive gene for phenylketonuria. *Amer. J. Hum. Genet.*, **10**, 53-60.
28. KRANZ, H., 1937. Untersuchungen an Zwillingen in Fürsorgeerziehungsan stalten. *Zeitschr. f. Indukt. u. Abstam. Vererbungslehre*, **73**: 508-512.
29. LANG, T., 1940. Genetic determination of homosexuality. *J. Nerv. Ment. Dis.*, **92**: 55.
30. LARSSON, T. and SJÖGREN, T., 1954. A methodological, psychiatric and statistical study of a large Swedish rural population. *Acta Psychiat., Kbh.*, Supp. 89.
31. LEJEUNE, J., GAUTHIER, M. and TURPIN, R., 1959. Les chromosomes humains en culture de tissus. *C. R. Acad. Sci. Paris*, **248**: 602.
32. McMENEMEY, W. H., 1961. Immunity mechanisms in neurological disease. *Proc. Roy. Soc. Med.*, **54**: 127-136.
33. ØSTER, J., 1953. Mongolism. *Opera Ex Domo Biologiae Hereditariae Humanae*, 32. Copenhagen: Danish Science Press.
34. PARE, C. M. B., 1956. Homosexuality and chromosomal sex. *J. Psychosom. Res.*, 1: 247-251.
35. PASQUALINI, R. Q., VIDAL, G. and BUR, G. E., 1957. Psychopathology of Klinefelter's syndrome: a review of thirty-one cases. *Lancet*, ii: 164-7.
36. PATAU, K., SMITH, D. W., THERMAN, E., INHORN, S. L. and WAGNER, H. P., 1960. Multiple congenital anomaly caused by an extra autosome. *Lancet*, i: 790-3.
37. PENROSE, L. S., 1955. Genetics and the criminal. *Brit. J. Delinq.*, **6**: 15-25.
38. 1960. Personal communication.
39. 1961. Mongolism. *Brit. Med. Bull.*, **17**: 184-9.
40. 1962. Paternal age in mongolism. *Lancet*, i: 1101.
40a. PENROSE, L. S., ELLIS., J. R. and DELHANTY, J. D. A., 1960. Chromosomal translocation in mongolism and in normal relatives. *Lancet*, ii: 409-10.

41. POLANI, P. E., BRIGGS, J. H., FORD, C. E., CLARKE, C. M. and BERG, J. M.'
    1960. A mongol girl with 46 chromosomes. *Lancet*, i: 721-4.
42. PRADER, A., SCHNEIDER, J., ZÜBLIN, W., FRANCES, J. M. and RÜDI, K., 1958.
    Die Haufigkeit des echten chromatin-positiven Klinefelter-Syndroms und
    seine Beziehungen zum Schwachsinn. *Schweiz. med. Wschr.*, 88: 917-920.
43. PRITCHARD, M., 1962. Homosexuality and genetic sex. *J. Ment. Sci.*, 108:
    616-623.
44. ROSANOFF, A. J., HANDY, L. M. and PLESSET, I. R., 1941. The etiology of
    child behaviour difficulties, juvenile delinquency and adult criminality,
    with special reference to their occurrence in twins. *Psychiat. Monogr.*, 1:
    187. Dept. of Institutions, Sacramento, Cal.
    1941. Authors' abstract of the preceding. *Amer. J. Psychiat.*, 97: 1479.
45. ROSANOFF, A. J., HANDY, L. M. and ROSANOFF, I. A., 1934. Criminality and
    delinquency in twins. *J. Crim. Law and Criminal.*, 24: 923-934.
46. RUNDLE, A., COPPEN, A. and COWIE, V., 1961. Steroid excretion in mothers of
    mongols. *Lancet*, ii: 846-8.
47. SCOTTISH COUNCIL FOR RESEARCH IN EDUCATION, 1949. *The Trend of Scottish
    Intelligence*. London.
48. SEAKINS, J. W. T. and COWIE, V., 1962. Urinary alanine excretor in a Hunting-
    ton's chorea family. *J. Ment. Sci.*, 108: 427-431.
49. SHIELDS, J., 1954. Personality differences and neurotic traits in normal twin
    schoolchildren. *Eugen. Rev.*, 45: 213-246.
50. SLATER, E., 1943. The neurotic constitution. *J. Neurol. Psychiat.*, 6: 1.
51. STEIN, M. H. and GARDNER, L. I., 1960. Possible site of a biochemical error
    in Gaucher's disease. *Lancet*, ii: 1254.
52. TJIO, J. H. and LEVAN, A., 1956. Chromosome number of man. *Hereditas*,
    42: 1.
53. WATSON, J. D. and CRICK, F. H. C., 1953. Genetical implications of the
    structure of deoxyribonucleic acid. *Nature*, 171: 964.

IV

PIAGET'S THEORY

MARY WOODWARD

B.A., PH.D.

*Lecturer in Psychology, University College of Swansea,
University of Wales*

1

Introduction

Piaget's theory is concerned with the way children think. Since the late 1920's he has worked with a group of colleagues and students at Geneva, and they have made intensive studies of the concepts which children of different ages have about the world around them. The aim has been to investigate in detail many aspects of various concepts by means either of a free-ranging interview or by observations of children's attempts to solve problems. Attention has been directed to the process by which the child's thinking becomes progressively adapted to the understanding of objective reality and freed from the distorting features of early childhood.

In order to trace this process, it was necessary to go back to the origins of adaptive behaviour in infancy. The theory thus begins with the formless world of the infant in which patches of light and sounds come and go, without permanence beyond the immediate present and without solidity or organisation in space. It considers how, from this, the child achieves stability in his view of the world, first on the level of perception and then in his thinking.

The relevance of this theory for child psychiatry is that it is a systematic account of a major aspect of child development, namely of intelligence. It suggests that it is characteristic of children at certain ages to be bound to the present, to distort reality in the interest of subjective needs, to consider one aspect of a situation and neglect others, to be animistic, egocentric, concrete and unable to deal with the abstract and hypothetical.

The concepts studied have included, for example, those of physical causality (19)[1], time (27), movement and speed (21) and the world (18).

[1] The bibliographical references are to English translations when these are available; otherwise the publications in French are given.

Mathematical concepts have been investigated in collaboration with Inhelder and Szeminska: number (23), space (28) and geometry (30). Adolescent thinking has been given particular attention by Inhelder; it is to her findings that Piaget has most extensively applied the logical analysis which is a feature of his approach (Inhelder and Piaget (8)). A less widely known interest of Piaget is in the developmental study of perceptual illusions in children, in which he has been associated with Lambercier and others.

Readers interested in a more detailed knowledge of this work are referred to the original publications. In this chapter an outline of the theory of intellectual development will be given, with more detail on those aspects that are most relevant to problems of child psychiatry. This account is of the psychological processes; the logical analysis of these, of which a short account can be found in Piaget (25), will not be dealt with. The work on perception, which also will not be considered, has been ably summarised by Wohlwill (34).

2

General Features of the Theory

The essential feature of the theory is that intelligence develops through a sequence of progressively more complex patterns of action and thinking, beginning with the reflexes present at birth and culminating in abstract thinking; the new patterns are organised out of the simpler ones of the previous phases. The steps in the sequence are considered to be stages of development: when a new type of behaviour pattern or of thinking appears it is generalised to other aspects of reality, though with some time-lag.

The process which Piaget describes is one of learning, in interaction with the material and social environment, within the limits set by maturation. The two main explanatory concepts used in the account of this process are assimilation and accommodation: the child applies his behaviour patterns to an increasing variety of objects, and modifies them in order to adapt to new aspects of reality. The child is however not passive in this process: it is through his active seeking (to repeat an experience or to solve a problem) that he develops organised patterns of action and thinking. The term *schema* is used for these patterns of action and thinking. An aspect of reality arouses a schema which has been acquired in relation to a similar object, and the new object is said to be incorporated or *assimilated* into that schema. For example, the child has acquired a schema of patting a doll which hangs near him in order to make it swing; he then pats other hanging objects, which are assimilated into this schema, i.e. perceived as objects to be patted. In this way new objects are linked with past experience.

Sometimes, however, the new aspect of reality is too dissimilar from those around which existing schemata have been developed. If a schema is modified in order to deal with it, Piagets peaks of *accommodation*. When the infant manipulates objects, the way they behave does not always fit in with his expectations; similarly the child's views about the world are frequently at variance with those of adults around him. Consequently the behaviour of objects and the concepts of adults are facts of reality which require the child to accommodate his schemata. He does so if he varies his action when existing ones are inadequate, and if he alters his beliefs in order to take account of new facts.

In adaptive action and in the development of more complex schemata there is a balance between the two processes: when there is little accommodation the assimilated reality is distorted; on the other hand without assimilation there cannot be comprehension.

3

The Methods of Investigation

Details of the methods used by Piaget and his co-workers will appear in the account of the theory. There are, however, one or two general points which should be made. In all but the earlier studies (16, 17, 18, 19, 20) children of 4 years and over are set tasks with concrete material. They are given the opportunity to experiment with it and see what happens, to try out their beliefs in action and to correct them by their observations. Detailed records are made of the methods used by children when they tackle problems; inappropriate responses resulting in failure are as illuminating as methods which lead to a successful solution. If the child arrives at an incorrect solution, he is presented with repeated trials of the problem in such a way as to draw his attention to the source of his error. This procedure gives him the opportunity to find out whether his inference is correct. The point of interest is whether he coordinates these successive observations, or whether he persists in his error. The term 'clinical' has frequently been applied by Piaget to his methods, particularly to those of the earlier studies, when the child was questioned in detail about his concepts.

4

The Stages of Development

Piaget distinguishes four main stages. During the *sensori-motor* stage the child acts in relation to objects that are perceptually present, and behaves as if the objective world is centred on his activities. In the *pre-operational* stage the child can manipulate words and mental images as representations of absent objects. though he is egocentric in his thinking and consequently has a distorted view of reality. With the stage of *concrete operations*, at about the age of 7 years, he is able to come to correct conclusions about concrete aspects of reality, though it is not until the advent of *abstract operations* in adolescence that he is able to deal with the possible and the abstract.

The Sensori-motor Stage (up to about 18 months)

To a certain extent the behaviour which Piaget observed during the sensori-motor stage has also been recorded by other investigators of infant behaviour, such as Gesell. Similarly others, for example Buhler, have studied the infant's attempts to solve the same kinds of problems. They, like Piaget, have been interested in how the child handles objects, what he does when he drops them and whether he can draw to him a toy that is attached to a piece of string.

Piaget's approach is, however, different in several respects from that of the normative studies. In the first place he has classified the items of behaviour on the basis of their similarity. For example, instead of recording such items as shaking a rattle, banging a brick, etc., he classified together those manipulations which are repeated in about the same form, producing each time the same effect on the object, such as banging a brick on the same surface, patting a hanging toy. Another group of similar manipulations were those in which the child varied his action and consequently the effect on the object, for example when he banged a toy successively on different surfaces or dropped an object from different heights. Behaviour patterns used for solving problems were classified in the same way.

One of the most important differences is that Piaget has interpreted the behaviour in terms of what it reveals about the way the world appears to the infant. Thus he observed behaviour and devised problems with a view to determining whether the child appeared to be aware of objects when he no longer perceived them, to what extent he regarded objects as organised in space, and whether he attributed the movements of objects to other agents besides himself.

Furthermore Piaget was interested in finding out how more complex patterns developed. This meant that he had to make observations at frequent intervals on a small number of children. For this reason he observed his own three children for this period.

Investigations were made of the development of intelligent adaptive behaviour by means of observations of spontaneous movements, manipulations of toys and problem-solving. The result of the classification of behaviour patterns is that six types were distinguished, giving six sub-stages (Piaget (24)). A second set of observations dealt with the child's construction of objective reality (awareness of the permanent object, spatial relations, causal interactions and the temporal sequence) (26). Correspondences were found between stages in this aspect and those in adaptive behaviour. The third set of observations concerned the development of imitation, and again correspondences were found with the other aspects (22).

The quality of the observations, the amount of detailed observation and the careful checks can be appreciated only by consulting the original works. The following outline is restricted to the main characteristic of each sub-stage. There are, of course, large differences between the ages at which infants develop various behaviour patterns, and those given are assumed average ages.

Sub-stage 1 (the first month). The first sub-stage is that of reflex schemata. Because the functions exist, the infant exercises them; he looks at light, attempts to grasp, etc. There is learning within each schema, but not coordination of schemata nor the formation of new ones. For example the child learns to recognise the nipple through repeated contact with the surrounding area, but he is unable to coordinate the movement of his head with that of his hand in order to direct his thumb to his mouth when it falls out. The extension of visual, sucking and grasping reflexes to a variety of objects depends on chance contact with them.

Sub-stage 2 (approx. 1 to $4\frac{1}{2}$ months). From the second sub-stage onwards, new schemata are acquired. Piaget accounts for their development in terms of Baldwin's concept of the circular reaction, namely that an action by chance leads to a certain result, and if the child perceives it, that result is the stimulus for the repetition of the action, and so on. The characteristic behaviour patterns (*primary circular reactions*) classified at the second sub-stage are concerned only with the child's functions and do not produce effects on objects. For example the infant fixates objects and follows moving ones; he develops various kinds of hand movements, such as opening and closing his fist and moving his hand about while looking at it; he repetitively utters sounds; he plays with his saliva.

The independent schemata are coordinated with one another during this sub-stage, through a process of accommodation and reciprocal assimilation. When the child grasps objects placed in his mouth as well as taking to his mouth objects that he grasps, there is reciprocal assimilation between the grasping and sucking schemata. These coordinations unify different experiences of the object: when the child is able to look in the direction of the source of a sound, the visual and auditory sensations are associated with the same object. Later, when the visual, sucking and grasping schemata are coordinated with one another, these different experiences of objects are related to the same object.

It cannot be inferred at this point that the infant is aware of the existence of objects when he does not perceive them. The infant of 2 to 3 months goes on gazing in the direction in which a person went out of his view, but if nothing happens he soon gives up. Piaget argues that if the child had an awareness of unperceived objects he would go on searching, at least with his eyes.

Sub-stage 3 (approx. $4\frac{1}{2}$ to 8 or 9 months). After the last coordination, when the child begins to use vision to direct his hands towards objects in order to grasp them, he is able to develop a new type of behaviour pattern, the *secondary circular reaction*, which characterises the third sub-stage. Unlike the schemata of the previous sub-stage, the new ones produce an effect on objects; unlike the tertiary circular reactions of the fifth sub-stage, they produce with each repetition the same sort of effect on the object. For example, while shaking his pram, the infant by chance on one occasion sees that the toys hanging from the hood swing. The sight of this stimulates him to repeat the same movement, which produces the effect again, and so on. Other examples of secondary circular reactions are banging a brick on the same surface, shaking a rattle, hitting a hanging object so that it swings.

The ability to acquire this sort of schema makes for progress in the child's construction of the world of objects, but it also imposes limitations on this. The continuation of an action or perception, as when the child retrieves an object he drops by following the line of fall with his hand, or visually follows one dropped by someone else, contributes to the development of subsequent schemata that will lead to an awareness of the permanence of objects. And when the infant pulls a string in order to make an object hanging from it swing, he is seeing two objects united in space. But at the same time these developments suggest to the child that the existence of objects and their spatial relations and movements depend on his actions and perceptions.

Even when highly motivated, children at this stage do not uncover a completely hidden object. For example, one child before a meal was shown the feeding-bottle, and then saw the observer's hand placed in front of it. She did not move the hand, although she could reach it. Instead she kicked with anger, and stared at it expectantly, with an expression of desire, as if the bottle would reappear. The existence of the bottle, for the child, appeared to be dependent on her perception of it.

The child also acts as if the spatial position of objects is related to himself. When a child was seated on his lap, Piaget spoke into her left ear, and she turned until she saw his face. He then spoke into her right ear, and she looked again to her left, although she was usually accurate in localising sounds.

The development of secondary circular reactions depends on the learning of an association between an action the child performs and an effect he perceives while doing so, such that the repetition of the action reproduces the effect. But there is incorrect generalisation when the infant acts as if any movement which he observes while he is making an action is the result of that action. For example, Piaget passed a toy to and fro in front of the child, who looked at it attentively and arched her back (her typical way of expressing pleasure). She did this each time the toy was passed to and fro (Piaget himself not being visible). Then it was held motionless and she again arched her back, as if her action were responsible for the movement of the object.

Imitation, which had previously occurred sporadically, became systematic with the development of secondary circular reactions. The models which the child then imitated were sounds already uttered by him, and movements in his repertoire which involved parts of his body that he could see.

Sub-stage 4 (8 or 9 months to 11 or 12 months). The coordination of the schemata formed in sub-stage 3 marks a new sub-stage. One schema is subordinated to another with the aim of achieving a goal, as when the child pushes aside an obstacle that prevents him from grasping a toy he can see behind it. The particular schemata which were utilised varied from child to child. In one instance the obstacle problem evoked the schema of striking hanging objects; this was applied to knocking down the screen, so that the child could grasp the toy he saw behind it. There is a similar coordination and attainment of a goal when the child uses the hand of another person as an instrument, for example when he takes an adult's hand and places it on the toy it had previously been shaking.

More complex manipulations (derived secondary circular reactions) are achieved through coordinating existing schemata; for example the child repeatedly picks up and drops an object from a height of a few inches.

Other manipulations are interpreted as indicating development in the objectification of the child's view of his immediate world. Hiding and finding games suggest that the infant is beginning to be aware of unperceived objects (which was confirmed by systematic observation). When the child holds a toy successively at different distances and angles, looking at it intently, apparently comparing its appearance, Piaget suggests he is learning to recognise the object in different spatial positions, despite differences in the retinal image. Experiments on the development of perceptual constancy in infancy are cited in support of this interpretation.

At this stage also the child frequently turned an object round and round, while looking at it intently; this suggested he was learning about the three-dimensional nature of objects, particularly of the reverse side. This interpretation was confirmed by other observations. When the feeding bottle had been presented with the bottom end towards the child in the third sub-stage, he did not rotate the bottle and find the nipple, even after it had been presented vertically and he had looked alternately at the top and bottom. Children had sucked the glass at the bottom end. Now, however, they quickly rotated the bottle.

Similarly with regard to awareness of causality, the children began to behave as if they were aware that objects may be moved by external agents.

This progress in adaptive behaviour and this partial detachment of the object from the child's actions and perceptions make possible the new developments that were observed in imitation. To begin with the child is still limited to imitating movements already in his repertoire, but the advance is that he can now imitate when he cannot see the part of his body that is involved. Later in this phase he begins to imitate new sounds and new movements, though the latter are again restricted to those he can see himself making. The imitation of new models is considered to result from the child's incipient awareness of objects as distinct from himself. New models are thus seen as different from and similar to his movements and the sounds he has already made. The familiar aspect of the model tends to induce the child to assimilate it to his schema in its entirety, but the unfamiliar aspect attracts his attention, because it is an obstacle to the reproduction of the sound or movement. The coordination of schemata in intelligent adaptive actions produces flexibility and increases accommodation. Thus the schemata that are aroused by the new models can be accommodated to them. This explains why the new models that are first imitated are analogous to the objects of the child's schemata; the totally unfamiliar model, which involves actions not developed by the child, are not imitated. Piaget gives a number of interesting examples of this process (22).

Sub-stage 5 (11 or 12 months to approx. 18 months). The fifth sub-stage is characterised by more complex manipulations (*tertiary circular reactions*), in which the movement, and consequently the effect on the object, is varied. Adaptive behaviour in problem situations is increased in that the child finds new means to achieve a solution by a trial and error process. There is corresponding progress in the construction of the objective world and in imitation.

These developments are attributed to increased accommodation and a greater differentiation of this process from the assimilating process: when an object or an aspect of it cannot be assimilated into existing schemata, the latter can now be accommodated to it, provided it is not too different from those assimilated in the schemata it evokes. In this way the tertiary circular reactions develop. Instead of replicating his previous manipulation, the child now varies the movement and discovers new effects on the object. For example he bangs an object successively on different-sounding surfaces, apparently listening to the sounds; he drops an object successively from different heights, and watches the result; he makes an object roll, slide or splash in water, and watches the result. He is thus learning more about the properties of objects through exploring them.

When familiar means are inadequate to deal with a situation, new schemata are now formed. Earlier, when a toy was placed out of his reach, on a cushion or atttached to string, the child had applied familiar schemata to the toy (reaching and grasping), failing to obtain it. At the present stage the child makes trial and error attempts, and from them discovers new means, and so draws the toy towards him by pulling the cushion or the string. The string problem evokes a systematic schema that was developed during the third sub-stage, namely pulling a string in order to make a toy hanging from it swing; the solution is discovered in the course of trying out this schema. Each successive attempt at such accommodation involves also the assimilation of the result (observation of the inadequacy of the schema), a balance between the two processes being necessary for the intelligent adaptation. Once the appropriate action is discovered, it is used rapidly on subsequent occasions.

The child's awareness of an unperceived object extends to taking account of changes of position which he sees. If he retrieves an object from under cover A, and then sees it hidden under cover B, he no longer looks for it under cover A as he did at sub-stage 4, but goes directly to B. But if the object is buried deeply or under several layers, he makes no attempt to uncover it, unless a sound from it indicates its presence.

Some repetitive manipulations indicate that children of this age are making new discoveries about the spatial relations of objects. They place a toy on supports at different levels, e.g. on tables of different heights; they put small objects in and out of larger ones, and place toys under a table; they begin to put objects on top of one another and range them in a line. But they cannot anticipate spatial relations which they do not perceive at the moment. A child at this stage who tries to obtain a long toy on the other side of his play-pen, when it is at right angles to the bars of the pen, cannot anticipate its correct position, and so instead of rotating it by 90 degrees, he tries to pull it through as it is, achieving success only by chance. The same mistake is made repeatedly.

Further awareness of causal agents outside himself follows from these developments. An example of this is that the child puts an object in such a position that it moves of its own accord, as when he lets it slide down a slope. Previously he had acted as if a push from him were necessary for the movement.

The child's ability to vary his actions in a trial and error way, and so form new schemata instead of being limited to applying existing ones, leads to new developments in imitation. He can copy new models, including those that involve movements by the child of parts of his body which he cannot see. The examples given of the imitation of unfamiliar movements and new sounds (words that are not identical with spontaneous babbles) indicate that these imitations of new models develop first through the coordination of familiar schemata, which are then progressively accommodated by trial and error.

Sub-stage 6 (18 months onwards). The new type of behaviour pattern, which is classified into the last sub-stage, is that the solution of a problem is achieved by the invention of new means instead of being discovered by trial and error. With the long toy and bars problem, the child at once turns the toy to the correct position in relation to the bars in order to pull it through them. Similarly he can immediately use one object as an instrument with which to draw in another which is out of his reach. Thus the child is able to foresee spatial relations of objects other than as he directly perceives them. The string and support problems did not require such anticipation for their solutions. Hence they could be solved (with sub-stage 5 schemata) after a relatively short period of trial and error and then generalised. The use of a stick to draw near another object was, however, achieved at that stage only after months of trials, and then it was not generalised, i.e. the child was unable to form the schemata necessary for this. The new development which makes possible the sub-stage 6 schemata is the ability to represent objects and their spatial relations in a way not given in the immediate perceptual situation. Mental trial and error can thus replace trial and error in action.

Ability of the child to represent to himself the object he no longer perceives is also evident in the child's persistent searching for hidden objects. He can now find an object that he has seen hidden under five successive layers of covers. He has thus achieved a concept of permanent objects, which exist independently of his activities.

If the pram in which the child is sitting is moved, he looks for an external cause; if he finds an adult's foot, he is satisfied. (Contrast this with the behaviour at sub-stage 3, when the child acts as if his own actions were responsible for the movements of objects.) As well as looking for the cause of an observed movement, he also correctly anticipates (i.e. represents) the consequence of an action. These developments also imply an awareness of the correct temporal sequence of events.

In imitation, the child now re-enacts an event of the previous day; he is no longer restricted to imitating a model immediately after seeing it.

The child has therefore completed the process of distinguishing between himself and objects. In his actions he now regards objects as having a separate existence, as being related in space rather than being centred spatially on him, and as being moved by other agents than himself. These developments also imply that the child is aware of himself as a separate object and as one object among others in a spatial field. In general the child has moved from action in relation to perceptually present objects to the representation of objects that are not perceptually present; in other words, in addition to schemata of action, he is now beginning to form representative schemata. With this the child has moved to a new plane, and Piaget distinguishes it by a new stage.

The Pre-operational Stage

(a) *The Symbolic and Pre-conceptual Stage* (approx. 1½ to 4 years). The developments at the end of the sensori-motor period indicate that the child responds to an object in the absence of direct sensory stimulation from it. This implies the ability to represent the object symbolically in some other form. Piaget suggests that the memory image is the vehicle of representation. Imitation is considered to give rise to the memory image, and hence it is the important link in the process from sensori-motor to representative schemata. Imitation involves the accommodation of an existing schema to a model. When the development of tertiary circular reactions makes possible the imitation of new models, each repetition gives rise to new anticipations, and these eventually give rise to the memory image, in the absence of the model (deferred imitation). Then symbolic activity is possible. This image represents the unperceived object, and it is combined with other objects and with words in make-believe play and in language respectively.

Since these various activities involving symbolism occur at about the same time, Piaget argues that a general symbolic function develops. This enables the child to form schemata of thinking in relation to represented objects, instead of merely schemata of action in relation to perceived objects. His world begins to extend in time beyond the present. This produces continuity and greater stability of the child's inner world, which is no longer limited to perceived objects, that come and go; awareness of the object is continued in a representative form.

The shift from the plane of action to the plane of representation by means of memory images and words does not mean that the child's thinking at once becomes rational and conceptual, and adapted to objective reality. As Piaget defines these terms, this does not begin to occur until about the age of 7 years and is not complete until adolescence. Between the end of the sensori-motor period and the beginning of conceptual thinking, the child's thinking is characterised by two features: by symbolic activity in make-believe play, in which the child uses individual symbols as he chooses, with no social usage involved; and by attempts at verbal reasoning, which in Piaget's terms is pre-conceptual in character.

These two aspects of early thinking will later develop into creative imagination and rational thinking respectively. These do not occur in early childhood because they require adaptation, namely a permanent equilibrium between the assimilatory and accommodatory processes. Since the child's horizon, through the ability to represent unperceived objects, is extended in time and space, the reality with which he is thereby faced is much wider than the reality he met in practical action, and it also includes the thinking of others, since this can now be communicated in suitable words. Hence the child must learn on the representative plane what he has learned on the plane of action: physical and social reality will keep presenting him with the unexpected. Equilibrium is only temporary in the young child, because it is continually being disturbed by some aspect of reality, which requires another adaptation. Hence, in order to preserve the stability of his inner construction of reality, the child is forced either to assimilate reality to his schemata without accommodating them to it, in symbolic play, or to imitate reality (accommodating) without assimilating it (e.g. in drawing). Without assimilation the new event is not linked with past experience, i.e. with analogous schemata; on the other hand if schemata are not modified by (accommodated to) new aspects of reality, then the reality that is incorporated into them must be distorted in order to fit into them. Thus to some extent the child is building up a view of the world which is more in accord with his needs and viewpoint than with the objective facts. But this does enable the child to consolidate his developing schemata, which he could not do if he were continually modifying them. Piaget therefore views the predominance of make-believe play in the activities of the pre-school child as the outcome of the nature of the child's thought at the time, which lacks permanent equilibrium.

The other reason for its early predominance is that memory images are readily available to be used symbolically in play, as words are not, since these have to be learned. Hence the young child can more readily express himself in symbolic play than in words.

Piaget distinguishes between 'symbolic play', occurring after the age of about 18 months, and the play before this which he terms 'practice play'. This he defines as the repetition, for the pleasure of exercising a function, of schemata already developed, without the accommodation or efforts at understanding that are involved in adaptive behaviour and the acquisition of new schemata. When an infant sucks his thumb after a meal, he satisfies the need to suck, but there are no grounds for assuming that this is symbolic, or that the infant has a memory image of his mother's breast. Practice play is therefore regarded as having the same relation to sensorimotor intelligence as symbolic play has to representative intelligence, the latter pair employing symbolic functions whereas the former do not. In both assimilation is predominant over accommodation.

The extent to which this is so in symbolic activities varies with the subject's degree of awareness of the significance of the symbolism he is using. A child who states that an object with which he is playing is something else (a shell on a box is a cat on a wall) is aware of what he is representing (the cat). When he relives a past experience in a way that makes it more acceptable (a fearsome dog as a friendly dog) he is presumably somewhat less aware of what he is doing, and may not recall the frightening episode. When he plays out scenes of jealousy or other intensely emotional situations, he is presumably not aware of the reality that his play represents, and so is not accommodating to it. With dreams the extreme of pure assimilation is reached, there being no possibility of any accommodation to reality since the subject is not conscious. He thus cannot be aware of the assimilating mechanisms and hence of the significance of the symbolism. Secondary or unconscious symbolism, whether in play or dreams, is thus seen by Piaget as the result of limited contact with reality, i.e. of accommodation. Repression may be operative in certain cases, when it is an additional particular factor contributing to lack of awareness of the significance of the symbolism, but it is not a general factor accounting for all unconscious symbolism.

Although no absolute distinction can be made between cognitive and affective schemata, since interest enters into all cognitive activity and cognition into affective activities, it is possible to consider separately affective schemata, these being, for example, ways of feeling or reacting to people. They are developed in the same way as motor or representative schemata, through the assimilation of present situations to previous ones, thereby giving rise to consistent ways of reacting and feeling. As with cognitive schemata, adaptation to reality is greater when affective assimilation and accommodation are in equilibrium: the predominance of one or the other produces imbalance, an excess of accommodation tending towards loss of identity and the primacy of assimilation to a false view of reality. Reacting subsequently to other adults in a similar way as to parents can be explained on the basis of generalisation.

Although Piaget distinguishes symbolic and pre-conceptual forms of early thinking for the sake of discussion, he points out that there are gradations between them, and in some instances it is difficult to categorise a child's behaviour as one or the other. However the pre-conceptual aspect is considered when the young child attempts to reason. Many examples of false conclusions are quoted. These are attributed to the child's lack of understanding of general class concepts, of the relation of individual members to a general class, and of classes to higher-order classes. An illustration of this is the oft-quoted example of the child out for a walk who saw a slug, on which she remarked. Ten yards further on there was another slug, whereupon she said 'There it is again.' When asked whether it was another one, she went back to look at the first one. Questions such as 'Is it the same one?', 'Is it another slug?' had no meaning for her; she answered 'Yes' to all.

For the discussion of pre-conceptual thinking, Piaget avoids examples of the child reasoning falsely when his conclusion is motivated by his wishes and desires; instead he analyses the reflective statements of the child when he comments on events. For example a child described as 'ill' a hunchback who had a hump. When told she could not go and see him because he had influenza, she called this 'ill-in-bed'. Some time later she asked whether he was still ill in bed, and on being told that he was not she answered 'He hasn't a hump now.' Thus the child failed to distinguish the illness that produced the hump from the illness that had produced the influenza, and to see their relation to the general class of illnesses.

Piaget uses the term 'transduction', borrowed from Stern, for these inferences. Since the representations are midway between the imaged symbol and the general concept, he calls them 'pre-concepts'. These will later develop into concepts and give rise to logical thinking.

In some cases at the pre-conceptual stage a correct conclusion may be achieved if class concepts in the sense of hierarchical classes are not involved, that is, when schemata are generalised in relation to individual actions through previous actions. When for example a child knew that her father had a jug of hot water in the bathroom and inferred that he was going to shave, the inference merely used past experience of a similar conjunction of events; no reference to general classes was involved. Hence the child can come to correct conclusions in practical situations.

When understanding of classes or relations is required for a correct inference, then the conclusion is false, as when an afternoon without a nap is considered by a child not to be an afternoon, or when a horse is called a cow because it is yellow. In these cases there is assimilation of the particular to the particular, or of a general class to one of its members, or confusion between the point of view of the child and that of the object, as when the child states that a baby cannot speak, so it has no name. There is a failure to generalise because the child 'centres' his thinking on his own interests, activities or point of view. In this situation there cannot be reciprocity between assimilated elements, because the child is centred on one of them, and reduces the other to this. When there is 'decentring' and reciprocal assimilation between the two elements, the child can conceive of a general class to which both belong (red triangles and green triangles to the general class of triangles).

When the situation allows little centring and hence distortion, there is correct reasoning. An example is quoted in which there was unavoidable decentring when the child defended her point of view against her father's, pointing out a distinction he had not made. This example also illustrates the importance of social influences in the development of children's thinking. When adults make statements contrary to the child's, the latter argues his point of view, and so matches his inferences against those of others, learning gradually to correct false ones and to point out the fallacies in the statements of others.

Progress towards general concepts and operational thinking is made in the intuitive stage, in which Piaget classifies a different type of pre-operational thinking, marked by a new structuring of schemata and by a decline in the features described in the symbolic and pre-conceptual period.

(b) *The Intuitive Stage* (approx. 4 to 7 years). Intuitive thinking is characterised by increased accommodation to reality and a partial decentring of assimilation. However the child still centres his attention on one aspect of a situation and is still dominated by his own viewpoint, with consequent distortion and incorrect inferences. But the tendency to increased accommodation to reality means that the child is made increasingly aware of discrepancies between his judgements of the way objects will behave and what he observes of their actual behaviour. This continual correction of false beliefs by the facts of reality eventually leads to correct judgements and operational thinking.

These developments may be illustrated by studies of the child's concepts at this period.

Given a group of counters in a row, circle, or any other arrangement, the child can pair them with counters of a different colour, one for one. Such an ability to make a one-to-one correspondence between two sets of objects underlies accurate object-counting (as opposed to the recitation of numbers) in which one word must match one object. Similarly by making use of spatial patterns the child at this stage can solve such a problem as making equal in number two unequal groups of counters, say 8 and 18.

He can arrange the smaller group in pairs and transfer counters from one group to the other in a trial and error manner until he has identical patterns in both groups. Also, by measuring sticks against one another in a trial and error manner, he can arrange in order a series of sticks that are graded in length.

These developments do not mean, however, that the child has a concept of number abstracted from the concrete elements, or of numbers as forming a series. The very feature which makes possible this new development is a hindrance to such concepts, and it leads to incorrect inferences: the child's thinking is dominated by the immediate spatial arrangements of objects which he perceives, and these override what he has perceived on successive occasions. The child who has placed a row of counters in a one-to-one correspondence below another row states that there is the same number of counters in both rows, as does the child who has made two equal groups of counters by matching them in patterns. But spread out the row and disturb the pattern of one group, and the child maintains that there are more counters in the group that covers the larger area. Despite repeated experiences of seeing the counters matched in the same spatial arrangement and then disturbed, he is unable to coordinate these successive experiences in order to arrive at a correct conclusion when faced with an immediate perceptual situation which contradicts it. In other words the child's concept of number at this stage is bound up with the spatial arrangements of the concrete elements; it changes with changes in these, and there is no conservation from one situation to another. The child is taking account of one feature of the situation and not of another: for example he takes account of the difference in total area taken up by the group of counters, but does not consider the differences in the size of the spaces between them.

Conservation may eventually be achieved in some situations, but it may break down when further generalisations are required. The child may believe in the equality of a ball of plasticene with an equivalent one when the latter is broken up into two smaller balls, but he denies the equivalence if the ball is broken up into four smaller ones.

Piaget's studies of the child's concepts of length, distance and area produced similar results from children of 5 to 6 years: a failure to conserve equivalence through changes of state. The same findings are reported for concepts of time and speed in children of this age. If two toy cars enter tunnels at the same time and travel over different distances in parallel lines, and then emerge and stop simultaneously, the child of this age does not concede that they stopped at the same time, or travelled for the same length of time; seeing them at rest in different places is a fact which cannot be coordinated with his knowledge that one came to rest when the other did. Only when the tunnels are removed, and the child sees one car over-take another, does he state that the overtaking car travelled faster.

The studies of concepts of space (Piaget and Inhelder (28)) show up the inability of the child of 5 to 6 years to take account of viewpoints other than his own. This is most clearly demonstrated with the task using a model of a scene of three mountains which are clearly distinguished by colour, position and size. The problem is to reproduce the model from various viewpoints. Children of 5 or 6 years could easily copy the model when looking at it, placing the mountains in the correct left-right and fore-aft positions in relation to one another. But asked to copy the model as it would be if they imagined themselves sitting opposite, they reproduced again the view as it was from the position in which they faced it, even after starting off by placing the mountains differently. Some of the older children in this age range succeeded in making the correct changes in fore-aft or left-right relations, but not in both changes at once.

It is during the pre-operational period that Piaget, from the results of his earlier studies, claimed that the young child's thinking tends to be animistic; early in this stage the child attributes life to everything that moves, later only to things that move spontaneously. In defining night the four-year-old is more egocentric than animistic: he states that it is night because people have gone to sleep. According to the six-year-olds a big black cloud, such as smoke from a train, comes over the sun. In another study Piaget (16) suggested that the young child's use of language tends to be egocentric, though to a decreasing extent as he progresses through the pre-operational period. He meant by this that, whether children at this stage talk to themselves or to one another, they are more inclined to follow their own line of thought, with little exchange of information on a topic.

Examples of egocentricity in the thinking of children of 5 or 6 years were found in the study of judgement and reasoning (17). A child can learn left and right in relation to himself, but cannot get it right in another person and refers left-right relations among three objects on a table to himself. Similarly, having stated that he has a brother, he denies that the brother has a brother; he cannot conceive of himself as such. A child says she has two sisters, X and Y. When asked how many sisters X has, she replies 'One.'

Three features of the intuitive period are important in the process of developing operational thinking: the child has an increasing tendency to seek to verify his statements by testing them in action; he shows increased accommodation to the facts of reality thereby observed; consequently assimilation becomes progressively freed or 'decentred' from the child's interests, focus of perception and point of view. In particular, extremes of distortion draw the child's attention to relations he had previously ignored. If the same amounts of water are compared in glasses which differ vastly in shape (e.g. one is short and wide and the other is tall and thin), the difference in the height of the two water levels is so great that the child is at some point forced to consider the compensating difference in width. When the child consistently takes account of two aspects of a situation in various examples, Piaget considers that a new type of thinking has developed.

Concrete Operational Stage (approx. 7 to 11 years)

The beginning of operational thinking is for Piaget a major turning-point in the child's development. Operations are understood as 'actions which are not only internalised but are also integrated with other actions to form general reversible systems' (Inhelder and Piaget (8), p. 6). The difference between concrete and abstract (or formal) operations is in the extent of the integration. The lesser integration at the level of concrete operations limits the child's organisation of the facts of reality to those in the immediate situation; with the more complex integration of schemata at the abstract level, the child can organise facts given in a hypothetical form.

The main change with operational schemata is that the child's thinking becomes reversible. By reversibility Piaget means 'the permanent possibility of returning to the starting-point of the operation in question' (Inhelder and Piaget (8), p. 272). An action once completed cannot be undone; the situation cannot be returned to its previous state. But an operation of thinking can be undone or reversed, so that a return is made to the starting-point. For example 6 can be added mentally to 4; 6 can then be subtracted from the result of 10, thus returning to the original situation. Two classes A and A' (red triangles and green triangles) can be combined mentally to form the more general class of triangles (B). Separating the one sub-class from the more general class involves a return to the starting situation.

With reversibility there is a permanent equilibrium between assimilation and accommodation. Hence intelligent adaptation can be made to more complex aspects of reality; understanding is increased.

A more specific difference between operational and pre-operational thinking, involving reversibility, is the ability to coordinate successive changes in time and space, as when counters are changed from one spatial arrangement to another, or one of two identical balls of plasticene is moulded into a different shape. The child is no longer dominated by the configuration which he perceives at a given moment.

Moreover the child's thinking is freed from the tendency to centre on one aspect of a situation, or on his own viewpoint, as it was in the previous stage. The child can now take account of two variables at once, realising that a change in one is compensated for by a complementary change in the other (increased height is compensated for by decreased width in the liquid and glasses problem; the larger area covered by one group of counters is compensated for by the larger space between them). And he can consider other spatial viewpoints besides his own.

There is greater objectivity, since objects are now assimilated to one another in schemata which are adapted to reality; they are no longer assimilated to the subject's interests, wishes, focus of attention or viewpoint. Thus he can organise the facts of immediately present reality in a way that accords with that reality. As we shall see later, he is not yet able to organise hypothetical statements about reality.

These changes can be seen in the development of various concepts in children. Conservation is achieved. The area of a model field is considered to be unchanged by the number of buildings in it. Length is conserved through changes of shape: straight, bent, etc. A number is believed to remain invariant despite changes in the spatial configuration. Numbers, moreover, are understood as forming a series. The child can not only place in order a series of graded sticks, without trial and error, but he can insert them in the appropriate place. If the sticks are disarranged he knows that, in order to find out the ordinal position of a given stick, he has to remake the series up to that stick.

The freeing of the child's thinking from the dominance of his own viewpoint may be illustrated by the study of spatial concepts. The child can now reproduce correctly the view of the model of mountains as it would be if he were opposite his present position, or to the side on his left or right. The difficulties experienced over problems of time and speed mentioned in the previous section are also overcome.

Piaget maintains that new general schemata underlie these various conceptual developments. The child now has schemata of thinking that enable him to classify objects when two variables (though not more) are involved, and to arrange ordered phenomena in a series. These can be applied to various problems. For example he can correctly sort objects that vary in two ways (e.g. form and colour) by one criterion (e.g. form) (Piaget and Inhelder (29)). Given the problem of finding out which rod is the most flexible among some that vary in material, length, thickness and form of cross-section, when different weights are placed on the tip, the child has not the necessary schemata for solving the problem. But, unlike the intuitive child, he can place the rods in order in terms of the limited number of effects he has observed, namely the extent to which they bend (i.e. he can use his schema of serialising).

This last example brings up some of the limitations of concrete operational thinking. The child has not the schema of 'all other things being equal' which would enable him to solve this problem. Piaget analyses these limitations in terms of the child's inability at this stage to integrate two forms of reversibility into a single system, though he can use either separately. He can undo an operation (reversibility by inversion or negation) and return to the original state; or he can compensate the original operation without cancelling it by a symmetrical operation (reversibility by reciprocity). For example, given the problem of a balance with a weight on one arm, the bar can be returned to the horizontal by removal of the weight (inversion) or by the placement of an equal weight at an equal distance from the centre on the other arm (reciprocity).

The younger child at the concrete operational stage can solve this problem by finding a weight equal to that on one arm and placing it at an equal distance from the centre on the other arm. When he has only unequal weights to deal with, he mainly tries to solve the problem by adding other weights on to one side, removing them and trying others. The older child at this stage attempts to make the bar horizontal by trying the weight he already has at different distances from the centre. He may even, in this trial and error manner, discover in a qualitative way that weight and distance have an inverse relation. The metric, proportional relation is discovered by children at the abstract stage.

Concrete operations are limited by the form of the operation, and in the content with which they can deal. They are restricted to organising immediately given data and do not extend to the hypothetical or possible. With regard to content, they are not immediately generalised. The schema of serialising can be applied more readily to lengths than to weights (Piaget found a time-lag of two years between the two).

Although permanent equilibrium is achieved for some aspects of reality, instability appears when two aspects have to be coordinated, as in the problem of balancing the horizontal bar with unequal weights, which involves weight and distance. Moreover the child at this level is limited to actions, recording the results of these and organising them. He does not formulate hypotheses and organise his observations in a way that could test them. When this does occur, Piaget classifies the thinking as abstract, and considers that more complex schemata and another equilibrium have been achieved.

Abstract Operational Thinking (approx. 11 years onwards)

The main characteristics of the abstract operational stage (the last in the sequence) are that the child can form abstract concepts such as infinity, and that he can reason from hypotheses, i.e. from verbal statements alone and in a propositional form (e.g. 'If a, then b'). He thus has the basis for scientific thinking. Inhelder and Piaget (8) have investigated this with a series of problems.

One of these has been previously mentioned. Children were provided with a set of rods, differing in material (brass, steel, etc.), in the form of the cross-section (round or square) and in thickness. Length could be adjusted on the apparatus, and three weights of different value could be placed on the tip. The rods could be fixed horizontally above a basin of water. Observations were made of the method the child used and of his comments on what he thought were the relevant variables influencing flexibility. In addition he was asked to prove his assertions.

Less advanced concrete operational children tackled the problem haphazardly; but the more advanced ones began to realise some relations, although they did not take account of all the factors; for example a child who found that the thinner of two bars of the same length was more flexible was asked to demonstrate the part played by thickness. He compared two bars that differed in thickness, without ensuring that they were of the same material, form of cross-section, etc., and he did not realise that a procedure of this sort was of no value.

Children using methods which were considered to involve abstract operations did control all the relevant variables. Moreover they chose rods to compare with a view to answering a specific question concerning the role of a given factor, unlike the child using concrete operational thinking, who compared any rod with any other, and then observed the effects. Thus children using the abstract method are formulating hypotheses before they observe, and are making observations in order to test the hypothesis. In addition the child using concrete operational thinking looks for an association between a factor and its result, whereas the child with abstract thinking makes an attempt to find out the consequences of decreasing or eliminating the factor.

Although children of 11 or 12 years show this advance in finding out relevant variables, they are less successful in attempts at verification of what they observe. By the age of 14 or 15 years, however, verification was systematised with a schema of 'all other things being equal' developed and generalised.

With their fourteen other problems Inhelder and Piaget found similar differences in approach by younger and older children.

At the abstract stage the process of assimilation is that of objects to one another and not to the subject, i.e. the objective facts which are observed are incorporated into the subject's logical and mathematical schemata which have been developed at this stage. The schemata of thinking are in turn modified in order to take account of objective facts. Intelligent adaptation again requires equilibrium between assimilation and accommodation: the assimilation of reality to the schemata of thinking, together with accommodation of the schemata to the objective facts and to the thoughts of others. Reflective thinking is possible.

The development at the abstract level of the other aspect of thinking, symbolical as opposed to conceptual, is in the direction of creative imagination.

5

Summary

In summary, Piaget's theory is an account of the process of the development of schemata of thinking that make possible increased understanding of the physical world. The first intelligent adaptations are actions in relation to perceived objects as the result of the gradual dissociation by the infant of the objective world from his own actions and perceptions. From then on the child is able to represent objects by means of memory images and to begin to form symbolic representations of the objective world; this happens at the time when he begins to acquire language systematically. At the sensori-motor stage the child is egocentric in action; at the representative level he is at first egocentric in thinking, being dominated by his interests, his own viewpoint and by what he perceives at a given moment. The next major step is when he is able to free his thinking from these influences. He is then able to develop conceptual, operational schemata, and to come to correct conclusions about concrete aspects of reality. Finally he is able to abstract his concepts from the concrete form and to reason from hypothesis, in fact to operate on the operations.

6

Piaget's Theory and current Criticisms

Current criticism of Piaget's work centres around the selection of his subjects, the presentation of his data, the absence of statistical analysis, the age of certain developments, the question of stages and the use of logical analogies for psychological operations. To what extent are these criticisms justified?

It is objected (e.g. by Braine (3)) that the groups of children are not representative, or at least that no details of the method of selection, of occupational class etc. are given and that the average age and scatter for the different types of thinking are not provided. This is so, though data on ages are given in a recent publication by Piaget and Inhelder (29). The absence of data on the numbers of children investigated has at times led to the conclusion by others that they are no more numerous than the number of illustrative examples quoted, an impression that proves to be erroneous when the number is indicated, e.g. 1,500 in the study of logical thinking (Inhelder and Piaget (8)) and 2,159 in the study of classification (Piaget and Inhelder (29)).

Piaget's main interest is in the process, not in normative aspects. The important part of his theory is the sequence of development and not the ages at which steps in it appear. For the educational and clinical application of Piaget's work the average ages at which different types of action and thinking occur need to be known, but the validity of the theory does not hinge upon them. The findings of Braine (2) with regard to one kind of operation which occurred much earlier when a different method was used is more relevant, and it suggests the need for further investigation of this point.

The influence of socio-economic and cultural factors on the rate of progress through the sequence is of obvious interest, but such findings are not evidence against Piaget's views, unless he is misrepresented as postulating a sequence which is entirely due to the unfolding of maturational influences.

The important aspects of the theory are (1) the distinction of different types of thinking and action, (2) the sequence for particular concepts, and

(3) stages, namely that one kind of behaviour pattern or thinking characterises action or thinking for a given period.

Other investigators have no difficulty in classifying the responses to
problems into Piaget's categories of action and thinking (unlike those who
replicated the earlier work for which mainly verbal methods were used),
and most of them have confirmed the sequences for particular concepts
(Lovell (9, 10); Lovell and Ogilvie (12); Lovell, Mitchell and Everett (11);
Peel (15); Hood (6); Hyde (7); Woodward (35, 36, 37)).

When investigators have examined whether children show the same
type of action or thinking for a variety of problems, results are more
divergent, though few studies have as yet been carried out. Considerable
consistency has been found by Lovell (10) between the concrete operational
and abstract operational levels, children tending to show one or the other
type of thinking for various combinations of four of the Inhelder and Piaget
problems. At the other end of the scale, Woodward (35) found a high
degree of correspondence between aspects of sensori-motor development,
using severely subnormal children. In between there appears to be less
consistency, concrete operational thinking being shown for one concept
and intuitive thinking for another (Hyde (7) and Woodward (36)). And
Lovell and Ogilvie (12, 13) even found variations for the same concept
when different material was used: some of the children who thought that
the amount of plasticene changed with a change in shape (intuitive response)
thought the amount invariant when a rubber band was shown stretched
and unstretched.

These results suggest that, even if it is subsequently found that children show the same type of thinking for all concepts for a period, there is a
transitional period during which they have achieved a higher type of
thinking for one concept while having a less advanced kind for another.
Further research is required before the question of stages of development
is settled.

Criticisms have been made of the method of logical analysis (Parsons
(14)), but these are outside the scope of this summary.

7

The Implications of Piaget's Theory for Child Psychiatry

Before considering Piaget's theory and child psychiatry, it may be as well
to place it in relation to general and child psychology. Although maturational factors influence the rate of progress through a sequence such as
that described by Piaget, they cannot at present be observed; it is the
individual's interactions with the environment that can be traced in detail,
namely the learning process. Hence it is relevant to examine the relation
of Piaget's investigations to studies of learning. The main difference seems
to be that the latter are concerned with the details of the learning process
at any one time, whereas Piaget's studies span the period of time from

birth to maturity. Learning theory is concerned with the conditions affecting the acquisition and retention of particular habits. Piaget's theory deals with the coordination and differentiation of behaviour patterns and their organisation into more general patterns. The principles of learning are required to explain the details of a particular learned response to physical and social stimuli. An approach such as Piaget's is needed for the investigation of the process by which new and more complex cognitive functions develop, for example the development of symbolic functions from motor patterns or the transition from concrete to abstract concepts.

In a similar way Piaget's approach is complementary to factorial studies of intelligence. These, or at least the interpretations favoured by Burt (4) and Vernon (33), indicate a hierarchical structure; such a view is implied in Piaget's account of the development of more general and complex schemata, which arise out of but do not supersede earlier behaviour patterns, which remain in the individual's repertoire.

Piaget's importance for child psychology is undoubted. His methods of investigation have given new insight into children's concepts. And he has presented the only systematic and comprehensive theory of the process of intellectual development. Recently his work has become recognised as a major contribution to general psychology (Berlyne (2)).

Since it deals with observations and theory concerning a major aspect of child development, it is relevant also to child psychiatry. Its importance lies, in the first place, in the hypothesis of an orderly succession of increasingly complex developmental events in the cognitive sphere and, secondly, in the fact that these events can be qualitatively described. Furthermore the scheme provides a framework for a bridge between the intellectual and motivational-emotional aspects of development, which on the whole have been treated separately in the study of children. The sequence of developmental steps gives an indication of what kinds of thinking may be expected of children at various age ranges. For example, although the two-year-old shows some capacity for recall of past events in his actions in play, he has not the necessary verbal structures for understanding a promise; the young child may be expected to be egocentric and animistic and unable to coordinate successive events in time or two aspects of a spatial situation; before the age of about 11 years concreteness in thinking may be expected.

These differences in cognitive development help to explain the varying emotional reactions of children of different ages. This is very well illustrated by reactions to hospital admission. Schaffer (32) found differences in babies of under and over 7 months in age. The former on their return home showed a preoccupation with their physical environment; the latter showed a disturbed relation with the mother. He attributed this to changes in the development of awareness of permanent objects around this time.

Similarly the fact that in the Prugh et al. (31) study the most marked reactions in hospital and on the return home were observed in the 2–4 year age group may be explained by the combination of a strong emotional tie to the mother with an inability to understand promises. The tendency of the 6–8 year old children in this study to regard their illness as a magical retribution for their bad behaviour is in accord with Piaget's results on the concepts of the world and the moral judgements of children of this age (18, 20).

At the level of theoretical analysis, it is possible to apply the concepts of assimilation and accommodation to affective phenomena. Piaget discusses the role of wishes, interests and the dominance of the subjective viewpoint in false reasoning in the pre-operational period, and considers this to be the nature of the child's thinking at this time, when he can achieve only brief adaptations to objective reality. But he does not continue this analysis to the period after the development of operational thinking, to cover instances in which the influence of motivational-emotional factors lead to a distortion of reality, when the available operational schemata necessary for correct inferences are not applied because of interference from subjective interests. These instances, for example, in cases of rationalisation, could also be described in terms of an assimilation of reality which is distorted because there is little accommodation: the facts of reality are distorted to fit into the subject's beliefs when the latter are not altered to accommodate the facts.

These concepts can equally be applied to adaptation or maladaptation to social situations, i.e. to inter-personal relations, an aspect which is mentioned only briefly by Piaget in terms of 'affective schemata' or ways of reacting to people. Adaptation to a social situation involves a balance between assimilation of the facts and accommodation to them. If one of the two is predominant, the action is maladaptive. When an individual attempts to use an established pattern of action, which has been learned in previous actual situations, in a situation where it is inappropriate, this might be described as excessive assimilation at the expense of accommodation, in that new patterns of behaviour demanded by the situation are not developed because the individual refuses to accommodate his existing patterns. On the other hand the individual who changes with every wind that blows might be described as excessively accommodating without absorbing his experiences.

A further point of interest is the examination of theories of early emotional development in the light of Piaget's account of the appearance of cognitive functions, particularly of memory and other symbolic activities. The observations suggest that, up to about the age of 18 months, the infant's inner world and actions are bound by perceived objects and hence by the immediate present; the capacity to represent unperceived objects in the form of memory images or words does not develop until half-way through the second year, nor does the capacity to represent one object symbolically by another. Although there is development in the direction of awareness of objects that are no longer perceived towards the end of the first year, the length of time that the object can be out of sight and then recovered is extremely limited. Piaget's findings are thus at variance with theories which attribute to the infant a capacity for recall, as distinct from the modification of behaviour through learning without awareness of the process.

Similarly Piaget's observations on the appearance of symbolic play are not in accord with theories which depend on the child's having a capacity for the symbolic representation of one object by another in the first year. His interpretation of the early manipulations of infants is that they are learning about the objects they handle (intelligent adaptation), or exercising for pleasure a behaviour pattern they have acquired (practice play). He therefore considers that symbolic representation of matters of emotional significance is ruled out by the nature of the child's cognitive functions at this time: the child playing at hiding and finding is investigating the disappearance and reappearance of the particular object he is playing with, not symbolising other events.

In his discussion of symbolism in general, including that in dreams, Piaget (22) contrasts his views with those of Freud on the role of repression in unconscious symbolism. While recognising repression as operative in certain instances, Piaget considers that the general factor giving rise to degrees of lack of awareness of what is being represented by the symbol is the degree of contact with reality, i.e. the extent to which assimilation dominates accommodation. The extreme of pure assimilation is reached in dreams, since the sleeper is cut off from reality, and from any possibility of accommodating to it.

A final point which may be mentioned is the practical value of the techniques devised by Piaget and Inhelder as tools in psychological research concerned with subnormal and emotionally disturbed children. Their usefulness for research in the field of subnormality has been discussed by the writer in a recent publication edited by Ellis (5). The investigation of the concepts of children with learning difficulties is a promising line of study for examining the influence of emotional factors on the process of thinking.

REFERENCES

1. BEARD, RUTH, 1957. *An Investigation of Concept Formation among Infant Schoolchildren.* Unpublished Ph.D. Thesis, University of London.
2. BERLYNE, D. E., 1957. Recent developments in Piaget's work. *Brit. J. Educ. Psychol.*, 27: 1-12.
3. BRAINE, M. D. S., 1959. The ontogeny of certain logical operations: Piaget's formulation examined by non-verbal methods. *Psychol. Monogr.*, 73, No. 5.
4. BURT, C., 1940. *The Factors of the Mind.* London: Univ. of London Press.

5. ELLIS, N., 1963. *Handbook of Mental Deficiency.* New York: McGraw-Hill.
6. HOOD, H. B., 1962. An experimental study of Piaget's theory of the development of number in children. *Brit. J. Psychol.*, **53**: 273-286.
7. HYDE, DORIS M., 1959. *An Investigation of Piaget's Theories of the Development of the Concept of Number.* Unpublished Ph.D. Thesis, University of London.
8. INHELDER, BARBEL and PIAGET, J., 1958. *The Growth of Logical Thinking from Childhood to Adolescence.* Trans. by A. Parsons and S. Milgram. London: Routledge & Kegan Paul.
9. LOVELL, K., 1959. A follow-up study of some aspects of the work of Piaget and Inhelder on the child's conception of space. *Brit. J. Educ. Psychol.*, **29**: 104-117.
10. 1961. A follow-up study of Inhelder and Piaget's 'The Growth of Logical Thinking'. *Brit. J. Psychol.*, **52**: 143-153.
11. LOVELL, K., MITCHELL, B. and EVERETT, I. R., 1962. An experimental study of the growth of some logical structures. *Brit. J. Psychol.*, **53**: 175-188.
12. LOVELL, K. and OGILVIE, E., 1960. A study of the conservation of substance in the junior school child. *Brit. J. Educ. Psychol.*, **30**: 109-118.
13. 1961. A study of conservation of weight in the junior school child. *Brit. J. Educ. Psychol.*, **31**: 138-144.
14. PARSONS, C., 1960. Inhelder and Piaget's 'The Growth of Logical Thinking': II. A logical viewpoint. *Brit. J. Psychol.*, **51**: 75-84.
15. PEEL, E. A., 1959. Experimental examination of some of Piaget's schemata concerning the child's perception and thinking, and a discussion of their educational significance. *Brit. J. Educ. Psychol.*, **29**: 89-100.
16. PIAGET, J., 1926. *The Language and Thought of the Child.* Trans. by M. Warden. London: Routledge & Kegan Paul.
17. 1928*a. Judgment and Reasoning in the Child.* Trans. by M. Warden. London: Routledge & Kegan Paul.
18. 1928*b. The Child's Conception of the World.* Trans. by T. and A. Thomlinson. London: Routledge & Kegan Paul.
19. 1930. *The Child's Conception of Physical Causality.* Trans. by M. Gabain. London: Routledge & Kegan Paul.
20. 1932. *The Moral Judgment of the Child.* Trans. by M. Gabain. London: Routledge & Kegan Paul.
21. 1946. *Les Notions de Mouvement et de Vitesse chez l'Enfant.* Paris: Presses Universitaires de France.
22. 1951. *Play, Dreams and Imitation in Childhood.* Trans. by C. Gattegno and F. M. Hodgson. London: Routledge & Kegan Paul.
23. 1952. *The Child's Conception of Number.* Trans. by C. Gattegno and F. M. Hodgson. London: Routledge & Kegan Paul.
24. 1953*a. The Origins of Intelligence in the Child.* Trans. by M. Cook. London: Routledge & Kegan Paul.
25. 1953*b. Logic and Psychology.* Manchester: Manchester Univ. Press.
26. 1955*a. The Construction of Reality in the Child.* Trans. by M. Cook. London: Routledge & Kegan Paul.
27. 1955*b.* The development of time concepts in the child. *In* Hoch, P. H. and Zubin, J. (eds.), *Psychopathology of Childhood.* New York: Grune & Stratton.
28. PIAGET, J. and INHELDER, BARBEL, 1956. *The Child's Conception of Space.* Trans. by F. J. Langdon and J. L. Lunzer. London: Routledge & Kegan Paul.
29. 1964. *The Early Growth of Logic in the Child: Classification and Seriation.* Trans. by E. A. Lunzer and D. Papert. London: Routledge & Kegan Paul.

30. PIAGET, J., INHELDER, BARBEL and SZEMINSKA, A., 1960. *The Child's Conception of Geometry*. Trans. by E. A. Lunzer. London: Routledge & Kegan Paul.
31. PRUGH, D. G., STAUB, E. M., SANDS, H. H., KIRSCHBAUM, R. M. and LENIHAN, E. A., 1953. A study of the emotional reactions of children and families to hospitalization and illness. *Amer. J. Orthopsychiat.*, **23**: 70-106.
32. SCHAFFER, H. R., 1958. Objective observations of personality development in early infancy. *Brit. J. Med. Psychol.*, **31**: 174-183.
33. VERNON, P. E., 1961. *The Structure of Human Abilities*. London: Methuen.
34. WOHLWILL, J. F., 1960. Developmental studies of perception. *Psychol. Bull.*, **57**: 249-288.
35. WOODWARD, MARY, 1959. The behaviour of idiots interpreted by Piaget's theory of sensori-motor development. *Brit. J. Educ. Psychol.*, **29**: 60-71.
36. ———— 1961. Concepts of number in the mentally subnormal studied by Piaget's method. *J. Child Psychol. and Psychiat.*, **2**: 249-259.
37. ———— 1962. Concepts of space in the mentally subnormal studied by Piaget's method. *Brit. J. Soc. and Clin. Psychol.*, **1**: 25-37.

V

THE DEVELOPMENT OF PERCEPTION

M. D. Vernon
M.A., Sc.D.

Professor of Psychology in the University of Reading

1
Maturation and Learning in the Development of Perception

If one is to understand how the child establishes and maintains contacts with the world around him, it is clearly important to study the development of his perceptual capacities. Only when these have become extensive, rapid and accurate can he obtain a thorough knowledge of his environment such as will enable him to react effectively to its continually changing aspects. However, when this is achieved, he does not have to wait passively for the environment to change and then adjust to it, but anticipates the type of variation and modification in it which may occur at various times and in various places. He is able to foresee what is likely to happen, and to set himself to observe the occurrence of certain types of event which are the more readily and accurately perceived in consequence. Thus he seldom perceives single isolated stimuli, but rather groups and sequences of stimuli related together in space and time, often originating in more than one sensory mode. Indeed it may be difficult for him to perceive single events, still more single stimuli, independently of each other and of the total spatial and temporal setting of which they form part. Thus immediate sensory perceptions are supplemented and integrated by means of other cognitive processes—memories and ideas which link them together and give them meaning, which meaning is in turn a guide to appropriate action. It should therefore be realised that perceptions, although they may not lead immediately to direct action, are nevertheless continually checked and tested according as to whether reactions to them have proved ultimately successful. For instance, if I imagine that I perceive a friend walking towards me and greet him with a smile, and he responds with a blank stare, I know that my perception was faulty. In the excessively complex scenes with which we are continually confronted in our natural environment, we may frequently be obliged to correct inaccurate perceptions in the light of actions which have proved inappropriate. In this manner also we learn to adjust rapidly to significant aspects and changes in the environment, while overlooking those which have no importance for us.

Now it is clear that the infant and the young child are incapable of perceiving extensively and accurately the world around them. They lack both the capacity to discriminate and identify objects and people, and also the knowledge of what to expect, and the memories and ideas which give meaning to their perceptions. For adequate perception, the capacity must be developed and the knowledge acquired. Clearly the latter is a matter of learning. But the former depends partly on the maturation of the sense organs, nervous system and intellectual abilities, and partly on the continual exercise of their functions. There has been much controversy about the extent to which perceptual development depends on maturation or on learning, but clearly both are essential for normal development. It is true that a temporary or more prolonged retardation in perceptual development may be produced by exposing a young child to restricted environmental conditions which do not permit the normal exercise of the perceptual functions. Thus Schaffer (38) noted that infants of 2–7 months of age who were hospitalised for a week or two seemed excessively bewildered when they returned home. They did not respond normally to people, even to the mother, but were continually preoccupied in scanning their surroundings, as if they had forgotten what these looked like. Schaffer attributed this setback in normal perception to the perceptual deprivation experienced in the hospital environment, where the infants were confined in cots or cubicles from which they could see little or nothing of their surroundings. However, their condition did not persist for more than a few days. Other psychologists have found certain retardations in perceptual development to result from a more prolonged exposure to the restricted surroundings of institutional life. Even if children in institutions have normal physical surroundings, their social milieu is usually impoverished. We shall note some of these effects below.

There is no evidence, however, to prove that such cases cannot recover and develop normal perceptual capacities if later their circumstances improve. Thus the lack of experience may have only a temporary effect. More severe appear to be the results of prolonged deprivation of one of the senses, particularly that of sight. Von Senden (39) collected a number of observations relating to adults, blind since birth or shortly afterwards, whose sight had been restored by operational removal of cataracts. Many of these patients were very slow to learn to identify objects by sight, and even to perceive shapes. Some never did so with any facility.

Another type of deprivation which may have serious consequences is that of speech. Thus cases have been reported, such as that of the 'wild boy of Aveyron', of children who have lost all human contact and grown up among animals, and who have never learnt to use language in any way. Their capacity to perceive, when they were ultimately discovered as adults, appears to have been similar to that of the year-old child whom we shall consider subsequently. Nor did they ever recover. These cases are of course very rare, and we should not rely too heavily on the descriptions which have been given of them.

We may conclude that prolonged failure to exercise the perceptual capacities may permanently prevent them from developing normally. But clearly also their rate of development is limited by the general maturation of the organism. We shall give evidence to show that before a certain age the child is incapable of perceiving, or even of learning to perceive, in the same manner as do older children and adults. He is also incapable of understanding the nature of the world around him and of the objects it contains.

2
Difficulties in the Study of Children's Perceptions

But when we endeavour to trace the development of the perceptual capacities in infancy, we are inevitably handicapped by the fact that the infant cannot describe his perceptual experience. Thus although we possess experimental data relating to the infant's direction of gaze, we can infer only that he is orientated towards certain parts of the field of view rather than others, and we cannot be at all certain to what extent and in what manner he is aware of them. So later when it appears that he is able to discriminate between two objects, shapes or colours, and learns to repeat this discriminative response, we may conclude that he observes a difference between them but not that he perceives them as separate objects, shapes and so on. Again, as I shall discuss below, Piaget has described a succession of typical reactions to objects and situations which suggest the manner in which perception and understanding of these develop during infancy and early childhood. But the nature of the understanding is conjectural. Even when the child is a little older, and can use language to name objects, we cannot be certain that the meaning he attaches to his identifications is the same as that ascribed by adults; indeed probably this is not so. So also when he makes apparently inexplicable mistakes in the perception of form and relationship, it is difficult to be certain whether he has failed to attend to these, whether he is incapable of perceiving them if he does attend to them, or whether he cannot respond in such a way as to demonstrate the nature of his perceptions.

It is perhaps because perception cannot be overtly demonstrated in early childhood as easily and as precisely as can response and activity that the literature on the subject is meagre and rather unsatisfactory. Numerous experiments were carried out in the third and fourth decades of the century on topics such as shape and colour discrimination, but such experiments then became comparatively infrequent, presumably because they did not contribute very much towards our knowledge of how the child's perception of his ordinary everyday-life surroundings developed. We are largely indebted to Piaget's work for such understanding as we possess. Yet it must be pointed out that his hypotheses as to the nature of perception in infancy were based on the inferences drawn from observations of behaviour in his own three children. These observations were undoubtedly carried out with great care and objective accuracy, and were repeated a number of times. Successive observations appeared to present a coherent and comprehensible picture of development. But it would certainly be desirable to have more corroboration from other sources of both observations and hypotheses.

3

Attention in Infants

It would perhaps be generally agreed, however, that during the early part of the first year of life the infant has little capacity to perceive or understand the world around him. Undoubtedly from birth or shortly afterwards he reacts promptly to a number of reflex stimuli. He retracts his limbs from painful stimuli, blinks at bright lights, sucks the nipple or sweet-tasting objects put in his mouth while attempting to spit out anything bitter. Thus we may if we wish say that he perceives these, though it is difficult to tell whether he is aware of them. It seems probable that he is aware that something is happening to him, pleasant or unpleasant, but that he has no idea what is stimulating him. He may not even discriminate between the effects of stimuli external to the body, and those of internal stimuli, for instance, fullness, emptiness, colic and so on. But during his first year he learns to attribute the source of external stimulation to perceived objects and events in the environment, and to discriminate these from internal events.

Within the first week of life there is some evidence that the infant 'attends' to external stimuli unrelated to reflex responses. This occurs during the state called by Bühler (9) 'positive quiet wakefulness', when he shows signs of orientation towards and perhaps awareness of such stimuli. Gesell, Ilg and Bullis (20) noted that from time to time the neonate fixated certain objects with his eyes—or rather, with one eye, since he could not coordinate the two eyes. Sporadic bodily activity declined and there was a rudimentary postural 'set' of the body indicating orientation and attention. The infant followed with his eyes objects moved across his field of vision such as a dangling ring. Chase (11) found that at about 15 days such pursuit movements of the eyes occurred in response to moving coloured patches of light. The infant followed with his eyes a patch of colour moving across a background of equal brightness but of another colour, suggesting that even at that age he could discriminate between the primary colours red, green and blue. These observations indicate that at a very early age the infant's attention may be directed primarily towards changing and moving stimuli rather than towards stationary ones. Moreover the pursuit move-

 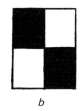 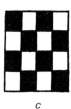

a   *b*   *c*

FIG. 1

ments and the resulting perceptions become increasingly more accurate with increasing age.

But the infant may also attend to stationary objects. Bright objects become particularly attractive from about 8 weeks of age (20). But Fantz (18) found that even from about one week infants seemed to prefer patterned to plain surfaces, and looked at them longer. Such a preference was well established by three months, according to Berlyne (6), who found that of three surfaces Fig. 1c was looked at first consistently more often than were Figs. 1a and 1b. At this age also Staples (43) showed that infants looked longer at coloured than at grey discs, even when these were motionless.

Particularly interesting are the responses made by infants to perception of the human face. Ambrose has recently discussed work on this topic (2), and has investigated it further himself. Fantz had noted that at two months infants looked longer at a representation of the human face than at other patterns. But the characteristic response of infants to the human face is not mere attention, but smiling. Ambrose found that infants began smiling in response to a stationary unsmiling face at about 14 weeks, but their smiles soon disappeared unless the face moved. Smiles increased in frequency up to a maximum at about 18 weeks, and thereafter decreased. But earlier experimenters had found that smiling could be stimulated by mere schematic representations of the human face. Kaila (24) noted smiling at 2–3 months in response to two glass balls in the same positions as two eyes. Ahrens (1) found that at about the fifth week infants would smile at a drawing of two eyes, and even sometimes at two large black dots. Later, at about the third month, other parts of the face were necessary to produce smiling, particularly the mouth. But Spitz and Wolf (42) showed that for a time a grimacing mouth was as effective as a smiling one, particularly if it moved. From the sixth month the smiling response became increasingly discriminative, occurring only to a smiling face, and later to a familiar face. Without entering into the social implications of these findings, we may conclude that a specific perception of a particular type of configuration,

crude at first but later becoming increasingly precise, develops spontaneously in children. But it may appear rather earlier in infants brought up at
home, according to Ambrose, than in the infants he mainly studied who
were brought up in institutions. This suggests that some learning through
experience with smiling adults is important for the development of the
smiling response.

4

Development of Perception of Objects

It seems probable that in early infancy there is no awareness of the relationship of different sensory patterns as originating in one and the same object,
but that each is perceived in isolation, perhaps leading in each case to a
specific response. However, as he continues to attend to these, the infant
becomes aware that certain sensory patterns recur periodically at the same
time and in the same position as each other. It is usually supposed that the
earliest association of sensory patterns of which the infant becomes aware
is that between the tactile, gustatory, visual and auditory sensations
provided by the mother. But detailed observations have been made by
Gesell *et al.* and by Piaget of the development of such associations, as
shown by the reaching, grasping and handling of objects while they are
examined visually. Piaget (31) observed that at about 3–4 months an infant
seized and examined something which had touched his hand. Gesell *et al.*
(20), from observations on a large number of infants, noted that at 16
weeks an infant looked to and fro from his hands to a cube placed on the
table before him. At 20 weeks he flung out his arms and grasped a dangling
ring, and put it in his mouth if he could. At about 28 weeks he turned it
about in his hands, fingered it all over and examined it carefully with his
eyes. But it is interesting to note that, according to Dennis (15), infants
reared in institutions in which their environmental contacts had been
severely restricted did not make reaching movements until as much as
three months later than did children reared at home. Presumably this was
because the former did not have the experience necessary to develop these
movements.

It seems probable that by means of the coordination of visual and
tactile sensory data the infant gradually learns not only the characteristics
of shape of objects, but also those of solidity and permanence. He finds that
solid objects can be turned about in space, thus changing their visual
appearance while their identity remains unchanged. This realisation does
not, according to Piaget (31), develop until the 7th or 8th month. Thus,
before then, if the infant's bottle is presented to him with the nipple
turned away from him he does not reach for it, since he does not recognise
the total visual pattern and identity of the bottle from one part of it.
He also realises only gradually that objects retain their existence and
identity when they are hidden from sight. At 6 or 7 months an infant may

look for something which has just dropped from his hand, because he wants to continue playing with it. But there is no active search, and he does not seem to think that the object still exists. At 8 or 9 months he begins to search actively for something which has been hidden, thus apparently expecting it still to be in existence, though somewhat vague as to where it is. Even at more than one year of age, one of Piaget's children expected that particular people were always to be expected in particular places. For instance she looked for her sister, who had been ill in bed, in the bedroom immediately after playing with her downstairs. This seems to indicate that to the young child particular objects belong to certain settings, and are not easily divorced from these and perceived independently of them.

Long after the child has become quite adept in the recognition and identification of objects, he may still be slower than the adult in doing this. Thus Taylor (44) exposed six toys for a period of three seconds to children of about four years of age (and of high intelligence), and found that the mean number they could name subsequently was two. The number varied with age and mental age, but did not increase with practice. Adults shown ten such toys could subsequently name six, on the average. Of course the difference between adults and children may have been due in part to differences in immediate memory. But it also seems likely that the original perception and identification were slower in children.

5

Development of Perception of Shape

We noted that the ability to discriminate between shapes seemed to develop at an early age before children could be said to perceive shape as such. Thus Ling (26) found that children of six months could discriminate between solid blocks shaped as a circle, oval, square, triangle and cross, and could learn, though slowly, to pick up one of these which was detachable and tasted sweet when put in the mouth, rejecting another which was fastened down. The rate of learning increased rapidly up till 12 months, and correct choice was unaffected by changes in size and position. Gellerman (19) found that at two years children could perceive immediately, or almost immedaitely, and remember simple shapes such as a triangle and a cross, and could recognise these in different positions, and placed on different-shaped backgrounds. But shape relationships are apparently more difficult to perceive, possibly because it is necessary to observe the relative shapes of spaces as well as of objects. Thus Meyer (29) showed that when children aged under three years were required to place boxes belonging to a nest inside one another they adopted a random procedure, banging the boxes together and clearly not appreciating their relative sizes. The same behaviour occurred in trying to pull objects through holes of different shapes. At 3–4 years the children were able to work out the shape relations by trial and error; but not until after this could they perceive the shape relations visually with sufficient accuracy to manoeuvre them without actually handling them.

It seems that in general children learn to perceive shapes more easily if they can manipulate them as well as view them. This is the manner in

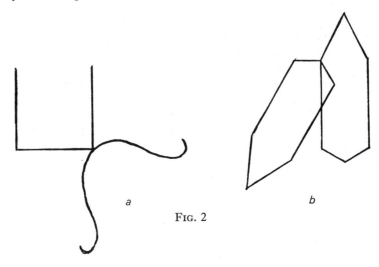

a

b

Fig. 2

which they learn in infancy. Luria (27) found that even at the age of five children could discriminate more accurately between shapes if they could handle them than if they merely looked at them. Again, at 3–4 years they could do tasks involving the use of levers if they could manipulate these, but not if they only looked at pictures of them. This was in all probability, as we shall discuss below, partly because to children of this age pictures do not represent objects as completely and convincingly as they do to older children and adults, but also because it seems that for young children several corroborative sensory patterns may be necessary even for the identification of objects. As they grow older, they no longer need tactile and kinaesthetic patterns but can rely almost entirely on the more accurate and sensitive visual patterns, Again, at a very early age, at 3–4 months, manipulation by the mouth is used in exploring objects (31); but this is soon abandoned, presumably because the tactile sensory patterns of the mouth are less accurate than those obtained from the fingers.

That children are relatively slow to perceive shapes by means of vision alone appears in the difficulty which children have in copying shapes accurately. Of course it may be maintained that this difficulty results from lack of skill in drawing. The shapes, however, which they can copy seem not much easier to draw than those which they cannot copy. Thus the diamond is not reproduced correctly until about two years later than the square. The diamond would not appear to be more difficult to draw than the square, but children find it harder to perceive correctly the orientation of the inclined lines than of the horizontal and vertical (34).

More complex shapes and combinations of shapes are even harder for the child to perceive correctly. Slochower (41) found a tendency to make such figures simpler, more regular and more symmetrical than the originals. Again, with the Bender Visual Motor Gestalt test, correct reproduction varied from 7 years for Fig. 2*a* to over 11 years for Fig. 2*b* (5). Brain-injured children may have particular difficulty with this test, since its correct performance depends on the careful analysis of shape relations, the capacity for which has apparently failed to develop in them.

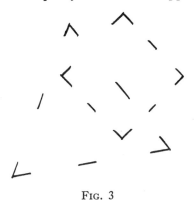

FIG. 3

Other experimental findings which demonstrated children's slowness in perceiving complex shape relations include that of Piaget and Stettler-Von Albertini (36), who showed that 4–5 year old children had some difficulty in perceiving overlapping geometrical figures; and six-year-olds could not do this when the outlines of the shapes were dashed instead of solid (see Fig. 3). Ghent (21), however, found that even four-year-old children could recognise overlapping shapes, but that numerous errors were still made at eight years in tracing out simple figures embedded in more complex ones (see Fig. 4).

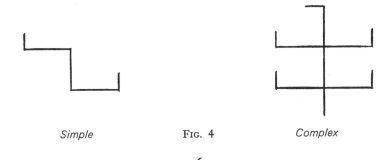

Simple   FIG. 4   *Complex*

6

The Analysis of Shape

It appears from these data that the child only gradually acquires the capacity to perceive the details of shapes as such, and their relationship within the whole. To do this he must cease to perceive 'syncretically', with all details merged in a whole, in the way that even adults tend to perceive illusions such as the Müller-Lyer illusion. It should be noted in passing that 'syncretic' perception is not necessarily the perception of the outline alone; as Osterrieth (30) showed, it may be the perception of dominant and striking details rather than of the outline. But for accurate perception of complex shapes the whole must be analysed into its constituent parts, each of these perceived independently, and their relationship to each other observed. This in turn necessitates the active and systematic direction of attention towards successive aspects of the shape. So also for the correct perception of the complex scenes such as we habitually encounter in ordinary life: attention must be systematically directed from one feature to another, and in particular objects must be differentiated from their background and perceived as having an existence independent of it. We noted that children at a year old were sometimes unable to do this.

In his recent book *Les Mécanismes Perceptifs* (33) Piaget has discussed the gradual development of 'perceptual activity' and the direction of attention in children. He has suggested that in the first year of life infants, as they explore and manipulate objects with their fingers, direct their attention to the contours of shapes, their angles and corners, and also to their solidity and three-dimensionality. But it is not until they are about six years or over that they can explore systematically with their eyes alone. Before that they tend either to let their eyes wander at random over the field of view, or to remain fixated upon particular parts of it. Thus they tend to overestimate the larger part of, for instance, a line divided into two unequal parts, because they fixate it for longer; again, they perceive the horizontal-vertical illusion to an exaggerated extent, because they look longer at the upper than at the lower part of the field. Older children and adults, however, scan the field more regularly and systematically, fixating the important parts of figures and comparing them together until they can judge their relative sizes more accurately. It should be noted that, although Piaget undoubtedly obtained characteristic differences between the illusions perceived by young children and by adults, his evidence as to direction of fixation was somewhat weak. Piaget and Vinh-Bang (37) did record actual eye movements and fixations in viewing these illusions, but the number especially of the younger children on whom observations were made was very small. It is indeed quite likely that young children do not attend very carefully to figures such as these which have no particular appeal for them. It seems that the regard of the young child is attracted and held by certain features in his environment, for instance those which are novel or unusual, or appeal to his interest, and also perhaps by certain patterns which are striking in themselves though devoid of meaning. He tends to fix his gaze on these and to ignore the remainder of the field. When the field contains little to interest or attract him his attention is vague and haphazard; and he does not yet possess the capacity to control it voluntarily and direct it systematically.

7

Development of Auditory Perception and the Use of Language

We must now consider the development of auditory perception, and its relationship to the child's understanding of the environment. Particularly important is the child's reaction to and understanding of human speech. It seems probable that he perceives this type of auditory pattern before any other. Thus specific responses to speech appear early in infancy. Piaget (31) observed that an infant turned his head towards the source of a voice at about two months; and a little later he looked attentively at the person who spoke. Hetzer and Tudor-Hart (23) noted a smiling response to the human voice at 2–4 months. This suggests that the infant is aware of it in much the same way as he is aware of the face, namely as some kind of pleasurable social stimulus. But before long he develops the capacity to react with the appropriate emotional responses to the intonational patterns of speech expressing emotion. This occurs before the phonetic patterns of speech are perceived and understood. But according to Seth and Guthrie (40) the child does attach some meaning to words before he can utter them; and he can understand simple sentences and commands by the 9th–12th month. However, he probably does not understand the words separately, but rather the general gist of what is spoken to him. Indeed it is difficult to decide whether single words mean much to the child until he uses them himself. Possibly they act mainly as signals by means of which his attention is drawn to objects and events in his surroundings. In this manner he begins to link particular word sounds with particular objects, and during his second year to enunciate these himself, using a process of trial and error to discover from adults whether he is correct or not.

It is clear from the work of numerous psychologists that the first names are used for several different objects which have a general similarity to each other. Hence the use of 'dada' and 'mama' for any familiar adult, and of 'bow-wow', etc. for a number of different animals. Piaget (32) noted that 'tch-tch', first applied to a train, was then used for any vehicle passing the window. Other words such as 'no more' were used for anything which had disappeared from view. 'Panana' applied not only to 'grandpapa' but also to anything which the child wanted and which grandpapa might have given her. Lewis (25) quotes similar misconceptions, resulting mainly from the tendency to class together objects and situations which have the same significance or emotional appeal for the child.

On the other hand children may be relatively slow to adopt the adult type of classification, in which generalisation is based on more abstract resemblances. Thus Lewis reported that at about nine months his son understood the word 'ballie' to refer to a small white ball, but did not respond to this word in relation to a larger coloured ball until he was a year old. Again, Piaget (32) noted that even at over two years of age a child used the name 'slug' for one particular slug encountered on the path, and did not realise that there were many different slugs in existence. Thus it is clear that the child at first is uncertain how to generalise his percepts as conceptual classes, and how to name these. Luria and Yudovitch (28) studied twins of five years who had not developed normal speech and could not understand speech unless it referred directly to some immediately perceptible object or situation. They were unable to classify objects by grouping similar ones together, presumably because such classification requires the use of language.

In normal children the use of naming and verbal description becomes increasingly precise as they grow older, and it may then be of considerable assistance in a number of perceptual tasks. Thus Cantor (10) showed that children aged 3–5 years could recognise faces more correctly when they had first been taught to name these than when they had merely been shown the faces and their attention drawn to various features of them. Again, Luria (27) found that the children who could not solve the lever problem when it was presented pictorially were often able to do so if they could talk about it to an adult.

It does not follow, however, that children cannot perceive relationships unless they can formulate them verbally. Braine (8) found that children aged 4–5 years could perceive and understand the size relationships of objects when these were demonstrated by means of a measuring stick, without being able to verbalise them. Indeed, verbalisation when it was achieved did not seem to facilitate the understanding of the relationships. Again, in a comparatively simple task such as colour matching, Cook (12) showed that children could match primary colours with fair accuracy at four years, but could not always name them correctly even at six years. It seems probable that children are helped by their use of language to achieve more accurate perception, especially when generalisation and judgement are involved. But much immediate perception, especially of the simpler sort, takes place without the use of words; and indeed, if the child is required to formulate precisely what he has perceived, these may hinder rather than help him.

8

The Understanding of Pictures

One type of perception which is of some interest as demonstrating the difficulty which children have in understanding a complex presentation is that of pictures and representational drawings. The sensory data provided even by a good reproduction of an object are so different from those emanating from the object itself that one might suppose that children would be slow to associate the drawing with the object. However, they begin to understand such drawings only about a year after they can identify the objects themselves. Thus in the Terman-Merrill test (45) an average child of three years can name 12 out of 18 simple clear outline drawings of familiar objects such as a chair, table, fork, cup, etc., and the average child of four can name 16. It seems probable that he learns to recognise shapes from their contours alone partly by handling them; and it is likely that frequent experience of looking at pictures which are named and described to him is important also.

If, however, the outlines of the reproduction are not clear and obvious, the child is considerably handicapped. Thus Gollin (22) found that children of under 4½ years were much less able than older children to recognise drawings of familiar objects with dashed outlines than with solid outlines; but over this age they did as well as adults. Draguns and Multari (16) presented blurred pictures of familiar objects for a period of 10 seconds only, and found that even children of eight years could not perceive them as well as older children could. And Ghent (21) showed that under eight years numerous omissions were made in perceiving overlapping drawings of familiar objects. Thus it may be concluded that with this type of material also children require fuller and clearer perceptual data than do adults.

The ability of children to describe complex pictures of scenes also develops slowly. Many years ago Binet (7) noted that at 3 years children merely enumerated the objects shown in a picture. At 7 years they described the pictures and their more obvious aspects, including some description of the actions of people. But a real understanding of a picture and the ability to interpret what was happening in it did not develop fully until 15 years. Now the ages at which these procedures appear differ according to the nature of the pictures and the familiarity and comprehensibility of their contents. The author (46) showed that, with pictures of fairly obvious meaning, interpretation and understanding developed at about 11 years. Amen (3) found enumeration to begin to disappear even at 3 years, and description of overt activities to appear in about half the children of that age. Some interpretation of the meaning of activities, and even of feelings and intentions, was observed at 4 years. However, in all the responses of children of 2–5 years there was a tendency to report unrelated details, such as the dog in one picture. The younger children were liable to concentrate on one particular part of the picture, not necessarily the most relevant and important, and to ignore the remainder. This finding is similar to that of Piaget with visual illusions.

Now clearly, in describing pictures, much cognitive activity is necessary in addition to immediate perception. But the young child does not know how to direct his attention appropriately, or to select those aspects of the field of view which are important and which give meaning to the total experience. One cannot assume that young children are equally inept in perceiving and understanding the scenes of everyday life; although it is probable, as we noted above, that in these also they perceive mainly what first catches their attention and appeals to their interest, overlooking other aspects, and fail to understand the whole significance of events and situations. But in everyday life their perception and understanding may be considerably assisted by the three-dimensionality of objects in space, and still more by their movement. It may be noted in passing that even with adults Wallach and O'Connell (49) have shown that shadows of three-dimensional objects thrown on a screen appear quite flat when the objects are motionless, but are seen as the shadows of solid objects when these are in continuous movement. The author (47) also found that for adults television scenes appeared much more 'real' when they depicted objects and people in motion. It may be that movement is even more important to children's perceptions and understanding of events. But the findings in relation to the perception of pictures are interesting in that they suggest once again that children require more and fuller corroborative data than do adults for adequate perception, and are less able to perceive and understand 'impoverished' material and situations.

9

The Perception of Space

One very important type of perception which develops only gradually in children is that of the space relations of objects and the manner in which their spatial positions are related to each other, to the observer and to the surrounding environment. Although in the adult all spatial percepts are integrated together and related to ideas about space and spatial relations, these spatial 'schemes', as Piaget called them (31), develop only slowly and to some extent independently. In the first place, perception of distance of near objects depends largely upon the binocular disparity (unlikeness) of the retinal images in the two eyes, and upon the convergence of the eyes during binocular fixation. It is somewhat doubtful when this type of perception develops in infants. It must of course be preceded by binocular coordination, the ability to fixate a single point with both eyes. According to Gesell et al. (20) this is well established by about four months, though Piaget (31) considered that it was not completely accurate until nine months. Now an experiment by Walk and Gibson (48) showed that infants could perceive distance at the age of about eight months, or possibly even younger. In this experiment there was a large horizontal sheet of glass which had a checkered surface immediately below half of it, and another checkered surface four feet below the other half. Each infant was placed on the glass on the midline, and the mother beckoned to it from the farther edge of the shallow or the deep side. Most of the infants from eight months upwards crawled across the former, but would not crawl across the latter. Walk and Gibson, however, obtained similar results with animals which do not possess binocular vision, and therefore concluded that factors other than binocular disparity must have been responsible for the infants' perception of the drop on the deep side.

Undoubtedly data other than those afforded by binocular disparity and convergence are utilised in the fully developed perception of space and distance. Among the most important are the changes in size of the retinal image as objects recede from or advance towards the observer, though it appeared that these were not of great importance to the infants in Walk and Gibson's experiment. Normally we perceive the size of the objects to remain constant, while their distance changes, an effect known as 'size constancy'; and the change in size of retinal image is therefore utilised in judging the distance of the object. The perception of size constancy begins to develop during the second half of the first year. By six months the infant can apparently discriminate between what is within his reach and what is not. Thus Cruikshank (13) found that a six-months infant reached for a rattle which was close to him, but not for one three times as far away, outside his reach, even when the latter was three times as large as the former and therefore projected an image on his retina equal in size to that of the nearer rattle. However this does not prove that the infant yet perceived size constancy. Piaget (31) found that by 8–9 months infants could reach for objects in the near distance with fair accuracy, and paid little attention to far distant objects such as the moon. Infants learned gradually to improve the accuracy of their judgements of distance by moving towards and away from objects and observing how their visual impressions (disparity, retinal size, etc.) changed as the distances changed. During the early part of the second year, the child also experimented continuously with the positions of objects in space relative to each other, and thus acquired the ability to judge relative distances.

By 8–9 months infants appeared fully to realise that objects retain their identity in spite of change in size of retinal image with change in distance, at least over short distances. But again it was possible that they did not actually perceive real size as unchanged. Piaget and Lambercier (35) found that up to six years children could make more accurate judgements of projected (retinal image) size than adults could, but that they were liable to underestimate real size. This result was confirmed by Zeigler and Leibowitz (50), who showed that even children of 7–9 years increasingly underestimated the sizes of stakes, of unknown height, as their distance increased from 10 to 100 ft. Denis-Prinzhorn (14) found that children aged 5–7 years also underestimated the lengths of farther distances by comparison with nearer ones. Thus when required to bisect the distance between two objects, one situated at 34 cm. and the other at 200 cm., they consistently underestimated the farther half.

It should be noted that these judgements were made in 'impoverished' situations. The sizes of the objects were unfamiliar, and there were no very obvious clues to the distance at which they were situated. On the other hand Dukes (17) found that a six-year-old child could make fairly accurate judgements of the real size of familiar objects at various distances in natural surroundings. However, it may be concluded, as Denis-Prinzhorn argues, that the young child does not perceive distant space with the same clarity and accuracy as adults do. Perhaps he does not attend to it much, and therefore he underestimates its size and the size of objects in it. Of course when it is a matter of judging the size of really distant objects, such as people and houses seen across a lake or from the top of a mountain, immediate perception is unreliable even in adults. They perceive these objects as tiny, and judge their distances and real sizes by using the ideas they have acquired about the appearance of objects at a great distance. It is clear from the work of Piaget and Inhelder (34) that children only slowly develop such ideas on the nature of spatial relations. But to discuss these would go beyond the scope of this chapter. We may note, however, that they are probably linked in the first place to the appearance and use of words about space and spatial relations. Ames and Learned (4) showed that children begin to use such words at quite an early age, though primarily in relation to comparatively short distances and in rather a vague manner. Whereas up to the age of three the child localises objects by pointing at them, from this age onwards he begins to use words such as 'here' and 'there' to denote their position; and he can also describe locations which are not actually visible at the moment. For instance he can answer the question 'What is above the ceiling?' Words relating to far distance appear last.

10

The Nature of Perceptual Development

It may be argued that from the information given here it is difficult to derive an overall picture of the child's developing perceptions of his natural environment, from the rudimentary stages in early infancy to their virtual identity with those of adults at the age of 8–9 years. Indeed it *is* difficult, for several reasons. Firstly, as I have said, we cannot be certain exactly what young children do perceive, still less what they understand from their perceptions, before they can tell us this clearly in words. Piaget has given us masterly expositions of the manner in which he considers that perception develops, which are based upon careful observations of the reactions of his children to various perceived situations. But for the reasons described above his views should not be accepted without further evidence. And unfortunately most of the evidence adduced by other psychologists was obtained in carefully controlled but essentially limited and 'impoverished' situations. However, it does seem justifiable to conclude that perception develops piecemeal, from a vague awareness of certain sensory patterns which at first mean little to the child. By coordinating these together he gains some understanding of the nature of solid objects, and particularly that they are solid and permanent, and retain their identity unchanged, in spite of modifications, lawfully coordinated together, in visually perceived shape and size, and even when they are out of view. The child learns gradually to perceive these more accurately, and to recognise them from rapid glimpses of parts only of their complete three-dimensional appearance, such as two-dimensional outlines. But this is more difficult for him than for adults, and in general he requires more and fuller corroborative data for adequate perception of objects. He may discriminate between abstract geometrical shapes at an early age, but he is slower to perceive these shapes as such with sufficient clarity to reproduce them accurately. He is also slow to learn how to analyse complex shapes into their constituent parts, first perceiving these independently of each other, and then coordinating them in relation to one another and to the whole. Thus the full development of shape perception of the adult type is gradual and piecemeal. Again, the child must learn how to view a complex field, directing his attention appropriately and extracting its essential and significant features, until he is able not only to perceive readily those parts which are interesting and important to him, but also to compare and assess the sizes and distance of objects in surrounding space. He must also acquire the capacity to perceive and understand significant changes in the environment while ignoring those which are relatively unimportant, such as changes of shape in the outlines of objects rotated into various positions. In doing this he is assisted firstly by his manipulation of objects, when he grasps, fingers and handles them and moves them about in space; and later by reasoning about them, their functions and interrelationships, in words. But the greater the degree of reasoning required and the more complex and abstract the concepts and ideas involved, the later the age at which perception becomes accurate and effective. Clearly intelligence is involved; and the performance of many of the tasks described above has in fact been found to be correlated with mental age as well as with chronological age.

REFERENCES

1. AHRENS, R., 1954. Beitrag zur Entwicklung des Physiognomie und Mimikerkennens. *Zeit. f. exper. u. ange. Psychol.*, II: 412 and 599. Quoted in (2).
2. AMBROSE, J. A., 1960. *The Smiling Response in Early Human Infancy*. Unpublished Ph.D. Thesis, University of London.
   1961. The development of the smiling response in early infancy. In *Determinants of Infant Behaviour*, ed. B. M. Foss. London: Methuen.
3. AMEN, E. A., 1941. Individual differences in apperceptive reaction. *Genet. Psychol. Monogr.*, 23: 219.
4. AMES, L. B. and LEARNED, J., 1948. The development of verbalized space in the young child. *J. Genet. Psychol.*, 72: 63.
5. BENDER, L., 1938. *A Visual Motor Gestalt Test and its Clinical Use*. New York: American Orthopsychiatric Association.
6. BERLYNE, D. E., 1958. The influence of the albedo and complexity of stimuli on visual fixation in the human infant. *Brit. J. Psychol.*, 49: 315.
7. BINET, A., 1905. Interpretation. *Ann. Psychol.*: 11.
8. BRAINE, M. D. S., 1959. The ontogeny of certain logical operations. *Psychol. Monogr.*, 73: No. 5.
9. BÜHLER, C., 1945. *From Birth to Maturity*. London: Kegan Paul.
10. CANTOR, G. N., 1955. Effects of three types of pre-training on discrimination learning in pre-school children. *J. Exper. Psychol.*, 49: 339.
11. CHASE, W. P., 1937. Color vision in infants. *J. Exper. Psychol.*, 20: 203.
12. COOK, W. M., 1931. Ability of children in color discrimination. *Child Developm.* 2: 303.
13. CRUIKSHANK, R. M., 1941. The development of visual size-constancy in early infancy. *J. Genet. Psychol.*, 58: 377.

14. DENIS-PRINZHORN, M., 1960. Perception des distances et constance des grandeurs (étude génétique). *Arch. de Psychol.*, **37**: 181.

15. DENNIS, W., 1941. Infant development under conditions of restricted practice and of minimum social stimulation. *Genet. Psychol. Monogr.*, **23**: 143.

16. DRAGUNS, J. G. and MULTARI, G., 1961. Recognition of perceptually ambiguous stimuli in grade school children. *Child Developm.*, **32**: 541.

17. DUKES, W. F., 1951. Ecological representativeness in studying perceptual size-constancy in childhood. *Amer. J. Psychol.*, **64**: 87.

18. FANTZ, R. L., 1961. The origin of form perception. *Scient. Amer.*, **204** (5): 66.

19. GELLERMAN, L. W., 1933. Form discrimination in chimpanzees and two-year-old children. *J. Genet. Psychol.*, **42**: 3 and 28.

20. GESELL, A., ILG, F. L. and BULLIS, G. E., 1949. *Vision: its Development in Infant and Child.* New York: Hoeber.

21. GHENT, L., 1956. Perception of overlapping and embedded figures by children of different ages. *Amer. J. Psychol.*, **69**: 575.

22. GOLLIN, E. S., 1960. Developmental studies of visual recognition of incomplete objects. *Percept. Motor Skills*, **11**: 289.

23. HETZER, H. and TUDOR-HART, B. H., 1927. Die frühesten Reaktionen auf die menschliche Stimme. *Quellen u. Stud. z. Jugendk.*, **5**. Quoted in (2).

24. KAILA, E., 1932. Die Reaktionen des Sauglings auf das Menschliche Gesicht. *Annales Universitatis Fennicae Åboensis*, Ser. B, Humaniora. Quoted in (2).

25. LEWIS, M. M., 1936. *Infant Speech.* London: Kegan Paul.

26. LING, B. C., 1941. Form discrimination as a learning cue in infants. *Comp. Psychol. Monogr.*, **17**, No. 2.

27. LURIA, A. R., 1961. *The Role of Speech in the Regulation of Normal and Abnormal Behaviour.* London: Pergamon.

28. LURIA, A. R. and YUDOVICH, F. I., 1959. *Speech and the Development of Mental Processes in the Child.* London: Staples Press.

29. MEYER, E., 1940. Comprehension of spatial relations in pre-school children. *J. Genet. Psychol.*, **57**: 119.

30. OSTERRIETH, P. A., 1945. Le test de copie d'une figure complexe. *Arch. de Psychol.*, **30**; 205.

31. PIAGET, J., 1955. *The Child's Construction of Reality.* London: Routledge & Kegan Paul.

32. ———— 1951. *Play, Dreams and Imitation in Childhood.* London: Heinemann.

33. ———— 1961. *Les Mécanismes Perceptifs.* Paris: Presses Universitaires de France.

34. PIAGET, J. and INHELDER, B., 1956. *The Child's Conception of Space.* London: Routledge & Kegan Paul.

35. PIAGET, J. and LAMBERCIER, M., 1951. La comparaison des grandeurs projectives chez l'enfant et chez l'adulte. *Arch. de Psychol.*, **33**: 81.

36. PIAGET, J. and STETTLER-VON ALBERTINI, B., 1954. Observations sur la perception des bonnes formes chez l'enfant par actualisation des lignes virtuelles. *Arch. de Psychol.*, **34**: 203.

37. PIAGET, J. and VINH-BANG, 1961. Comparaison des mouvements oculaires et des centrations du regard chez l'enfant et chez l'adulte. *Arch. de Psychol.*, **38**: 167.

38. SCHAFFER, H. R., 1958. Objective observations of personality development in early infancy. *Brit. J. Med. Psychol.*, **31**: 174.

39. VON SENDEN, M., 1960. *Space and Sight.* London: Methuen.

40. SETH, G. and GUTHRIE, D., 1935. *Speech in Childhood.* Oxford Univ. Press.

41. SLOCHOWER, M. Z., 1946. Experiments on dimensional and figural problems in the clay and pencil reproductions of line figures by young children. II. Shape. *J. Genet. Psychol.*, **69**: 77.

42. SPIZT, R. A. and WOLF, K. M., 1946. The smiling response. *Genet. Psychol. Monogr.*, **34**: 57.
43. STAPLES, R., 1932. The responses of infants to color. *J. Exper. Psychol.*, **15**: 119.
44. TAYLOR, C. D., 1931. A comparative study of visual apprehension in nursery school children and adults. *Child Developm.*, **2**: 263.
45. TERMAN, L. M. and MERRILL, M. A., 1937. *Measuring Intelligence*. London: Harrap.
46. VERNON, M. D., 1940. The relation of cognition and phantasy in children. *Brit. J. Psychol.*, **30**: 273.
47. 1953. Perception and understanding of instructional television programmes. *Brit. J. Psychol.*, **44**: 116.
48. WALK, R. D. and GIBSON, E. J., 1961. A comparative and analytical study of visual depth perception. *Psychol. Monogr.*, **75**, No. 15.
49. WALLACH, H. and O'CONNELL, D. N., 1953. The kinetic depth effect. *J. Exper. Psychol.*, **45**: 205.
50. ZEIGLER, H. P. and LEIBOWITZ, H., 1957. Apparent visual size as a function of distance for children and adults. *Amer. J. Pychol.*, **70**: 106.

VI

THE APPLICATION OF LEARNING THEORY
TO CHILD PSYCHIATRY

H. J. Eysenck
B.A., Ph.D.
Professor of Psychology, Institute of Psychiatry, University of London

AND

S. J. Rachman
M.A., Ph.D.
Lecturer in Clinical Psychology, Institute of Psychiatry, University of London

Introduction

Learning theory is that part of modern psychology which deals with the modification of behaviour through experience, and attempts to formulate the laws according to which such modification takes place. As almost all behaviour is modified by experience, the processes of learning and conditioning are obviously so fundamental to psychology that the wider title 'behaviour theory' has sometimes been applied to this body of knowledge. Most of the concepts used stem from the experimental and theoretical work originally done by Pavlov on what is now called 'classical conditioning', but there has been a considerable degree of interest also in another type of learning originally investigated by Pavlov's great rival Bechterev, and now mainly studied by Skinner and his students under the title of 'instrumental conditioning'. The typical paradigm of 'classical conditioning' is the dog that learns to salivate to the sound of a bell because this bell has in the past been presented in temporal association with food; the typical experiment of the 'instrumental conditioning' type is that of the sheep which learns to raise its fore-leg because whenever it does so a suitable reward is administered. For an introduction to modern learning theory Hilgard's (1) and Kimble's (2) monographs are perhaps the most suitable guide.

The application of modern learning theory to child psychiatry is mediated by a postulate which can be put in several different ways, but which essentially maintains that *neurotic and personality disorders are essentially learned reactions* rather than being *directly* inherited or being produced by demonstrable lesions. Granted this, and few psychiatrists will be found to disagree with this very wide statement, it must follow that whatever knowledge psychologists may have acquired regarding the acquisition and extinction of habits, behaviour patterns, conditioned autonomic responses and the like, must be relevant to aetiology, nosology and treatment of these disorders in children as well as in adults.

Even where the hypothesis that learning has been responsible for the main part of the aberrant behaviour pattern is difficult to maintain, as in the case of autistic, schizophrenic or brain-damaged children, nevertheless it will be clear that rehabilitation, as far as this is possible, must occur through the use of whatever capacities for learning they may possess; thus learning theory will provide hypotheses and suggestions for the optimal use of those capacities, both cognitive and non-cognitive, which remain to the individual. It will be found that this distinction between neurotic disorders largely produced by environmental influences, and psychotic and other disorders due to specific defects of the nervous system, metabolism, et cetera, tends to be mirrored in the methods of treatment recommended and used by psychologists: the former tend to be treated by means of some derivative of Pavlov's type of 'classical conditioning' where the latter tend to be treated rather by means of Bechterev's type of 'instrumental conditioning' (sometimes called 'operant conditioning', following Skinner). The distinction is not absolute but is sufficiently striking to be worth mentioning. As far more work has perhaps been done with the neurotic type of disorder, we shall in our theoretical analysis concentrate more on this aspect rather than on the other types of disorder, where aetiological factors are in any case outside the field of the psychologist.

REFERENCES

1. HILGARD, E. R., 1958. *Theories of Learning.* New York: Appleton-Century-Crofts.
2. KIMBLE, G., 1961. *Conditioning and Learning.* Revised ed., Hilgard and Marquis. London: Methuen.

Part I. PERSONALITY

In dealing with the so-called neurotic, or nervous, or behaviour disorders of children, it may be useful to start from the nosological point of view in order to delineate more precisely just what the problem is to which an aetiological theory will be required to provide an answer. Suppose we were to take a very large random group of children coming to a child guidance clinic, and suppose that we note down for each child the presence or absence of a large number of different items of behaviour, ranging from rudeness to depression, from seclusiveness to fighting behaviour, from disobedience to sensitiveness, from laziness to egocentricity and from stealing to irritability; we could then, by means of the statistical method of correlation analysis (Eysenck (9)), discover the empirical tendencies of these various items to cohere together in the same child. Thus we might find a high correlation between swearing, destructiveness and rudeness, or between seclusiveness, absent-mindedness and irritability. Having collected large numbers of correlations of this type we could then attempt to bring some order into this large body of data by the statistical method of factor analysis, the main purpose of which is to reduce a large number of separate correlations to a few more inclusive guiding principles or factors. The results of a typical study of this kind are shown in Fig. 1. It will be seen there that the factor analysis of our data results in a perfectly clear-cut and simple picture. All the behaviour traits included tend to correlate together and define a factor variously named neuroticism, abnormality, emotionality or instability. Cutting across this factor is another one which divides the 'conduct problems' from 'personality problems'[1]; we may perhaps call this by the not altogether appropriate but well-known terms 'introversion-extraversion'. The introverted neurotic child is characterised by *personality problems*: he tends to be depressed, seclusive, absent-minded, irritable, to have daydreams, inferiority feelings, mood swings and mental conflict. The extraverted neurotic child, on the other hand, tends to have *conduct problems*: he is egocentric, rude, violent, disobedient, destructive; he has temper tantrums, is given to fighting, stealing and truanting. This division appears with girls as well as with boys, and it does so at various ages (Collins *et al.* (2)); it clearly is a very fundamental type of division. It is also identical with what has been found in very many researches conducted on adults, both normal and neurotic; Fig. 2 shows in summary form results of many studies run along similar lines with adults. It will also be seen from Fig. 2 that these relatively recent factor analytic discoveries were adumbrated by Galen and his successors when they framed the well-known humoral theories of personality (Eysenck (3)).

Granted that this description is reasonably accurate, how can we account for these divisions? There is much evidence to show that underlying the 'neuroticism' variable lies an inherited tendency[2] of the autonomic system to react strongly and lastingly to stimuli; children and adults whose autonomic nervous systems possess this strong lability are much more likely to develop neurotic disorders than are children and adults in whom this lability is relatively slight. This inherited tendency, of course, is only a predisposition; whether this predisposition will actually issue in symptoms

---

[1] In a recent study of 831 children, this analysis received strong confirmation: " . . . the two factors emerged with remarkable invariance ". (Peterson (12).)

[2] For a discussion of the influence of heredity on neurotic and extraverted or introverted behaviour, see Shields (13).

will depend very much on environmental influences and events. It was observed during the war that in military personnel referred to the psychiatric hospitals there was a distinct inverse correlation between predisposition and the strength of the traumatic event which precipitated the illness; it is to be surmised that in civilian life too such an inverse correlation is to be found.

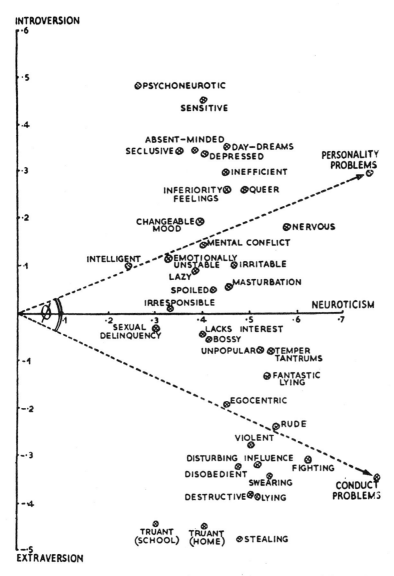

FIG. 1. Diagram showing grouping of neurotic symptoms in children into *personality problems* and *conduct problems*. The grouping is established on an objective basis, being based on observed relationships in large samples of children. (From Eysenck, H. J., *The Structure of Human Personality*.)

When we come to the difference between the extraverted and introverted patterns of behaviour, i.e. between conduct problems and personality problems, we must have recourse to another set of predisposing

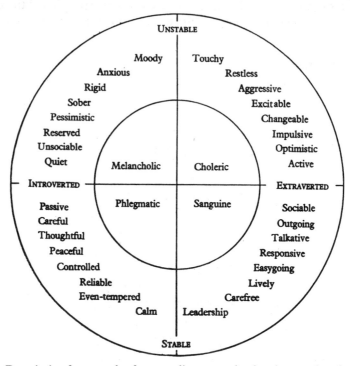

FIG. 2. Descriptive framework of personality research, showing results of modern
nosological research in relation to the old 'four temperaments' of Galen.
    (From Eysenck, H. J. and Eysenck, S. B. G., *Manual of the Eysenck Personality
Inventory*.)

factors, this time related to the speed and strength with which conditioned
responses are formed in the individual (Eysenck (3)). It is well known
that there are very marked individual differences in this respect, and a
theory has been put forward to the effect that introverts form conditioned
responses more quickly and lastingly than do extraverts. (As we shall see,
this statement should really be inverted; it would then read that individuals
who condition quickly tend to develop introverted personality patterns,
whereas individuals who condition slowly tend to develop extraverted
personality patterns.) Fig. 3 shows the results of an experimental study
in which extraverted and introverted individuals, both normal and neurotic,
were compared with respect to the speed with which they acquire conditioned eye-blink reflexes; the conditioned stimulus was a tone, the
unconditioned stimulus a puff of air to the eyeball. It will be seen that the
introverted subjects conditioned twice as well as did the extraverted ones,
and that is typical of many other studies (Eysenck (6)).

Consider now the ways in which differences in conditioning may be crucial in determining the direction which the neurotic behaviour will take. We would suggest that anxieties, phobias, reactive depressions, obsessions and compulsions are essentially maladaptive emotional responses which

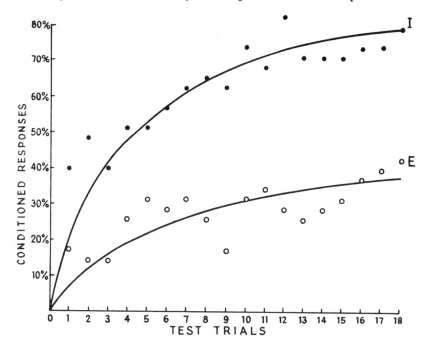

FIG. 3. Eye-blink conditioning in introverted and extraverted subjects. It will be seen that the former show roughly twice as many conditioned responses at any stage as do the latter.
(From Eysenck H. J., Conditioning and Personality. *Brit. J. Psychol.*, 1962, 53: 299-305.)

have been acquired through the process of Pavlovian conditioning. There may have been either a traumatic event or a series of sub-traumatic events playing the role of the unconditioned stimulus; the strong emotional reactions appropriate to this unconditioned stimulus have now become transferred through conditioning to a previously neutral and logically irrelevant conditioned stimulus or set of stimuli. The evidence in favour of this hypothesis will be discussed later; let us simply note here that other things being equal this acquisition of a conditioned autonomic response will be enormously facilitated in individuals who form conditioned responses quickly, strongly and lastingly, whereas individuals who condition poorly would be effectively protected against the acquisition of these maladaptive behaviour patterns. Hence we would predict a strong relationship between the *dysthymic* group of neurotic symptoms, introversion and conditionability, and indeed the evidence is very strongly in favour of such a link (Eysenck (3)).

A high degree of conditionability would appear to be a disadvantage, but it should not be concluded that the absence of conditionability would be found to be advantageous. It has been argued by Mowrer (11) and others that the whole process of socialisation is essentially mediated by Pavlovian conditioning: the child's misdemeanours are immediately punished by a slap or in some other way, thus associating the conditioned stimulus (the nefarious behaviour pattern) and the unconditioned stimulus (the punishment). Through a process of generalisation, which itself is aided by parental labelling of all such behaviour patterns as 'bad' or 'naughty', the child soon builds up a conditioned autonomic reaction towards all acts of this class, thus introjecting the moral precepts of his parents, his teachers and his peers (Eysenck (5)). We will not here argue about the truth of this hypothesis, which is strongly supported by experimental research; we will instead draw attention to the consequences that would follow if a particular child formed conditioned responses weakly and slowly. Clearly in such a person the process of socialisation would proceed only to a very limited degree, and if his failure to condition were to be particularly severe, then he would grow up into a 'moral imbecile', a psychopath or more generally a 'conduct problem'. Again we have evidence that in actual fact psychopathic and hysterical behaviour, extraversion and lack of conditionability, are quite strongly correlated, so that there is factual support for our general theory (Eysenck (3, 6)).

We now have a nosological and aetiological model which enables us to understand the growth and existence of behaviour patterns as they are observed in the clinic: these behaviour patterns arise from environmental influences, but individuals are predisposed towards one type of behaviour or the other in terms of inherited structures in the central nervous system (particularly the ascending reticular formation) and the autonomic nervous system (particularly the sympathetic branch). We may now proceed to apply these notions to the *reversal* of the learned maladaptive responses which constitute the neurotic behaviour pattern. Before doing so, however, we would like to draw attention to a fundamental difference between the 'personality problems' and the 'conduct problems' presented by children. The former essentially constitute a set of conditioned autonomic responses, together with the skeletal and muscular consequences thereof; the task of the therapist is to *decondition* the individual and to get rid of all these maladaptive behaviour patterns. Exactly the obverse is true of our 'conduct problems'; here we are dealing with a *failure* on the part of the individual to acquire adaptive autonomic responses and behaviour patterns, and it is the task of the therapist to inculcate these in the individual and thus socialise him through conditioning. As we shall see, the second of these tasks has always been found to be much more difficult, and one of us has argued that disorders of the first type will tend to have a much higher spontaneous rate of remission than disorders of the second type (Eysenck (8)). Most applications of learning theory to treatment have been in terms of deconditioning, i.e. of treating personality problems, and the success which has been reached has certainly indicated that in this connection behaviour therapy has a considerable contribution to make. Less has

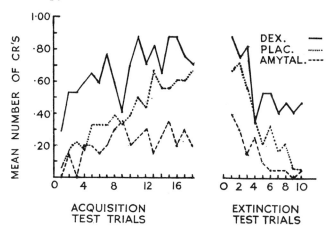

Fig. 4. Eye-blink conditioning under drug conditions. Stimulant drugs increase, depressant drugs decrease rate of conditioning, as compared with placebo conditions.

(Results reported by Franks, C., reprinted from Eysenck, H. J., *Dynamics of Anxiety and Hysteria*.)

been done in relation to 'conduct problems', but we may perhaps be allowed a suggestion which may go a long way to reverse this situation. As this suggestion involves the use of drugs, and is in many other ways dissimilar to the main line of argument followed in our discussion of treatment, it may be permissible to discuss it here in relation to our general theoretical formulations.

It has been shown that the position of an individual on the extraversion-introversion dimension can be altered by the use of drugs; so-called CNS stimulation drugs have an introverting effect while CNS depressant drugs have an extraverting effect (Eysenck (7)). Thus it has been found that stimulant drugs increase conditioning while depressant drugs decrease the rate of conditioning; Fig. 4 shows the differences produced by the application of a stimulant and a depressant drug as compared with placebo reactions. It will be seen by comparison with Fig. 3 that normal people, neither extremely extraverted nor introverted, condition as well as introverts when given a stimulant drug and condition as poorly as extraverts when given a depressant drug. This knowledge can obviously be applied with advantage to our extraverted 'conduct problem' cases. According to our theory these individuals, although subjected to a process of conditioning by society, have failed to benefit by virtue of their inability to form conditioned responses.

Application of stimulant drugs over a period of weeks or even months should render their nervous system more susceptible to the associative process of conditioning, and should make any kind of 'socialisation treatment' more successful than it would otherwise have been. Indeed it might be quite sufficient to rely on the ordinary conditioning processes going on in the individual's everyday life, without having to have recourse to special treatment designed to produce the relevant conditioned responses.

There is a considerable degree of evidence to show that this hypothesis contains at least a certain amount of truth. Bradley and Bowen (1), Lindsley and Henry (10) and Shorvon (14) have all shown that the administration of stimulant drugs over a period of time to psychopathic children does indeed produce a remarkable decrease in their antisocial behaviour, even when no other treatment is attempted besides the drug administration. These effects are not purely transitory but have been found to be long-lasting, and in some cases quite long follow-ups have failed to show any return of the original difficulty. It is surprising that these reports have been rather neglected, and that treatment of conduct problems is seldom accompanied by the appropriate prescription of drugs; the reason for this neglect may lie in the absence at the time these studies were done of a theoretical basis justifying the action taken. Much further research with this particular type of behaviour therapy would seem to be indicated. It is curious to note that most behaviour therapists as well as most psychotherapists have tended to fight shy of the use of drugs in spite of the obvious advantages of being able to control a person's position on the extraversion-introversion continuum, or of being able to control his autonomic reactions to a given stimulus by suitable administration of drugs.

REFERENCES

1. BRADLEY, C. and BOWEN, M., 1961. Amphetamine (benzedrine) therapy of children's behaviour disorders. *Amer. J. Orthopsychiat.*, **11**: 92-103.
2. COLLINS, L. F., MAXWELL, A. E. and CAMERON, K., 1962. A factor analysis of some child psychiatric clinic data. *J. Ment. Sci.*, **108**: 274-285.
3. EYSENCK, H. J., 1957. *The Dynamics of Anxiety and Hysteria*. London: Routledge & Kegan Paul.
4.   1960a. *The Structure of Human Personality*. London: Methuen.
5.   1960b. Symposium: The development of moral values in children. VII. The contribution of learning theory. *Brit. J. Educ. Psychol.*, **30**: 11-21.
6.   1962. Conditioning and personality. *Brit. J. Psychol.*, **53**: 299-305.
7.   1963a. (ed.) *Experiments with Drugs*. Oxford: Pergamon Press.
8.   1963b. Behaviour therapy, spontaneous remission and transference in neurotics. *Amer. J. Psychiat.*, **119**, 867-871.
9.   1963c. Funktion und Anwendung der Statistik in der Psychiatrie. In *Psychiatrie der Gegenwart*, Band 1, Feil 2, 249-273. Berlin: Springer.
10. LINDSLEY, D. B. and HENRY, C. E., 1942. The effects of drugs on behaviour and the electroencephalograms of children with behaviour disorders. *Psychosom. Med.*, **4**: 140-9.

11. MOWRER, O. H., 1950. *Learning Theory and Personality Dynamics*. New York: Ronald Press.
12. PETERSON, D., 1961. Behavior problems of middle childhood. *J. Consult. Psychol.*, **25**: 205-9.
13. SHIELDS, J., 1962. *Monozygotic Twins Brought up Apart and Brought up Together*. Oxford Univ. Press.
14. SHORVON. H. J., 1947. Benzedrine in psychopathy and behaviour disorders. *British J. Addict.*, **44**: 58-63.

Part II. CLINICAL

The applicability of modern learning theory to clinical problems has now been established. Progress in the investigation and treatment of behaviour disorders in adults has not however been accompanied by a similar rate of advance in child psychology. With the exception of the problems of enuresis, and to a lesser extent of phobias, there has been little systematic research conducted in this field by learning theorists. On purely historical grounds this uneven development is a little surprising. The first experimental demonstration of the genesis of neurotic behaviour in a human being was carried out in 1920 by Watson (139) on a young boy, Albert. Watson produced a phobia in Albert by presenting a disturbing loud noise when a white rat was brought into the boy's presence. After a few repetitions of this association Albert developed a phobia for small white furry objects (see p. 118 below). In addition to Watson's classical demonstration, the first attempt at treatment based on learning principles was also carried out on a child. In 1924 Mary Cover Jones (63, 64) used deconditioning methods to eliminate a rabbit phobia in a 3-year-old boy, Peter. The techniques she employed were a precursor of some of the new methods used by contemporary behaviour therapy; in particular, Wolpe's (142) systematic desensitisation method has an affinity to Jones's early study. The next significant advance in the application of learning theory to children's disorders was Mowrer and Mowrer's (100) work on the conditioning treatment of enuresis. This disorder has continued to receive the attention of behaviour therapists, but the progress made in the treatment of adults since 1948 has not been reflected in child psychology and psychiatry.

The reason for this discrepancy is probably an important difference in the nature of behaviour disturbances in children and adults. Many behaviour problems in children (especially in the early years) are associated with inadequate or inappropriate responses. These deficits usually centre around the activities of eating, sleeping, elimination and speaking. In most instances the problem arises because (in a learning theory sense) the child has failed to develop an adequate way of responding (e.g. enuresis, aphemia, anorexia, dyslexia). In adults on the other hand most problems seem to be concerned with unadaptive behaviour, and the purpose of therapy is generally directed at eliminating the unwanted responses (e.g. phobias, anxiety states, compulsions, perversions). Most often the aim in therapy with adults is to break down a behaviour pattern, whereas in children the therapist usually has to build up an adequate behaviour pattern.

The recent infiltration of operant conditioning procedures into clinical psychology seems to provide a tool for building up deficient responses in children. Lindsley (82, 83) followed up the proposals of Skinner (122) and of Skinner, Solomon and Lindsley (123), and has already produced extremely interesting analyses of the behaviour of acute schizophrenic patients. The clinical application of this technique in child psychology is foreshadowed by the work of Ferster (37), Lovaas (91, 92), Baer (11), Spradlin (126) and Bijou (16) among others.

The established methods of behaviour therapy, such as Wolpe's (142) reciprocal inhibition technique and the extinction procedures used by Gwynne Jones (62) and Yates (146), have already been successfully used on child patients and are described first.

Desensitisation, Conditioned Inhibition, Negative Practice

In his book Wolpe (142) describes the treatment of eighty-eight patients. Of these, two were children. An 11-year-old boy, suffering from interpersonal anxiety and tic-like movements, was treated by desensitisation and was markedly improved after eight treatment sessions. The second patient, a 14-year-old stammerer, relapsed under stress after showing considerable improvement in the first few months of treatment. Further treatment was only able to counteract the relapse to a limited degree. The methods used in this case consisted of relaxation and breathing exercises. In a later series of thirty-nine cases treated by desensitisation Wolpe (143) describes two further child patients. An 11-year-old boy was successfully treated for his fear of authority figures in six sessions, while another stammerer (aged 13) failed to respond. This boy, being unable to obtain vivid visual images, was unable to comply with the requirements of desensitisation therapy. While the lack of success with two cases of stuttering is not conclusive, there are grounds for believing that some of the methods used in treating this condition in adults may prove more successful. The work of Case (25) on negative practice, of Sheehan (116) and Sheehan and Voas (117) on non-reinforcement, and of Cherry and Sayers (27) on shadowing, are among the most promising.

White (140) describes the successful treatment of a 5-year-old girl who suffered from anorexia. The child's feeding difficulties started at the age of 3, and worsened after the death of her father when she was 5 years old. She had been deeply attached to her father and was extremely disturbed by his illness and death. Her father had fed her from an early age. Attempts made by her mother, relations, doctors and nurses to feed her were mainly unsuccessful. 'The immediate problem', writes White, 'was formulated in terms of simple conditioning, with father as the conditioned stimulus upon which the conditioned response of eating had come to depend.' The reinforcement was 'supplied by the satisfaction of hunger as well as by anxiety-reduction through sitting on the father's knee and being fed by him'.

The method of treatment was based on this analysis and bears a strong resemblance to M. C. Jones's (63) treatment of Peter. 'The first step', says White, 'was to provide a substitute for the father and to arrange a series of experiences that might gradually approximate those obtaining before the father's death.' Initially the psychologist attempted to replace the conditioned stimulus provided by the father. When this was accomplished, generalisation to selected relatives was undertaken (aunts, uncles and mother). This general plan of treatment (with some additions during the course of therapy) was followed for 7 months. Some marked improvements were evident after only 3 to 4 weeks, and when treatment concluded at the end of 7 months the girl was very much improved. This improvement has been maintained over a 3-year follow-up period. White's formulation of the problem in 'terms of simple conditioning' is not entirely satisfactory. His description of the child's eating as a conditioned response is questionable, and the analysis fails to account for the onset of the feeding difficulties before the father's death. It may be more useful to re-set the treatment programme in terms of an operant conditioning process in which the psychologist 'shaped' and expanded the range of the child's eating behaviour. While a clear theoretical explanation would be valuable, the successful outcome of this difficult case is encouraging.

Walton (137) describes how an 11-year-old boy, who suffered from a complex of severe tics, was successfully treated by negative practice and conditioned inhibition methods. The treatment was carried out over 36 sessions ranging in duration from 15 minutes in the early stages to 30 minutes at the closing stages. A follow-up conducted a year later showed that the improvements had been maintained and that the boy's general adjustment had been highly satisfactory. The essence of the treatment is that the repeated evocation of the tics produces an inhibitory effect which eventually 'exhausts' these movements. Williams (141) treated temper tantrums in a 21-month-old child by a process of experimental extinction. The child displayed tantrum behaviour whenever he was put to bed in the evening. Williams argued that this unadaptive behaviour was being maintained, or reinforced, by the parental attention which it produced. The parents were instructed to refrain from re-entering the bedroom after the child had been placed in bed, and to record the duration of each tantrum. The duration of the tantrums gradually decreased, and in less than 2 weeks had almost ceased. Spontaneous recovery of the tantrum pattern was later observed when one evening the maternal grandmother entered the bedroom before the child had stopped crying. The tantrum behaviour was then reinstated for another few days, but persistent non-reinforcement (i.e. refraining from re-entering the bedroom) brought the disturbance to an end after nine days. A 2-year follow-up of this case revealed no further behaviour difficulties. Boardman (20) reported the successful treatment of a rebellious and defiant child by manipulating the home environment in such a way as to inhibit his anti-social, unacceptable behaviour.

Enuresis

The first systematic investigation of therapy derived from learning theory was Mowrer and Mowrer's (100) famous study of enuresis. Despite its efficiency this method was neglected for many years. Serious interest in this so-called 'bell-and-pad method' has revived in the past five years, and a comprehensive evaluation of the available evidence was carried out by Gwynne Jones (61), who concluded that 'if widely adopted, the specific conditioning method of treatment is capable of significantly reducing the incidence of *enuresis nocturna* at the later ages of childhood'. (See Table 1.)

TABLE 1

The Effects of Conditioning Treatment of Enuresis
(Reproduced from H. G. Jones (1960), by permission of
Pergamon Press)

Author	No. of cases	Age range	% cured	% markedly improved	% failures
Mowrer . . .	30	3–13	100	100	0
Davidson and Douglass	20	5–15 (+2 adults)	75	25	0
Crosby . . .	35	3½–10½	88	3	9
	23	11–28	83	5	12
Sieger . . .	106	3–15 (+4 adults)	89	7	4
Geppert . . .	42	5–10	74	16	10
Baller and Schalock .	55	Median 9·5	70	30	30
Wickes . . .	100	5–17	50	24	26
Gillison and Skinner .	100	3½–21	88	5	7
Freyman . . .	15	5–14	33	40	27
Murray . . .	33	–	75	9	16
Martin and Kubly .	118	3½–18½	56	18	26
Lowe . . .	322	5–10	88	12	12
	276	10–16	88	12	12
	171	16+	85	15	15

This view is borne out by the recent work of Lovibond (93, 94), who carried out a well planned and executed investigation. He showed that the Mowrer, Crosby and his own Twin-Signal technique of conditioning were all highly effective in arresting enuresis. The mean number of trials required to arrest the enuresis was 13·5, but the relapse rate for all three methods was unsatisfactorily high. Consequently Lovibond tried some variations of the method in an attempt to increase the stability of the newly learnt ability. He eventually developed a refined Twin-Signal method used on an intermittent reinforcement schedule. None of the fourteen subjects had experienced a relapse at the time of Lovibond's writing (i.e. from 1 to 9 months after treatment). This result is already an improvement on the earlier procedures and deserves further field trials. Lovibond's work recommends itself for two reasons. His developments of the technique promise improved results, and his theoretical analysis is more convincing than either Mowrer's or Crosby's. The conditioning paradigms proposed by Mowrer and by Crosby are both subject to criticism (Jones (61), Lovibond (93)), and Lovibond's reformulation of the problem in terms of conditioned avoidance training seems able to accommodate all the available information:

Reflex contraction of the detrusor and relaxation of the sphincter are followed by the noxious stimulus, electric shock or loud noise. After a number of such conjunctions the stimuli arising from sphincter relaxation become the conditioned stimuli for the avoidance response of sphincter contraction. In other words, the conditioned stimulus is not bladder distension but the pattern of stimuli arising from the response of sphincter relaxation and urination. When conditioning reaches the stage where the first indication of the stimulation gives rise to the antagonistic response of sphincter contraction, the child does not wet the bed and the noxious stimulus is avoided . . . (Lovibond (93).)

This analysis and its implications provided the basis for the design of a modified conditioning technique. Two essential considerations which determined the form of the new Twin-Signal were:

1. The critical function of the unconditioned stimulus is to produce a sudden relaxation of the detrusor and contraction of the sphincter.
2. The child's response must 'turn off' or permit escape from the unconditioned stimulus, thus facilitating the formation of a conditioned avoidance response.

The Twin-Signal apparatus consists of a pad electrode, a strong auditory stimulus (240-volt signal similar to a car hooter, suitably attenuated) and a mild buzzer. When the pad is wet, the strong stimulus sounds for one second. After a minute of silence, the buzzer sounds—in order to summon the attendant.

During the acquisition (training) period, the apparatus is switched off for 50% of the trials (intermittent reinforcement). The presentation or non-presentation of the unreinforced stimulus is randomly determined so that the child may experience 'runs' of hooter and no-hooter, e.g. wet—hooter, wet—hooter, wet—hooter, wet—no hooter, wet—no hooter, and so on. The purpose of this intermittent patterning is to enhance the stability of the developing habit of continence (Lovibond (94)).

Does the conditioning treatment of enuresis produce unfavourable emotional changes in the child? This notion appears to be unsupported by the evidence (Jones (62)). The only change noted by Lovibond (93), for example, was that his enuretic group displayed improved self-evaluation after successful treatment.

Phobias

Apart from enuresis, the only other disorder which has been subjected to systematic consideration is phobia. A theory to account for the genesis and treatment of children's phobias was proposed in 1959 by Wolpe and Rachman (144) and by Rachman and Costello (109). The present account is a development of earlier versions, and only the alterations and additions will be discussed in detail.

In terms of the behaviour theory, phobias may be regarded as conditioned anxiety (fear) reactions.

Any neutral stimulus, simple or complex, that happens to make an impact on an individual at about the time that a fear reaction is evoked acquires the ability to evoke fear subsequently. If the fear at the original conditioning situation is of high intensity or if the conditioning is repeated a good many times the conditioned fear will show the persistence that is characteristic of neurotic fear; and there will be generalization of fear reactions to stimuli resembling the conditioned stimulus. (Wolpe and Rachman (144).)

The experimental evidence supporting this view of phobias is discussed in Wolpe (142), Wolpe and Rachman (144) and Rachman and Costello (109), and is derived from studies of the behaviour of children and of animals. The classical demonstration of the development of a phobia in a child was provided by Watson and Rayner (139) in 1920. Having first ascertained that it was a neutral object, the authors presented an 11-month-old boy, Albert, with a white rat to play with. Whenever he reached for the animal the experimenters made a loud noise behind him. After only five trials Albert began showing signs of fear in the presence of the white rat. This fear then generalised to similar stimuli such as furry objects, cotton wool, white rabbits. The phobic reactions were still present when Albert was tested 4 months later.

The process involved in this demonstration provides a striking illustration of the manner in which phobias develop, and may be represented in this way:

1. Neutral Stimulus (rat) $\longrightarrow$ Approach R
2. Painful noise stimulus (UCS) $\longrightarrow$ Fear (UCR)
3. Rat (CS)+noise (UCS) $\longrightarrow$ Fear
4. Rat (CS) $\longrightarrow$ Fear (CR)
5. Rabbit (GS^1) $\longrightarrow$ Fear (GCR).
6. Cotton Wool (GS^2) $\longrightarrow$ Fear (GCR).

The essentials of the theory may be summarised in nine statements:

1. Phobias are learned responses.
2. Stimuli develop phobic qualities when they are associated temporally and spatially with a fear-producing state of affairs.

3. Neutral stimuli which are of relevance in the fear-producing situation and/or make an impact on the person in the situation are more likely to develop phobic qualities than weak or irrelevant stimuli.
4. Repetition of the association between the fear situation and the new phobic stimuli will strengthen the phobia.
5. Associations between high-intensity fear situations and neutral stimuli are more likely to produce phobic reactions.
6. Generalisation from the original phobic stimulus to stimuli of a similar nature will occur.
7. Noxious experiences which occur under conditions of excessive confinement are more likely to produce phobic reactions.
8. Neutral stimuli which are associated with a noxious experience or experiences may develop (secondary) motivating properties. This acquired drive is termed 'the fear-drive'.
9. Responses (such as avoidance) which reduce the fear-drive are reinforced.

Each of these nine statements is based on experimental evidence and would also appear to be consistent with clinical experience (Wolpe (142); Eysenck (34)). It can be legitimately argued in fact that these propositions are supported by the full weight of almost all the evidence accumulated in research on the learning process. Some sources of this evidence include Metzner (96); Wolpe (142); Eysenck (34, 35); Liddell (81); Gantt (41); Kimble (65); Mowrer (99).

In considering the aetiology of a patient's phobia, it is often difficult to determine the nature of the original causal experience. Is it possible to trace phobias back to a single experience or even to date the onset of the disorder? Allport's (1) view is that 'an experience associated only once with a bereavement, an accident or a battle may become the centre of a permanent phobia or complex, not in the least dependent on a recurrence of the original shock'. He also points out that tracing a phobia back to its origin is not necessarily a profitable enterprise. Evidence suggesting the occurrence of one-trial learning of fear was obtained by Woodward (145). Of 198 children who had suffered severe burns two to five years previously, 81% showed 'signs of emotional disturbance, according to their mothers'. Their most prominent symptom was described as 'fear and anxiety'. Only 7% of the siblings of these children showed similar symptoms.

Nevertheless it is likely that the great majority of phobias develop after cumulative traumatic or sub-traumatic experiences. Even in Watson's experiment with Albert, five trials were required before the boy first showed fear in the presence of the neutral stimulus. In a replication of Watson's findings, H. E. Jones (60) confirmed the cumulative effect of repeated trials. This cumulative effect has also been observed in experiments with animals. Repeated mild shocks 'which by themselves do not elicit great emotional disturbance' can eventually produce neurotic behaviour' (Metzner (96)). Similarly Kurtz and Walters (71) demonstrated that 'experiences of intense fear predispose animals to react with increased fear in subsequent encounters[1] with aversive stimuli'. Furthermore one of the firmest conclusions that research on the psychology of learning has yielded is that repetition fosters learning.

The importance of repeated exposures to noxious stimulation lies mainly in the relationship between the frequency of traumata and the *strength* of the fear. The mechanism which is thought to be primarily responsible for the *persistence* of the fear is the secondary fear-drive.

Determinants of Strength of Fear. Miller (97) noted that the factors which determine the strength of fear-drives are similar to those which operate in generating and sustaining other learned drives. He accordingly proposed six major determinants which contribute to the strength of a fear. These factors may be summarised as follows (for present purposes we have changed the emphasis from fear as a drive to fear as a response):

(i) Repetition of exposures to the fear-inducing situation will increase the strength of the fear.

(ii) Strong noxious stimuli will produce strong fears (e.g. a powerful shock will produce greater fear than a weak one).

(iii) Stimuli which are closely associated, temporally and spatially, with a noxious experience will produce strong fears.

(iv) Generalised fear stimuli which closely resemble the original noxious stimuli will produce strong fears.

(v) The summation of fear-inducing stimuli will increase the strength of the fear.

Fear as an Acquired Drive. Thus far we have considered fear primarily as a *response*. Fear can, however, also act as a drive to motivate the learning of new responses. In 1938 Mowrer formulated the idea of fear as a learned, anticipatory response to painful stimulation. He argued that the presence of the conditioned pain response (fear) motivates 'escape' behaviour and that those responses which bring about a reduction of the fear are reinforced or strengthened. The development of an agoraphobic syndrome illustrates this process quite clearly. The patient undergoes painful experiences (in a public place), which then give rise to a conditioned anticipatory fear-drive. The fear-drive persists or increases when he enters the noxious (public) situation. He indulges in various attempts to escape from the fear, and only obtains relief when he reaches his home. The response of returning home will be reinforced because it is followed by a reduction of the fear-drive. Further attempts to travel towards public situations result in a re-activation of the fear-drive. Returning home reduces the fear-drive and this behaviour

---

[1] Under carefully controlled experimental conditions, however, the gradual and graduated exposure of animals to sub-traumatic stimulation can lead to the acquisition of a type of immunity to later stresses (Miller (98)).

pattern is reinforced still further. Eventually this process, if not checked, will restrict the person's movements to a narrow environment surrounding the home or make him entirely housebound.

The critical importance of the fear-drive in *sustaining* phobic (and other) patterns of behaviour is amply supported (Mowrer (99); Metzner (96); Yates (147); Miller (97)). Neurotic behaviour patterns persist, paradoxically, because they are unpleasant. Once the child has acquired an unpleasant reaction to a particular situation, he will then tend to avoid further contact with that situation. As learned patterns of behaviour can only be extinguished by repeated unreinforced (or inhibited) evocations, the tendency to avoid the noxious situation often precludes the 'spontaneous' disappearance of the neurotic behaviour. This analysis would lead one to predict, for example, that the spontaneous remission rate in agoraphobic conditions would be lower than in most other phobias.

The typical reaction of a phobic person when he comes into contact with the phobic situation is to retreat. This withdrawal is generally followed by a reduction of the fear-drive, which in turn reinforces the avoidance behaviour. This then is what has been described as 'the vicious circle which protects the conditioned fear response from extinction' (Eysenck (34)).

The development of phobias may be summed up in this way: the fear is *generated* by a painful experience (or experiences) and is *sustained* by the operation of the acquired fear-drive.

A Note on the Effects of Confinement. Research on the production of experimental neuroses in animals has shown that the restriction of the subject's behaviour plays an important part in the development of these disorders (Liddell (81) ;Wolpe (142)). The probable explanation of this finding is that confinement reduces the animal's chances of making an adaptive response in the face of noxious stimulation. If the experimental subject is prevented from making a response which will terminate the noxious stimulus, a greater degree of fear is observed (Mowrer and Vieck (101)). The role of restriction in the aetiology of phobias is summarised by Metzner (96) thus:

The factor of confinement works (*a*) by preventing an escape response, (*b*) by restricting . . . fear-conditioning to a few cues, and (*c*) by not allowing any consistent response to control shock. All of these factors would make for more fear and hence more severe neurotic breakdowns.

Obviously, in considering the significance of these experimental findings for children's phobias, it is necessary to interpret confinement in a broad manner. It is psychological confinement rather than actual physical restraint which is the important influence to be considered. Psychological confinement is no less real than physical confinement. The barriers which prevent a child from carrying out a particular response may as easily reside within himself as in an external object. A simple example of psychological confinement may be found in the relations between a child and her school-teacher. The number of responses which the child can make in reply to a scolding is very limited. She cannot shout back, nor can she kick, scream, bite or run away. If she is subjected to frequent verbal attacks of this kind, the child is likely to develop social anxiety. The degree of generalisation of the anxiety to situations outside the school will, of course, depend on the general circumstances of her life and her previous social experiences.

Normal and Abnormal Fears

During infancy, children's fears develop in response to pain and to 'any intense, sudden, unexpected or novel stimulus for which the organism

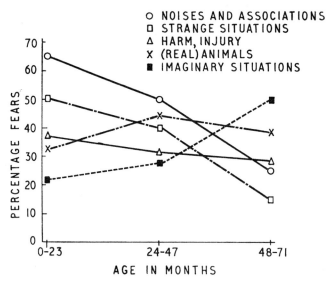

FIG. 5. The relative frequency of fear responses in children of differing ages. (Adapted from Jersild and Holmes, Child Develop. Monogr., 1935.)

appears to be unprepared' (Jersild (56)). With increasing age the child's range of fears widens. He can recall past events and anticipate future dangers; he can also respond to imaginative impulses and images, such as ghosts and bogy-men. As the child graduates to more complex fears, however, he also learns to cope with the earlier sources of fear—he is less likely to fear sudden noises, for example.

Jersild and Holmes (58, 59) described the fear responses of children at different ages. They demonstrated an overall change from *immediate, tangible* fears to *anticipatory, less tangible*[1] fears with increasing maturity. Most 2-year-old children, for example, respond fearfully to loud noises and to events associated with noise (see Fig. 5). Only a minority of 6-year-old

---

[1] This difference in the source and nature of the stimulus has sometimes been used to discriminate between *fear* and *anxiety*. Fear is a response to a tangible source of danger; anxiety is a response to an intangible danger.

children show this response. On the other hand, 6-year-old children are inclined to fear imaginary situations or objects far more frequently than two-year-olds.

Twni oa ortant sources of fear which do not vary noticeably with age are: realmpmals, and the possibility of harm or bodily injury. Both of these sourceso if stimulation are potentially painful and children are likely to receive intermittent reminders of this fact. For this reason they do not decrease during the early years. As the child's physical strength increases[1] and he gains experience, he should overcome the fear of most animals. Most noises cease to elicit fear because of general adaptation, and the majority of fearful *associations* with noise disappear through a process of stimulus

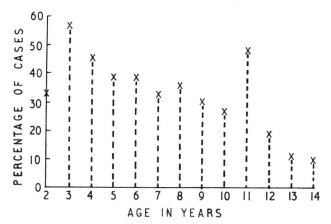

FIG. 6. Fears of normal children: percentage frequencies by age.
(Adapted from MacFarlane *et al.*, 1954. University of California Press.)

discrimination and extinction. The hissing of steam or the roar of a motor-cycle receive reinforcement of a noxious kind and will retain the power to provoke fear. The proportional increase in fears concerning imaginary situations and objects can best be accounted for by the fact that the conditions which eliminate fears are difficult to 'arrange' if the feared situation cannot be manipulated in ordinary circumstances; it is difficult to reduce a child's fear of a bogy-man who is intangible and cannot be easily recalled or re-created. The fear of *new situations* is gradually eroded by the very nature of the child's day-to-day experiences. Frequent exposures to a new situation will usually be followed by positive rewards or simply the absence of unpleasant stimulation; consequently the fear of new situations will tend to extinguish 'spontaneously'. It should be possible, by extending this type of analysis, to predict which sort of fear stimuli will persist and which ones will disappear spontaneously during the various periods of childhood.

MacFarlane *et al.* (95), in their survey of some 200 normal children,

---

[1] MacFarlane *et al.* (95) report a correlation of 0·63 between fear and physical timidity in 3-year-old boys.

found in fact that a second peak occurs at about eleven years of age (see Fig. 6). Their findings for the *younger* age groups are strikingly similar to those reported by Jersild and Holmes. In particular they confirmed these observations: (i) the fears of young normal children are extensive; (ii) these fears undergo a steady natural decline; (iii) the quality of the fears changes from tangible to intangible with increasing age.

The decline of fears with increasing age is demonstrated by the experimental findings of Holmes (52). She exposed more than fifty children (ages 2–6 years) to numerous experimental situations of a provocative nature. The percentage of children in whom fear responses were elicited by the presence of a strange person decreased from 31% in the 2-year-old group to 22% in the 3-year-old group, 7% in the 4-year-old and 0% in the 5-year-old group (see Table 2). Other examples include the fear of being placed in a darkroom (declines from 46% of two-year-olds to 0% of five-year-olds) and the fear of being left alone (12% of two-year-olds to

TABLE 2

Percentage of Children showing Fear in Experimental Situations
(Adapted from Holmes, Child Development Monogr. No. 20, 1935)

	Percentage showing fear			
	2–3 yrs.	3–4 yrs.	4–5 yrs.	5–6 yrs.
I Being left alone	12	15	7	0
II Falling boards	24	9	0	0
III Dark room	46	51	35	0
IV Strange person	31	22	7	0
V High boards	35	35	7	0
VI Loud sound	22	20	14	0
VII Snake	34	55	43	30
VIII Large dog	61	43	43	12
TOTAL	32	30	18	5·2

0% of five-year-olds). As far as tangible fears are concerned, the most striking trend is the sharp decrease in the number of fearful children found in the 5-year-old group (and also the decrease in the number of fear-provoking situations). As we have seen, however, older children do acquire other less tangible fears after they have overcome these more direct stimuli.

The development of fears is, of course, influenced by the child's history and the setting in which the noxious stimulation occurs. For example, children are less likely to develop fears when in the company of trusted reassuring adults than when they are alone (M. C. Jones (64)). Again, they are less likely to develop fears in the presence of unafraid children than in the presence of frightened children. The social facilitation or inhibition of fear was also noted in a study on the effects of air raids on children's behaviour.[1] It was found that the fear (or lack of fear) displayed

[1] JOHN, E., 1941. *Br. J. Educ. Psychol.*, **11**: 173.

by the mother was an important determinant of the child's fears. It is well known that there is 'a good deal of correspondence between frequency of fears of children of the same family'—the correlations between fears displayed by siblings range from 0·65 to 0·74.[1] Similarly Hagman (46) found a correlation of 0·667 between the gross number of fears exhibited by children and their mothers. The probability of a child acquiring fears (by social learning) is directly influenced by the fears which he observes in his parents, siblings and peers.

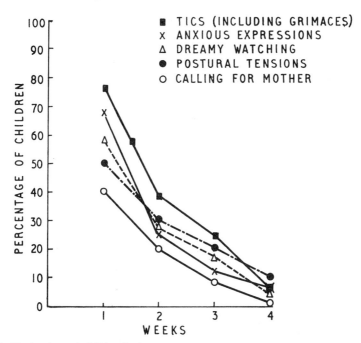

FIG. 7. Extinction of children's fear responses in nursery school. (Adapted from Slater, 1939, *Monogr. Soc. Res. Child Developm.*)

Prevention. An important demonstration of the extinction of fear responses in non-clinical circumstances was provided by Slater (124). Forty children aged 2–3 years were observed during their first four weeks of attendance at nursery school. During the first week the majority of children displayed signs of uneasiness and apprehension. By the end of the fourth week all but three of the children had adapted to the new situation successfully (see Fig. 7). Apart from providing an instructive study of the process of spontaneous remission, Slater's results indicate the necessity for providing children with a gradual and gentle introduction to nursery school. Many nursery schools prevent the development of school phobias and related problems by careful planning of the child's early days.

---

[1] MAY, R., 1950, *The Meaning of Anxiety*. New York: Ronald.

The Holmes experiment (52) showed that at least 30% of 2-year-old children display fear in the presence of a strange person. Consequently it is safer to introduce the child to the teacher and allow him to warm to this stranger in the presence of the mother or some other known and trusted person. Allowing the child to become acquainted with the new (school) *situation* in the presence of a trusted person is also advisable. For example, a headmistress of a London nursery school encourages the parents to bring the child on visits to the school even before he has reached the starting age. By this and other similar means it has been possible virtually to eliminate school phobias in the infant and primary sections and also to ensure a simpler and happier introduction to the long business of schooling. The first day of a new school year is no longer dreaded by the staff, and very few children now show signs of distress on this occasion (crying, for example, has all but disappeared).

In a different setting the graded and gradual desensitisation of a child's fears (or expected fears) is also practised with apparent success. The children's section of at least one London dental hospital uses this method in an endeavour to prevent fear and avoidance reactions developing in a situation of objective discomfort and pain. No actual treatment is commenced on the child's first visit; if he is comfortable in the chair, a dental inspection is conducted and his teeth charted. Depending on the child's reactions, treatment may begin on the second or even the fifth visit. If he is anxious on the first visit the full inspection is postponed until he is adequately desensitised.

The value of adequate preparation and careful handling in the prevention of fear and anxiety is also attested to by Prugh's (106) study on the effects of hospitalisation. Those children who were prepared for the experience and given fear-reducing care in hospital made better adjustments to the experience of hospitalisation and showed less disturbances after returning home.

Treatment. The most common method used by parents in attempting to quell their children's fears is rational explanation (Jersild (56)). This method is relatively useless unless supplementary means are used.[1] Jersild describes the effective methods of overcoming children's fears:

(i) social imitation of adults and/or other children who display fearlessness in the noxious situation;
(ii) reconditioning;
(iii) acquiring experience and skill in handling the feared situation.

The last two methods, reconditioning and acquiring experience, can legitimately be subsumed under the label 'desensitisation'. The power of

---

[1] In a study by Hagman (46), mothers reported that explanation *and* gradual exposure to the feared situation was the most effective combination.

these methods can be illustrated by two experiments (Holmes, 52). It was observed that fourteen out of twenty nursery school children were afraid to enter a dark room to retrieve a ball. The children were then exposed to the situation in gradually increasing doses. After a few practice sessions, thirteen of the initially frightened children went into the room without hesitation and recovered the ball. The second experiment concerned two children who were afraid of walking along an elevated plank. After a series of graded exercises had been successfully completed, they were able to walk the plank fearlessly.

The effectiveness of reconditioning was also demonstrated by Jones in 1924. She compared the effects of six different methods of overcoming the fears of a large group of children in temporary care. Only reconditioning and social imitation produced 'unqualified success'.

The conclusions drawn from these experiments are supported by case history material, animal experiments and controlled therapeutic experiments with adults.

The therapeutic experiments of Lazowik and Lang (79) and of Lazarus (76) both dealt with the effects of the desensitisation technique. In these experiments matched groups of adults with excessive fears were investigated. The results of the experiments indicated that the groups treated by desensitisation improved significantly more than the control groups.

Various experimenters have attempted to treat experimentally induced neuroses in animals. It has been shown that improvements can be obtained with a selection of methods. The most systematic study of desensitisation, however, was that conducted by Wolpe (142), who obtained encouraging results. These experiments were in fact an important influence in the development of his methods of behaviour therapy.

Most of the case reports available to date which deal with the treatment of children's phobias involve the use of Wolpe's 'inhibitory therapy'. He defines the principle of reciprocal inhibition psychotherapy:

'If a response antagonistic to anxiety can be made to occur in the presence of anxiety-evoking stimuli so that it is accompanied by a complete or partial suppression of the anxiety responses, the bond between these stimuli and the anxiety responses will be weakened.'

The method may be illustrated by referring to some case reports which we summarise briefly here.

A 3-year-old boy, Peter, evinced fear of white rats, rabbits, fur, cotton wool and other stimuli along this continuum. He was treated by Jones (1924), using deconditioning methods. It was decided to work on the rabbit phobia, as this seemed to be a focus of Peter's fears. Peter was gradually introduced to contacts with a rabbit during his daily play period. He was placed in a play group with three fearless children and the rabbit was brought into the room for short periods each day. Peter's toleration of the rabbit was gradually improved. The progressive steps observed in the process included: 'rabbit in cage 12 feet away tolerated . . . in cage 4 feet away tolerated . . . close by in cage tolerated . . . free in room tolerated . . . eventually, fondling rabbit affectionately'. Another measure employed by Jones involved the use of feeding responses. 'Through the presence of the pleasant stimulus (food) whenever the rabbit was shown, the fear was eliminated gradually in favour of a positive response.'

Using these techniques Jones overcame not only Peter's fear of rabbits but all the associated fears. The follow-up of this case showed no resurgence of the phobia.

A 9-year-old boy (R. R.) was referred for treatment of a bee phobia. The phobia, which was intense and interfered with many of his activities (e.g. playing in the garden), had been present for 3 years. Although the boy could not remember ever having received a bee sting, he knew of several people who had been stung and/or displayed excessive fear of bees. After a full investigation had elucidated the nature of his fear, a hierarchy of anxiety-provoking situations was constructed. The techniques chosen for generating conditioned inhibition were social approval, encouragement, and feeding responses.

The desensitisation began with exposures of small photographs of bees, and then went through the following phases: large photographs, coloured photographs, dead bee in bottle at far end of room, dead bee in bottle brought gradually closer, dead bee out of bottle, dead bee on coat, gradually increasing manipulation of dead bee, introduction of several dead bees, playing imaginative games with dead bees. In addition to these densensitisation sessions, the parents were encouraged to take R. R. on brief, controlled visits to a natural history museum. The boy made gradual and systematic progress and after eight sessions he and his mother both reported a considerable improvement. His mother stated that he was 'very much improved. He no longer has a physical reaction; he used to go white, sweaty, cold and trembling and his legs were like jelly. He can play alone in the garden quite comfortably.' A 3-month follow-up showed no recurrence of the phobia.

The third case, reported by Lazarus (75), deals with an 8-year-old boy who developed a fear of moving vehicles two years after having been involved in a motor accident. Initially the therapist rewarded the boy whenever he made a positive comment concerning vehicles by giving him a piece of his favourite chocolate. By the third interview the boy was able to talk freely about all types of moving vehicles. Next, a series of 'accidents' with toy motor-cars was demonstrated. The boy, John, was given chocolate after each accident. Later John was seated in a stationary vehicle and slow progress (with chocolate feeding reinforcements used at each point) was made until John was able to enjoy motor travel without any anxiety.

In the same paper Lazarus recounts the successful treatment of a case of separation anxiety and a case of dog phobia, and mentions another 15 successfully treated cases. Additional case reports are provided by Landreth (73), by Bentler (15) and by Lazarus and Abramovitz (77). Numerous descriptions of adult cases treated by behaviour therapy are presented by Wolpe (142) and by Eysenck (34).

Reciprocal Inhibition. The success of reciprocal inhibition therapy depends on the appropriate choice and skilful manipulation of the inhibitory response. The inhibiting response which has been most commonly used in the treatment of adult phobics is relaxation. For obvious reasons it is not possible to use relaxation with many children, especially very young ones.

The three inhibiting responses which seem to be the most promising alternatives are: affection, feeding and social reassurance (imitation). Affection and comforting are among the methods frequently used by parents in assuaging their children's fears. Therapists can advise the parents in order to foster the effective application of affection as a direct inhibitor of anxiety. The treatment of an infant with a bath phobia reported by Bentler (15) is an illustration of this procedure. The effectiveness of social reassurance is demonstrated by the studies of Mary Cover Jones (63, 64), and indirectly by the work of Jersild (1957) and Hagman (1932). A less obvious inhibitor of anxiety (and one which is rarely used by parents) is feeding.

Anxiety and feeding responses can be mutually inhibitory. Some of the evidence which supports this statement is presented by Metzner (96), Wolpe (142) and Gantt (41).[1] Massermann and Lichtenstein reported experiments in which animals were shocked while feeding. The effect of the shock was to inhibit feeding—often for long periods. In the case of the dog described by Lichtenstein the feeding inhibition lasted for several months. Conversely, Gantt, Wolpe, and Farber were able to suppress anxiety and associated responses in their experimental animals by the careful introduction of food.

Clinically, feeding was one of the very first 'inhibitors' used by Jones (63) in her treatment of Peter's rabbit phobia. More recently Lazarus published an account of the successful treatment of a phobic child by means of feeding responses (see p. 128 above). The use of feeding responses has, of course, to be carefully controlled. If the process of desensitising is accelerated unduly there is a danger that the anxiety evoked may inhibit the child's eating.

Fear In Children: Summary and Conclusions

Mention has been made of Mary Cover Jones's (63, 64) classic studies in which she described her attempt to develop techniques for eliminating children's fears. The significance of this early work is only now becoming recognised. She gave an account of several methods of treatment, five of which appear to be promising, practical and in accord with present-day learning theory. They are the methods of:

1. Direct conditioning; 2. Social imitation; 3. Systematic distraction; 4. Feeding responses; 5. Affectional response.

The fruitfulness of the behaviour theory approach to phobias is well

---

[1] See also: FARBER, E., 1948, *J. Exp. Psychol.*, **38**: 111. LICHTENSTEIN, P., 1950, *J. Comp. Physiol. Psychol.*, **43**: 16. MASSERMAN, J., 1943, *Behaviour and Neurosis*.

demonstrated if we add to Jones's list the new methods which have been or could be used in overcoming children's phobias.[1]

6. Systematic desensitisation (Wolpe); 7. Assertive responses (Wolpe); 8. Relaxation responses (Wolpe); 9. 'Pleasant 'responses in the life situation —with drug enhancement (Wolpe).

In a suggestive article by Jersild and Holmes (58), further possible methods for treatment of children's fears are discussed. From their survey of parents' experiences in dealing with children's fears Jersild and Holmes suggest these techniques (among others): prompting the child to acquire skills which will enable him to cope with the feared situation; progressive contact with, and participation in, the feared situation; verbal explanation and reassurance; practical demonstration of fearlessness.

Some of these techniques are already employed by prevailing therapies without receiving explicit acknowledgment. All these methods certainly provide therapists with a formidable range to begin with. What is now required is careful, thorough investigation of these methods and, above all, a major project to establish the degree and permanence of improvements which may be obtained by these techniques.

In the meantime, active therapists may consider conducting their own investigations of these methods when faced with children suffering from phobic conditions. Obviously the choice of the method will depend to a considerable extent on the nature of the phobia. It is worth remembering also that these methods are not mutually exclusive and it is probable that in many cases a combination of these techniques may offer the most promising approach.

School Phobia

A fairly common childhood phobia is school phobia. For this reason, and also because a good deal has been written on the subject, we have chosen to re-examine school phobia in learning theory terms.

The first point to emerge from an examination of the literature on this subject is that most writers regard the term 'school phobia' as a misnomer. It is argued that the child does not really fear the *school* but that his persistent refusal to attend is a manifestation of some other, deeper disturbance. Eisenberg (30) described 26 cases of school refusal, and concluded that 'systematic study of these children reveals that, almost without exception, the basic fear is not of attending school but of leaving mother or, less commonly, father'. No details of the study beyond the clinical descriptions are provided, and this precludes an independent, external assessment of Eisenberg's rating system. Similarly, Waldfogel *et al.* (135) insist that school phobia 'is invariably found to originate in

---

[1] Naturally many of these methods are equally applicable in the treatment of adults' phobias.

the child's fear of being separated from his mother'. The clinical impressions of Klein (69) however led him to affirm the essentially sexual nature of the complaint. He offered a psychoanalytic view which suffers from the weakness of Freud's original proposals (Wolpe and Rachman (144)), and there is no serious evidence for the view that in school phobias 'an increase in sexual longing' reactivates the oedipal or pre-oedipal fear of sexual injury of the mother (Klein, (69)). Like Eisenberg and Waldfogel et al., Klein supports the position that the school-phobic child is not basically frightened of school.

None of the major proponents of this view give adequate details for supporting their clinical impressions on this matter. It seems unlikely that a systematic examination of the child's school adjustment was conducted, for, as we will indicate below, there are more than a dozen possible sources of school phobia in the school itself. Unless all of these possibilities are firmly excluded in each case, a diagnosis of separation anxiety seems justified only on (dubious) theoretical grounds—that is, Jimmy Brown cannot be school-phobic because there is no such disorder. In one of the few studies to provide at least some basis for an external judgement, Hersov (47, 48) was able to detect separation anxiety in only 36% of his cases of school refusal; 22% of his cases were confirmed as school phobias.

Even more convincing evidence of the role of the school situation in the development of school phobias is provided by Chazan's recent study (26). It was found for example that many of the children with this condition were experiencing severe educational difficulties. The scholastic progress of 24 school-phobic children was assessed by several attainment tests and a school report. Four children were shown to be slightly backward and another 13 (mean IQ 98·7) were 'very backward, i.e. they were experiencing great difficulty with their work, and were in need of special educational treatment'.

It cannot be concluded from the evidence and arguments presented that school phobias, in their original and precise sense, do not occur. In fact it is probably more reasonable and safer to begin one's inquiry with the belief that children who refuse to commence attending school or who refuse to continue such an attendance are displaying an avoidance reaction to a noxious or potentially noxious school situation. In other words, one should begin by regarding a school refusal at its face value: the child is attempting to avoid attendance at school. Secondly, the presence or absence of anxiety concerning school should be assessed, and this assessment should include a full analysis of all aspects of the child's experience of school. Some possible sources of anxiety at school are: the child's relations with his teachers and schoolmates; his intellectual ability and educational attainments; parental pressures and ambitions; examination stresses; specific learning disabilities; the size and routine of a new school; loss of close friends; experience(s) of educational failure; specific experience(s) of a disturbing nature (see Table 3).

TABLE 3

School Worries of Sixth Grade Children
(Adapted from Jersild *et al.*, *J. Experimental Education*, 1941)

	% (often or sometimes)
Failing a test	90
Being late for school	66
Scolded by teacher	68
Left back in school	56
Poor in spelling	55
Asked to answer questions	50
Poor in reading	44
Poor report card	76
Reprimanded by pupils	46
Not doing as well as other pupils	67
Giving report in class	44
Poor in arithmetic	67
Poor at drawing	45

If the clinical investigations (including a school visit) fail to reveal possible sources of anxiety at school, then one must avoid using the term 'school phobia'. An alternative possibility is that the child is suffering from separation phobia or, as it is more commonly known, separation anxiety. Some obvious test can be applied in these cases: Will the child attend school if he is accompanied by his mother/father? Is the child unable to go on excursions without his mother/father? Does the child get disturbed if left alone at home? If these behaviour patterns are present in a child who refuses to attend school, then it is preferable to call this condition *separation anxiety in a school situation*. It is necessary to specify the 'school situation' in this description if the refusal to attend school is the reason for referral and is in fact a prominent feature of the child's disorder.

As we have noted, some writers avoid using the term 'school phobia' because their theoretical orientation demands that the manifest phobic object is merely a symbol of some other, more important fear. Even if one accepts the questionable view that the manifest phobic object is merely symbolic, this is insufficient reason for displaying such a fastidious attitude to the term 'school phobia'. On similar grounds objections could be made to the use of terms like agoraphobia, claustrophobia and so on. It is suggested therefore that the term 'school phobia' be retained ,and employed to describe a persistent refusal to attend school which can be attributed primarily to anxiety regarding some aspects of the school situation. In those cases where school refusal is based upon or closely related to a fear of separation, the description 'separation anxiety in a school situation' should be used in preference. A distinction of this type is important because of its implications for therapy. Separation anxiety and school phobia require different treatment plans.

Personality Factors. A great deal has been written about the personality of school-phobic children (and their mothers). Regrettably most of this literature consists of generalisations which are seldom supported by adequate evidence. For example, very few of these generalisations are drawn from investigations with control groups of similar children who are not school-phobic. Even the inclusion of a satisfactory control group does not, unfortunately, prevent over-generalised conclusions. Hersov (47) for example states that children who refuse to attend school 'are passive, dependent and overprotected, but exhibit a high standard of work and behaviour at school'. In fact only 52% of his group of school-phobics were rated as being passive and dependent. Moreover, 28% of his group of truants and 28% of his control subjects were similarly rated. The statement that all school-phobics exhibit a high standard of work at school has been corrected by Chazan (26).

Studies (such as Hersov's) which attempt to tease out the personality differences between truanters and school-phobics are likely to prove fruitful. Levitt has suggested that children's disorders which have elements of anti-social or asocial conduct may be more resistant to therapeutic changes than disorders with 'identifiable behaviour symptoms' (e.g. enuresis, phobias). Truancy and school phobias present a potentially valuable testing ground because they are both concerned with the child's reactions to school—truancy is an 'extravert reaction' and school phobia an 'introvert reaction' (see pp. 104-112 above).

Treatment. Lippman (86) asserts that 'treatment of this condition has not been very satisfactory except when the child has been analysed'.

In one of the most successful series of cases (Talbot (132)) the treatment was carried out primarily by social caseworkers. Of the 24 children treated for this condition, 20 showed marked improvements. Most of these children were treated by social caseworkers, who in spite of their dynamic orientation used a behaviour therapy type of treatment programme. After interviews with the child, the parents and the school personnel had prepared the way, the child was gradually reintegrated into the school. Talbot's 'temporary plans' are reminiscent of the familiar anxiety-hierarchy used in behaviour therapy. When the child was ready, the following 'temporary plans' were worked through: 'mother sits in the classroom, father remains in the car; child helps in the school office; child sits near a friend; child remains in school a brief period each day, gradually increasing the time' (Talbot (132)). This outline programme seems more suitable for the treatment of cases of separation anxiety in a school situation, but could with some modifications be employed in the management of sheer school phobias.

Chazan (26) also reports success in excess of 80%. Twenty-nine out of 33 school phobia cases were successfully treated within five months. Five major measures were used (often in combination). Unfortunately Chazan does not include an analysis of the relation between the type of treatment provided and the outcome of the case. Sixteen of the 33 cases received individual psychotherapy (details not provided), 19 cases were moved to another school, 9 cases received remedial education, 9 received group therapy and 5 were given sedatives. When a change of school was carried out the child was generally placed in a smaller, more protected, special school. Two of the children recovered spontaneously. In Waldfogel's report (136) the spontaneous remission rate was more marked. Seven out of 16 cases receiving no treatment showed improvements (i.e. 44%). The recovery rate in this report was extremely good—18 out of 20 cases were successfully treated (90%). Eisenberg (30) similarly reported a high recovery rate of 80% in a group of 26 cases. Hersov (47, 48) reported 58% successes in 50 cases.

Is it possible that there is a large spontaneous remission effect here? In other words, do these children recover irrespective of the treatment applied? The answer to this remarkable possibility must await a properly controlled investigation which includes a group of school-phobic children who receive no treatment whatever during the specified period. One coincidence (?) is worth noting en passant. According to Chazan, the peak age for the occurrence of school phobias is 11. The peak age for general fears in older children (as shown by the MacFarlane survey: see Fig. 6 above) is also 11 years of age. The MacFarlane data indicates in addition that there is a sharp decline in fears after 11 years of age.

Most writers agree, however divergent their theoretical positions or brand of psychotherapy, that a gradual reintroduction to the school situation is at the very least helpful. In Talbot's (132) successful series of cases the 'temporary plans' appear to have provided the basis for treatment. Waldfogel et al. (135) also employed the method of gradual reintegration ('temporary compromises') as part of their treatment programme; even Lippmann (86) was 'impressed by these devices used to lessen the child's anxiety'. Eisenberg (30) recommends that 'if necessary he may be permitted to begin by spending his day in the principal's or counsellor's office or by having his mother with him, but he must at any event be in the school building'. Chazan (26) also reports the use of this method in some cases.

The most useful outline plan for treating school phobias would appear to be that proposed by Chazan. Depending on the information revealed by a thorough psychological and psychometric investigation, various procedures can be followed. Remedial education can be provided when necessary, a change of class or school can be arranged and individual therapy can be applied. The cooperation of the parents and the school is of course of great importance. The type of individual therapy programme to be instituted will naturally be determined by the exact nature of the disturbance. In most cases it is to be expected that some form of graduated desensitisation programme will be called for.

Operant Conditioning

Operant behaviour usually affects the environment and generates stimuli which 'feed back' to the organism. Some feedback may have the effects identified by the layman as reward and punishment. Any consequence of behaviour which is rewarding or, more technically, *reinforcing* increases the probability of further responsing (Skinner (122)).

From this acorn very large oaks indeed are growing. After nearly two decades of persistent laboratory investigations (mostly with animals) Skinner and his colleagues are now exploring the applications of operant conditioning in diverse areas of human behaviour. The topics which they have probed include the affects of drugs (Dews (28)), attention (Holland (51)), learning (Spiker (125)), psychotic behaviour (Lindsley (82, 83)), motor behaviour (Verplank (134)), verbal behaviour (Skinner (121); Krasner (70); Salzinger (112)), therapy and the effects of therapy (Lindsley (84, 85); King *et al.* (68)), psychological functioning in retarded children (Orlando and Bijou (105); Spradlin (126, 127); Ellis (31)), personality (Staats *et al.* (130); Brady *et al.* (23).)

As an introduction to the research on clinical problems in child psychology, it is necessary to consider first the work of Lindsley, King and Brady on adult psychopathology. Lindsley (82, 83, 84, 85) has made protracted observations of the operant behaviour of chronic schizophrenic patients. His research has already yielded important findings (such as the relationship between vocal hallucinatory symptoms and motor perform-ance) and has prepared the path for detailed functional analyses of schizo-phrenic behaviour. Lindsley's experiments were conducted in an indes-tructible room which contained only one chair and a manipulandum panel on the wall. The panel contained a lever and a small aperture through which the rewards were automatically presented. All recordings were made automatically, and the *E* (in an adjoining room) observed the patient's behaviour through a periscope or one-way screen. By using this basic situation imaginatively, Lindsley was able to investigate 'motivations ranging from food to social altruism, and discriminations ranging from simple visual to time estimation and complicated concept formation'. This method has already produced clinically useful results. It can be used as a sensitive evaluative device (e.g. insulin coma produced its greatest effect on operant behaviour at the time of the first insulin reaction— Lindsley (82, 83)). It can elucidate the characteristics of psychotic behaviour (e.g. schizophrenics develop low, erratic response rates and display stereotyping—Lindsley (82)). Further advantages which this method offers to the experimentally minded clinician include the possibility of tight control of experimental variables, freedom from verbal instructions, exclusion of variables associated with the clinician himself, the possibility of controlled investigations of a single case, and the possibility of thera-peutic control. An 'unseen' advantage is provided of course by the sub-stantial body of evidence concerning learning in human beings and operant conditioning in particular (for example the effects of intermittent reinforce-ment). Each of the advantages listed here are of direct interest to child psychologists: evaluative procedures, analysis of disturbed behaviour, non-verbal instructions, control of variables, exclusion of 'clinician variables', therapeutic control, single-case studies. This technique also provides the child psychologist with a suitable environment for response-building in cases of behavioural deficit, such as for example mutism and anorexia.

The possibilities of response-building are illustrated by the study of King *et al.* (68), who shaped the behaviour of adult schizophrenics (of extreme pathology) in a Lindsley-type situation. They were able to develop the initial lever-pulling response into relatively complex problem-solving and social behaviour. In this and other studies (King (66); King *et al.* (67)) attempts were made to relate operant behaviour to clinical status. The early indications are that clinical conditions and operant rate are related in a curvilinear rather than inverse manner.

While there have been no reports of behaviour disorders in children treated by operant methods, the fine case study described by Brady and Lind (22) is worth noting. They cured a man suffering from hysterical blindness by means of operant conditioning (see p. 142 below). An interesting combination of reward and punishment was employed by Barrett (14) in her treatment of an adult patient suffering from a multiple tic. As mentioned earlier, there are no reports of children being treated by operant methods for specific clinical problems. The work however of Flanagan *et al.* (40), Baer (11), Spradlin (126), Salzinger *et al.* (114) and Ferster and de Meyer (38, 39) has a direct bearing on such problems.

Flanagan *et al.* (40) attempted to bring the stuttering of three patients under operant control. Their preliminary analysis is encouraging, as they were able to produce total suppression of the stutter in one patient and partial suppression in the other two patients. The suppression of the stutter, which was achieved by aversive control, lasted slightly longer than the period of aversive stimulation. This stimulation was similar to that used by Barrett (14) in her study of a patient with multiple tics, and consisted of a loud 1-second blast of noise which was triggered off by the occurrence of a stutter. Spradlin (126) conducted a pilot study to explore the possibility of modifying the behaviour of severely retarded children by operant conditioning techniques and was able to train three children in such difficult tasks as detour, verbal and alternation behaviour. Spradlin's study also provides valuable information about procedures for adapting the children to the experimental room and about the role of different types of reinforcers. Salzinger *et al.* (114) applied conditioning methods 'to the vocalizations of a 4-year-old boy who had never learned to say any words at all and who had initially been hospitalized for autism'. In daily sessions over 9 months it was possible to increase his vocalisations and 'shape' at least a dozen words.

Ferster (37) and Ferster and de Meyer (38, 39) have made a study of the performance of autistic children in an operant behaviour environment. Ferster and de Meyer conducted a prolonged investigation of the development of performance in two autistic children aged 8 and 9½ years respectively. The experimental environment consisted of vending machines, a pinball machine, gramophone, kaleidoscope and a trained pigeon. The experimenters were able to shape the behaviour of the children in relation to all these objects, and obtained information about the effectiveness of different training schedules and different reinforcers. 'Both subjects emitted more of the experimentally developed behaviour with continual exposure to the automatic equipment. Conversely, they spent less time in tantrums of inactivity while in the experimental room.' This finding recalls Lindsley's observations on adult psychotics, in which he noted an inverse relationship between operant performance and psychotic episodes.

This important study by Ferster and de Meyer shows that the behaviour of autistic children can be brought under experimental control. The next step is to develop situations and techniques of this type which can be used to induce *therapeutic* control and, in a general sense, to find ways of developing the behavioural repertoire of children with deficit disorders. Salzinger, Spradlin, and Ferster and de Meyer, have clearly demonstrated that such a programme is conceivable even with the most severe cases. Ferster and de Meyer have also demonstrated that a range of reinforcers (candy, food, music) can be used effectively, that both fixed and variable schedules of reinforcement are effective, and that certain objects (e.g. coins) can generate a variety of other reinforcers in the manner of a generalized reinforcer. They are careful to point out, however, that their study was not designed for therapeutic purposes and that it 'cannot be assumed that performances developed in the experimental room will have general effects elsewhere'. They suggest that social reinforcers may prove valuable in developing extra-experimental performance. These two topics, social reinforcement and the spread of experimental changes in behaviour, are likely to occupy the centre of the stage for some time and are discussed below.

The application of operant methods to clinical problems has been explored in a limited manner at the Institute of Psychiatry, London. To date, attempts have been made to use operant methods in cases of reading disabilities, speech problems and encopresis, and in the analysis of the behaviour of a child suspected of experiencing auditory hallucinations. The remedial reading method was partly derived from the work of Staats and Staats (128, 129) on the teaching of reading to very young children. The procedure (Rachman (108)) is, briefly, as follows. The child is rewarded for correctly read words on a fixed ratio of 1 : 6.[1] Correct pronunciation of a word is signalled on a small panel consisting of 6 lights; when the sixth light is reached, a buzzer sounds and a sweet is automatically delivered. Words which are incorrectly pronounced are analysed phonically by

---

[1] This ratio is steadily increased, from about the third session, up to approximately 1 : 50. Later on a variable ratio of reinforcements is substituted.

the psychologist, who then demonstrates the correct pronunciation; the child is then required to say the word correctly. The wrongly pronounced words are placed on a subsidiary list for re-presentation at the end of the lesson. Naturally the choice of reading material and rewards are tailored to the needs of the individual child. This remedial technique, like all operant methods, is extremely flexible. Provided that the requirements of *the learning process* are met, the particulars of the training technique can be freely manipulated.

One child, M.R., 9½ years old, was unable to read more than half of the letters of the alphabet despite four years of ordinary schooling and several attempts at remedial coaching. He quickly warmed to the operant situation, and in the first twenty sessions (each lasting 20 minutes) spread over 5 weeks he learnt 235 new words. The operant training was continued for another 22 sessions until his psychiatric discharge (he was initially referred for treatment of general behaviour disorder). At the completion of training he had learnt more than 500 new words and read two elementary books. Another child, C.E., aged 9 years and 3 months, was unable to identify many of the letters of the alphabet when training commenced. After 7 months of remedial teaching (for 20 minutes, twice a week) he was able to read books at an 8-year-old level. His Schonell GWRT scores increased from 0 to 24 (Reading Age 7 years 5 months) during this period. Obviously it is not yet possible to assess the effectiveness of operant methods in remedial reading, speech training and so on, but the preliminary results are not discouraging. Clinicians who are interested in the application of conditioning methods to problems of reading, and of speech, are recommended to read the lucid analysis offered by Staats and Staats (129) and the account of experiments on the conditioning of continuous speech in young children by Salzinger *et al.* (113).

Varying degrees of success have been obtained with operant methods in speech training (Salzinger (113); Robertson (111); Ferster and de Myer (38)). In the case of a 5-year-old autistic child seen at the Maudsley Hospital, the attempt to condition speech responses was abandoned after a few sessions as it proved impossible to control the child's behaviour sufficiently to introduce the planned programme. A second case has met with a measure of success so far. This child suffered a fairly sudden deterioration at the age of 12 years and became virtually mute. The cause and nature of the illness is not clear, but an operant speech training programme was able to restore some communicative speech.

Operant training methods were successfully applied in the treatment of 3 out of 4 encopretic children (Neale (104)). The general approach was to ignore all failures (soiling) and to give a prompt reward for successes (defaecation in the lavatory). The case of G.M. illustrates the method used:

This 9-year-old boy had been encopretic for nearly 18 months. After m onths of weekly out-patient treatment had failed to produce improvements either in his encopresis or his aggressive behaviour. G.M. was admitted to hospital. Six months after admission his general behaviour was somewhat improved but the encopresis persisted.

Treatment was then aimed at developing a normal pattern of defaecation in the lavatory and at the same time attempts were made to withdraw all rewards (e.g. attention) or punishments when the incorrect, soiling response occurred. The procedure was carefully explained to the child by a trusted nurse, who ensured that G.M. did not regard the training as coercive or punitive. He was encouraged to go to the toilet at four specified times during the day and to report his successes. These were immediately rewarded by praise and a desired sweet and also recorded in a special book in the boy's presence. If the boy failed to defaecate within 5 minutes of entering the lavatory he was told not to persist. When soiling occurred he was given a clean pair of pants without comment.

As the training progressed, the four-times-daily routine was stopped and he was told to go to the lavatory whenever he felt the sensation of rectal fullness, which had returned by this stage. Successes in the lavatory continued to be rewarded. 'The response to treatment was rapid and complete in that he had become continent of faeces by day and night . . . the slow improvement in other aspects of his behaviour continued unchecked and he was discharged 3 months after completion of bowel training . . . after 3 months back in his own home there has been no relapse in bowel habits or in general behaviour, . . .' (Neale (104)).

In the substantial body of information on operant conditioning, there are four topics which seem to have particular relevance for clinicians dealing with children. These selected topics are: social reinforcement, intermittent reinforcement, the generalisation of responses and the shaping process.

Social Reinforcement

The important role of social reinforcement in child development is emphasised by some of the findings on operant conditioning. In this context social reinforcement may be regarded as any event mediated by a person which has the effect of increasing the strength of the behaviour which immediately preceded it. By definition, then, most reinforcers would be social in nature. Ferster (36) provides a detailed discussion of the nature and significance of social reinforcement in terms of operant conditioning, and Rheingold *et al.* (110) have shown its effectiveness in altering the behaviour of infants.

The exploratory studies reported by Ayllon (2) and Ayllon and Michael (5) indicate some of the possible applications of social reinforcers in handling disturbed patients. Although their reports deal with adult psychiatric patients, some of their techniques have a direct bearing on the care and management of both normal and disturbed children. Ayllon (2) describes, for example, how they were able to overcome an eating difficulty in a catatonic schizophrenic patient by operant training methods. The ward staff withheld attention when the patient displayed unadaptive eating behaviour (e.g. they ceased fetching her when she failed to walk to the dining-room) and reinforced satisfactory eating actions (e.g. placing candy on her tray when she served herself). These exploratory investigations are significant because they demonstrate the possibility of transferring laboratory findings into the ward, the clinic or the home. They also demonstrate that social reinforcers can be controlled and measured (albeit loosely so far) in extra-laboratory settings.

Experiments on the operation of social reinforcement in children have been reported by Gewirtz and Baer (43, 44) and Gewirtz, Baer and Roth (45). They examined two variables affecting social reinforcement: brief social deprivation and the social availability of an adult. Their results showed that the 'frequency of attention-seeking responses was greater under Low Availability than under High Availability' and that the 'frequency of behaviours for approval was reliably increased by the Deprivation condition' (Gewirtz, Baer and Roth (45)). The studies of imitative behaviour discussed by Bandura and Walters (13) are closely related to these findings. For example, the transmission of social behaviour by imitation is facilitated by providing models of high prestige (Bandura (12)). Individual differences in susceptibility to social influences have also received some attention. Dependent children are more easily influenced by social reinforcers than independent children (Jacubczak and Walters (54)), and children with a history of failures are more likely to display social imitation and to respond to social reinforcement (Lesser and Abelson (80)). Research along these avenues will eventually become incorporated in clinical work and child care.

Baer (9, 10) and Ferster (36) have in fact already started the process of integration. Baer (10) emphasises the 'reinforcement history' of the child, and indicates how the analysis of individual children may be used in designing techniques for promoting their development. He also outlines some methods which can be used to present social reinforcers. In addition to the pointers derived from the research discussed above on imitation, prestige, deprivation and availability, Baer describes some gadget-like aids. One of these 'gadgets' is a mechanised puppet which appeals to children and permits the experimenter to introduce and control simple and uniform social reinforcers. Lovaas (92) used the puppet to manipulate the eating habits of nursery school children, and further investigations are being conducted.

The broad guide that emerges from the available evidence is that social reinforcers should be presented intermittently, and preferably by an adult of high prestige. The use of social reinforcers in eliminating undesirable behaviour should follow a pattern of non-reinforcement rather than aversive conditioning. At the risk of over-simplifying, we may state it in this way: an undesirable response is more likely to be eliminated if it is met by no reaction at all than if it is met with a negative or punishing reaction.

Intermittent Reinforcement

It has been found in numerous experiments on animals and humans that intermittent (partial) reinforcement produces greater resistance to the extinction of the response than does continuous reinforcement (Jenkins and Stanley (55)). This effect may be illustrated by two recent examples from the literature. Spradlin (127) investigated the effects of different reinforcement schedules on the operant behaviour of 20 severely retarded children. The children were divided into four equivalent groups and trained on a Lindsley-type task with candy acting as the reinforcer. As predicted, the group which received 100% reinforcement (i.e. a reward for every correct response) showed faster extinction rates than the other groups of children who received intermittent rewards. Similarly Lovibond (94) found that the unsatisfactory relapse rate which occurs in the conditioning treatment of enuresis could be offset by the introduction of intermittent reinforcement; in other words, the high extinction rates (relapses) could be countered by altering the reinforcement schedule. In a different context Salzinger *et al.* (113) showed that it was possible to condition continuous speech in young children, and that the stability and rate of such speech was enhanced by an intermittent reinforcement schedule.

Long *et al.* (89) have published extensive findings on the intermittent reinforcement of operant behaviour in over 200 children. Their monograph details the effects of various rewards and schedules of reinforcement on children's behaviour in a Lindsley-type operant environment, and provides a wealth of important details for child psychologists who propose to use this technique. For example they show that small fixed-ratios rapidly produce satiation and cessation of response, while very large fixed-ratios made experimental control difficult to obtain. They suggest that an introductory session of small fixed-ratios should then proceed gradually to ratios of up to 1 : 100. Additional technical suggestions of this nature are provided in two further papers by Long (87, 88).

The theoretical value of intermittently reinforced operant behaviour derives from the fact that this type of reinforcement schedule generates stable and prolonged performance. Bijou (16) argues persuasively that the experimental analysis of the behaviour of individual children is made feasible by this method, 'since a clear functional relationship has been shown between a stable baseline performance and the introduction of a special stimulus condition'. If this claim is borne out by research results it will be of considerable value to clinical psychologists, who are constantly faced with the dilemma of group norms and individual patients (Shapiro (115)). Stable operant responding certainly lends itself to investigations designed to evaluate therapeutic (or drug) effects, or indeed any specific effect. Baer (9) has, in fact, demonstrated its value in an experiment on the effects of reward and punishment.

Generalisation of Responses

These experimental learning techniques would be of limited interest if the changes they produce failed to generalise or spread into the patient's ordinary life and behaviour. Changes produced by the reciprocal inhibition method do spread to the patient's out-of-clinic behaviour. This is well documented, particularly in the treatment of adults (Wolpe (142); Eysenck (34)).

The clinical application of operant conditioning has not yet progressed to the point where one can reach a firm conclusion. Baer (10), for example, was able to reduce thumb-sucking in three children during experimental sessions but the habit promptly returned when the relevant conditions were withdrawn. King et al. (67), however, were able to record significant general improvements in a group of (adult) acute schizophrenics who were treated by operant methods. By comparison with three control groups, the operant-treated patients improved in the following areas: 'levels of verbalization, motivation to leave the ward, less resistance to therapy, more interest in occupational therapy, decreased enuresis, and transfers to better wards'. In an earlier study, King (66) reported a 'positive relationship between rate of operant motor response in schizophrenic patients and another measure of manipulative responsiveness, i.e. energy displayed in regard to the various crafts of occupational therapy'.

A spread of experimentally induced changes in behaviour was noted by Salzinger et al. (113) in their study on the operant training of speech in young children. They found that 'the application of reinforcement to the response class of first person pronouns produced an increase not only in the specific class itself but also in general speech rate'. Brady and Lind (22) obtained a dramatic change in an adult patient who had been suffering from hysterical blindness for more than two years despite numerous attempts at treatment. The patient was awarded points on a counter when he responded correctly to the presence of a light. These counter-points were exchanged for canteen vouchers after each training session and the patient gradually learnt to respond only when the light was on. This ability then transferred to situations other than the experimental room. The patient regained his sight. This cleverly designed and simple (but highly effective) experimental procedure is a vivid example of the spread of effectiveness from the laboratory clinic to the 'outside world'.

The experimental work of Lovaas (90, 91, 92) promises to elucidate the relationship between the particular response which is being conditioned and the person's general behaviour. So far Lovaas has shown that operant conditioning of verbal behaviour can transfer to other behaviour and hence influence eating habits (92), motor behaviour (90) and aggressive behaviour (91). The trend of these results encourages the assumption that the effects of operant conditioning in the clinic will spread to the child's ordinary behaviour and environment.

Before leaving the topic of generalisation of responses, it should be pointed out that there is also a technique which can be used in promoting the irradiation of newly acquired responses. If the gap between the clinical and social environments is not surmounted spontaneously, the bridge of 'successive approximation' can be used. The patient can be taught intermediate responses which will enable him to cope with non-clinical situations. A theoretical account of this technique is provided in a paper by Skinner, Solomon and Lindsley (123), and Ayllon (2), Orlando and Bijou (105) and Spradlin (126) used it in the early stages of the conditioning process. Spradlin for example used successive approximations in order to adapt his retarded patients to the experimental situation.

Shaping and Successive Approximation

The technique of shaping is best illustrated by examples from clinical experiments such as those of Spradlin (126), Ayllon (2, 3, 5) and Ferster and de Myer (38). In the initial stages of his study on the operant conditioning of severely retarded children, Spradlin found it necessary to train the children to use the experimental manipulanda. The first step in the shaping process was to teach the child to retrieve the rewards (candy) from the goal box. The psychologist first retrieved the candy for the child. After this demonstration the psychologist withdrew from the situation and controlled the instruments remotely.

Initially, the experimenter reinforced any approach to the goal box. Once the child was spending most of his time near the goal box, the experimenter withheld reinforcement until the child moved his hand toward the manipulandum. Soon the child would touch the knob. After the knob-touching response was firmly established, the experimenter withheld reinforcement until the child made a grasping motion toward the knob—this was then reinforced. Later, reinforcement was withheld until the child shook the knob of the manipulandum, and still later until the child made an outward movement of the knob. Once this stage was reached, independent activation of the Lindsley manipulandum followed readily, . . . (Spradlin (126).)

The effectiveness of shaping procedures in ameliorating the condition of chronic (adult) psychotic patients is admirably demonstrated by the work of Ayllon (2, 3, 5). One aspect of behaviour which he has shaped with considerable success in adult patients is feeding, and his reports suggest methods of dealing with similar difficulties as they occur in children. A striking success in the shaping of speech was reported in 1960 by Isaacs and Goldiamond.[1] The patient, a catatonic schizophrenic, had been mute for 20 years. During a group session, the psychologist accidentally dropped a packet of chewing-gum on the floor. This provoked a slight eye-movement in the patient and the psychologist immediately rewarded the

[1] *J. Speech (and Hearing) Dis.*, 1960, **25**: 8-12.

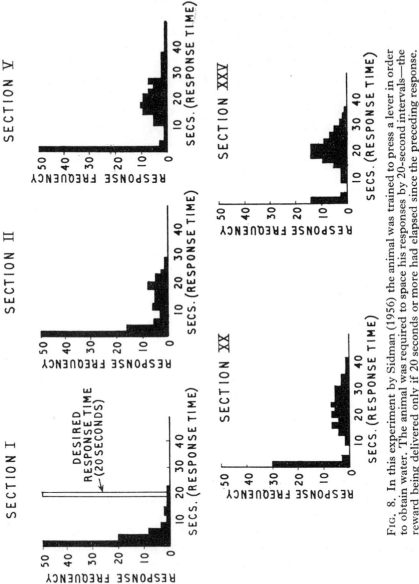

Fig. 8. In this experiment by Sidman (1956) the animal was trained to press a lever in order to obtain water. The animal was required to space his responses by 20-second intervals—the reward being delivered only if 20 seconds or more had elapsed since the preceding response. As the training progresses, the animal's behaviour becomes more accurate and efficient, session by session. (Adapted from Sidman, *Ann. N. Y. Acad. Sci.*, 1956.)

patient with a piece of gum. Thereafter, the psychologist gradually shaped more frequent and more extensive eye movements. He then made the reward contingent on vocalisations, until eventually the patient regained his speech.

The shaping process begins by utilising responses which the subject is capable of making (e.g. an eye movement in the case mentioned above.) The learning is 'most easily established by starting with the reinforcement of responses that only generally resemble the one that you ultimately seek to establish, then gradually increasing the strictness of your definition of a correct response, i.e. the one that will be reinforced, . . .' (Lawson (74)). The same procedure is used in training the organism to discriminate between stimuli. 'Ultimately, only a very precise response is being reinforced, and only when it occurs in the presence of a very specific stimulus pattern, . . .' (Lawson (74)). The shaping of increasingly accurate responses is neatly illustrated in an experiment by Sidman (119). He trained rats to make a lever press every 20 seconds by withholding the reward if the animal responded before the 20-second time period had elapsed (see Fig. 8).

Summary and Conclusions

Advances in the application of learning theory to clinical problems in adults have not been accompanied by development at a similar rate in child psychology. A probable reason for this uneven progress lies in the fact that behaviour therapy is more obviously applicable to adult disorders. Behaviour therapy has so far provided more techniques for the elimination of unadaptive behaviour than for the development of desired behaviour, and the disturbances of behaviour in childhood are more often of the deficit type. Consequently it is likely that the methods of operant conditioning will increase the applications of behaviour therapy to the clinical problems of child psychology.

Operant conditioning methods can be used to generate and/or sustain stable behaviour patterns. The advantages of operant methods are that they permit when required (i) non-verbal operations, (ii) strict control of variables, (iii) quantification of operations, (iv) exclusion of 'clinician-variables' and (v) single-case studies. The disadvantages are both of a practical nature: operant methods usually demand special equipment and experimental rooms, and can be time-consuming. These two factors are probably inversely related—better equipment provides for more automatic control and saves time.

In regard to further research, the four selected topics discussed above (social reinforcement, intermittent reinforcement, shaping, generalisation of responses) all require further investigation. Another difficult problem concerns the effects of punishment—a subject which seems to become more complicated with the accumulation of each new piece of evidence (see Broadbent (24) and Metzner (96), for example). What is needed above all, however, are clinical trials of operant methods. With very few exceptions, operant conditioning has not been used as a *clinical* procedure.

Both operant conditioning and the more familiar methods of behaviour therapy are likely to make a significant contribution to child psychology in the coming years.

REFERENCES

1. ALLPORT, G., 1951. *Personality*. London: Constable.
2. AYLLON, T., 1960. Some behavioural problems associated with eating in chronic schizophrenic patients. Paper read at A.P.A. meeting, Chicago.
3. ——— 1963. Treatment of chronic schizophrenia by operant conditioning. *Behav. Res. Ther.*, 1. (In the press.)
4. AYLLON, T. and HAUGHTON, E., 1962. Control of the behaviour of schizophrenic patients by food. *J. Exp. Anal. Behav.*, 5: 343-352.
5. AYLLON, T. and MICHAEL, J., 1959. The psychiatric nurse as a behavioural engineer. *J. Exp. Anal. Behav.*, 2: 323-324.
6. AZRIN, A. H. and LINDSLEY, O. R., 1956. The reinforcement of cooperation between children. *J. Abnorm. and Soc. Psychol.*, 52: 100-2.
7. BACHRACH, A. I., 1962. (Ed.) *Experimental Foundations of Clinical Psychology*. New York: Basic Books.
8. BAER, D. M., 1960. Escape and avoidance response of pre-school children to two schedules of reinforcement withdrawal. *J. Exp. Anal. Behav.*, 3, 155-159.
9. ——— 1961a. Effect of withdrawal of positive reinforcement on an extinguishing response in young children. *Child Developm.*, 32: 67-74.
10. ——— 1961b. Modes of presenting social reinforcers. Paper read at A.P.A. meeting, New York.
11. ——— 1962. Laboratory control of thumbsucking in three young children by withdrawal and re-presentation of positive reinforcement. *J. Exp. Anal. Behav.* (In the press.)
12. BANDURA, A., 1961. Psychotherapy as a learning process. *Psychol. Bull.*, 58: 144-159.
13. BANDURA, A. and WALTERS, R., 1962. Deviant response patterns. To be published.
14. BARRETT, B. H., 1962. Reduction in rate of multiple tics by free-operant conditioning methods. *J. Nerv, Ment. Dis.*, 135: 187-195.
15. BENTLER, P. M., 1962. An infant's phobia treated with reciprocal inhibition therapy. *J. Child Psychol. and Psychiat.*, 3, 185-9.
16. BIJOU, S. W., 1961. Discrimination performance as a baseline for individual analysis of young children.
17. BIJOU, S. W. and BAER, D., 1961. *Child Development*, Vol. I. New York: Appleton-Century-Crofts.
18. BIJOU, S. W. and OBLINGER, B., 1960. Responses of normal and retarded children as a function of the experimental situation. *Psychol. Rep.*, 6: 447-454.
19. BIJOU, S. W. and STURGES, P. T., 1959. Positive reinforcers for experimental studies with children—consumables and manipulatables. *Child Developm.*, 30: 151-170.
20. BOARDMAN, W., 1962. Rusty: A brief behaviour disorder. *J. Consult. Psychol.*, 26: 293-7.

21. BRADLEY, C. and BOWEN, M., 1961. Amphetamine (benzedrine) therapy of children's behaviour disorders. *Amer. J. Orthopsychiat.*, **11**: 92-103.
22. BRADY, J. and LIND, D. L., 1961. Experimental analysis of hysterical blindness. *Arch. Gen. Psychiat.*, **4**: 331-9.
23. BRADY, J., PAPPAS, N., TAUSIG, T. and THORNTON, D. R., 1962. MMPI correlates of operant behaviour. *J. Clin. Psychol.*, **18**: 67-70.
24. BROADBENT, D., 1961. *Behaviour*. London: Hodder and Stoughton.
25. CASE, H. W., 1960. Therapeutic methods in stuttering and speech blocking. In H. J. Eysenck (ed.), *Behaviour Therapy and the Neuroses*. Oxford: Pergamon Press.
26. CHAZAN, M., 1962. School phobia. *Brit. J. Educ. Psychol.*, **32**: 209-217.
27. CHERRY, C. and SAYERS, B., 1960. Experiments upon the total inhibition of stammering. In H. J. Eysenck (ed.), *Behaviour Therapy and the Neuroses*. Oxford: Pergamon Press.
28. DEWS, P. B., 1956. Modification by drugs of performance on simple schedules of positive reinforcement. *Ann. N. Y. Acad. Sci.*, **65**: 268-281.
29. DUNSWORTH, A. D., 1961. Phobias in children. *Canadian Psychiatric Ass. J.*, **6**: 291-4.
30. EISENBERG, L., 1958. School phobia. *Amer. J. Psychiat.*, **114**: 712-8.
31. ELLIS, N., 1962. Amount of reward and operant behaviour in mental defectives. *Amer. J. Ment. Def.*, **66**: 595-9.
32. ERICKSON, M., 1962. The effects of social deprivation and satiation on verbal conditioning in children. *J. Comp. and Physiol. Psychol.*, **55**: 953-8.
33. EYSENCK, H. J., 1957. *The Dynamics of Anxiety and Hysteria*. London: Routledge and Kegan Paul.
34. —— 1960a. (Ed.) *Behaviour Therapy and the Neuroses*. Oxford: Pergamon Press.
35. —— 1960b. Symposium: The development of moral values in children. VII. The contribution of learning theory. *Brit. J. Educ. Psychol.*, **30**: 11-21.
36. FERSTER, C. B., 1958. Reinforcement and punishment in the control of human behaviour by social agencies. *Psychiat. Res. Repts.*, **10**: 101-118.
37. —— 1961. Positive reinforcement and behavioural deficits of autistic children. *Child Developm.*, **32**: 437-456.
38. FERSTER, C. B. and DE MEYER, M., 1961. The development of performances in autistic children in an automatically controlled environment. *J. Chronic Dis.*, **13**: 312-345.
39. —— 1962. A method for the experimental analysis of the behaviour of autistic children. *Amer. J. Orthopsychiat.*, **32**: 89-98.
40. FLANAGAN, B., GOLDIAMOND, I. and AZRIN, N., 1958. Operant stuttering—The control of stuttering behaviour through response-contingent consequences. *J. Exp. Anal. Behav.*, **1**; 173-7.
41. GANTT, W. H., 1944. Experimental Basis for Neurotic Behaviour. *Psychosomat. Med. Monogr.*, 3.
42. GEWIRTZ, J., 1956. A programme of research on the dimensions and antecedents of emotional dependence. *Child Developm.*, **27**: 205-222.
43. GEWIRTZ, J. L. and BAER, D. M., 1958a. The effect of brief social deprivation on behaviours for a social reinforcer. *J. Abnorm. and Soc. Psychol.*, **56**: 49-56.
44. —— 1958b. Deprivation and satiation of social reinforcers as drive conditions. *J. Abnorm. and Soc. Psychol.*, **57**: 165-172.
45. GEWIRTZ, J. L., BAER, D. M. and ROTH, C., 1958. A note on the similar effects of low social availability of an adult and brief social deprivation on young children's behaviour. *Child Developm.*, **29**: 149-152.
46. HAGMAN, C., 1932. A study of fears of children of pre-school age. *J. Exper. Psychol.*, **1**: 110-130.

47. HERSOV, L., 1960a. Persistent non-attendance at school. *J. Child Psychol. and Psychiat.*, 1: 130-6.
48.   1960b. Refusal to go to school. *J. Child Psychol. and Psychiat.*, 1: 137-142.
49. HILGARD, E. R., 1958. *Theories of Learning.* New York: Appleton-Century-Crofts.
50. HINDLEY, C., 1957. Contributions of associative learning theory to an understanding of child development. *Brit. J. Med. Psychol.*, 30: 241-9.
51. HOLLAND, J. G., 1957. Technique for behavioural analysis of human observing. *Science*, 125: 348-350.
52. HOLMES, F., 1935. An experimental study of fears of young children. *In* Jersild, A. T. and Holmes, F., *Children's Fears.* Child Developm. Monogr., No. 20.
53. HULL, C. L., 1943. *Principles of Behavior.* New York: Appleton-Century-Crofts.
54. JACUBCZAK, L. and WALTERS, R. H., 1959. Suggestibility as dependency behaviour. *J. Abnorm. and Soc. Psychol.*, 59: 102-7.
55. JENKINS, W. O. and STANLEY, J. C., 1950. Partial reinforcement: A review and critique. *Psychol. Bull.*, 47: 193-234.
56. JERSILD, A. T., 1957. *Child Psychology.* New York: Prentice Hall.
57. JERSILD, A. T., GOLDMAN, B. and LOFTUS, J., 1941. A comparative study of the worries of children. *J. Exper. Educ.*, 9: 323-6.
58. JERSILD, A. T. and HOLMES, F. B., 1935a. Children's fears. *J. Psychol.*, 1: 75.
59. JERSILD, A. T. and HOLMES, F., 1935b. *Children's Fears.* Child Developm. Monogr., No. 20.
60. JONES, H. E., 1930. The galvanic skin reflex in infancy. *Child Developm.*, 1: 106-110.
61. JONES, H. G., 1960a. The behavioural treatment of enuresis nocturna. *In* H. J. Eysenck (ed.), *Behaviour Therapy and the Neuroses.* Oxford: Pergamon Press.
62.   1960b. Learning and Abnormal Behaviour. *In* H. J. Eysenck (ed.), *Handbook of Abnormal Psychology.* London: Pitman.
63. JONES, M. C., 1924. A laboratory study of fear: The case of Peter. *Pedagog. Sem.*, 31: 308-315.
64.   1925. A study of the emotions of pre-school children. *School and Soc.*, 21: 755-780.
65. KIMBLE, G., 1961. *Conditioning and Learning.* Revised ed., Hilgard and Marquis. London: Methuen.
66. KING, G. F., 1956. Withdrawal as a dimension of schizophrenia: An exploratory study. *J. Clin. Psychol.*, 12: 373-5.
67 KING, G. F., ARMITAGE, S. and TILTON, J., 1960. A therapeutic approach to schizophrenics of extreme pathology. *J. Abnorm. and Soc. Psychol.*, 61: 276-286.
68. KING, G. F., MERRELL, D., LOVINGER, E. and DENNY, M., 1957. Operant motor behaviour in acute schizophrenics. *J. Personality*, 25: 317-326.
69. KLEIN, E., 1945. The reluctance to go to school. *Psychoanal. Study of the Child*, 1: 263-292.
70. KRASNER, L., 1958. Studies of the conditioning of verbal behaviour. *Psychol. Bull.*, 55: 148-170.
71. KURTZ, K. and WALTERS, G., 1962. The effects of prior experiences on an approach-avoidance conflict. *J. Comp. and Physiol. Psychol.*, 55: 1075-8.
72. LANDIS, C., 1938. Statistical evaluation of psychotherapeutic methods. In *Concepts and Problems of Psychotherapy*, (ed. Himie, S. E.). London: Heinemann.
73. LANDRETH, C., 1958. *The Psychology of Early Childhood.* New York: Knopf.

74. LAWSON, R., 1960. *Learning and Behavior*. New York: Macmillan.
75. LAZARUS, A., 1960. The elimination of children's phobias by deconditioning. *In* H. J. Eysenck (ed.), *Behaviour Therapy and the Neuroses*. Oxford: Pergamon Press.
76. 1961. Group therapy of phobic disorders. *J. Abnorm. and Soc. Psychol.*, **63**: 504-512.
77. LAZARUS, A. and ABRAMOVITZ, A., 1962. The use of 'emotive imagery' in the treatment of children's phobias. *J. Ment. Sci.*, **108**: 191-5.
78. LAZARUS, A. and RACHMAN, S., 1960. The use of systematic desensitization in psychotherapy. *In* H. J. Eysenck (ed.), *Behaviour Therapy and the Neuroses*. Oxford: Pergamon Press.
79. LAZOWIK, A. and LANG, P., 1960. A laboratory demonstration of systematic desensitization. *J. Psychol. Stud.*, **11**: 238-247.
80. LESSER, G. and ABELSON, R., 1959. Personality correlates of persuasibility in children. In *Personality and Persuasibility* (ed. Janis, I. L. and Hovland, C. I.). New Haven: Yale Univ. Press.
81. LIDDELL, H., 1944. Conditioned reflex method and experimental neurosis. In *Personality and the Behavior Disorders* (ed. Hunt, J. McV.). New York: Ronald Press.
82. LINDSLEY, O. R., 1956. Operant conditioning methods applied to research in chronic schizophrenia. *Psychiat. Res. Repts.*, **5**: 118-139.
83. 1960. Characteristics of the behaviour of chronic psychotics as revealed by free-operant conditioning methods. *Dis. Nerv. System.*, **21**: 66-78.
84. 1961*a*. Free-operant conditioning, persuasion and psychotherapy. Paper read at A.P.A. meeting, Chicago.
85. 1961*b*. Direct measurement and functional definition of vocal hallucinatory symptoms in chronic psychosis. Paper read at 3rd World Congress of Psychiatry, Montreal.
86. LIPPMANN, R., 1957. Quoted by Waldfogel *et al.* (1957).
87. LONG, E. R., 1959. The use of operant conditioning techniques in children. In *Child Research in Psychopharmacology* (ed. Fisher, S.). Springfield: Thomas.
88. LONG, E. R., 1962. Additional techniques for producing multiple-schedule control in children. *J. Exp. Anal. Behav.*, **5**: 443-455.
89. LONG, E. R., HAMMACK, J. T., MAY, F. and CAMPBELL, B. J., 1958. Intermittent reinforcement of operant behaviour in children. *J. Exp. Anal. Behav.*, **1**: 315-339.
90. LOVAAS, O. I., 1960. The control of operant responding by rate and content of verbal operants: Preliminary report. Unpublished paper.
91. 1961*a*. Interaction between verbal and non-verbal behaviour. *Child Developm.*, **32**: 329-336.
92. 1961*b*. The control of food-intake in three children by reinforcement of relevant verbal behavior. (To appear.)
93. LOVIBOND, S. H., 1963*a*. The mechanism of conditioning treatment of enuresis. *Behav. Res. Ther.*, **1**: 17-22. (In the press.)
94. 1963*b*. Intermittent reinforcement. *Behav. Res. Ther.* (In the press.)
95. MACFARLANE, J. W., ALLEN, L. and HONZIK, M., 1954. *A developmental study of the behavior problems of normal children*. Berkeley: Univ. of California Press.
96. METZNER, R., 1961. Learning theory and the therapy of the neuroses. *Brit. J. Psychol. Monogr. Suppl.* 33.
97. MILLER, N., 1951. Learnable drives and rewards. In *Handbook of Experimental Psychology* (ed. Stevens, S. S.). New York: Wiley.
98. 1960. Learning resistance to pain and fear. *J. Exp. Psychol.*, **60**: 137-142.

99. Mowrer, O. H., 1960. *Learning Theory and Behavior.* New York: Wiley.
100. Mowrer, O. H. and Mowrer, W., 1938. Enuresis: A method for its study and treatment. *Amer. J. Orthopsychiat.*, **8**: 436-459.
101. Mowrer, O. H. and Viek, P., 1948. An experimental analogue of fear. *J. Abnorm. and Soc. Psychol.*, **43**: 193-200.
102. Munn, N. L., 1954. Learning in children. In *Manual of Child Psychology* (ed. Carmichael, L.). New York: Wiley.
103. Neale, D., 1962. Maudsley Hospital case data.
104. Neale, D. H., 1963. Behaviour therapy and encopresis in children. *Behav. Res. Ther.* (In the press.)
105. Orlando, R. and Bijou, S. W., 1960. Single and multiple schedules of reinforcement in developmentally retarded children. *J. Exp. Anal. Behav.*, **33**: 339-348.
106. Prugh, D., 1953. A study of the emotional reactions of children and families to hospitalization. *Amer. J. Orthopsychiat.*, **22**: 70-106.
107. Rachman, S., 1958. Objective psychotherapy: Some theoretical considerations. *S. Afr. Med. J.*, **33**: 19-21.
108.   1962. Learning theory and child psychology: Therapeutic possibilities. *J. Child Psychol. and Psychiat.*, **3**: 149-163.
109. Rachman, S. and Costello, C. G., 1961. The aetiology and treatment of children's phobias: A review. *Amer. J. Psychiat.*, **118**: 97-105
110 Rheingold, H., Gewirtz, J. and Ross, J., 1959. Social conditioning of vocalizations in the infant. *J. Comp. and Physiol. Psychol.*, **52**: 68-73.
111. Robertson, J. B. S., 1958. Operant conditioning of speech and drawing in schizophrenic patients. *Swiss Rev. Psychol.*, **17**: 309-315.
112. Salzinger, K., 1959. Experimental manipulation of verbal behaviour: A review. *J. Gen. Psychol.*, **61**: 65-94.
113. Salzinger, S., Salzinger, K., Pisoni, S., Eckman, J., Mathewson, P., Deutsch, M. and Zubin, J., 1962a. Operant conditioning of continuous speech in young children. *Child Developm.*, **33**: 683-695.
114. Salzinger, K. *et al.*, 1962b. Verbal behaviour of schizophrenic and normal subjects. Unpublished manuscript.
115. Shapiro, M. B., 1961. The single case in fundamental clinical psychological research. *Brit. J. Med. Psychol.*, **34**: 255-262.
116. Sheehan, J., 1951. The modification of stuttering through non-reinforcement. *J. Abnorm. and Soc. Psychol.*, **46**: 51-63.
117. Sheehan, J. and Voas, R. B., 1957. Stuttering as conflict. Comparison of therapy techniques involving approach and avoidance. *J. Speech and Hearing Dis.*, **22**: 714-723.
118. Shepherd, M. and Gruenberg, G. M., 1957. The age for neuroses. *Millbank Mem. Quart. Bull.*, **35**: 258-265.
119. Sidman, M., 1956. Drug-Behavior Interaction. *In* Dews and Skinner, B. F. (ed.), *Ann. N.Y. Acad. Sci.*, **65**: 281-295.
120.   1962. Operant Techniques. In *Experimental Foundations of Clinical Psychology* (ed. Bachrach, A. J.). New York: Basic Books.
121. Skinner, B. F., 1957. *Verbal Behaviour.* New York: Appleton-Century-Crofts.
122.   1959. *Cumulative Record.* New York: Appleton-Century-Crofts.
123. Skinner, B. F., Solomon, H. C. and Lindsley, O. R., 1954. A new method for the experimental analysis of the behaviour of psychotic patients. *J. Nerv. Ment. Dis.*, **120**: 403-6.
124. Slater, E., 1939. Responses to a nursery school situation. *Monogr. Soc. Res. Child Developm.* No. 4, Vol. 2.

125. SPIKER, C. C., 1960. Research methods in children's learning. In *Handbook of Research Methods in Child Development* (ed. Mussen, P. H.). New York: Wiley.

126. SPRADLIN, J. E., 1961. Operant conditioning of severely retarded children. Unpublished paper.

127. —— 1962. Effects of reinforcement schedules on extinction in severely mentally retarded children. *Amer. J. Ment. Def.*, **66**: 634-640.

128. STAATS, A. W. and STAATS, C. K., 1962a. Personal communication.

129. —— 1962b. A comparison of the development of speech and reading behaviour. *Child Developm.*, **33**: 831-846.

130. STAATS, A. W., STAATS, C. K., HEARD, W. G. and FINLEY, J. R., 1962. Operant conditioning of factor analytic personality traits. *J. Gen. Psychol.*, **66**: 101-114.

131. STEVENSON, I., 1961. Processes of 'spontaneous' recovery from the psychoneuroses. *Amer. J. Psychiat.*, **117**: 1057-1064.

132. TALBOT, M., 1957. Panic in school phobia. *Amer. J. Orthopsychiat.*, **27**: 286-295.

133. TOLMAN, E. C. and HONZIK, H. C., 1930. Introduction and removal of reward and maze performance in rats. *Univ. Calif. Publ. Psychol.*, **4**: 257-267.

134. VERPLANCK, W. S., 1956. Operant conditioning of human motor behaviour. *Psychol. Bull.*, **53**: 70-83.

135. WALDFOGEL, S., COOLIDGE, J. C. and HAHN, P., 1957. The development, meaning and management of school phobia. *Amer. J. Orthopsychiat.*, **27**: 754-8.

136. WALDFOGEL, S., TESSMAN, E. and HAHN, P. B., 1959. A programme for early intervention in school phobia. *Amer. J. Orthopsychiat.*, **29**: 324-332.

137. WALTON, D., 1961. Experimental psychology and the treatment of a ticqueur. *J. Child Psychol. and Psychiat.*, **2**: 148-155.

138. WARREN, A. H. and BROWN, R. H., 1943. Conditioned operant response phenomena in children. *J. Genet. Psychol.*, **28**: 1-14.

139. WATSON, J. B. and RAYNER, R., 1920. Conditioned emotional reactions. *J, Exp. Psychol.*, **3**: 1-14.

140. WHITE, J. G., 1959. The use of learning theory in the psychological treatment of children. *J. Clin. Psychol.*, **15**: 229-233.

141. WILLIAMS, C. D., 1959. The elimination of tantrum behaviour by extinction procedures: Case report. *J. Abnorm. and Soc. Psychol.*, **59**: 269.

142. WOLPE, J., 1958. *Psychotherapy by Reciprocal Inhibition*. Stanford: Stanford Univ. Press.

143. —— 1961. The systematic desensitization treatment of neuroses. *J. Nerv. Ment. Dis.*, **132**: 189-203.

144. WOLPE, J. and RACHMAN, S., 1960. Psychoanalytic evidence: A critique based on Freud's case of little Hans. *J. Nerv. Ment. Dis.*, **131**: 135-143.

145. WOODWARD, J., 1959. Emotional disturbances of burned children. *Brit. Med J.*, i: 1009-1013.

146. YATES, A., 1959. The application of learning theory to the treatment of tics. *J. Abnorm. and Soc. Psychol.*, **56**: 175-182.

147. YATES, A., 1962. *Frustration and Conflict*. London: Methuen.

Part III. RECOVERY AND RELAPSE

The Effects of Psychotherapy

In a recent article Rosenthal (25) recalled the observation of a group of psychologists that psychotherapy is 'an unidentified technique applied to unspecified problems with unpredictable outcomes. For this technique we recommend rigorous training.'

There is no satisfactory evidence that psychotherapy benefits people suffering from neurotic conditions. Examinations of the effects of psychotherapy on adults (Eysenck (4, 6)) have shown that there is no reason to suppose that this technique is capable of producing relief from neurotic illnesses. A similar examination of the evidence concerning the effects of psychotherapy on children was carried out by Levitt (17) in 1957. He reached the same conclusions as Eysenck—there is no proof that psychotherapy with children is effective. Of the 3,000 child patients included in this survey, two-thirds were improved when treatment ended (see Table 4). This statistic is no greater than that obtained from children who had received no psychotherapy; if anything, the treated group showed fewer improvements.

TABLE 4

Summary of Results of Psychotherapy with Children at Close
(From E. Levitt, *J. Consult. Psychol.*, 1957)

No.	Much improved	Partially improved		Unimproved		Per cent improved
57	16	18	12	8	3	80·7
100	13	18	42	26	1	73·0
70	12	29	19	10		85·7
250	54	82	46	68		72·8
196	76	52		68		65·3
50	15	18		17		66·0
126	25	54		47		62·7
290	75	154		61		79·0
814	207	398		209		74·3
72	26	31		15		79·2
196	93	61		42		78·6
27	5	11		11		59·3
31	13	8		10		67·7
23	2	9		12		47·8
75	35	22		18		76·0
80	31	21		28		65·0
522	225			297		43·1
420	251			169		59·8
3,399	1,174	1,105		1,120		67·05
100·00	34·54	32·51		32·95		

Levitt (18) has now brought his examination of the evidence up to date and the reports on the effectivness of psychotherapy which have appeared in the past 6 years bring no comfort. He concluded that there still 'does not seem to be a sound basis for the contention that psychotherapy facilitates recovery from emotional illness in children'. Once again the overall recovery rate shows that two out of three children are improved when treatment ends (see Table 5). Psychotherapy does not produce more recoveries than might be expected to occur without treatment.

TABLE 5

Summary of Evaluation Data from Twenty-four Studies
(From E. Levitt, *Behav. Res. Ther.*, 1963)

Type of disorder	No. of studies	Much improved		Partly improved		Unimproved		Total No.	Overall % improved
		No.	%	No.	%	No.	%		
Neurosis . .	3	34	15	107	46	89	39	230	61
Acting-out . .	5	108	31	84	24	157	45	349	55
Special symptoms .	5	114	54	49	23	50	23	213	77
Psychosis . .	5	62	25	102	40	88	35	252	65
Mixed . .	6	138	20	337	48	222	32	697	68
TOTAL . .	24	456	26·2	679	39·0	606	34·8	1741	65·2

It will be seen that in his second assessment Levitt attempted to analyse the results in diagnostic groups. He reached the tentative conclusion that 'the improvement rate with therapy is lowest for cases of delinquency and anti-social acting-out, and highest for identifiable behavioural symptoms like enuresis and school phobia'. This suggestion is interesting in the light of the prediction that 'extinctions occurring naturally during the life history of the individual should produce spontaneous remissions in patients suffering from dysthymic conditions' (Eysenck (8)).

Until substantial evidence is produced, the use of psychotherapy will continue to be viewed with serious misgivings. Clearly, *behaviour therapy* will have to do better than this. In view of the failure of psychotherapists to produce justifiable grounds for the continued use of a dubious technique, the proper exploration of behaviour therapy is overdue. The clinical investigation of behaviour therapy also seems to be recommended for more positive reasons. It has been developed from a broad background of information about the nature of learning processes in both normal and disordered organisms. Secondly, its applications have already achieved an encouraging degree of success, notably in the treatment of adult neurotics (Wolpe (29); Eysenck (5)). It has now to be demonstrated unequivocally that behaviour therapy produces more and/or quicker improvements than might be expected to occur spontaneously.

Behaviour Therapy, Spontaneous Remissions and Relapses

It has been argued elsewhere (Eysenck (7)) that a satisfactory theory of neurotic behaviour must account for the main phenomena in this field. The fact that approximately two out of three people with neurotic illnesses can be expected to recover without receiving any formal treatment cannot be ignored by any serious theory.

Levitt (17) calculated that the overall improvement rate for 160 cases who defected from the clinic before receiving treatment was 72·5%. This spontaneous remission rate was derived from two reports, in one of which disturbed children who had received no treatment were reassessed one year later and in the other 8-13 years later. Additional information about spontaneous improvements is provided by MacFarlane *et al.* (20). In their survey of the behaviour disorders of *normal* children, they found that the frequency of most disorders declines with increasing age. Some of their findings are reproduced here (see Figs. 9, a-f). Further data on the spontaneous remission of children's fears is provided by Holmes (see Table 2, p. 124).

One of the highest spontaneous remission rates ever recorded was that obtained by Clein (2) in a study carried out at the Maudsley Hospital. Thirty-eight non-attenders were traced 3-5 years after applying for treatment. None of these children had received psychological treatment in the interim, but 86·9% of them were found to be improved or much improved at follow-up. It should be pointed out however that the composition of this group of non-attenders was slightly atypical.

Spontaneous remission, although probably the best documented fact in the whole field of neurotic disorders, has received very scant attention from theoreticians; this is possibly because according to psychoanalytic theory the phenomenon itself simply should not happen. If neurotic disorders are always due to oedipal and other early conflicts in the child's history, which are repressed and required to be 'uncovered' before the nefarious symptom-producing results can be undone, then clearly spontaneous remission cannot take place, or if it does cannot be lasting. Indeed the demonstration that spontaneous remission occurs in the great majority of cases, even of very severe illness, and does not normally result in relapse, is a very powerful argument against the psychoanalytic interpretation (Denker (3)).

The improvement of neurotic patients without treatment appears to be a function of time. Eysenck (6) has suggested the following formula as descriptive of the situation:

$$X = 100 \ (1 - 10^{-0.00435N})$$

where X stands for the amount of improvement achieved expressed as a percentage and N for the number of weeks elapsed. He comments that 'while the exact values in this formula should not be taken too seriously,

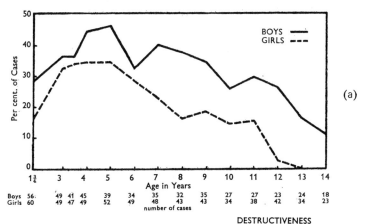

OVERACTIVITY
Percentage Frequencies by Age and Sex

(a)

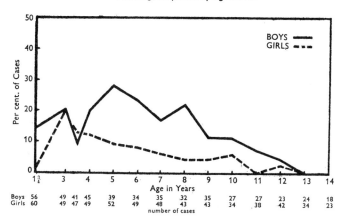

DESTRUCTIVENESS
Percentage Frequencies by Age and Sex

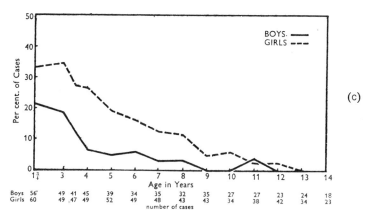

THUMBSUCKING
Percentage Frequencies by Age and Sex

(c)

FIGS. 9 (a to f). The decline of behaviour disorders in normal children.
(Reproduced from MacFarlane *et al.*, 1954. University of California Press.)

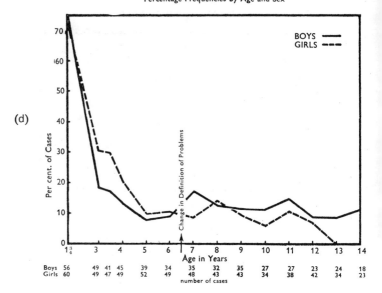

NOCTURNAL ENURESIS
Percentage Frequencies by Age and Sex

(d)

	1¾	3	4	5	6	7	8	9	10	11	12	13	14
Boys	56	49	41	45	39	34	35	32	35	27	27	23	24	18
Girls	60	49	47	49	52	49	48	43	43	34	38	42	34	23

number of cases

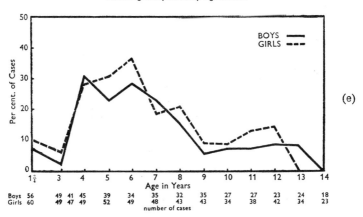

INSUFFICIENT APPETITE
Percentage Frequencies by Age and Sex

(e)

	1¾	3	4	5	6	7	8	9	10	11	12	13	14
Boys	56	49	41	45	39	34	35	32	35	27	27	23	24	18
Girls	60	49	47	49	52	49	48	43	43	34	38	42	34	23

number of cases

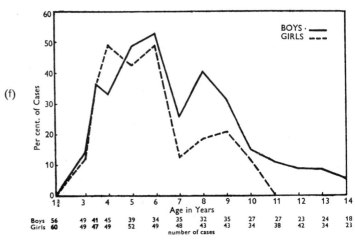

LYING
Percentage Frequencies by Age and Sex

(f)

	1¾	3	4	5	6	7	8	9	10	11	12	13	14
Boys	56	49	41	45	39	34	35	32	35	27	27	23	24	18
Girls	60	49	47	49	52	49	48	43	43	34	38	42	34	23

number of cases

its general form is of course that of the typical learning curve with which psychologists are familiar' (p. 711).

It may be worth while to take a closer look at the phenomenon of spontaneous recovery from a theoretical point of view in order to determine possible causative factors; it is clearly impermissible to implicate 'time' as such, because it can only be *events* happening in time which can exert a causal influence, and our formula does not tell us very much about the possible nature of these events.

How does behaviour therapy deal with spontaneous remission? In order to answer this question we must first state the main tenets of the general theory, without however being able here to bring forward all the supporting evidence; this task has been attempted elsewhere (Eysenck (5); Metzner (21); Wolpe (29)). For convenience we may number the points in order. (*1*) Neurotic behaviour consists of maladaptive conditioned responses of the autonomic system and of skeletal responses made to reduce the conditioned (sympathetic) reactions. (*2*) While the term 'symptom' may be retained to describe neurotic behaviour, there is no implication that such behaviour is 'symptomatic' of anything. (*3*) It follows that there is no underlying complex or other 'dynamic' cause which is responsible for the maladaptive behaviour; all we have to deal with in neurosis is conditioned maladaptive behaviour. (*4*) Treatment consists of the *deconditioning*, by reciprocal inhibition, extinction, conditioned inhibition or in some other way, of the maladaptive behaviour, and the *conditioning*, along orthodox lines, of adaptive behaviour. (*5*) The treatment is a-historical and does not involve any 'uncovering' of past events. (*6*) Conditioning and deconditioning will usually proceed through behavioural channels, but there is no reason why verbal methods should not also be used; there is good evidence that words are conditioned stimuli which have an ascertainable position on the stimulus and response generalisation gradients of the patients (Eysenck (6)).

Our theory of spontaneous remission is a direct development of our theory of neurosis as a form of maladaptive autonomic conditioning (Eysenck (7)). More specifically, spontaneous remission may be seen to be a simple example of the well known mechanism of *extinction* which occurs in laboratory experiments on conditioning whenever the conditioned stimulus is applied without reinforcement, i.e. without the application of the unconditioned stimulus. The dog acquires the habit of salivating to the bell because of the simultaneous presentation of the bell and the food; if the bell is presented alone he will salivate to the bell. Each time the bell is presented alone, however, the habit is weakened, and requires to be strengthened again by the pairing of tone and food. If no such strengthening takes place and if the bell is given alone a number of times, then extinction takes place and finally the position is reached where no salivation follows the sounding of the bell.

Consider now a typical case history involving the establishment and cure of a cat phobia (Freeman and Kendrick (10)). A traumatic event involving the patient's favourite cat produces a conditioned fear of cats; this develops to such an extent that she is effectively homebound for many years, refusing to go out for fear of encountering cats. Treatment is by means of graduated presentations of cats (first symbolically, i.e. by words and pictures, then bodily but at a distance, etc.) under conditions of relaxation and parasympathetic stimulation (desensitisation, reciprocal inhibition). After a few weeks treatment is completely successful, and a permanent cure achieved (no relapse for several years). In this case history there is no spontaneous remission, and we may inquire (a) why such a remission might have occurred, and (b) why in fact it did not do so.

First, we have a traumatic event which, by means of classical conditioning, produces a conditioned fear reaction to a previously neutral set of objects, i.e. cats. It is easy to see how this conditioned fear arose, but it is not so easy to see just why it should have persevered so long. Solomon and Wynne (26), on the basis of their work with dogs, have offered the principle of 'partial irreversibility' in avoidance conditioning, but it should be noted that the aversive stimuli in their case were probably stronger than in the case of the patient, and also that they report no single-trial learning, as seems to have occurred in this patient. On general learning theory principles one would have expected the gradual *extinction* of the conditioned fear response in the course of time. Each time the patient saw a cat (the CS) without a recurrence of the traumatic events which precipitated her original fear (the UCS), this unreinforced presentation of the CS should lead to an increment of inhibitory potential, leading to extinction. Similarly, each time she discussed her troubles with a sympathetic listener this should have had an effect similar to that of 'reciprocal inhibition', also leading to extinction of the fear response. In other words, behaviour theory seems to have no difficulty in explaining the extinction of neurotic symptoms by 'spontaneous remission', for this extinction is the natural result of the inevitable recurrence of the CS in the absence of reinforcement. We may thus reinterpret our formula for the time-course of spontaneous remission by saying, not that it resembles the typical learning curve, but rather that it resembles (and indeed is nothing but) the typical extinction curve. Our hypothesis, then, is that *all neurotic symptoms are subject to extinction*, and that this process of extinction is reflected in observable behaviour in the form of 'spontaneous remission'. The theory would appear to fit the facts reasonably well, but it would also appear to assert too much: not all cases of neurosis do in fact remit, and a theory predicting universal remission is clearly in need of an extension.

Such an extension is indeed implied in the first of our numbered postulates of behaviour therapy, given above, in which attention was drawn to the importance of 'skeletal responses made to reduce the conditioned (sympathetic) reaction'. What is asserted here is that in many cases of neurosis the original stage of classical conditioning is followed by a stage of instrumental conditioning, and that it is this secondary development which makes impossible the process of extinction by removing the conditions of its occurrence, i.e. the presentation of the CS under conditions of non-reinforcement. Consider the events in the laboratory during the extinction of a conditioned response. The dog, lashed to his stand, is presented with the CS a number of times; his conditioned responses get weaker and weaker until finally they cease altogether. This paradigm differs profoundly from that of our patient encountering a cat in the street after her conditioned fear has been established. The patient is not lashed to a stand, and thus forced to witness the conjunction CS—non-reinforcement; she is free to turn her back and run away. This course of conduct produces an entirely different paradigm, one favourable to the growth of an instrumental response of running away from cats. Simplifying the situation grossly, we may say that what happens is something like this. The patient approaches the cat and experiences a conditioned sympathetic response (fear) which is profoundly disturbing and (negatively) reinforcing. She turns and runs, thus excluding the cat from her field of vision, and also increasing the distance between herself and the feared object. This behaviour reduces the sympathetic arousal, and is thus reinforced by the resulting lessening of fear. The next time the patient encounters a cat, the newly acquired habit of running away will again, and more easily, be brought into play, until finally an instrumental conditioned response of running away is developed to such an extent that it permanently excludes the possibility of encountering the CS at all. In this way the secondary process of instrumental conditioning 'preserves' the primary conditioned response; putting the whole matter into psychiatric terminology, instrumental conditioning makes impossible the 'reality testing' of the classically conditioned response.

There is no doubt of course that in most cases the situation is much more complex than this. The original conditioning is not always, and perhaps not even usually, a traumatic, single-trial event; repeated subtraumatic trials may produce an even stronger conditioned fear response than a single traumatic event. Little is known about the precise dynamics of this process in individual cases, largely because psychiatric attention has not usually been directed at these events from the point of view of learning theory. Again, few neuroses are mono-symptomatic, and there may be a very complex interweaving of several different habit-family hierarchies (Hull (14); Wolpe (29)) each subject to extinction at different rates and by exposure to different events (CS's). Lastly, experience indicates, and theory suggests, that extinction of conditioned fear responses in one habit-family hierarchy facilitates (through a process of generalisation) extinction in others, whether this extinction is occurring during 'spontaneous remission' or during behaviour therapy. To mention these complications, to which many others could have been added, is simply to remind the reader that, while in principle the explanation of spontaneous remission here given is perhaps correct, nevertheless much experimental and observational work remains to be done before the details of the process can be said to be at all well understood.

We may use this theory of spontaneous remission in trying to deal with the problem often raised by psychotherapists, namely that of relapse. On the hypothesis that neurotic symptoms are merely the outcrop of repressed complexes, it would seem to be argued that no treatment of the symptoms alone could possible have any long-term beneficial effects, since either a recrudescence of the old symptoms or the growth of new symptoms would be predicted to follow. This is a case where there appears to be complete agreement between all psychoanalysists on a specific behaviourally testable outcome, and the disconfirmation of this prediction (Eysenck (8, 9)) is therefore of considerable theoretical as well as practical importance. The position seems to be that in the great majority of cases there is no relapse; it is also true, however, that under certain circumstances the neurotic who apparently has been cured does later on develop similar or different symptoms again. How can this fact be explained?

There are several points to be borne in mind here. The first and most obvious perhaps is that behaviour therapy is sometimes carried out by individuals not properly trained in the procedures, and without a proper background in modern learning theory; they may fail to carry the process through to its proper conclusion, they may break off treatment too early or they may make other mistakes which may lead to undesirable consequences. Eysenck (8) has drawn attention to the more obvious faults committed by some writers in the literature, and it must be obvious that where treatment is carried out under conditions which violate the laws of learning theory the results cannot be held to be damaging to the claims of behaviour therapy.

The second point to be considered is this. Let us assume that there is a one-in-ten chance of any particular individual undergoing a severe neurotic attack. If this occurs on a purely random basis, then one person in a hundred will contract two serious neurotic illnesses in the course of his life, one in a thousand will contract three, and so on. These calculations are of course not to be taken too seriously, as predisposition is known to weight the balance against any kind of random distribution; nevertheless the point remains that a person may contract the same illness twice during the course of his life without this being in any case a relapse. A rugby player may break his nose in 1959, and after it has been completely healed may break it again in 1962; this is not to be regarded as a relapse. Similarly a child prone to neurotic disorders may reproduce symptoms as a result of a certain conditioning process involving his parents, say, and he may after cure produce another set of symptoms on another occasion as a result of a new conditioning process involving, say, his girl friend. This does not necessarily constitute a relapse. It is clearly necessary to define with considerable care and accuracy precisely what is meant by a 'relapse', and how it is to be distinguished from a new and entirely separate breakdown.

However there is a third consideration, which suggests that certain types of neurotic disorder should hardly ever result in relapse after treatment while others are very much more likely to do so (Eysenck (8)). Let us first of all make a distinction between two types of neurotic disorder. When the symptom is of a dysthymic character (anxieties, phobias, depression, obsessive-compulsive reactions, etc.) it is assumed that the disorder consists of conditioned *sympathetic* reactions, and the treatment consists of reconditioning the stimulus (or stimuli) to produce *parasympathetic* reactions, which being antagonistic to the sympathetic ones will weaken and finally extinguish them. These disorders we will here call 'disorders of the first kind'.

When the symptom is of a socially disapproved type in which either the conditioned stimulus evokes parasympathetic responses (alcoholism, fetishism, homosexuality) or there is an entire absence of an appropriate conditioned response (enuresis, psychopathic behaviour), treatment (aversion therapy) consists of the pairing of the stimulus in question with strong aversive stimuli producing sympathetic reactions. These disorders we will call 'disorders of the second kind'. (In putting the distinction between these two types of treatment in this very abbreviated form, we have used the terms 'sympathetic' and 'parasympathetic' in a rather inexact shorthand notation to refer to hedonically positive and negative experiences respectively; the reader familiar with the complexities of autonomic reactions will no doubt be able to translate these blanket statements into more precise language appropriate to each individual case. We have retained this use of the terms here because it aids in the general description given, and indicates the physiological basis assumed to exist for the hedonic reactions.)

Let us now consider the role which extinction should play in these two types of disorder. It is our belief that, in tracing the fate of those conditioned responses we call neurotic symptoms, too little attention has been paid to the facts of extinction, and to the conditions giving rise to them. It is suggested that extinction affects in a profoundly different manner neurotic disorders of the first and second kind respectively, and that the problems of relapse cannot be discussed in any satisfactory manner without paying attention to these differences.

Consider neurotic disorders of the first kind, i.e. the dysthymic disorders. Here it is hypothesised that the original cause of the symptom is a conjunction of a single traumatic event (or several repeated subtraumatic experiences) with the presence of a previously neutral stimulus. Through the process of classical conditioning the previously neutral stimulus (CS) now itself acquires the properties properly belonging to the traumatic event (UCS), and produces the autonomic disturbances originally produced by the UCS.

Extinction, as explained above, should lead to spontaneous remission in cases of this type, and it is clear that in neuroses of the first kind extinction works in favour of the therapist and may even unaided lead to improvement and cure. Where the random events of life, acting in this fashion, do not produce a cure, the therapist can aid the process along the lines laid down by Wolpe (29) and others. Relapses should not occur in the ordinary way unless a new, repeated traumatic event occurs to produce a new symptom and a new neurotic disorder. This, of course, could not be considered a relapse, just as we would not consider it a relapse if a patient with a broken scapula should years after recovery suffer a Pott's fracture. Cure from one set of symptoms does not confer immunity on the patient.

Now consider the situation in relation to disorders of the second kind. Here the situation is clearly exactly the opposite to that which we have encountered so far. The patient is suffering from a maladaptive habit which is either itself an unconditioned response, as in enuresis, or where the conditioned stimulus has become associated with consequences which are immediately pleasurable to the patient, although they may be socially undesirable and highly unpleasant in their long-term consequences for the individual himself (fetishism, alcoholism and the like). Some types of disorder, such as homosexuality, may pertain to either one or the other of these two categories, i.e. homosexual disorders may be entirely due to an accidental conditioning process, or they may be innate response tendencies, or they may be a mixture of both. In any case what is true in all these types of disorder is that a strong bond has been created between a previously neutral stimulus and a strong positive reinforcement. Ordinary events of life occurring randomly are not likely to lead to extinction, as they are not likely to associate the conditioned stimulus with lack of reinforcement.

It might be objected that surely punishment in its various forms has been designed specially by society to produce precisely such a dissociative effect, so that by imprisonment, beating or torturing homosexuals, fetishists etc. we are substituting a negative reinforcement for a positive one. That such an objection is not tenable has been shown in practice by the failure of these methods throughout recorded history; no one nowadays assumes that the habits of the homosexual are altered by putting him into prison, even though such punishment may restrain the expression of these habits for a while. Even more important, Mowrer has shown, both theoretically and experimentally '. . . that the consequences of a given act determine the future of that act not only in terms of what may be called the quantitative aspects of the consequences but also in terms of their temporal pattern. In other words, if an act has two consequences—the one rewarding and the other punishing—which would be strictly equal if simultaneous, the influence of those consequences upon later performances of that act will vary depending on the *order* in which they occur. If the punishing consequence comes first and the rewarding one later the difference between the inhibiting and the reinforcing effects will be in favour of the inhibition. But if the rewarding consequence comes first and the punishing one later the difference will be in favour of the reinforcement.' (Mowrer (22).)

It is with respect to this temporal sequence that aversion therapy differs from punishment in the ordinary sense of the term. Punishment is a relatively arbitrary and long delayed consequence of action, which according to the principle just considered should have very little if any influence upon the habit in question. Aversion therapy attempts to apply the aversive stimulus *immediately* after the conditioned stimulus, and in such a way that it eliminates, or at least precedes, the positive reinforcement resulting from the act. This is often difficult to do, as clearly split-second timing is of the utmost importance; as has been pointed out before, many people who attempt aversion therapy do so without a full appreciation of the complexities of conditioning, and failure easily results from the haphazard manipulation of time relationships.

Consider now a case where aversion therapy has been successful and where the conditioned stimulus has been successfully linked with the aversive stimulus; we will call this link 'aversive conditioning'. Now clearly aversive conditioning, like all other types of conditioning, is subject to extinction, and we must consider how extinction can arise, and how it would influence the future course of the symptom. The first point to be borne in mind is that aversive conditioning tends to stop when conditioning has only just been achieved, i.e. without any considerable degree of over-learning. As an example, take the treatment of enuresis by means of the 'bell and pad' method. According to the theoretical analysis of Lovibond (19), urinating in bed is the conditioned stimulus which becomes linked with the aversive stimulus, the bell, which in turn produces the immediate reflex cessation of urination. Now it is clear that conditioning can only proceed while the patient still produces the conditioned stimulus, i.e. while conditioning is still far from complete. The moment the patient ceases to urinate in bed, further conditioning becomes impossible. With modifications the same argument would hold for other types of aversion therapy. Where the conditioned stimulus can be voluntarily applied, as in the case of consumption of alcoholic beverages, consideration of time, expense and the great discomfort produced usually limits the number of conditioning trials to a relatively small proportion of what may be required to produce any considerable degree of over-learning.

After successful aversion therapy, the patient emerges with a central nervous system into which has been built a certain amount of 'aversive conditioning', which is subject to what has been called oscillation by Hull (14). Oscillation is a feature of all biological systems and produces random variations in the strength of inhibitory and excitatory potential; these oscillations may be quite considerable in relation to the total amount of potential under consideration.

Consider now an individual who has submitted to a course of aversion conditioning, and whose degree of conditioning is just at the point where the original behaviour does not occur in relation to the stimuli which used to set it off before the course of aversive conditioning. Owing to the process of oscillation the effectiveness of aversive conditioning will be much weaker on certain occasions than on others, and if by accident the original stimuli are present at a time when the excitatory potential of the aversive conditioning is low, the individual will be liable to give way to temptation. If he does, then the extinction process phase of the aversive conditioning will have begun, because the conditioned stimulus has been presented without the (negative) reinforcement. It would follow that on subsequent occasions the excitatory potential would already be weaker to begin with, even without the action of oscillation, so that further extinction trials are even more likely to occur. We thus find that in neurotic disorders of the second kind the random events of everyday life, far from leading to spontaneous remission, will rather lead to relapse, other things being equal. Thus on theoretical grounds our prediction would be that relapse should be rare or even non-existent in disorders of the first kind, but relatively frequent with disorders of the second kind. There are no empirical studies the results of which could be used to support this deduction in any conclusvie manner, but it is noteworthy that those who have denied the importance of relapse, like Wolpe (29), have concentrated largely on disorders of the first kind, whereas writers dealing with disorders of the second kind, like Gwynne Jones (15), Oswald (23), Freund (11) and others, have drawn attention to the frequency of relapse in patients of this type. It would seem, therefore, that the distinction made is a potentially fruitful one, although the difference in relapse rates may be attributable, in part at least, to other causes as well. Thus the symptoms of disorders of the first kind are usually such as to motivate the patient very strongly to undergo a process of therapy in order to get relief from these symptoms. The symptoms of disorders of the second kind, however, are much less painful to bear as far as the individual is concerned; indeed they may appear quite pleasant and agreeable to him. It is society, through one of its various agencies, which provides the motivation for therapy, and this imposed drive is likely to be much weaker. This is important, because it is well known that the strength of conditioned responses is very much determined by the strength of the drive under which the individual is working. Here we may have, then, an additional principle accounting for the high relapse rate predicted for disorders of the second type.

There are, of course, several ways in which we can overcome the difficulty presented by disorders of the second type. Eysenck (8, 9) has suggested over-learning, partial reinforcement and repeated 'booster' doses of re-conditioning as weakening the forces of extinction, and there is evidence to show that either alone or in combination they may be sufficient to counteract the difficulties of conditioning treatment in cases of this kind.

Latent Learning

On the basis of observations made on therapeutic changes in children with behaviour disorders, it seems possible that a third learning process may also be involved in spontaneous remissions. This process, known as latent learning, may be responsible for spontaneous remissions in disorders which arise from the patient's failure to learn an adequate way of responding. These disorders are typified by enuresis, aphemia, dyslexia, encopresis and so forth and most commonly occur during childhood. They differ from the neuroses common in adults (e.g. phobias, obsessions) in an important respect. Phobias and obsessions for example are persistent, unadaptive and *surplus* response-patterns. Enuresis, dyslexia and encopresis on the other hand are persistent, unadaptive failures to respond adequately.

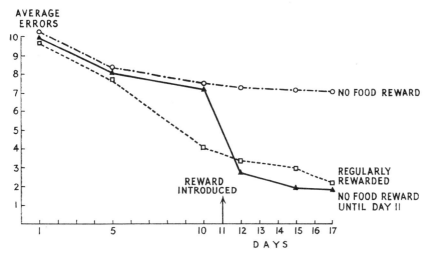

FIG. 10. Three groups of rats were run in a maze. Before receiving food rewards on day 11, the experimental group of rats had learnt very little. The introduction of an appropriate reward on day 11 produced a sudden, marked improvement in performance. The implication of this result is that some (latent) learning occurred during the first 10 days but only became apparent in the rats' performance when activated by the food reward.
(Adapted from Tolman and Honzik, 1930, *Univ. Calif. Publ. Psychol.*)

Latent learning was first studied by Blodgett (1) in 1929. It attracted the attention of numerous investigators because of its importance in the controversy between the learning theories propounded by Hull and by Tolman. The essence of latent learning is as follows. If, after a period of practice during which no improvement in performance occurs, an appropriate reward is introduced, sudden and large increments appear. The phenomenon is best described by reference to experimental findings such as those presented in Fig. 10.

Since Blodgett's early demonstration of latent learning the accumulation of experimental findings has given rise to five varieties of latent learning (Thistlethwaite (28); Hilgard (12)). The best substantiated and most germane varieties are: (i) unrewarded trials with the later introduction of appropriate rewards, (ii) free exploration followed by appropriate rewards, (iii) detection of rewards learned under satiation and re-located when the rewards become relevant. The occurrence of latent learning in children has been described by Stevenson (27), who showed that latent learning ability shows a striking increase during the pre-school years.

The laboratory evidence suggests a possible explanation for those sudden, striking improvements in performance which are often observed by clinicians. If the following three features are encountered when sudden

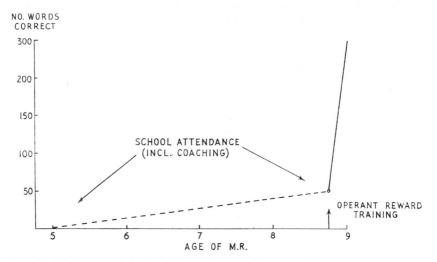

FIG. 11. M. R. attended school from the age of 5 years. When remedial training was started at age 8 yrs. 9 months he knew very few words. The dotted line is an estimate of his reading progress over the years. When he was changed to a rewarded operant training method, he acquired 257 words in 5 weeks.

improvements occur, we may with reasonable certainty conclude that latent learning has taken place:

(a) The patient has been exposed to the learning situation for a prolonged period—has had ample opportunity to learn the correct response.
(b) A new incentive has been introduced.
(c) The improved performance is of a rapid and/or sudden nature.

We may illustrate this process with a case of dyslexia (Rachman (24)). Despite his four years of ordinary school attendance and nine months of special coaching M. R., a 9-year-old boy, had learnt to read only a few simple words (condition (a) above is satisfied). He was then given a period of remedial training using an operant conditioning technique. Each correct word-recognition response was rewarded with a small piece of candy (condition (b) is satisfied). In less than nine hours of practice, spread over five weeks, he learnt 257 new words (condition (c) above is satisfied). M. R.'s extremely rapid acquisition of new words (despite the comparative absence of improvement in the preceding four years) was in large measure a reflection of the latent learning which had taken place before the start of the remedial training (see Fig. 11).

These sudden and striking improvements are very commonly seen in cases of enuresis. The case of D. H., a 7-year-old enuretic, is fairly typical. This boy had never been dry despite the application of parental pressures which ranged from stern rebukes to affectionate encouragement. A bell-and-pad conditioning technique was then tried and D. H. became dry overnight. He has remained completely dry for the past four years. This example of an 'incidental' cure of enuresis can be matched by any clinician, and no doubt explains why there are so many different types of folk and other remedies for this complaint. Kanner (16) comments on this state of affairs and lists some suggested remedies; they include 25 mechanical and surgical procedures, 23 types of drugs, 3 types of diet and endless psychological methods.

Sudden improvements are not restricted to cases of enuresis, however. If many of these improvements are the result of latent learning, we would then expect such rapid changes to occur in other disturbances which are reflections of inadequate learning. Apart from the case of dyslexia described above, other instances can be quoted. An encopretic child was recently put on an operant training procedure. While three other children required periods of training ranging from four weeks to four months before improving, the fourth child achieved almost total control in two days. Certain defects of speech comprise another group of disorders which can be expected to be subject to latent learning and should yield examples of sudden improvements. When confronted by a patient who has been cured by the application of leeches or a flash of lightning, one's customary reaction is to shrug and smile. If the operation of latent learning described here has any validity, we may in future be able to omit the shrug.

In conclusion, it is proposed that latent learning be added to the two processes (inhibition and extinction) which are presumed to effect spontaneous remissions. Latent learning may be presumed to be operating when clinical improvements are of a sudden and/or rapid nature and occur after the introduction of a new incentive. The presumption is strengthened if the patient has previously been exposed to the situation for a reasonable length of time and if the evidence indicates that the improvement is unlikely to have resulted from the effects of new practice. Remissions arising from the action of latent learning can be expected to occur most commonly in 'deficit' disorders where the complaint involves a failure to learn adequate responses (e.g. dyslexia, enuresis). It is probable that latent learning remissions can be cultivated by the introduction of new, powerful incentives when the disorder is of the deficit type and the patient has already experienced prolonged exposure to the learning situation.

Summary

We have attempted to indicate the fruits of applying learning theory in the consideration of personality, neurotic behaviour and clinical methods. Numerous applications of this analysis have been suggested, and attention has been drawn to those areas which require further clarification and development.

REFERENCES

1. BLODGETT, H. C., 1929. The effect of the introduction of reward upon the maze performance of rats. *Univ. of Calif. Publ. Psychol.*, **4**: 113-134.
2. CLEIN, L., 1959. *A follow-up of non-attenders at the Maudsley Hospital Children's Department.* Dissert., University of London.
3. DENKER, R., 1946. Results of the treatment of psychoneuroses by the general practitioner. *New York State J. Med.*, **46**: 2164-2170.
4. EYSENCK, H. J., 1952. The effects of psychotherapy. *J. Consult. Psychol.*, **16**: 319-324.
5. 1960a. (Ed.) *Behaviour Therapy and the Neuroses.* Oxford: Pergamon Press.
6. 1960b. The effects of psychotherapy. In *Handbook of Abnormal Psychology* (ed. H. J. Eysenck). London: Pitman.
7. 1962. Conditioning and personality. *Brit. J. Psychol.*, **53**: 299-305.
8. 1963a. Behaviour therapy, extinction and relapse in neurosis. *Brit. J. Psychiat.*, **109**: 12-18.
9. 1963b. Behaviour therapy, spontaneous remission and transference in neurotics. *Amer. J. Psychiat.*, **119**: 867-871.
10. FREEMAN, H. and KENDRICK, D. C., 1960. A case of cat phobia. *Brit. Med. J.*, ii, 497-502.
11. FREUND, K., 1960. Some problems on the treatment of homosexuality. In *Behaviour Therapy and the Neuroses* (ed. H. J. Eysenck). Oxford: Pergamon Press.
12. HILGARD, E. R., 1958. *Theories of Learning.* New York: Appleton-Century-Crofts.
13. HOLMES, F., 1935. An experimental study of fears of young children. *In* Jersild, A T. and Holmes, F., *Children's Fears.* Child Developm. Monogr. No. 20.
14. HULL, C. L , 1943. *Principles of Behavior.* New York: Appleton-Century-Crofts.
15. JONES, H. G., 1960. The behavioural treatment of enuresis nocturna. In *Behaviour Therapy and the Neuroses* (ed. H. J. Eysenck). Oxford: Pergamon Press.
16. KANNER, L., 1948. *Child Psychiatry.* Oxford: Blackwell.
17. LEVITT, E. E., 1957. The results of psychotherapy with children. *J. Consult. Psychol.*, **21**: 189-195.
18. 1963. Psychotherapy with children: A further evaluation. *Behav. Res. Ther.*, **1**: 45-52.
19. LOVIBOND, S. H., 1963. The mechanism of conditioning treatment of enuresis. *Behav. Res. Ther.*, **1**: 17-22.
20. MACFARLANE, J. W., ALLEN, L. and HONZIK, M., 1954. *A developmental study of the behavior problems of normal children.* Berkeley: Univ. of Calif. Press.
21. METZNER, R., 1961. Learning theory and the therapy of the neuroses. *Brit. J. Psychol. Monogr. Suppl. 33.*

22. MOWRER, O. H., 1950. *Learning theory and personality dynamics.* New York: Ronald Press.

23. OSWALD, I., 1962. The induction of illusory and hallucinatory voices. *J. Ment. Sci.,* **108**: 196-212.

24. RACHMAN, S., 1962. Learning theory and child psychology: Therapeutic possibilities. *J. Child Psychol. and Psychiat.,* **3**: 149-163.

25. ROSENTHAL, D., 1962. Book reviews. *Psychiatry,* **61**: 377-380.

26. SOLOMON, R. and WYNNE, L., 1954. Traumatic avoidance learning. *Psychol. Rev.,* **61**: 353-383.

27. STEVENSON, H. W., 1954. Latent learning in children. *J. Exp. Psychol.,* **47**: 17.

28. THISTLETHWAITE, D., 1951. A critical review of latent learning. *Psychol. Bull.,* **48**: 97-112.

29. WOLPE, J., 1958. *Psychotherapy by Reciprocal Inhibition.* Stanford: Stanford Univ. Press.

VII

THINKING, REMEMBERING AND IMAGINING

PETER McKELLAR

M.A., PH.D.

Senior Lecturer in Psychology, University of Sheffield

Happy people are not wicked.

—DUTCH PROVERB, quoted by Dollard *et al.*,
Frustration and Aggression, 1939.

1

Introduction

There are different kinds of thinking. And there are many different human activities to which words like 'thinking' and 'imagining' can be applied. In this consideration of some of these activities, both *subjective experiences* and *observable behaviour* will be discussed. Where it proves necessary, I shall draw upon adults' retrospections of their own childhood, as many investigators of avoidable childhood unhappiness have done. Moreover the influences of adult thinking itself will be considered: the thinking and the, at times, 'pathologically stable beliefs' (as Shapiro (34) has called them) to which adults who surround the child sometimes adhere can selectively inhibit or selectively reinforce the thinking and imaginative activities of the child. Four aspects will receive special attention:

1. *Adult and child differ in certain respects.* Childhood thinking is less intelligent, more concrete, and otherwise different in ways investigators like Piaget have elucidated. Remembering may differ between child and adult, and in particular the child's imagining may conflict with the exacting standards of adults in distinguishing subjective imaginings from external events.

2. *Individual human beings differ from one another.* Thus one of them, who happens to be a child, may exhibit to another, who happens to be an adult, what may seem to be a very odd form of subjective experience. The failures of communication thus resulting can give rise to anxiety and other avoidable unhappiness.

3. *These differences between people should be more widely known.*

Whether they are adults, children, or some expert like 'the doctor' to whom they may turn for advice, people need to be more fully aware of the variations that occur between normal individuals.

4. *A variety of kinds of 'thinking' can be distinguished.* Among these I shall deal with fantasy and other imaginative activity, and with both 'intelligent' and 'creative' forms of thinking.

This chapter will be specially concerned with the problem of achieving empathy with the mental life of the child. ·

2
Thinking, Remembering and Imagining

Empathy and Individual Differences

By empathy is meant an imaginative identification with another person of a kind which permits fuller understanding of his mental life and problems of adjustment. It implies curiosity, together with an implicit 'I see how you feel', though sometimes with the reservation 'even if I happen to think and feel differently myself'. The full implications of the differences between people are not always realised, even when they are comparatively obvious. In a symposium on 'The teacher and the learner', one speaker referred to a class of secondary school children who were learning the crawl stroke from their swimming coach (Birch (4)). As is usual with this swimming stroke, some were having difficulty with their breathing rhythm. For three individuals this problem was largely solved once they were allowed to breath with their heads turned to the left rather than the right. The swimming coach—aware though he was that there are left- and right-handed people—had not fully empathised with the problems of the left-handed learner in a right-handed world. This laterality difference influenced their preferred side for breathing in these three individuals: problems for them had arisen that need not have occurred.

There are many less obvious differences between people than those of laterality. Some can result in problems of adjustment whose very existence passes unnoticed by most adults. Sir Francis Galton (12, 13), in reporting his early studies of thinking, remembering and imagining, recorded that he had received 'many touching accounts of their childhood experiences' from people he had questioned.

They imagined at first that everyone else had the same way of regarding things as themselves. Then they betrayed their peculiarities by some chance remark that called forth a stare of surprise, or a sharp scolding for their silliness. (GALTON (13).)

Human beings are well equipped with an extensive repertoire of intolerances; prominent among these, in both adult and child, is intolerance of deviation from what is (or is believed to be) the norm. Much has been written about the *taboo on sexuality* which a child may violate by his questions or by talk about his own fantasies. To this may be added the *taboo on tenderness*, to which Suttie (38) has drawn attention: human beings can be very intolerant indeed of expressions of sentimentality or tender emotion. The taboo is stronger in some sub-cultural areas than others and may, as Suttie shows, become strong at certain stages of development; he instances the male child at the gang stage who rejects things feminine or girlish as 'soppy'. In addition to these two there is, firmly entrenched in many adults, what might be called a *taboo on enthusiasm*. In his fluent chatter, sometimes about his own mental life, a child may well exhibit the quality of enthusiasm and receive firm discouragement. Again, the taboo is stronger in some sub-cultures than others. In connection with it may be noted the child's lack of sophistication both in selecting and censoring what he says, and in distinguishing between fact and fantasy. Yet even if adults are sufficiently confident and well-disposed towards the happiness of children to control their own intolerances, it is not easy to empathise with the mental life of another person different from oneself. And there are some differences between individuals which a person may discover for the first time in middle life or even old age, to his own considerable surprise. It was to this problem that Galton drew attention, and I shall first discuss the variations in ways of thinking, remembering and imagining which he emphasised.

Imagery Differences

Most people can and do form visual images: their thinking, remembering and imagining occur in largely visual ways. Many such people do not realise that there are others whose 'mind's eye' is 'blind', and who do not understand them when they refer to their use of 'pictures in the mind's eye'. Some people visually image in colour, and some, but not others, three-dimensionally. Other people think predominantly in terms of auditory imagery: though they may also be able to form visual images, their tendency is to think about friends or others in terms of the imaged sound of their voices rather than of visual images of their faces. Yet again there are people whose imagery is largely verbal: they declare that they think mainly in words. But here again differences are to be found: one person may 'see' such words on a sort of mental blackboard, another may 'hear' them, while a third and a fourth imagine themselves 'speaking' or 'writing' them. Relations of such differences to problems of the school have been investigated from time to time, but too little is known about them. An experienced teacher recently wrote to me and said that in his opinion, first, 'the subject is very important indeed to education', and secondly, 'I would think that at present the number of teachers who appreciate mental differences in their pupils of the kind that you describe is negligible.'

With the problem of empathy between adult and child—whose imagery may be different—in mind, let us consider illustrative cases of extremes of imagery. The two individuals represent two categories of people, the first what seem to be the majority of people.

Good imagery. 'As visual imagery is the basis and the background, the bricks and tools of all my mental activity, I cannot conceive of the existence of thought without it.'

Poor imagery. 'My mental life is almost totally free from imagery. When I think about anything I suspect I mentally "use" the word for it, but I am not consciously aware of the word—certainly I don't "see" the word, and I doubt if I "hear" it.'

Sometimes attempts have been made to classify people in terms of their predominant kind of imagery as 'visiles', 'audiles' and 'motiles'. This typology stemmed from Lay (24), not from Galton himself; such a typology was too crude a simplification for an observer of Galton's stature, and it is certainly too gross an account of the subtle differences that actually occur. An attempt will now be made to examine some of these differences without resorting to the crude typology that has often been wrongly attributed to Galton. Three aspects of imagery will be distinguished: (1) Predominant kind; (2) Range of available imagery of different kinds; (3) Strength of imagery.

In elucidating these aspects I shall draw on several investigations of my own, especially upon a recent study of 500 adults representing a wide variety of occupations that require good intelligence. All were members of 'MENSA', an organisation concerned to assist scientific research, whose membership requirement is evidence of considerably better-than-average intelligence, as measured by standard intelligence tests. Since such a sample is unrepresentative I would stress that my purpose is not to establish other than very approximate incidences, but rather to elucidate different aspects of imagery. The fact may be kept in mind that two individuals, one a child and the other an adult, may differ in any of the ways to be enumerated.

By *predominant imagery* is meant the kind of imagery on which the person investigated declares he most relies for his thinking and related activities. Table 1 indicates data obtained.

TABLE 1

Predominant Imagery

	Cases	%
Visual	417	83·4
Auditory	130	26·0
Tactile	16	3·2
Olfactory	16	3·2
Motor	15	3·0
Gustatory	9	1·8
Pain	9	1·8
Temperature	9	1·8

(N = 500)

Since some individuals reported more than one kind of imagery as pre-dominant, these figures respectively add up to more than 500 and 100. The commonest responses were: for visual alone, 64%; visual and auditory, 14%; and auditory alone, 45%. Except in combination with the visual and auditory, predominance of any other kind of imagery was reported very rarely. Of the 500 people, two reported predominant motor imagery alone and one reported tactile imagery alone as predominant.

By *range of imagery* is meant the number of different kinds of which the individual declares himself capable, his repertoire of imagery. This proved to be rather unexpectedly extensive. The ability to have visual images was widespread, being reported by 486 or 97·2% of subjects. In support of this high incidence it may be noted that Carey (9), working on London elementary school children, failed to find *any* individuals who were totally bereft of visual imagery. My own data indicate that availability of auditory imagery is also widespread, it being reported by 464 or 92·8% of the subjects. But a fairly wide repertoire of other kinds of imagery also emerged: the most frequent number of available kinds was all eight of them. Frequency of mention was as follows: motor, 72%; tactile, 70%; gustatory, 67%; and olfactory, 66%. These figures, however approximate, indicate that a person who is predominantly a visual, or less commonly an auditory, imager may also have available to him a rather extensive number of other kinds of imagery as well.

Strength of imagery represents a third aspect of these differences of human thinking. We cannot of course equate what one person means by a 'strong' image with what another person means. Yet some distinction seems justified between those who say their imagery (or some aspect of it) is 'strong' and those who say it is 'weak' or 'fragmentary', particularly when the individuals concerned give supporting detail. Factorial work by Davis and Burt (Burt (6)) indicates a general factor of strength of imagery; in other words there is a tendency for strong imagery of one sense mode to go with strong imagery of other sense modes. In my own investigation more than half the subjects (52%) listed two, or three, kinds as 'reason-ably strong'; two was commoner than three. Eight kinds were listed as reasonably strong by 7% of subjects. As would be expected, the two kinds most often listed were the visual (86%) and auditory (69%). In order the others were: motor, tactile, olfactory, gustatory, pain, and tem-perature.

Three aspects of these variations of mental imagery have been eluci-dated, and I have quoted a teacher who expressed the opinion that such differences are not often appreciated by his colleagues in British schools. Some leading psychologists such as Burt, and Pear, have been aware of these differences and their relevances to problems of empathy between adult and child. And it may be noted that Soviet psychology has become interested in relations between visual vs. verbal imagery, and school performance in mathematics (see Krutetski in Simon, 1963 (23)). We may also keep in mind the parents. Of her own tendency towards thinking in strongly visual ways one wife and mother reported to me:

I thought everybody had this ability, but was astonished to discover that my husband had not. . . . And my son is also different, though both my brothers are like me.

When we are dealing with empathy with children's thought, imagination and scholastic problems of remembering, this late realisation is of some interest. And one wonders what proportion of parents *ever* achieve such insight.

Let us consider those individuals—a minority, the figures quoted would suggest—who are wholly or almost wholly without mental imagery. A good example is found in the psychologist W. H. R. Rivers (32), who reported:

I am one of those whose normal waking life is almost totally free from imagery, visual, auditory, tactile, or of any other kind.

In the investigation mentioned I reproduced this statement by Rivers and asked the subjects to indicate whether it applied to their own mental life.

TABLE 2

Absence of Imagery

	Cases	%
Does not apply	450	90
Does apply	50	10

(N = 500)

Thus we find that for these subjects the reported presence of mental imagery was commoner than its reported absence. But there were 10% who declared that they were relatively or totally lacking in such imagery. The influence of this upon recall of past events may be illustrated from the report of one of these people. Only recently had he realised that he differed from the majority, and had hitherto been puzzled by colleagues who returned to work and talked about the pleasure they had in being able to re-live their holiday experiences. Of himself he records:

When I have left a place after a visit I find that very little remains. . . . I feel underprivileged that a source of enjoyment open to so many people is closed to me.

By no means all people who lacked imagery felt this to be a handicap, for example to their work. But some emphasised how much it had impeded their school education; representative comments were: 'I have no drawing ability whatsoever', 'very poor at geography', 'poor at map work', and 'my lack of visual imagery handicapped by solid geometry'. In all those cases, and many more, the specific disadvantages were attributed to limitations of visual or other imagery.

Like teachers, parents are sometimes—perhaps not often—aware of these variations. One such parent, a woman with several children, happens to have a number of variations of her own image life of an interesting kind, including a capacity for crystal-gazing. These attributes were investigated a number of years ago, and she has as a result a sophisticated understanding of the variations that occur between people. (Compare McKellar (26), pp. 28 ff.) Recently she wrote:

It's so funny that 'but surely everybody thinks like me' feeling. It does cause quite a shock sometimes to find out that *nobody* in one's immediate environment does.

One encounters very much more naïve versions of the 'everybody is like me' reaction. I have found this reaction in individuals who have themselves had almost every conceivable variant of subjective experience of this kind, some common, some very rare indeed. These will be discussed below. Galton discovered at the turn of the century that such variations could be a source of considerable worry to the child and sometimes, if mentioned to others, an occasion of social disaster. I quote one of my own subjects who did learn early that he was different (in having several of the commoner variants of experience), and what happened. He is representative of many:

Once or twice in my youth I attempted to describe some of these phenomena but met with scoffing ridicule: I did think that perhaps I was not quite sane.

In this field we need not only tolerance, but also curiosity and much fact-collecting. What is needed is the spirit of the naturalist, as much patient work of observation, description, naming where necessary, and classification remains to be done. What is known needs to be more widely known, as it can help to minimise avoidable unhappiness and worry, and may assist empathy between adult and child and—we may add—between adult and adult.

Variations of Subjective Experience

All the variations that will be mentioned are compatible with sanity and good mental health. *Dreams* are a form of subjective experience which are socially recognised, named, and accepted. If a child reports happenings, however odd, which an adult can label 'only a dream', then nobody is excessively worried. We find much less acceptance for certain other types of subjective experience, particularly if they lack widely known names. Some of these experiences are a regular part of the mental life of the individual concerned, however disturbing this fact may be to others. As an example of one of the rarer variations, take *diagram forms*: a regular tendency to think of days of the week, numbers, months of the year etc. in terms of some spatial pattern. These diagram forms are sometimes coloured, and sometimes three-dimensional; estimates of their incidence vary from 5 to 7% of the population. Many people who have diagram forms reach adult life quite unaware of the fact that others don't have the experience. Alternatively a diagram former may think himself peculiar, or may be laughed at or otherwise discouraged for even such an innocent variation of thinking as this.

Some variants of subjective experience may be exceedingly frightening to a child who has them. As illustration I shall refer to certain phenomena relating to the *body image*. In the course of his life a person develops an impression of his own body as an object occupying space, with spatially related parts: his body image (or 'body schema'). When he is falling asleep, or at other times also, a quite normal individual may experience disturbances of his body image; he feels that his whole body, or one of its members, has changed in shape or size. Body image changes occur commonly in the falling asleep or 'hypnagogic' state, under conditions of fatigue, with migraine, and sometimes even with influenza. The fact that body image disturbances are a not uncommon variant of subjective experience should certainly be more widely known to adults, to children and to those they may come to anxiously for advice. This point was put to me rather strongly by a middle-aged woman who told of the misery of her own girlhood occasioned by body image changes:

It is terrifying enough for a small child to face alone in the dark . . . but when one is only five, and when it attacks one in a bus and people are looking, it is a bit much. One learned early to keep a dead-pan face, and to study one's bus ticket in one elephant-sized hand, *but I always thought it was the onset of madness.*

Another variant of experience, and a very common one, is called *colour association*. It is the tendency to associate colours with days of the week, numbers, letters, names or something else. Thus in one instance Monday was black, Tuesday yellow, Wednesday green, and so on. Problems of empathy and communication can stem from this variant. A correspondent writing in the *Listener* (11th April 1963) reported her own colour associations for numbers. Ten was for her a deep rust colour 'the colour of strong tea'. She told how, when about six, she explained to somebody that her brother liked 'ten tea', and of getting exasperated when told she was talking nonsense. Another person told me of her colour associations for different kinds of pain, and how—to her own surprise—this way of talking about pain would annoy her mother. As a way of thinking these colour associations were retained into adult life, but the child soon gave up trying to communicate in these terms. Yet many adults remain unaware of the fact that the colour associations they possess are not a universal phenomenon; 'I thought everybody was like me' is their frequent comment when they gain this insight. Somewhat more cautious was one with an elaborate system of colour associations, who remarked 'I *think* there *are* people who don't have it.' Alternatively the investigator encounters relief when a person with colour associations learns that his oddity of experience is known to science, and has a name.

A much commoner experience—and probably about 90 per cent of people have had it—is *déjà vu*. This is the illusion of recognition involving 'I feel as though I have lived through this before, though I know I haven't.' Yet even a nearly universal experience like this one can result in anxiety and worry over years because of the feeling one is 'different' in some undesirable way. 'Please don't tell me I'm going insane', wrote one adult to me, before relating a standard example of the *déjà vu* experience.

Because of the impressive and sometimes frightening forms it can take, another variant merits emphasis. When falling asleep some people, but not all, have visual or other imagery of a quasi-hallucinatory kind. This experience, *hypnagogic imagery*, is very common and occurs nightly for some people. The images seem to come and go of their own accord, and their character and content may seem to the imager quite foreign to his own personality: 'like pictures from the kind of travel book I don't read', wrote one such imager. Elsewhere I have suggested that hypnagogic images are like lantern slides shown at random and appropriate to the illustration of another lecture: for 'lecture' read 'the subject's other thoughts' to which they may seem so irrelevant. The visual kind sometimes occur open-eyed in a darkened room. Thus one 5-year-old 'saw' more or less nightly a large black dog which came and sat on her pillow! As in this case, children often need considerable reassurance because of such happenings. Moreover the imagery may possess peculiarities of colour and lighting, and has frequently been likened to surrealist paintings from the microscopic accuracy of detail and the strange juxtapositions that sometimes occur. Children may place their own interpretations on the imagery; thus one thought he was looking through someone else's eyes in the daylight on the other side of the world! An early investigator was Silberer (35), who arrived at the conclusion that the images were 'translations of thoughts into pictures'. Silberer found on systematic investigation that these pictorial comments were often surprisingly appropriate. For example, once he was thinking about the revision and polishing up of a piece of writing he was doing; suddenly, in the drowsy state, he had an image of himself planing a piece of wood. In hypnagogic imagery, as Silberer puts it, 'the tired consciousness switches to an easier form of mental functioning.' Investigations by my colleagues and myself indicate that hypnagogic images vary enormously in their content, and range from the terrifying, such as grotesque 'faces in the dark', to benign landscapes which the imager wishes he had the talent to paint, or amusing Walt Disney-cartoon-like happenings. The auditory images appear to be commoner even than the visual kind; they are frequently of music or voices, and sometimes mistaken for real sounds. Hypnagogic images whether visual, auditory, or of some other kind were reported by more than half the people studied (McKellar and Simpson (27); McKellar (26)). There is some evidence to suggest that the imagery is commoner in childhood than in adult life, and plenty to indicate that the imagery may be a source of avoidable worry to both children and adults.

Somewhat similar experiences may occur in the course of waking up, and are known as *hypnopompic images*. An example may be taken:

Recently just before waking up in the morning I distinctly heard my mother having a telephone conversation with a friend. . . . No such telephone call took place.

The hypnagogic imager sometimes rises from his bed to turn off the wireless, or to find out who is responsible for the non-existent voices he 'hears'. And similar things happen with the hypnopompic imager, as in the following case, which also illustrates hypnopompic imagery for smell:

I was dreaming that I was toasting bread, and awoke quite quickly only to smell toast cooking, I arose to check whether I had left the oven on, but I had not.

The person who reported this was a medical practitioner. An educated physician may accept this kind of confusion between subjective experience and reality in this way as a matter of course. It is otherwise with the child, particularly when he experiences, as one did on waking, an open-eyed hypnopompic image of 'a hand clutching a flaming torch'! Adults can be, and often are, upset by the content of their hypnopompic imagery when it takes such forms as 'the whole room was full of angels', or the recurrent appearance of shadowy ghost-like figures approaching the bed. As with hypnagogic imagery, the imagery of the hypnopompic state merits taking seriously if we would empathise with the problems of childhood imagination.

Children are known to be more subject than adults to *eidetic images*: vivid subjective experiences of a quasi-hallucinatory kind, that can give rise to confusions with reality because of their seemingly perceptual character. Jaensch (20) gives their incidence as 61% for children and 7% for adults; Peck and Hodges (31) reported eidetic imagery in 60% of white American children of 4 years of age. As one source of false testimony the imagery is thus of some interest to forensic psychology. A good illustration concerns myself at the age of 5, when I gave an entirely fictitious account to the investigating police officers of my own efforts to prevent some other children damaging my elder brother's car. Fortunately the officers were sensible enough neither to believe the eidetic images of a young child, nor to assess them as 'lying'. The distinction between eidetic imagery and hallucination is in practice not easy to draw in the case of the very young child, and eidetic imagery is one of the sources of behaviour that adults may assess as 'lying'.

Childhood Lying

In one of the great classics of modern psychology, *The Young Delin-*

quent, Sir Cyril Burt (5) repeatedly stresses the importance of individual differences. His discussion of childhood 'lying' demands special consideration. If a child produces a lie, or lies habitually, what kind of a lie is it? There are *all sorts* of childhood statements which adults may choose to call 'lying', and Burt distinguishes seven different kinds. These comprise: playful lies, lies resulting from confusions between mental experience and external events, lies of vanity, malevolent lies, lies which excuse oneself, lies for personal advantage, and lies of loyalty to others. Important among these is the excusive lie, which has been aptly defined as 'an abomination to the Lord, but an ever-present help in time of trouble'! In connection with such lies, and with the problem of adult reactions to childhood imagination, reference must be made to one important source of individual differences between children, emphasised by Burt: their punishment history. He distinguishes the over-punished, the under-punished and the inconsistently-punished child, and argues that what should be done to inhibit a given kind of behaviour like lying depends on *which kind* of child one is dealing with. Over-punishment and unpredictable punishment are likely to provoke fear and some of its unhappy by-products like excusive lies. A certain type of parent understands well the precise recipe for training his unfortunate child in the habit of excusive lying.

Let us now consider a different kind of behaviour which an obtuse and unimaginative adult may choose to label as 'lying': the phenomenon of *the imaginary companion*. This is comparatively common, and there is a known sex difference. In their study based on adult recall of childhood, Hurlock and Burnstein (18) found it reported by 31% of women and 23% of men, in a sample of 700 individuals. As an illustration I shall take the case of a child 'David', who in the period of $2\frac{1}{2}$ to 3 years had imaginary companions. One was a tiger he called 'Hallspeaker' of whom he was very fond; the other was a 'Mrs. Cornflake'. Mrs. Cornflake was a sort of imaginary kind aunt, and unlike Hallspeaker persisted until the child was five; she was an approachable, wise companion who knew all the answers, and well illustrates the usual characteristic of the imaginary companion of being a benign, helpful figure. Imaginary companions are, like eidetic imagery, mostly but not wholly specific to childhood, and have been known to persist into the adult life of normal people. Several of the characteristics of imaginary companions are illustrated in a detailed account summarised from the report of a psychologist colleague. As a child she had three imaginary companions, two of them dogs. The third, her main imaginary companion, was a blue fairy called 'Tinkerbell', whose origins my colleague was able to trace to a picture in a book she had seen as a very young child. In this case also the companion was a friendly figure, and relations between her and the child were invariably happy ones. Tinkerbell remained prominent in the child's life until 5. At this age the girl realised that Tinkerbell didn't really exist, but decided to have her anyway! And so the imaginary companion persisted as a kind of half-belief until about 9 or 10.

Elsewhere (25) I have discussed the *phenomenon of half-belief*: an attitude involving some of the features of belief together with some of those of disbelief, compatible with intellectual rejection but involving a sort of weakening of disbelief. A basis for empathy with childhood half-belief, whether in fairies, Father Christmas, imaginary companions or something else, can readily be found in certain adult behaviour. Many adults seem to have superstitious half-beliefs. Probably the majority of people in Britain don't fully believe that walking under a ladder will affect their future, yet systematic observations on a number of occasions reveal that the majority walk round the ladder and not under it! Adult half-belief seems to occur in relation to popular entertainers and certain characters of fictional literature. One viewer wrote to Cliff Michelmore of the Television programme 'Tonight', whom she had often seen in her room, and asked him how he liked the new wallpaper she now had in the room! Again, Conan Doyle had to deal with a good deal of correspondence addressed both to 'Sherlock Holmes' and 'Dr. Watson'. Adults give evidence on occasion of half-beliefs of their own, and may share the half-beliefs of children, as seems to have happened in the case of the Tinkerbell imaginary companion, who was more or less accepted as a member of the household. The child, now my adult colleague, herself acknowledges retention of a half-belief from 5 years onwards, and her mother seems both to have encouraged such half-belief and to have herself shared it to some extent.

Reasons for the occurrence of imaginary companions seem to be complex, and worried parents need not assume that they are signs of psychosis (which obviously they are not), nor reactions to loneliness, nor evidence of unsatisfactory attitudes to themselves. Such companions may indeed perform a distinctly positive function in a child's development, as he explores the realities of life and of inter-personal relations. In none of the instances I have studied was there evidence of actually 'seeing' the imaginary companion as an eidetic image.

Adult Thinking and the Child

Adults are not always so tolerant as those in the last instance discussed of what may seem to them deviations from the norm in the imaginative life of their children. For those who need reassurance or information, practical advice on how to deal with childhood fantasy and other problems is available from many sources, including an amusing but very sane pamphlet published by the National Association of Mental Health: *Do babies have worries?* (3). This publication discusses various problems of childhood, and in relation to each distinguishes three main types of parental attitude and resulting behaviour: those of duty, those of smothering love, and those of affection.

The sufferings children have, throughout history, experienced from *dutiful love* at its worst are an exceedingly grim story. Adult thinking may be dominated by a kind of righteousness which manifestly lacks insight into the resentments it expresses. Building on the work of Freud, Flugel (11) and others have produced a penetrating analysis of some of the forms of moralised aggression which can occur. Certain adults seem only too readily to mistake their hostility and ambivalence towards children for the call of duty. Apart altogether from any long-term effects of this kind of thinking upon children, there remains the question of here-and-now suffering for individuals too small to defend themselves. *Smothering love* creates problems of a different kind, and may find support from what the adult uncritically thinks are the doctrines of some system of child upbringing. One disadvantage of great thinkers is the rigid application of misconceived versions of their thought by uncritical disciples; Freud has had such disciples. Melitta Schmideberg (33), a New York psychoanalyst, has produced a remarkable series of cases of children who had been allowed to become unmanageable because of misguided parents who believed they were applying what 'psychiatry' and 'psychoanalysis' taught. Thus one such child was repeatedly expelled from a series of progressively more 'progressive' schools, and, in all cases reported, it took the efforts of a skilled psychoanalyst to undo the harm that had been done by misguided tolerance. With cold dutiful love, and misconceived over-indulgence, may be contrasted *affectionate love*: this is discriminating, efficient and realistic. What Bingham calls 'affectionate love' embraces much of what has been said in this chapter about empathy with childhood thinking and imagining, appreciation of differences, and understanding of the underlying problems of adjustment.

Perhaps the thinking of psychiatrists, psychologists and psychoanalysts has, on occasion, been a little too preoccupied with *long-term effects* of different practices upon the sexual and toilet training of the child, and too little concerned with his *immediate unhappiness*. Whatever these long-term effects on the personality, the immediate effect of certain kinds of thinking upon the unhappiness of individual children is perfectly obvious. The taboo on sexuality, for instance, is extremely strong. The distorted and sometimes quasi-pathological thinking of adults, encouraged at times by certain kinds of theology—whose content of Christianity seems to be minimal—and even by out-of-date textbooks, has resulted in a quite terrible chapter of human suffering. Those interested in the problems that adult thinking has itself created over the sexual development of the child may be referred to the almost unbelievable cruelties reported by Huschka (19). One kind of fantasy merits particular mention since it is likely to evoke adult disapproval, sometimes of the 'dutiful love' kind: I refer to fantasy of a sexual kind and the masturbatory activity that may accompany it. From reviews of the literature, Kanner (22) concludes that at puberty and early adolescence masturbation 'occurs in such high proportions that for practical purposes it can be considered a usual phenomenon'. This earlier *Text-Book of Child Psychiatry* adds that 'treatment' for childhood autoeroticism, which has given rise to so much dutiful aggression against the child, is needed 'only if adult attitudes have instilled into him feelings and preoccupations injurious to his emotional well-being'.

Mention may also be made of certain forms of adult thinking in relation to toilet training. I quote one individual:

My grandfather and grandmother were against corporal punishment but my grandmother was in favour of castor oil as a form of punishment.

Moreover toilet training matters can become a vehicle of expression of adult hypochondriasis as well as of adult hostility for the child. Some people are excessively preoccupied in their thinking about constipation, and of this a child may be the victim. Kanner (22) instances the case of 'Judy', who until her sixth year suffered from what seems to have been her mother's pathologically stable belief that the child could not have bowel movements without artificial aids. The mother had herself been constipated. And so the unfortunate child, an extreme case admittedly but representative of a category of avoidable suffering, was raised on special diets, made to submit to the indignity of enemas, and cascara and castor oil were stuffed into her. Eventually a normal life, for a normal child, was secured through the common sense of a physician who stood up to the mother and insisted on the abandonment of these superfluous aids disturbed adult thinking was forcing on the child. As in this instance, 'the doctor'—if alerted to the existence of these problems—can sometimes perform an important function of protection of the child against irrational adult thinking. Punishment, sexuality and constipation represent three areas in which such thinking seems liable to occur.

Even at best, empathy between adult and child is not easy, because their concepts and ways of thinking are different. As the child grows older additional differences may develop, and may help to intensify what has been called 'the younger generation-older generation conflict'. The process of the child's education may itself create problems, with new barriers of both speech and thought. As schooling continues or education is resumed elsewhere, the child learns new facts and new ways of thinking which the parent may neither share nor understand. Thus an intelligent adolescent or young adult may develop an awareness of the social, intellectual or educational limitations of his own parents. His ideas, his concepts and the way he thinks have become very different from theirs. For their part, and quite understandably, parents, who have themselves perhaps made sacrifices for the very education that is creating this additional barrier, may react with hostility and resentment. Both parent and child very often seem to conceal their hostility and guilty uneasiness; they find it difficult to acknowledge even to themselves, let alone others. Thus hostility expresses itself in disguised ways. One version of this problem concerns the girl child whose schooling may conflict with the ideas and expectations of her mother about the daily life of the house, e.g. help in dish-washing, care of clothes, bed-making etc. Her wish to read or otherwise pursue her studies may be assessed as 'laziness', and education itself something 'undesirable'. Alternatively parental pressure for educational achievement may be quite excessive in its demands on a child for achievements which are beyond his natural abilities.

Some examination may now be made of differences of ability between children, and the measurements and assessments that can be made in this area, about which there are many misconceptions. In considering these I shall discuss the intellectual and creative aspects of childhood thinking.

Intelligence and Childhood Thinking

The concept of IQ or 'intelligence quotient' is probably more discussed today by laymen than by psychologists. Any idea that it is the principal function of clinical or educational psychologists to 'test IQs' is evidence of out-of-datedness. Good accounts of the acquisition of knowledge about human intelligence are now available (e.g. Jenkins and Paterson (21)), and reference may be made to other statements of modern thinking on this complex and much misunderstood subject (see e.g. Vernon (40), Guilford (16) and Bereday and Lauwerys (1) for important but different statements of the problem).

Intelligence is not a thing. It is a word which has its uses in describing certain attributes of human thinking. Three aspects of intelligence may first be mentioned: (1) that the child's thinking differs from the adult's in some attribute for which 'intelligence' is, at times, an appropriate word; (2) that individual children differ from one another in this attribute; (3) that the same individual may exhibit more intelligent and less intelligent kinds of thinking on different occasions. In this field highly sophisticated techniques are now available, which may be used by those trained to use them to measure intelligence or one or other of its components.

In the study of intelligence we again encounter Galton. Galton's own personality is also of interest in that it provides a good illustration of the phenomenon of unusually high intelligence. In December of 1828 a visitor to the household recorded that young Francis Galton was a prodigy. To indicate what this visitor meant I shall quote what the child had written the previous year to his sister:

My dear Adele,
I am 4 years old and I can read any English book. I can say the Latin Substantives and Adjectives and active verbs besides 52 lines of Latin poetry. I can cast up any sum in addition and can multiply by 2, 3, 4, 5, 6, 7, 8, 10.
I can also say the pence table. I can read French a little and know the clock.

Francis Galton,
Febuary 15th, 1827.

In the reference to multiplication '9' and '11' were included, but crossed out, presumably because Francis thought he might be claiming too much. 'Febuary' is the only spelling error.

In 1904 a certain Dr. Blin and his pupil, Dr. Demayne, were concerned with the other end of the intelligence scale of differences between people. They sought and found a technique for classifying the community of 250 intellectually defective people in their care, employing a prearranged set of questions on twenty topics. Their work impressed Alfred Binet and Theophile Simon (2) as having the advantage of providing a test 'whose questions fixed in advance do not suffer from the bad humour or bad digestion of the examiner'. Binet and Simon themselves evolved a scale of measurement, involving items of increasing difficulty; this they administered to inmates of the Salpêtrière, and to both normal and subnormal children of the Paris schools. Intelligence was defined by Binet and Simon in these terms: '. . . judgment . . ., to judge well, to comprehend well, to reason well, these are the essential activities of intelligence.'

Binet and Simon's test, still in use in forms revised by Terman and others, exerted an important influence on subsequent work. Major investigators in this field have included Spearman, Burt, Thomson, and Vernon in Britain, and in the United States Thurstone, Terman, Kelly, Guilford and Cattell. Major works of these and other authorities may be consulted, and it would be inappropriate here to attempt more than mention of the fact that some highly complex issues surround the analysis of intelligence and its measurement.

Some of the main developments may be mentioned as illustrative. First, there are a large variety of different types of test used in this field. Their use may involve quite different tasks of assessment. If one wishes to determine whether a given child lies in the top 10%, the average group or the bottom 10%, one type of test will be used. If one is dealing with a child of superior intelligence and wants to know its placing within the top 10%, this is a different task requiring a different instrument. Other tests are appropriate to other problems, for example the assessment of subnormal children and their placing within the lower 10% range. Again, a single figure (e.g. an 'intelligence quotient' or IQ, the ratio of mental age to chronological age) may be appropriate for certain purposes; for other purposes one may wish to use a battery of tests which yield a number of figures, allowing one to map the profile of the individual's intellectual mental life, with its strengths and weaknesses. At the lower end of the intelligence scale it may be noted that both 'subnormality' and 'severe subnormality' have found their way into British law in the 1959 Mental Health Act, and that neither are defined in terms of IQ. Today psychologists themselves make increasing use of figures other than the IQ, and often prefer to place the child on a percentile scale within its own age group.

Important studies have been made in such fields as the growth of intelligence as the child develops, and of the subsequent history of individuals assessed as of high intelligence in early life. The respective influences of genetic and environmental influences on intelligence (the latter including schooling) have been much investigated. A frequently used method has been 'twin studies', on the basis of which Burt (7) reports the following correlations:

TABLE 3

Twin Studies

Identical twins reared apart	0·876
Fraternal twins reared together	0·553
Ordinary siblings	0·538

Such figures suggest the importance of genetic influences upon intelligence. Others, e.g. Hebb (17), have shown how experimental control of the environment of young organisms can affect their problem-solving ability at maturity advantageously or otherwise. The same investigator has shown, in investigations with human subjects, that while brain lesions or operations can greatly affect the intelligence of developing organisms, once maturity is reached such lesions or operations may have remarkably little influence on measurable intelligence.

An important field of investigation is the analysis of 'intelligence' into its components. On the whole most of the leading American investigators have adopted the view that intelligence is best considered as composite in this way, e.g. a series of primary mental abilities (compare Thurstone (39), whose standpoint is summarised by Eysenck (10)). A statement of a development of this position is to be found in the article by Guilford already mentioned (16), and Guilford and his colleagues have distinguished fifty different intellectual components or factors. On this doctrine there are, as Guilford puts it, 'at least fifty ways of being intelligent'. In connection with this work I shall now examine another aspect of thinking, 'creative talent', and the vigorous attempts now being made to measure this and its components.

Creative Talent

Burt (8) has argued strongly that, if we take creativity to mean useful creative activities, then intelligence is one essential component: 'Creativity *without* general intelligence produces nothing of interest or value.'

Numerous investigators have worked on the problems of creative thought, but an important impetus to this stemmed from Guilford's Presidential Address to the American Psychological Association in 1950 (15). In this he opposed attempts to account for creativity in terms of general intelligence. Guilford distinguished 'convergent thinking', measured by the usual type of intelligence test, from 'divergent thinking', which plays an important part in creative talent and which is concerned with invention and innovation. Subsequently he distinguished a number of the more important components of this other aspect of thinking, and had much to do with the design of tests for their measurement. In the 1962

Yearbook of Education considerable attention is paid to this problem of assessing creativity, and many of the leading investigators in this field wrote chapters. In one of these Burt develops the view that creativity should not be regarded as a primary faculty, but as a compound with various aspects. Among these he distinguishes: (1) fluency, e.g. unusual flow of ideas; (2) capacity for divergent associations, namely variety of ideas; (3) receptivity to new problems; (4) insight, in the sense of ability to recognise the relevant and essential. These components exhibit different trends of development; for example fluency appears early, diminishes in the primary school period, and revives again in early adolescence. To these it may be suggested can be added the possible relevance of differences of mental imagery that have been examined above. Recently Mednick (28) has reminded investigators of creativity that imagery differences, notably the visualiser-verbaliser dimension, may partly account for differential aptitudes in differing fields of thought. Burt himself has been interested in the imagery variables in relation to reading, and it may be noted that recent Russian work (Krutetski (23)) has concerned itself with the differential abilities of visualisers and verbalisers in relation to mathematical thinking.

The influence of schooling and the educational process upon the creative thinking of the child has engaged the attention of leading investigators. Thurstone (39), for instance, suggests that sometimes we are in danger of confusing 'scholarship' with 'intellectual docility'. As illustration of the adverse influence of the educational system upon divergent thinking, rather than blaming anybody else I shall take an instance involving myself as a university teacher.

Some years ago a former student was writing a laboratory report for me on the subject of intelligence testing. Her report included the following: 'The mental tester is like a little boy fishing, who throws his line with a bent pin on the end of it (his test) into the dark recesses of the mind.' Fortunately my discouragements as a teacher were unsuccessful, creativity prevailed, and the woman in question is now a poetess of some note. But she shouldn't really have written this in a laboratory report!

Some recent researches have opened up this problem of adverse effects of education upon creative talent. The study in question was conducted at Chicago by Getzels and Jackson (14). Two groups of children were investigated: *group A* consisted of those who were in the top 20% for intelligence (mean IQ, 150), but below the top 20% on tests of creativity; *group B* were in the top 20% on creativity tests, but below the top 20% on intelligence tests (mean IQ, 127). Studies were made of the values, aspirations, attitudes, and thought products of the two groups. The 'intelligence' group emerged as distinctly conformist, the 'creative' group as distinctly non-conformist in this analysis. Both groups of children did equally well on attainment tests. Yet when asked to assess the children as to how much they enjoyed having each child as a member of the class, teachers assessed the 'intelligence' group more favourably and the 'creativity' group less favourably than the average pupil. In other words the teachers distinguished between equally high achievers, favouring high intelligence but not high creativity. In many other respects also, emerged evidence of how conflict, and thus pressures from adults (notably teachers and parents), could result in the discouragement of creative talent. Research in this field is progressing vigorously. We need to know a great deal more about socially useful aspects of thinking of all kinds—including the divergent as well as the convergent—and about the best strategies for their encouragement and reinforcement.

3

Soviet Research

Brief mention may be made of the approach of Soviet developmental psychology, which is in certain respects different from that of leading investigators in Britain and America. As O'Connor has pointed out, the Russians do not accept the view of 'a given quantum of intelligence present from birth or from an early age'. Their concepts are different, and general or specific backwardness is dealt with on another basis, with something of the implication that 'intelligence differences' is an explanation that Western psychologists may have somewhat carelessly overworked. One suspects that what the Russians affirm is worthy of more serious attention than what they deny; although it is being vigorously developed in Britain and the United States and elsewhere, psychometric measurement is essentially (and officially) non-existent in the Soviet Union.

What has happened instead? A great deal of work is, in fact, going on in Russian child psychology. This merits mention, less to record its achievements to date than to alert the reader to notice subsequent work developing in this other tradition. Some translations of researches by leading Soviet investigators are now available and may be mentioned, e.g. Simon (36, 37), O'Connor (30), and Mintz (29). Soviet psychologists in rejecting methods of psychometric measurement have devoted themselves to other things, including studies of the unsuccessful learner and of ways of overcoming his backwardness (compare Simon (37)). Studies have been made of arithmetical thinking, of the general development of comprehension in the child, and of how children develop the concepts necessary to understanding such subjects as physics and biology. The important researches of Piaget in Geneva have been excluded from this chapter, as they have already been discussed in an earlier one. But it may be noted that there are similarities between Piaget's studies and the work that is being pursued in the Soviet Union; Piaget himself in 1956 wrote of the 'rich and varied' researches into thinking of the Russian investigators. An intellectual framework for much of this was provided by a major influence on contemporary Russian psychology, Vigotsky (see (36 and (37)), who pointed out in 1954: 'Schooling never begins in a vacuum. All the learning the child meets with in the school has its pre-history.' To illustrate, Fleshner has investigated how, in learning to think with the concepts of scientific physics, the child builds on or overcomes his earlier concepts; he has for example to give up his earlier notions and realise that 'weight' is a property of all objects, not just of those objects he has himself weighed on a scales. Even at 12 to 13 years Fleshner found that children had difficulty in achieving this more abstract way of thinking.

Another aspect of Soviet psychology may be mentioned: its concern with the subject of 'defectology'. Defectology embraces research into all kinds of abnormality in children: blindness, deafness, the deaf-blind child, motor, speech, emotional, and intellectual defects. The Institute of Defectology in Moscow gives a five-year course of training in this subject; an example of its equipment is a device which scans print and transmits tactile signals to the finger-tips of the blind or deaf-blind child. Backwardness, defectology, and the educational psychology of the normal child have, studied in this way, some points of contact. An illustration may be taken in Slavina's work on the intellectually backward child, who is viewed as intellectually passive. Slavina's conception of this child is that he lacks the skills, habits and knowledge needed for successful work; her hypothesis is that this is the result of environment; her method of overcoming this passivity is to carry out didactic tasks in the form of a game in which the child 'wins' when he learns and 'loses' otherwise. Success in overcoming intellectual passivity is claimed on the basis of such methods.

In placing emphasis upon Soviet developments in child psychology, I do not wish to imply that similar work does not go on elsewhere. But the orientation of the Russians is different from our own, and their exploration of familiar issues from their different standpoint may, particularly in interaction with British and American researches, provide some interesting points of growth. Soviet psychology is much concerned with the understanding of thinking, and with the problems of the individual learner in the school, and it is fortunate that some of its findings are now available in translation.

4

Conclusion

In conclusion I would like to reiterate the central theme of this chapter individuals differ from one another, it is not easy to empathise with the mental life of another person, and additional barriers exist to such empathy. Three illustrations may be given as reminders of these differences; they were provided by three adults all of whom today hold responsible posts providing some evidence of intelligence and psychiatric normality. They relate respectively to thinking, remembering, and imagining.

Childhood thinking. At the age of about 5 the child, who was born and reared overseas, could not understand how Dick Whittington came to London 'in a wagon'. This was impossible since people must go to London in a ship. The parents, perhaps more understanding than most, agreed with this piece of concrete, childish thinking: yes, the story teller had made a mistake, and Dick had, of course, come to London in a ship, not a wagon.

Unusual powers of remembering. 'When I was a schoolgirl my mother used to tell me to "study" and, since I had read the lesson and knew it, I simply didn't know what she meant. *She* seemed to think that one learned by reading a thing over and over, and going through some process of iteration called "studying".'

Fluency of imagination. (This is not a case of hypnagogic imagery, which the individual in question also has, but recognises as different.) 'I don't really understand how my imagination works, it is a thing completely beyond my control. . . . I used to shut my eyes and let my mind go free and into it would come what I used to call my "night stories" . . . all kinds of imaginings in story form. . . . I thought all children had the same night stories and was amazed one day when I found they hadn't.'

Much more needs to be ascertained in this field, but a wider awareness of what is already known will reduce avoidable unhappiness, and may assist understanding of thinking, remembering and imagining in childhood.

REFERENCES

1. BEREDAY, G. and LAUWERYS, J., 1962. *The Yearbook of Education, 1962.* London: Evans.
2. BINET, A. and SIMON, TH., 1905. The development of intelligence in children. *L'Année Psychologique*, **11**.
3. BINGHAM, J., 1955. *Do babies have worries?* Pamphlet. London: National Association of Mental Health.
4. BIRCH, L. B., 1963. The teacher as learner. In Symposium on 'The teacher and the learner'. *Bull. Brit. Psychol. Soc.*, **16**: 50.
5. BURT, C., 1925. *The Young Delinquent*, 4th edition, 1957. Univ. of London Press.
6. —— 1938. Factor analysis by sub-matrices. *J. Psychol.*, **6**.
7. —— 1962a. Critical notice: the psychology of creative ability. *Brit. J. Educ. Psychol.*, **32**.
8. —— 1962b. The gifted child. In Ref. No. 1, *q.v.*
9. CAREY, N., 1915. Factors in the mental processes of school children. *Brit. J. Psychol.*, **7**.
10. EYSENCK, H. J., 1953. *Uses and Abuses of Psychology*. London: Penguin Books.
11. FLUGEL, J. C., 1945. *Man, Morals and Society*. London: Duckworth.
12. GALTON, F., 1880. Statistics of mental imagery. *Mind*, **5**: 19.
13. —— 1904. *Inquiries into Human Faculty*. Everyman Library edition, 1919. London: Dent.
14. GETZELS, J. W. and JACKSON, P. W., 1962. *Creativity and Intelligence*. New York: Wiley.
15. GUILFORD, J. P., 1950. Creativity. *Amer. Psychologist*, 444-454.
16. —— 1959. Three faces of intellect. *Amer. Psychologist*, 469-479.
17. HEBB, D. O., 1949. *The Organisation of Behaviour*. New York: Wiley.

18. HURLOCK, R. and BURNSTEIN, A., 1932. The imaginary playmate: a question-
    naire study. *J. Genet. Psychol.*, **41**.
19. HUSCHKA, M., 1944. The incidence and character of masturbation threats in a
    group of problem children. *In* Tomkins, S. S. (ed.), *Contemporary
    Psychopathology*. Harvard Univ. Press.
20. JAENSCH, E. R., 1930. *Eidetic Imagery*. London: Kegan Paul.
21. JENKINS, J. J. and PATTERSON, D. G., 1961. *Studies in Individual Differences:
    the Search for Intelligence*. New York: Appleton-Century-Crofts.
22. KANNER, L., 1935. *Child Psychiatry*. Springfield, Illinois: Thomas.
23. KRUTETSKI, V. A., 1961. Some characteristics of the thinking of pupils with
    little capacity for mathematics. *In* Simon, B. (ed.), 1963, Ref. No. 37, *q.v.*
24. LAY, W., 1898. Mental imagery, experimentally and subjectively considered.
    Psychol. Rev. Monogr. Suppl.
25. McKELLAR, P., 1952. *A Text-book of Human Psychology*. London: Cohen &
    West.
26.   1957. *Imagination and Thinking: a Psychological Analysis*. London: Cohen
    & West.
27. McKELLAR, P. and SIMPSON, L., 1954. Between wakefulness and sleep:
    hypnagogic imagery. *Brit. J. Psychol.*, **45**.
28. MEDNICK, S. A., 1962. The associative basis of the creative process. *Psychol.
    Rev.*, **69**: 3.
29. MINTZ, T., 1958; 1959. Recent developments in psychology in the U.S.S.R.;
    Further developments in psychology in the U.S.S.R. *Ann. Rev. Psychol.*,
    Vols. **8**; **9**.
30. O'CONNOR, N., 1961. *Recent Soviet Psychology*. Oxford: Pergamon.
31. PECK, L. and HODGES, R., 1937. A study of racial differences in eidetic imagery
    of pre-school children. *J. Genet. Psychol.*, **51**.
32. RIVERS, W. H. R., 1920. *Instinct and the Unconscious*. Cambridge Univ. Press.
33. SCHMIDEBERG, M., 1957. Tolerance in upbringing and its abuses. *Internat. J.
    Soc. Psychiat.*, **5**: 2.
34. SHAPIRO, M. B. and RAVENETTE, A. T., 1959. A Preliminary experiment on
    paranoid delusions. *J. Ment. Sci.*, **105**: 439, 295-312.
35. SILBERER, H., 1909. Report on a method of eliciting and observing certain
    symbolic hallucination phenomena. *In* Rapaport, D. (ed.), *The Organisa-
    tion and Pathology of Thought*, 1951. New York: Columbia Univ. Press.
36. SIMON, B., 1957. *Psychology in the Soviet Union*. London: Routledge.
37. SIMON, B. and SIMON, J., 1963. *Educational Psychology in the U.S.S.R.*
    London: Routledge.
38. SUTTIE, I. D., 1935. *The Origins of Love and Hate*. London: Kegan Paul.
39. THURSTONE, L. L., 1952. Creative talent. *In* Thurstone, L. L. (ed.), *Applica-
    tions of Psychology*. New York: Harper.
40. VERNON, P. E., 1955. The psychology of intelligence and 'G'. *Bull. Brit.
    Psychol. Soc.*, **26**.

VIII

EXCEPTIONAL CHILDREN

E. M. BARTLETT

O.B.E., PH.D., F.B.Ps.S.

Formerly Psychologist to the Essex Education Committee

1

Introduction

In identifying the group of children to be discussed here, something must first be said concerning the meaning to be attached to the word 'exceptional'. It will not be used here in the sense in which American educationalists take the term, i.e. as including all types of handicapped children, but as indicating those children who are exceptional in virtue of their superior intelligence. Furthermore although something will be said about special talents, particularly in so far as these give an early indication that a child is of outstanding ability, on the whole the discussion will be confined to the nature of high general intelligence, to the ways in which it reveals itself in the development of children, and to the kinds of problem it is liable to produce in their education and development.

One difficulty here is that almost all the research on this subject has been American, and what is true of the family and social background of highly intelligent children in an American setting and of the effects of their education on their development may not be applicable to English children. To give one example. In a discussion of the records of children referred to the New York Counselling Centre for Gifted Children, it is stated:

> The role that the mothers of highly gifted children frequently play in this family picture is pertinent. They are, in general, women of superior intelligence and unusual drive. They are members of a generation of women for whom innumerable conflicts and frustrations have been created by the rapidly changing role of women in our culture. These conflicts and frustrations present greater problems to these mothers because of their intelligence, superior education, ambition and drive. Many of them show more or less rejection of the traditional feminine role. This rejection is likely to complicate relationships with their children, contributing to two problems that repeat themselves: the mother's rejection to some degree of the child, with the familiar aftermath of guilt,

anxiety and overprotection; and the attempt by the mother to compensate for personal frustration by identifying her own life too closely with that of the gifted child (11).

It is doubtful whether this is equally true of highly intelligent mothers and their children in this country. There is also the problem that fashions change. Many American studies of gifted children state that these children are almost invariably found in very small families, and that this may have an adverse effect on their development because it results in too much attention being focused on them. Until comparatively recently this was probably true of the families of intelligent parents in this country too. But there seems to be a clear trend, even as recently as the last ten years or so, for these parents to desire larger families, four children seeming to be the optimum number, and this may have marked effects on the development and adjustment of the highly intelligent child.

A further difficulty arises from the fact that it is not easy to obtain information about the highly intelligent child unless something has gone wrong with his development or his education. One of the few studies of gifted children made in this country, for example, is that by Mildred Neville, of seventy-eight children with IQs ranging from 140–180 on the Terman Merrill individual test of intelligence who had been referred to a Psychological Centre. Of these seventy-eight children, thirty-five were considered 'difficult' (7). The fascinating information about highly gifted children which is locked up in the files of Child Guidance and Child Psychiatric Clinics up and down the country would also, even if it could be got at, provide rather a biased sample, although it is probably true that some of the difficulties for which these children were referred arose not so much from inherent defects of personality in the children themselves as from misunderstanding and poor handling on the part of the adults concerned in their upbringing.

I have been fortunate, therefore, in that my own studies of gifted children have not been based solely on children presenting problems of one kind or another. My interest in these children was first aroused by their educational problems. As part of my work as psychologist to a Local Education Authority I was given the assignment of advising the Education Committee on the future placement of children in their second year at a Grammar or Technical School who, in the opinion of the Head of the school, were failing to justify the award of a place to them. I have in the past fourteen years interviewed and assessed some eight hundred of such children. A pilot investigation was first carried out, partly to try out the suitability of the battery of tests which it was proposed to use, but also to get some information on the type of children whom the Heads considered 'misfits' and on those whom they considered of average educational proficiency and of outstanding performance as pupils. The selected battery of tests proved to be quite useful and, with certain modifications, was employed during the ensuing years. (More will be said of the findings of these investigations in a later section of the chapter.) I have therefore over the past fourteen years had exceptional opportunities of studying why the gifted child fails to realise his potentialities in the educational field at the secondary school stage.

I have also had very valuable opportunities of studying such children in circumstances where they are using their gifts successfully, since another of my assignments as a psychologist has been concerned with children in the third year of their Junior School life who are considered by their teachers to be so intelligent and outstanding in their school work that they ought to be allowed to begin their secondary school studies a year earlier than the general run of children. During the past six years I have interviewed well over a hundred of these children and discussed them with their teachers and parents, and have examined the records and school work of several hundred more. Follow-up studies have also been carried out on two of the earliest groups of these under-age transfers. Besides this I have, as opportunity occurred, filled out the picture of what highly gifted children are like, by observing and making notes on the very early development of children whose parentage and inheritance would lead one to expect them to be of exceptional ability, and have in some instances been able to follow their development through childhood and into maturity. The present study is therefore based not only on the findings of other researches, but on first-hand contact with the children themselves.

2
Assessment

Demarcation of the Group

Where one draws the line between the exceptional and the normal groups is, of course, arbitrary, partly because intelligence is a continuum and partly because of the inherent unreliability in any one test score. The matter is further complicated by differences in the ways in which the scores on various tests are calculated. If one administers an Intelligence Test such as the Moray House tests of Verbal Reasoning, or the Wechsler Individual Test with its Verbal and Performance Scales, where the scores are arrived at through Percentiles (i.e. by comparing a child's score with that of the whole range of children of his own age), one cannot easily discriminate among the children comprising, say, the top 1% of the population, and will rarely obtain Quotients above 145. On tests such as the various Revisions of the Binet-Simon Scale on the other hand, where the child is given a Mental Age arrived at by a comparison of his performance with that of children both older and younger than himself and even with that of average and superior adults, this Mental Age being finally compared with his own Chronological Age, the 'ceiling' of the test is much higher. It differs moreover at different ages, probably being highest at about the age of ten years.

If one thinks of the group of Exceptional Children as that which is most commonly selected by Local Education Authorities for education in Grammar and Technical Schools, one would draw the line, in terms of general ability, at or near an Intelligence Quotient of 116, cutting off the top 20% of the school population. If one thinks of the group as composed of that top 5% which Sir William Alexander considers is alone genuinely suited for an academic type of education involving advanced study of mathematics and languages, one would draw the line at an Intelligence Quotient of 125. If however one wishes to include only the 'high fliers', one would draw the line at an Intelligence Quotient of 134 or thereabouts, cutting off the top 1% of the population. (These alternative lines have been given in terms of Percentiles, and with reference to quotients based on a Standard Deviation of 15.) If one uses a test such as the Terman Merrill individual test of intelligence one can discriminate quite widely within this top 1%, and can, at certain ages, obtain Quotients which can only be described as astronomical. I have from time to time, in my own testing of children of nine and ten years who were put forward as candidates for early transfer to a selective secondary school, obtained Intelligence Quotients of the order of 180, 185, 195, 197, and even on one occasion of 212, while this group of children have quite commonly obtained Quotients in the 160s and 170s. Quotients of this magnitude have perhaps very little meaning in terms of statistics, but a great deal of meaning in terms of the kind of mental operation which these highly gifted children can perform, and the test results of these children can most profitably be used in this way.

It was this top 1% which Terman selected for his studies of exceptional children. In the first volume of the *Genetic Studies of Genius*, 'The Mental and Physical Traits of a Thousand Gifted Children' (10), he took an IQ of 140 as the lower limit for inclusion in the group where the Terman individual test had been used, and one of 135 on the Terman Group Test. From a school population of about a quarter of a million he identified some 1,470 of these highly gifted children. He later made a more intensive study of those who obtained IQs of 170 or over. Leta Hollingworth also made a special study of children obtaining exceptionally high scores on individual tests of intelligence, and at the time of her death was preparing a book on the subject which was later issued under the title of *Children Above 180 IQ* (5).

Children obtaining IQs of this magnitude are so rare that it is doubtful whether conclusions drawn from a study of them are of very general application to the larger group commonly known as the highly intelligent, fascinating as the facts revealed by such a study are. There is, however, some evidence to support the view that the mental health of children of this degree of intelligence is at greater risk and that they are likely to be referred for psychiatric help in greater numbers, proportionate to the size of their group, than are children of less outstanding ability. Herbert Carroll, for example, in his book *Genius in the Making*, in which he summarises a good deal of research into the characteristics of the highly gifted, concluded that such children have a relatively poorer chance of making good social adjustment than have less brilliant children, and that 'although many children with IQs above 170 succeed in making satisfactory play adjustments, the chances are great that they will not.' (1).

Leta Hollingworth's studies led her to the concept of a socially optimum range of intelligence, above which the individual was likely to be poorly adjusted and socially isolated:

> The psychologist who has observed the development of gifted children over a long period of time from early childhood to maturity, evolves the idea that there is a certain restricted portion of the total range of intelligence which is most favourable to the development of successful and well-rounded personality in the world as it now exists. This limited range appears to be somewhere between 125 and 155 IQ. Children and adolescents in this area are enough more intelligent than the average to win the confidence of large numbers of their fellows which brings about leadership, and to manage their own lives with superior efficiency. Moreover, there are enough of them to afford mutual esteem and understanding. But those of 170 IQ and beyond are too intelligent to be understood by the general run of persons with whom they make contact. They are too infrequent to find many congenial companions. They have to contend with loneliness and with personal isolation from their contemporaries throughout the period of immaturity. . . . There is thus an 'optimum' intelligence from the point of view of personal happiness and adjustment to society, which is well below the maximum. . . . Intellectually gifted children between 130 and 150 IQ seem to find the world well suited to their development. . . . Above this limit, however, the deviation is so great that it leads to special problems of development which are correlated with personal isolation (5).

A good deal of reference, therefore, in the present study will be made to the characteristics and problems of children well up in the top 1% of the school population.

Reliability of Assessments

Two questions about Intelligence Tests remain to be considered. One concerns the reliability of any test results obtained for these exceptional children. There is, as stated earlier, a statistical unreliability in any test result, and as the standard error of a score is directly related to its magnitude, deviations between a child's scores on two similar tests of equal standard deviation and reliability are likely to be the greater, the more intelligent the child. This is not likely however to be so great as to give a false impression, except perhaps in the very early years, and such variations are not of practical significance, since if a child's scores consistently put him in the top 1% of the population, or even in the top 5%, variations within this band of ability are comparatively unimportant. What is more important is whether the test results of these exceptional children are likely to vary, at some ages, by a degree so much greater than the statistical expectation that one misjudges the ability of the child in question. Another way of putting this is: how much prognostic value has the test result of a highly gifted child, and has it the same prognostic value at all ages? How early in life, especially, can one detect, by means of tests, the child who is of exceptional ability? Tests of intelligence given at an early age are likely to be less reliable for all children than those given later. Rating scales based on observation of performance in various fields may also give quite misleading results unless one takes into account the fact that young children, as they develop, have a wide range of skills to try out and perfect. A highly intelligent young child may be caught at a moment when he is concentrating so intensely on the perfection of one skill that he is unresponsive to stimuli designed to assess his level of performance in other directions. Even speech is not always developed unusually early in highly intelligent children. There is the classic example of Carlyle, who was completely dumb until the age of three years, and was thought to be of poor ability because of this, but who startled his parents by a first essay at talking which took the form of 'What ails wee Jock?' when he heard a young visitor crying. Indeed there is some evidence that *not* to develop speech early may be a safeguard where the highly intelligent child's stability and adjustment are concerned (see later, in the section *Mental Health and Adjustment*). It is difficult also, when assessing the abilities of very young children, to exclude the element of sheer 'time in the world', especially where physical and manual skills are concerned. For this reason children of, say, five or six who are of very poor ability may, if tested on a scale such as the Merrill Palmer, which is intended for the first years of life, give too optimistic a picture of their intelligence on the practical side of the test simply because they have had a longer time during which to perfect these physical skills. For the same kind of reason highly intelligent children will sometimes fail to show their true quality on a test such as the Terman Merrill scale, which is very much 'school loaded', because they have not had the opportunity or been in the world long enough to cope with certain of the items. A boy of four, for example, who passed the vocabulary item of this test at a ten-year-level, obtained an IQ much below what such a performance would suggest was the correct one for him (which he later attained) because, not having been to school, and not having been forced in any way by his parents, he was quite unable to deal with some of the items. Another boy, of three years, gave a quite false impression of his ability when tested on the same scale because he happened at the time of testing to be absorbed in the development of speech and was fascinated by the ideas of 'nothing' and 'something'; faced with the picture vocabulary cards, for example, he would only say that they were of 'something' or, in the case of the less realistic items, of 'nothing'. The same boy was also at that time concentrating on perfecting his physical skills and had developed outstanding deftness in manipulating his tricycle in all directions. Much to the disappointment of his mother, he was completely uninterested in books. But three months later he turned from physical skills to more intellectual ones, and showed equally outstanding concentration and interest where books were concerned. It is perhaps this element of concentration that is the most prognostic in the behaviour of gifted children when they are very young. It has been said, for example, that the mentally defective child can be detected at a very early stage by such things as the listless, flabby quality of his sucking, whereas the intelligent baby concentrates well on the business of sucking and co-ordinates all the necessary responses in an unusually competent and advanced way. The same concentrated attention is seen in the way in which such a baby sucks with his eyes riveted on his mother's face; and this intense identification with the mother, if it meets with an equally intense response, may be yet another safeguard against later difficulties of adjustment and one of the surest guarantees of stability in childhood and maturity. It would appear to be intensity, then, rather than precocity, which marks out the highly intelligent child at a very early age, and this almost passionate quality of his thinking and functioning makes it easy to understand why Spearman defined the general element in ability as 'mental energy' (8). A characteristic of this type cannot however be assessed by formal tests, and in general the prognostic value of standardised tests for gifted children is not likely to be high at an early age. But by the age of eight or nine one can obtain a clear indication, through a test situation, of the genuine and lasting quality of the child's intelligence, and by the age of ten or eleven its manifestation is unmistakable.

Genius and Special Gifts

The second of the two remaining questions arising from this discussion of intelligence tests as they concern the highly gifted is whether the assessing of all-round ability is the most useful or the most relevant way of delineating the group. Are we concerned here at all with Genius and with special abilities? If so, what is their relation to general intelligence? Spearman thought that the influence of the general factor in ability diminishes as the individual matures, the specific factors becoming more and more important in successful achievement (9). He considered moreover that this is even more characteristic of people of high intelligence than of the average group. It is certainly true that with the emergence of special bents and the canalisation of interests which comes in adolescence it is increasingly difficult to find tests of general intelligence which give an accurate assessment of outstandingly able individuals, and the exceptional child probably under-tests in adolescence as he does in early childhood.

Spearman also considered that the importance of the general factor in superior functioning varies with the nature of the special ability, being of the order of 4 : 1 in Classics and of 1 : 4 in Music. This raises very interesting questions. To what extent can an individual do outstandingly well in any one direction while possessing only moderately high general intelligence? How far is the outstanding quality of his performance the result of abnormal persistence, of a concentration of all his energies in one direction, and of an unshakeable determination to succeed? Is this exceptional concentration of energy in one direction itself one aspect of high intelligence? One is reminded of the hackneyed definition of genius as an abnormal capacity for taking pains. An interesting light is thrown on this subject by the studies of the early mental traits of three hundred geniuses given in Vol. II of the *Genetic Studies of Genius*. Catherine Cox in that study concludes that, although these outstanding individuals had, in general, heredity above average and superior advantages in their early environment, and were distinguished in childhood by behaviour which indicates an unusually high IQ, they were also characterised by 'persistence of motive and effort, confidence in their abilities, and great strength of character' (2). Yet their probable intelligence, as estimated from an analysis of biographical material, letters, paternal standing and so on, was not invariably high (although of course an IQ arrived at in this way must to some extent be suspect). Two estimates of intelligence were made, one from material referring to the life of the individual up to the age of seventeen, and the other from records concerning the years between seventeen and twenty-six. And it is interesting that the second estimate is usually considerably higher than the first. (This may be additional evidence of the increasing influence of special gifts on performance as maturity is achieved.) Examples of this relatively low pre-maturity rating in terms of IQ are: Gluck 110, Murillo 110, Goldsmith 115, Harvey 120 and Jenner 125.

In certain types of genius, notably in the sphere of music, where the relations to be understood and utilised are relatively abstract and formal and where experience of life is not so essential for successful achievement as it is for example in literature, special gifts may appear very early. But in general it is all-round proficiency, rather than early precocity in any one direction, which would appear to be characteristic of the exceptional child.

3
Some Characteristics

Precocity

In what sense are these exceptional children 'precocious', taking this as meaning that they are outstandingly advanced in their general development in very early childhood, and in particular that they learn such formal school subjects as reading at a very early age? Any conclusions on this matter must, I think, be related to the pattern of nurture and education customary at the time being considered. Terman, in the preface to Vol. II of the Stanford *Genetic Studies of Genius*, supports the conclusion of the author that there is always evidence of very superior abilities in the early childhood of the genius, and says that 'the traits which make for prodigious performance in manhood are probably in evidence as budding capacities in the child'; and the case studies which follow give many examples of the extraordinary early performances of the selected geniuses. Galton, for example, whose IQ was estimated as 200, could point to all the letters of the alphabet before he could speak, and when he was two-and-a-half years old had read a book called 'Cobwebs to Catch Flies'. John Stuart Mill, estimated to have an IQ of 190, 'had no childhood; his interests and activities were mature from the first'. He began to learn Greek at three, read Plato at eight, and at six-and-a-half wrote a history of Rome. Coleridge went to school at the age of two, and by the age of six was considered ready for a Grammar School, where he outstripped everyone. Before he was five he had read the *Arabian Nights* (and after it was 'haunted by spectors'). Tasso is said by the historians to have done 'incredible things at the age of six months', expressing his wants in sentences and answering questions. He studied grammar at three years, and by the age of seven was 'pretty well-acquainted with the Latin and Greek tongues'. In considering facts such as these one must of course take into account that in former centuries only those children who were from cultured homes and who were therefore presumably of good inheritance had any education at all, and that for all such children education began very early and was entirely formal and academic. But the Terman studies ((10), p. 271) also found very early proficiency in school subjects, particularly in reading, among children at the time the investigations were made; of 552 children, 1·6% learnt to read before the age of three, 6·1% before the age of four, and 20·5% before the age of five. Parallel evidence for English children is very scanty, but although doubtless some, if not all, highly gifted children in this country *could* learn to read at this very early age, my impression is that on the whole they do not. There is a healthy tendency today not to force formal learning on young children, and even the most gifted of them seem on the whole, if left to themselves, not to want to learn to read much before the age of five or six years. Some of them moreover, even at that age, do not seem particularly quick at learning. By the age of six or seven however almost all of them read fluently and with avid pleasure, sometimes disliking school because, as one boy put it, 'They don't let you do enough reading there. You see, reading is my hobby.'

Apart from formal learning, the exceptional child picks up an enormous amount of incidental knowledge and often pursues one interest along very unusual lines. Fossils and prehistoric animals are two that come to mind, both in boys of five years. My own feeling is that undue precocity of an intellectual type is not to a child's ultimate advantage. Indeed, as was stated earlier, some of these exceptional children seem stubbornly to resist any attempt to force them or to teach them prematurely, as if some unconscious mechanism is at work to safeguard them from early and harmful exploitation.

An interesting example of the dangers of too early forcing is afforded by the experience of John Middleton Murray. His early history also illustrates very clearly the frustrations and difficulties affecting the brilliant child of a generation ago born into a family in poor circumstances and with few cultural advantages. In his book *Between Two Worlds* he describes how he suffered as a very small child by being made the victim of his father's thwarted ambitions, and how his precocity and only too sensitive response to teaching led to anxiety, nervousness and resentment, ending in complete hostility and rejection of his father, and to a feeling of 'belonging nowhere'. He had learnt to read at the age of two, and at two-and-a-half went to school, where he surprised his teacher by his ability to 'pipe the multiplication table up to twelve times without a mistake'. At seven he was in Standard Ex-seven (the highest in the school) and was learning 'algebra up to quadratics, a good deal of chemistry, and geology', and had written impromptu an essay on Gothic architecture. This grim education, in his own words, 'involved the complete obliteration of a child's childhood' and produced 'a timid little boy who would not sleep without a knotted towel for company' to save him from nightmares (6).

Family Background

Both in the Terman studies of gifted children in the nineteen-twenties and in the analysis made by Catherine Cox of the records of three hundred geniuses of the past, emphasis is placed on the superior heredity and family background of the outstanding individual. The great majority of the children and adults who were studied came from distinguished or professional families, in which the cultural level was high and in which the child had every encouragement to satisfy his growing curiosity, develop intellectual interests and mature along a wide front. My own studies confirm this. Many, indeed almost all, of the children who did outstandingly well at school at the primary stage were not only exceptionally intelligent but came from families where there was either a tradition of education and culture or where these things were valued even if the parents did not have the chance of extended education themselves. On the other hand, where this was not so, the child, although doing well at the primary school stage, often seemed to peter out later on in the secondary school. This raises the important question of how far, given good innate potential, the exceptional *development* of the gifted child depends on environmental and cultural factors. The American psychologist Hebb emphasises the importance of these environmental factors, and distinguishes what he calls 'Intelligence A', which he defines as 'innate potential, the capacity for development, a fully innate property that amounts to the possession of a good brain and a good neural metabolism', from 'Intelligence B', which is 'the functioning of a brain in which development has gone on, determining an average level of performance or comprehension by the partly grown mature person'. He adds, 'If the effects of early experience are more or less generalised, one can concede a major effect of experience on the IQ', and adds that 'an innate potential for development is not logically a guarantee that the development will occur' (4). Most English psychologists would support this conclusion, and the contemporary view of the nature of intelligence is shown in such things as the change of title in the Moray

House and other Group Tests from 'Tests of Intelligence' to 'Tests of Verbal Reasoning'. My own research suggests that, in the early stages, the effects of unfavourable environment and nurture upon innate potential are damaging in inverse ratio to the degree of a child's inborn intelligence. Children of less intelligence, born into families of equally poor ability where they receive little stimulation or cultural encouragement, seem held back in the development of even that degree of innate potentiality which they possess; in the highest reaches of the ability scale, on the other hand, the effects of a poor family background do not seem so damaging in the early stages, and by the time the Junior School stage is reached these clever children seem to have made up through reading, the radio and perhaps above all through television for the deficiencies of their environment. In the later stages of education these adverse effects are undoubtedly extremely severe, especially during early adolescence when the child has to make the vital transition from the possession of general all-round intelligence to the development of intellect and of special gifts. One can moreover sometimes see the shadow of things to come even before adolescence. Some of the children I interviewed as candidates for early transfer to a selective secondary school came from homes which were obviously lacking in culture and intellectual stimulus, and even at the age of nine this was often reflected in the children's general attitude to education. One girl, for example, said that she wanted to go to a technical school and take a commercial course (although she could easily have succeeded in a grammar school course leading to an honours degree at a University) because she thought it was 'better for a poor man's child'. Another girl from a similar background had no ambition higher than hairdressing, while an exceptionally able boy had not grown beyond the childish stage of wanting to be an engine-driver. This choice of a career seems a quite significant pointer, at the age of nine or ten, not only to the child's present state of maturity but also to the likelihood of his continuing to develop in accordance with his potential. Several of those children who professed ambitions not in keeping with their ability did not fulfil their early promise, in some cases to such a degree that the Heads of the secondary schools doubted the accuracy of the earlier assessment. There may be several factors at work here. The choice of a career may itself be only another reflection of the cultural level of the home, at least where the child is identifying with that level and with the interests of his parents. The children from cultured, professional backgrounds certainly expressed ambitions which on the whole reflected this. One boy, for example, wanted to be an archeologist. TV may have had something to do with this, but why did he select archeology from all the other possible ambitions? His explanation was that it was because 'I like digging up old bones'. Another boy wanted to be a research scientist, and had rigged up a complicated system of floodlighting for his bedroom. He told me regretfully that it had to be run off an old car battery 'because, of course, I'm not allowed to fiddle with the mains'. Yet another boy, who at the age of nine obtained an IQ of 212 on the Terman Merrill individual test, said that he wanted to design motor cars, and that he knew that for this he would have to study aerodynamics, which he explained as 'the behaviour of the wind when it passes over a car'. Other expressed ambitions were: a commercial artist, a famous violinist, an author, an explorer. When a child at the age of eight or nine is identifying to this extent with the adult world, and is moreover carrying out his ambition in his practical activities, it obviously indicates a good level of emotional maturity. It may also be a guarantee of later stability and satisfactory development in that it is already providing the child, before the stresses of puberty and adolescence overtake him, with an integrating, steadying interest and a satisfying motive for maturing.

Reasoning

A characteristic of highly gifted children which appears very early and which is probably one of the most reliable indications of later superiority is the capacity for reasoning. At an early age this capacity, like many others, cannot easily be assessed by formal intelligence tests, since these have necessarily to be embodied in 'situations' and so involve facets of experience which a particular child may or may not have run up against. But the exceptional child very clearly reveals his ability to use relations and arrive at relevant conclusions in the course of his natural, everyday experience, and particularly in the service of fantasy and play. Because it is in fantasy and play, his reasoning processes are often not recognised for what they are, so that it is said for instance that an average child is not capable of genuine ratiocination until the age of eight. There is, I think, something significant about the age of eight, where formal reasoning is concerned, even for the highly intelligent child, but it is an emotional significance rather than an intellectual one. The Raven Progressive Matrices test of reasoning, for example, requires a certain degree of emotional maturity in a child before it gives a reliable estimate of his ability. (Raven himself says that the scores of children under the age of eight are not reliable.) The reason for this seems to be that the test requires the child to detect what principle he must use in solving each set of problems, keep this in mind throughout, and apply it to increasingly difficult items. To do this demands a degree of maturity not found in the average child until the age of eight, and not, I think, often found even in the highly intelligent child much before this age. At the age of eight however a test such as the Matrices, which is relatively independent of experience and teaching, seems to give the same clear indication of exceptional ability as does the Terman Merrill test at the age of ten. I gave the Matrices test to a fairly large number of children of eight, nine and ten who were considered by the Heads of their schools to be the most outstanding in their year. They often obtained scores which were so high as to be right outside the scale—e.g. Raw Scores of 43, 50, 54 where the 95th Percentiles for the age group were

38, 41 and 48 respectively. (It is an interesting comment on the reasoning capacity of these exceptional children that an adult doctor of philosophy and research scientist who consented to do the test for me while his eight-year-old daughter was being tested achieved a score of only 56!) In view of this outstanding ability to reason, one wonders just how restricting and unstimulating the work in the primary school may sometimes appear to these children, and whether lack of adequate challenge to their abilities at this stage may not be one of the reasons why some of them fail to fulfil their earlier promise at the secondary stage (see the section on the Intelligent School Failure, p. 207).

If it were correct that the average child only becomes capable of genuine logical thought at the age of eight, it would follow that even the exceptionally intelligent child would not reach this stage until the age of four or five, whereas in the service of play and fantasy these children appear to use the fundamental concepts of logic even at the age of two, although they cannot use the language of logic and are not aware of the nature of the rules and principles they are using. A two-year-old boy, for example, whose brother of five had just begun school and who bitterly resented not being able to go with him, invented a school of his own, complete with a register of imaginary children possessing the most bizarre and intriguing names. When his brother, infuriated by the loss of prestige which this caused him, said desperately, 'You *don't* go to school; you *know* you don't', the younger boy replied blandly, 'You don't know what I do. You're always gone when I go.' A little later, in reply to an aunt who, hoping to call his bluff, said she would come to meet him after school one day, he stated with equal imperturbability and with no further comment, 'I've got two doors to my school.' One of the most fruitful ways, therefore, of detecting the child of unusual ability at an early stage will be to watch his spontaneous play and to assess the quality of the reasoning processes he employs in this and in his fantasy.

Vocabulary

There is some difference of opinion whether verbal facility is a special ability or merely a sign of good general intelligence. On the whole, the two would seem to go together. But in the early stages the breadth of a child's vocabulary is at least partly conditioned by the cultural level of his home, although he needs intelligence to profit from the opportunities it provides for him. It was suggested earlier that not all exceptional children develop speech precociously; by the age of three or four however they seem in general to be keenly interested in words and eager to try out new forms of phrase. This they often do by 'playing the sedulous ape', reproducing whole phrases without fully understanding the meaning of each word, but savouring with relish the feel of the whole on their tongue. A four-year-old, commenting on some paper witches' hats made for her sister and herself by an aunt, remarked, 'You know, she's really made these hats remarkably well, considering her age.' By the age of eight or nine the interest in language has often reached fever-heat, and the child goes about all the while with ear cocked for new words. A girl of this age, in the course of a tea-party, asked the meaning of 'indicative', 'pandemonium' and 'precocious', pouncing on them as they occurred in the conversation of the adults, finally shouting triumphantly, 'That's three new words I've learnt today.'

This superior verbal facility is seen at its clearest at the age of ten or eleven, and is probably largely responsible for the phenomenally high IQs which children can obtain at that age. Wide reading together with a maturing power of expression enable them to give surprisingly adult definitions of words, and extremely clear analyses of their mental processes. Examples of the former are 'harpy' defined as 'a legendary monster with a woman's head and with wings', 'flaunt' as 'to behave proudly', 'frustrate' as 'being prevented from doing something you've planned' and 'shrewd' as 'very much to the point in your answers'. One illustration of the latter must suffice. A boy of nine, having successfully solved the problem (in the Most Superior Adult group of the Terman Merrill test) of the growing tree, employing the more complex method of arithmetical progression, remarked casually, 'I could see it was a kind of series'.

4

Some Problems

Mental Health and Adjustment

Questions of mental health and adjustment belong more properly to chapters on psychiatry than to one on the psychology of highly gifted children. It is, however, relevant to the present chapter to survey those factors in the innate constitution and in the development of these children which make for good adjustment or bad.

On the credit side there is, firstly, the fact mentioned earlier that the intelligent baby usually sucks in a competent, energetic fashion. His obvious satisfaction in feeding is likely to evoke in his mother an answering pleasure and satisfaction as being a 'good provider', so that a warm, close relationship, favourable to a feeling of security, is established from the beginning. This is reflected in the way the baby sucks with his eyes riveted on the mother's face. Superior intelligence is also of great assistance to the child, as he grows up, in finding alternative and more mature satisfactions for the primitive and infantile ones he is constantly having to give up. This is particularly obvious in his play and in the exploration and mastery of his environment, each new conquest adding to his self-confidence and self-satisfaction. The easy and successful acquisition of speech also helps him to externalise, communicate and understand his feelings, thus freeing himself from their overwhelming intensity. Furthermore his superior powers of reasoning should help him to understand and generalise when situations of discipline and control arise, and thus to accept cheerfully the necessary limitations on his freedom and desires.

When the highly intelligent child goes to school he usually settles well because he welcomes the opportunity for new and more challenging experiences. He finds the work easy and so learns successfully, and wins the approval of his teachers. His confidence in his own powers leads him to trust adults and to expect to be liked, so that he is cheerful and easy to control. Whatever may be his relationship with others of his own age at a later stage, at the Junior School stage the intelligent child is usually popular and accepted as a leader, his success in school work and at sport winning for him the warm-hearted, generous admiration so characteristic of children at this stage.

In adolescence too the gifted child has many things in his favour. It is then, probably, that he first clearly sees himself as an exceptional person, and feels the full exultant force of the powers within himself. Many alternative routes to maturity lie open to him, and he has endless sources of consolation if things go wrong.

On the debit side, most of the highly intelligent child's difficulties in adjustment would seem to spring from what is perhaps an almost unavoidable imbalance between the varying facets of his development. Emotional maturity in particular is likely to lag behind intellectual growth, since in this sphere there would seem to be no substitute for time. The effects of this are the more severe because the child's superior vocabulary and reasoning ability make adults forget that he is really only a small child, so that they expect a greater degree of emotional control and maturity than he is capable of. His intellectual superiority and his sometimes sharp tongue, coupled with his small size, may make him unpopular with other children and lead to loneliness and bitterness, as he is bored by children of his own age yet not welcomed as a companion by those older than himself.

This imbalance is perhaps most likely to have an adverse effect on the child's growth and adjustment during the period, at about the age of two or three years, when he must solve the problems of love, hate and authority. The behaviour of children at this stage is often so exaggerated and bizarre that one easily accepts Freud's theory that human beings are born insane and only gradually become sane under the pressure of experience. Mercifully the ordinary child gets through this period with very little awareness, if any, of the kind of figure he is cutting, and so is able to repress his guilty feelings with the minimum of anxiety; but what of the greater self-awareness of the highly intelligent child? Is he already, at two or three, able to some extent to step outside himself and appreciate what kind of person he is presenting to the world? Does he metaphorically kick himself for a fool after one of his tantrums and find it difficult to recover his serenity, where the less intelligent child passes easily to some new and distracting experience?

Other difficulties in the adjustment of the highly intelligent may arise, particularly in adolescence and the early years of maturity, from their outstanding capacity to become absorbed in what is occupying their interest at the moment. This sometimes makes them unaware of the effect on others of what they say and do, with the result that they are thought callous, selfish and indifferent when they may be merely innocently single-minded. One of the most astonishing examples of this is the young Shelley, apparently completely unaware of the devastating effect which the public-ation of his pamphlet on the necessity for atheism would inevitably have on the Oxford of his day, and suggesting quite seriously to Harriet, his first wife, when he felt he 'must' abandon her for Mary Godwin, that she should come abroad with them and continue to live with him 'as a sister'.

Adolescence is also likely to bring especial problems to the highly intelligent because their intellectual superiority and sensitiveness lead them to worry about the 'state of the world' whereas their immaturity makes them helpless to do anything about it, while they lack the stability and cynicism of the adult which make injustice, insecurity and the like bearable. This sometimes leads to indecision, undue introspection, or even to com-plete withdrawal. One outstandingly intelligent boy in this state of mind refused to attend school or to go out of the house, but spent all his time trying to invent a 'device' which would make it impossible for opposing armies to attack each other.

Finally, a word about discipline during adolescence. The last few years at school are likely to be almost intolerable for the intelligent adoles-cent if he does not receive easy, sensitive handling. He feels himself mature intellectually, knows he is capable of managing his own affairs, and some-times sees no reason why he should obey rules which he thinks senseless or submit to the natural concern of his parents for his welfare. Left to himself he usually orders his affairs quite sensibly, but any attempt to advise or control him may be taken as a challenge to his maturity and lead to endless argument and bitter resentment. Difficulties of this kind will be the greater if, as sometimes happens, an exceptionally intelligent child is born of parents who are apparently of only average ability, or who even if intelligent have had no chance of prolonged education and are not interested in the things of the mind. Such a child, particularly during adolescence, will be bored, frustrated and unhappy, not understood by his parents and often despising them in return.

Underfunctioning

There is a good deal of concern in America at the present time about the failure of highly gifted children and young adults to function education-ally at a level appropriate to their ability, and the American system of education, with its emphasis on equality of opportunity, has been blamed for this. Professor Miriam Goldberg (3),[1] in a report on work carried out

---

[1] I am indebted for this information to Prof. A. H. Passow, of Teachers College, Columbia University.

at the De Witt Clinton High School, refers to these children as 'potential giants who perform like pygmies', and describes various steps which have been taken to help them realise their potentialities. The main conclusion drawn from these American studies is that the highly intelligent child who does not do well at school is usually either maladjusted or has been adversely affected by unfortunate home conditions. Miriam Goldberg found, for example, that the lack of a satisfactory father figure, through death or divorce or illness, was one of the most influential factors in the school failure of clever boys: 10% of the research group had this factor in their circumstances, as against 3% among the group doing well at school.

Is this equally true of English children? One has to distinguish here between the clever child who is not working up to his own capacity, and the clever child who is doing so badly as to be dubbed a school failure. It is probably true that the exceptional child rarely works to capacity in school, even though he may be quite successful there and is considered an outstanding scholar. This may simply be because it is in fact extremely difficult to 'stretch' him sufficiently in the earlier stages of school life, because of his lack of experience and of that 'time in the world' to which reference was made earlier. His Reading Age, for example, will usually lag behind his Mental Age simply because of the disparity between the vocabulary he could pronounce and read and the content which he could understand and be interested in. But this underfunctioning in the early stages, due to lack of challenge, may sometimes lead to underfunctioning in the second sense, particularly in clever children who are emotionally immature. In my own investigations into the causes of school failure among highly intelligent children at the secondary school stage there was a constantly recurring factor of this emotional immaturity, often coupled with an actual 'youngness' which in itself made the transfer to the less personal atmosphere of a selective school difficult. These children had had very little to contend with at the Junior School stage, particularly if this had been in a small rural Primary School, as they could be the outstandingly successful pupils there without much effort. On transfer to the Secondary School, where they had to compete with children as clever as or abler than themselves, they were unable to accept the challenge, taking refuge in such things as neurotic illness, truancy, resentment, laziness and ill-temper in order to 'justify' their failure.

My own studies also support the American view that, although high intelligence normally leads to success at school, it does not, in itself, guarantee it. Of 715 children in their second year at a Grammar or Technical school, doing so badly that a transfer to a less exacting type of education was considered necessary, seventy children obtained on an individual test IQs between 130 and 135, sixty-five between 135 and 140, seventy-three above 140 and a fair number in the 150 to 160 range. I found also the same recurring pattern of maladjustment and adverse home conditions. Each year a very high proportion of the children, amounting to some 37%, seemed so emotionally disturbed that a psychiatric investigation was necessary. The children showed their maladjustment in depression, anxiety, restlessness, day-dreaming and inability to concentrate, and their work was consistently poor, being untidy, inaccurate, meagre and badly spelt. They were almost all unpopular with the staff, and their behaviour was often so bad that it seemed as if they had some inner compulsion to bring down rebuke and punishment upon themselves. Their family circumstances also exhibited the common pattern of broken homes, loss of a parent (usually the father) through death or divorce, ill-health in one or other of the parents. The children themselves too, either as cause or effect of their failure, seemed often in poor health and lacking robustness and stamina. All these factors seemed more damaging in their effect if the child came from a family in poor financial circumstances and of a low cultural level.

Facts such as these emphasise the necessity for reasonably good nurture and favourable environmental conditions if the child of high intelligence is to realise his potential and maintain a sound state of adjustment.

REFERENCES

1. CARROLL, H. A. *Genius in the Making*. New York: McGraw-Hill Book Co. Quoted in Ref. 11, p. 93.
2. Cox, C. The Early Mental Traits of Three Hundred Geniuses. In Ref. 10, Vol. II: 216-8.
3. GOLDBERG, M. A Three Year Experimental Program at the De Witt Clinton High School to Help Bright Underachievers.
4. HEBB, D. O. *The Organization of Behaviour*: 294.
5. HOLLINGWORTH, L., 1942. *Children Above 180 IQ*: 264-6. New York: World Book Co.
6. MURRAY, J. M. *Between Two Worlds*, Ch. I.
7. NEVILLE, E. M. Brilliant children: with special reference to their particular difficulties. *Brit. J. Educ. Psychol.*, 7, Nov. 1937.
8. SPEARMAN, C. *The Nature of Intelligence and the Principles of Cognition*, Ch. IX.
9. *The Abilities of Man*: 219.
10. TERMAN, L. M. *et al. Genetic Studies of Genius*. Vol. I, Mental and Physical Traits of a Thousand Gifted Children. Stanford Univ. Press.
11. WITTY, P. (ed.). *The Gifted Child*: 100. The American Association for Gifted Children. Boston: D. C. Heath & Co.

IX

NORMAL CHILD DEVELOPMENT AND
HANDICAPPED CHILDREN

ELSPETH STEPHEN
M.A., DIP.ED.

Principal Psychologist, Fountain and Carshalton Hospital Group, Surrey

AND

JEAN ROBERTSON
B.Sc., DIP.PSYCHOL.

Senior Psychologist, Fountain and Carshalton Hospital Group, Surrey

---

1

Introduction

In this chapter we have attempted to outline a developmental approach to handicapped children. Our definition of a developmental approach is the application of the facts of normal child development to the guidance of handicapped children. The success of a developmental approach depends on two things:

1. That the facts of normal child development are established;
2. That the application of this knowledge to handicapped children does help them.

We propose to discuss knowledge of certain aspects of child development, and then to show some of the specific ways in which this knowledge can be applied to help groups of handicapped children.

We have chosen the areas of child development and the groups of children about whom we know most. Therefore this is neither a complete review of the literature on child development, nor an exhaustive demonstration of this developmental approach. We hope rather that it is an outline which will be further filled in and expanded by other people. As psychologists we are interested in psychological aspects of child development and the knowledge we discuss is derived from the work of psychologists and paediatricians. Yet it is clear that child development belongs to many disciplines. Already other specialists are realising the need to think developmentally in relation to children, and are establishing developmental norms in their own specialities.

In this chapter we have divided knowledge of child development into certain areas, i.e. perception, relationships, self-help and intelligence. This may be criticised as a fragmental and partial approach, since it cannot give the whole picture of a child's development. On the other hand there will be overlapping between areas, and we think that at present this is a useful way in which to approach the study of children, for although if one looks at each individual aspect one may miss some of the dynamic interrelationships, one will not go very far wrong provided one has considered all the essential areas. We have not attempted to describe the development of children psychoanalytically because this is covered in another chapter and it is outside our competence; but in applying our knowledge of normal child development we should be able to throw up any anomalies, as in the case of emotional disturbance in children, thereby allowing them to be referred to the appropriate experts.

2

Relationships

An important feature of the lives of a large number of handicapped children is that, even though they may not be permanently hospitalised, they spend many years either going into hospital for various periods of time or living in usually restricted conditions at home. Because of this the frequency and nature of their contacts with others differ in various degrees from those experienced by a non-handicapped child living in a normal environment. The question arises, therefore, to what extent these variations disrupt the pattern of development of social skills and relationships. If some disrupting influences can be demonstrated, in what ways can their effects be prevented or counteracted, and to what extent remedied at a later date?

In a normal environment the child is handled most frequently by one person, usually the mother. As he grows older he learns to distinguish between the members of his family and to learn what to expect of them and what they expect of him. His knowledge of people gradually widens, both his emotions and the type and intensity of his relationships become differentiated, and he learns to inter-act with his peers. By the time he is of school age he is beginning to deal with others in a wide variety of social situations, has acquired a number of skills, particularly that of verbal communication, and shows capacity for differential emotional attachments to other individuals.

General Effects

This pattern is in many ways altered for the handicapped child. If he is in hospital throughout, he may have little opportunity of getting to know a few people well and of differentiating their roles. In a hospital the complexity of his environment is not easily reduced, and he himself may be required to cope with only a limited number of situations, so that he may be totally unequipped for the complexity of everyday life. It can be seen that loss of vision and hearing will directly interfere with the establishment of communication and the differentiation and subsequent integration of the environment, while locomotor difficulties may prevent the child from investigating his surroundings freely. Because of difficulties in moving them, or because they look or behave oddly, many such children are restricted to the home and thus deprived of a wide variety of experiences. The way in which a handicapped child is penalised by his appearance is often far-reaching. Abercrombie (1) notes how talking to a child with disordered eye movements often disturbs the listener, which in turn upsets the speaker. The restrictions on the parents imposed by these children, together with ambivalent feelings towards them, may severely disrupt the relationships within the family. Tizard and Grad (46), in a survey of the effects of mentally backward children on family life, conclude that 15% of families with a defective child living at home have 'severely limited' social contact, and quote the following as a typical case:

A young mother, 6 months pregnant, with two young children, one of them a mongol, had not been out of the house for 2 months. She could not manage the children in the pram since they fought so much. She was unwilling to ask relatives to look after the mongol, who was excitable, difficult and demanding, and who would not be parted from his mother. The shopping was done by the husband and the woman was lonely and unhappy.

The attitudes of the parents are clearly very important for the emotional adjustment of the child and his subsequent ability to cope with his handicap, and the importance of help and support to the family as a whole must be stressed.

Verbal Communication

One of the most important skills for normal social development is the ability to communicate verbally. Two main questions must be considered. To what extent do the earlier experiences of the child affect his acquisition of speech? And is it necessary for him to have close contact with a single or at the most two or three individuals, as opposed to the relatively large and constantly changing staff on a ward?

In one of a series of studies Lyle (26) compared the speech development of two matched groups of imbecile children at the Fountain Hospital, 21 with traumatic home experiences and 21 without. He found that disturbances in mother/child relationships before entry to the institution were negatively associated with present verbal ability. Some of the factors included among traumatic experiences were: the child had been placed in a residential nursery before being placed in the hospital; the child was officially classified as a neglected child; the social worker stated that the child was being seriously neglected or ill-treated by the mother; or the mother was definitely disturbed (psychotic or neurotic) and had sought psychiatric treatment for these disorders.

In general it is easier to learn any skill from one fairly consistent teacher giving intensive stimulation than from a number of people with whom one spends only a short time. This will apply for example to toilet training and feeding, where regular patterns of reinforcement are most easily carried out by one person. In addition, particularly where speech is involved, the desire and incentive to learn will be important, and will most probably be strongest where the child is involved in a close relationship. In an experiment on methods of residential care of mentally handicapped children (Tizard (44)), a group of imbeciles were placed in a small unit in which the aim was to make their environment as much like a normal nursery school as possible. There was no formal curriculum but group activities were encouraged, and the children were divided into 'families' and cared for by house-mothers; both increased social interplay between the children themselves and close relationships with one adult resulted. Lyle (27) showed that, over a period of 18 months, this group made significant gains in verbal ability as compared with a matched group remaining in ordinary hospital wards. Any programme which decreases the number of people dealing with an individual child and allows nurses to care for particular children would be expected to be beneficial.

Co-operation

Besides inter-acting with and learning from adults, the child inter-acts with other children and gradually through his play learns to co-operate, a skill basic to becoming integrated in any group. Piaget (35) traces the way in which, from the age of 7 years onwards, the child begins to appreciate the true functions of rules in enabling games to be played. From 3–7 years he obeys rules because they are 'obligatory and sacred', as contrasted with the 12-year-old who regards the same rules as valid only after they have been mutually agreed upon and as existing in order to render co-operation and reciprocity possible. Parten and Newhall (34) present a play scale which traces the degree of social participation and the growing interest of the child in others. At first he plays independently with his interest centred on his own activity; next he watches others play (onlooker behaviour), and then chooses behaviour which brings him amongst other children but which does not influence their activity. Eventually he begins to play with others, he borrows and lends, but each child does as he wishes; only later he plays in a group organised for some goal (co-operative play).

If importance is attached to the role of group play, care must be taken to provide opportunities not only for children actually to play together but also for them to go through the earlier stages, where their inter-action is not so obvious to the observer. Physically handicapped children or children confined to bed rely a great deal on adults to provide such situations. Those who cannot move themselves can be sat facing each other; close proximity will be particularly important to children who cannot see; children who cannot hear must have specially good chances of seeing others, although, as with all other children, seeing from a distance is not enough.

Emotion

Along with the ability to co-operate successfully in a group, the capacity for normal emotional response is of major importance both in early development and in later life. A good deal of work has been done on the effects of maternal separation and hospitalisation on the development of these capacities. Many handicapped children face a whole series of short-term admissions, to enable operations and investigations to be carried out, whereas for others the problems are those of long-term hospitalisation.

The general picture of distressed and disturbed emotional behaviour presented by a young child coming into hospital has been extensively described. Bowlby (6) claims that it is primarily a reaction to the stress and frustration of separation from the mother, while Woodward (51) has suggested that repeated experience of the unfamiliar is the essential way in which adverse circumstances make an impact on the child: he has inadequate information with which to deal with the situation in which he is placed, and is constantly faced with uncertainties.

Schaffer (41) has described post-hospitalisation syndromes appearing in young infants on their return home from hospital. He studied 76 normal infants admitted for a variety of medical and surgical reasons, with ages on admission ranging from 3–51 weeks and duration of stay ranging from 4–49 days. Two distinct syndromes emerged, each closely associated with a particular age range, with a cutting point of approximately 7 months, and comparatively little overlap. Under 7 months the baby showed extreme preoccupation with his environment, while over 7 months the central feature was over-dependence, including continued clinging to the mother and fear of strangers. The mean duration for the latter syndrome was 14·69 days but its range from 1–80 days. Schaffer links this change of pattern to the cognitive stage reached, referring to Anthony (2) who had previously deduced from Piaget's material (36, 37) that the infant's reaction to separation from the mother after 7 months would take on a new quality different from that observed previously. The cognitive changes occurring at this period will be discussed more fully in the section dealing with perception and the development of the body image (and see p. 220).

It seems likely that these problems can be tackled fairly directly by allowing the mother to be with the child as much as possible, or, failing this, by arranging for one or two nurses to deal with him so that at least he is not confronted by a constant flow of strangers. It is probably justifiable to doubt the existence of important long-term effects on the majority of children experiencing a single admission to hospital, although clearly one would wish to avoid even temporary stress. However other information is needed; a series of admissions may present a very different picture, and the occurrence of longer-lasting effects in a minority of cases cannot be precluded. There is also the possibility of disturbances arising when the child returns home if the parents have not been prepared for his unusual behaviour, or are very distressed by it.

The additional problems of the long-stay patient must now be considered. Bowlby (6) concluded that prolonged separation from the continuous care of a mother or mother substitute causes a variety of personality disturbances, of which the 'affectionless character' is the most characteristic and the most serious. Goldfarb (13) found marked differences between a group of foster-children who had spent most of the first 3 years of their lives in an institution, and a group who had from their early months lived with foster-families. These differences he attributed to the lack of opportunity for developing relationships with adults during the early years. Munday (29) points out that the hospitalised individual usually finds it best to behave quietly and inconspicuously, which in the long run probably limits drives and aspirations. The more normal a person's intelligence, the more frustrating this is likely to be; and, as she says (and this might well apply to many of the physically handicapped), one would expect a child 'growing up with inadequate affective contacts, insufficient opportunities to learn and exposed to frustrating experiences, to function at a more primitive level'.

The quality of social and emotional responses shown by children living in hospital, however, does vary a great deal. Woodward (51) described the responses of 90 hospitalised severely subnormal children, with levels of intellectual development similar to normal children up to the age of 2 years. Those who reacted to a social approach with distressed or avoiding reactions were significantly differentiated from the rest of the group by their pre-admission experiences: 73% of the former had lived in adverse material or emotional circumstances, while only 30% of the latter had suffered in this way. A subsequent study (52), with more advanced severely subnormal children with mental ages of between 2 and 6 years, yielded similar results. Here too the source of the behaviour disorders appeared to be in the pre-admission experiences of the children.

Nevertheless, as is discussed later, improvements in behaviour can often be brought about, and it seems likely that the effects are prolonged by the continuation of other adverse experiences. One of the main criticisms of the hypothesis of maternal deprivation has been that the subsequent care of the children in the studies originally quoted was far from adequate. A hospital environment is not thought to provide sufficient opportunities for normal emotional development. This among other things is acknowledged when small units are recommended, and out-patient treatment rather than admission. The superiority of small units for imbecile children has already been described in the section on verbal communication. In this experiment Tizard (44) found that 'the most striking and pleasing effect of this ordered but free regimen upon the children has been in their social and emotional behaviour.' On coming into the unit from an ordinary ward many had been unable to play with other children or bear frustration, and most had violent rages. They made only superficial and fleeting contacts with adults, showing no preferences, and were both destructive and aggressive. Eighteen months later:

... the old 'pathological' behaviour has largely gone; nearly all the children can enjoy simple group play with other children for long periods, . . . they are affectionate and happy children, usually busy and interested in what they are doing. . . . They are for the most part docile and easy to manage and they are fond of the staff and the staff of them.

Reversibility of Effects

Bowlby has suggested that, if deprivation has come at critical periods, its effects are likely to be irreversible. The evidence for this will not be discussed further as it has been reviewed in detail by O'Connor (32), who has contested the necessarily permanent nature of the damage. Murphy too (30) states that 'there is increasing evidence that later gratification may go far towards offsetting the effects of early frustration'.

Tizard's work (44) which showed great improvements in the behaviour of young imbeciles has already been considered, while Clarke and Clarke (9) have extensively reviewed the literature on adolescent and adult subnormals. Clarke and Clarke have also carried out a number of investigations in which they have studied IQ changes, on the grounds that intelligence is one important aspect of personality which is known to be affected by adverse circumstances, and which can be measured fairly well. The results of a number of studies may be summarised briefly by saying that, on an average, IQ increments were greater where the individual had suffered the most serious deprivation, and that a larger proportion drawn from exceptionally adverse conditions underwent larger changes. An important feature of these improvements was that 'they tended to be long term, and after a period of eight years improvement had not ceased'. One of their conclusions, that 'the most adverse social conditions characterised by cruelty and neglect . . . retard intellectual development by at least 16 points (SD 6 points) on the average', might well apply to other groups, since the essential feature of the subnormals chosen was the fact that they had been severely deprived rather than that they were of low intelligence.

In a further study conducted by Clarke and Clarke (8) over a period of 4 years, a group which had enjoyed specially stimulating conditions and which was working in the community was compared with a group which had been stimulated but which remained in the institution. Although IQ increments were similar, the social changes were far greater in the former group.

3

Perception

To a large extent our perception of the world around us is learned. Learning proceeds in combination with physical maturation, and although occasionally one is aware of applying specific methods in order to develop some perceptual skill, such as the judgement of height, usually the stimulation and experience received from the environment is adequate for the attainment of all essential perceptual abilities.

In considering the development of perception in the handicapped child it can be seen that the usual physical maturational processes may not occur, and that the limitations thus arising may prevent full use being made of the environment, or alternatively that we may have to deal with children for whom the environment itself is restricted in some way. There are some features of the situation therefore about which we can do little—we may not be able to restore normal movement to a spastic limb or to give full sight to the partially blind—but we can consider in detail the results of the handicap on the ordering of the child's experience of the world, and look for ways in which to compensate for any deficiencies. In order to do this it is important to know how perceptual skills develop and how they are involved in a variety of tasks; defects may be present which are not recognised in themselves but only in as far as they are shown in general inadequacies of performance.

Sensory deficiencies associated with other handicaps are common. 'Over half of infantile hemiplegics have sensory defects' (Tizard (45)). Dunsdon (11) found that, of a group of 27 cerebral palsied children (23 of whom were receiving speech therapy but none of whom had had audiometry), only 2 had normal hearing and one of these showed slight unilateral loss. 'In imbeciles the prevalence of sensory handicaps though largely unknown is probably high' (Hilliard and Kirman (15)). In mongolism, 'The eye proper is also very frequently abnormal, some degree of squint, often gross, is the rule. Nystagmus is also common . . . gross cataract is rare but small opacities visible with the slit lamp are exceedingly common.' Birch and Matthews (4), in an audiometric survey of all patients in a mental deficiency institution with ages ranging from 10–19 years and mental ages of approximately 5 years and over, showed that only 44% had no hearing loss in either ear, while 5% suffered sufficient loss to handicap them in ordinary life activities and 28% sufficient to handicap them in many life activities.

The defects found are not necessarily straightforward ones. Tizard (45) discussing hemiplegics states that

the sensory loss does not usually involve simple sensations such as touch, pain and temperature etc. . . . it is powers of discriminatory sensation . . . that are affected—i.e. the ability to appreciate shape and texture, the position and movement of joints, and the ability to differentiate between touch of one or two points.

The Body Image

One of the major steps in establishing concepts of the world is the child becoming aware of the separation of himself from his environment. This differentiation, which enables relationships to external objects to be established, occurs during the second half of the first year (Piaget (36, 37)), and from it arises in the individual an image of his own body. The body image system has been defined by Ritchie Russell (40) as 'that which makes it possible for appropriate bodily movements to be performed in relation to afferent stimuli'. In order for these appropriate reactions to take place in response to stimulation an intact bodily image system is essential: there must be an awareness of the position of the body in space. Any deficit may affect the ability of the child to fulfil the most basic functions of walking feeding, dressing and washing.

There are a whole range of sensory handicaps that might be expected to slow down the achievement of this concept. For example, Gesell (12), referring to the blind child, states that he

has more difficulty than the seeing child in attaining the perception of his physical self. His physical self is ambiguously involved with garments and with blankets and with furniture. He has not the assistance of sight to make the fundamental distinction between his anatomical self and all these appurtenances.

Willison, quoted by Ritchie Russell (40), has suggested that if motor control is defective, as in children developing athetosis, faulty afferents from the movements made may lead to a faulty development of the body image. This could clearly become self-perpetuating, which raises the possibility that if suitable training were given before the abnormal movements were fully developed, athetosis might be to some extent prevented. Woods (50) draws attention to the importance of movement and the subsequent impulses from the muscles, joints and vestibular system. If this partially explains, as she suggests, the difficulties encountered by poliomyelitis cases and spastic children, similar effects would be expected in a wide variety of instances where children are confined to bed and their movements restricted.

Various modalities are involved in establishing the body image, and usually if one area is defective other sources of information will compensate. When the handicap is severe, however, as in cerebral palsy, children must be assisted in using all the experience they can get. They must be encouraged to roll and crawl, to feel their own bodies and to be aware of all their movements. The aim is not to teach the form of the body, but to provide basic experience from which the concept can develop.

Motor Handicap and Spatial Ability

As the child grows older, the awareness of perceptual constancies develops. Size, distance etc. can be judged, culminating in the ability to deal with spatial relationships. Detailed information about the development of these skills is scanty, but we do have information about the cues ultimately used in making judgements. The use of these cues must develop through long periods of trial and error, of having one's expectancies more and more frequently confirmed. If however the individual is not free to explore and manipulate the environment, it might be expected that development would not take place in the normal fashion.

Berko (3) suggested that the limited sensori-motor experience of cerebral palsied children could be regarded as the cause of the difficulties in perceptual tasks which have been recognised in this group. Wedell (47, 48, 49) in a series of studies compared athetoids, bilateral, left-sided and right-sided spastic groups, and a group of non-brain-injured children without motor handicap. He demonstrated the importance of cortical damage in producing these deficiencies, but agrees 'that both motor and visual handicap contribute to perceptual impairment' although they are not sufficient to determine it. He also found in all groups improvement with increased mental and chronological ages, and feels the improvement with age 'might very largely be due to the accumulation of limited sensori-motor experience and also to the unravelling of confused kinaesthetic and other sensations'. It should be possible to look at the sort of experience that the child is deprived of, both in relation to stages of sensori-motor development and to the development of specific skills such as the judgement of distances, and to substitute other ways of providing this experience. For example, unless a child is moved around frequently it may take longer for a distant and 'visually' small object to be recognised as possibly larger than the child himself. The amount of experimentation involved in the discovery of depth will be realized by anyone watching the play of a child putting things in and out of each other.

Abnormal Eye Movements

One very important modality, the impairment of which seriously disturbs the development of the child's ability to deal with his environment, is that of vision. Abercrombie (1) has demonstrated by electro-oculographic studies that cerebral palsied children show greater inefficiency in very simple-version eye movements than normal schoolchildren, so that when a child is asked to look at a target the image is received for only part of the time, and exposure to the learning situation is thereby reduced. She states:

Eye movements as erratic as some of those in cerebral palsy must present the child with a fragmentary and inconsequential series of images of the world, and by whatever processes of suppression or inhibition the sensory input may be monitored, it is difficult to believe that adjustments are not made at the cost of loss of cerebral efficiency.

Similarly the absence of binocular vision will have great importance for the child who already has other handicaps, since the latter may deprive him of the wide variety of cues which are normally used when dealing with space perception, shape recognition, etc. A successful operation would be particularly beneficial for such cases, although unfortunately it is not always possible to achieve good results. Again, however, with the difficulties of the child in mind, methods of training in infancy can be considered.

The General Approach

As has already been mentioned, it seems that the emphasis should not be placed directly on teaching but on providing opportunities to learn, on allowing children to formulate and to test out their hypotheses. This should be related to stages of maturation and development; and in considering this, the question of the age at which training should begin arises. While there is not always evidence for critical learning periods in man, it is most important to realise that functions do not develop in isolation: although, for example, a child may learn to use an appliance efficiently when he is older, the loss of experience he would have gained in other areas had he used it sooner may not be so easily compensated for.

General retardation resulting from lack of stimulation is recognised in both physically and mentally handicapped children. Reference to its effect on the mentally handicapped is to be found elsewhere in this chapter, but the findings of Norris, Spaulding and Brodie (31) give an illustration of the general point. In an intensive survey of 66 blind pre-school children followed up for 5 years, they found that achievements were not very closely correlated with the degree of blindness, but that opportunities for learning were very important with regard to prediction of the child's total capacities. Even the ability to get about was not directly related to the degree of vision but to the general level of the child's functioning. It should be realised that a child hospitalised for any reason is deprived of normal stimulation by the reduced intensity of contact with other people, and also by the lack of variety in his surroundings and the limitations put on his own movements. Particularly if he is lying down, his view of the world is very restricted; unless he is sitting up, the way in which he becomes accustomed to view things is an abnormal one. The effects of these restrictions probably contribute considerably to the distress experienced by children coming into hospital.

A Developmental Approach to Hospitalisation in Babies

The way in which a child is disturbed by any change depends upon the stage of development he has reached. The importance of knowing the features of particular stages, if one is to explain reactions and behaviour, is illustrated in a hypothesis put forward by Schaffer (41) in connection with the effects of hospitalisation on babies of under 7 months. In this study, described in more detail in the previous section (p. 214), he relates the behaviour of the children to the stage they have reached in perceptual development.

On their return home they showed an extreme preoccupation with the environment. 'For hours on end sometimes the infant would crane his neck, scanning his surroundings without apparently focusing on any particular feature and letting his eyes sweep all over objects without attending to any particular one.' Where this behaviour was extreme the infants were quite inactive apart from the scanning movements, did not vocalise, and disregarded toys. Some degree of this behaviour was shown by about two-thirds of babies from 9–12 weeks to 7 months old. It was quite different in intensity and duration from the child's normal reactions to a change in surroundings, and no trace of any behaviour resembling it had been observed at the time of admission, whereas after the child had been hospitalised any change, even within the hospital, elicited it. At this age the cognitive structure is still at the stage of 'adualism' described by Piaget (36, 37), in which the self is merged with the environment in one functional whole. Under normal circumstances the variations in the individual's surroundings keeps his perceptual field in a relatively 'fluid 'state, but when he comes into hospital the rate of change is drastically reduced. Many of the children were confined to bed and the general physical nature of the environment was restrictive, the amount of human stimulation was reduced as they were rarely handled except when it was necessary to relieve their physical needs, and in addition many could not sit up and consequently their sensory range tended to be limited. Schaffer postulates that, under these conditions of 'perceptual monotony', in the infant 'in whom the self has not yet emerged as a differentiated unit . . . the natural tendency to merge with the environment is emphasised. It is as though under the conditions the perceptual field would tend to become "set".' When the child is moved, 'the "set" perceptual field is disrupted and distintegrates, and such disintegration may be experienced as a stress situation—hence the somatic upset found in many of the infants. A new perceptual field must now be formed, and the infant's acute awareness of new sensations is reflected in the intense concentration with which he regards his new surroundings.' If this explanation proves to be correct the situation should not be a prohibitively difficult one to remedy.

4

Orthopaedically and Mentally Handicapped Children

In this section it is proposed to relate knowledge of certain aspects of child development as specifically as possible to ages and stages in two groups of handicapped children. The two groups considered are children with orthopaedic handicaps and those with severe mental handicaps. Here the developmental approach does emphasise the usefulness of thinking in terms of severity of handicap as well as of type of handicap.

In discussing physically handicapped children the main emphasis will be on the usefulness of child development scales, particularly sub-scales of daily living activities. In relation to mentally handicapped children the main emphasis will be on the knowledge we have of speech and of total care, which is not so clearly defined in terms of ages as the knowledge contained in the child development scales. There will be a certain amount of overlapping between the two, and also with earlier sections.

Orthopaedically Handicapped Children

An example of the developmental approach to the total problem of young children with cerebral palsy and their parents is demonstrated by Lawson (21) in his description of the Cerebral Palsy Unit at Queen Mary's Hospital for Children:

New patients are seen with their parents at a diagnostic clinic. . . . The prognosis, both physical and mental, is then explained to and discussed with the parents and the services of the advice clinic are offered to them.
They are told that the day-to-day management and guidance of these children does not need any special technical facility and that affected children will make better and faster progress if they are looked after by their parents. The day-to-day continuity of treatment needed is such that nobody but the parents can carry it out, unless the child has to be admitted for a very long period to a heavily staffed unit, and thus separated from his home for long periods during his formative years. . . . One of the most serious practical problems arises from the late age at which children are referred to the diagnostic clinics.

Lawson adds later, pin-pointing one of the uses of developmental diagnosis:

Early diagnosis is not always followed by immediate measures of management. Commonly, when cerebral palsy has been correctly diagnosed in the first year of life, the parents are told that nothing can be done until the child is three or five years of age. By this time failure to provide day-by-day guidance of the child's developing physical activity has resulted in avoidable abnormalities of function and structure.

The neuro-paediatricians are also thinking developmentally. For example Zappella, in an unpublished study, writes, 'In the human infant and in the child, we have no information about the cerebral mechanisms involved in the management of the placing reaction: it might well be that these vary with the increasing maturation of the central nervous system.'

Perhaps the clearest description of a physiotherapist's use of this approach is given by Spiers and Saunders (43). This short treatment note is not only a guide to present practice in the treatment of 'Thalidamide babies', but also suggests the general lines on which further work should proceed. They point out that even quite small babies can become frustrated at their inability to suck their own fingers and play with rattles, and at seeing the world from only one position of lying on their backs. 'Our aim at Chailey Heritage (Craft School and Hospital) has therefore been, as soon as they are the right age, to see that they are able to sit up and play with toys to suit their particular ability, and to meet the normal developmental stages.' They also recognise the interplay of skills, e.g. that the ability to move about in a chair with special castors not only strengthens the baby's trunk and spinal muscles in preparation for the fitting of lower limb prostheses, but also gives pleasure to the baby or young child, and makes other normal experiences available to them.

Developmental Scales. Paediatricians and psychologists have been studying areas of normal child development for many years. Their study has led to the development of scales of behaviour. These scales are based on the normal behaviour of a sample of children at age levels from a few weeks to five years at the most. The general rationale is that an item is assigned to an age level if it is achieved by 50–60% of the children of that age and if it discriminates between age levels, i.e. is achieved by few children below the age level and the majority of children above. In actual fact it is sometimes difficult to discover from the authors the nature of their samples and their method of scale construction.

These scales are concerned with aspects of behaviour relevant to child development, e.g. speech, motor development, manipulation, and social development. Although they are constructed to give total performance age scores, or quotients, similar to mental ages or IQs, many of the items are themselves direct measures of meaningful behaviour and are therefore of interest to the clinician. The fact that items are assigned to age levels is useful to people working with babies and young children, and this will be discussed in more detail later. In this connection Tizard wrote, in an unpublished report:

The psychometrician tends to be primarily interested in comparing one person's scores with another's. The clinician is sometimes interested in this, but for many purposes (for example for assessing the effects of treatment) he wishes to follow the performance of a single person over a period of time. Again, perhaps because so much of psychological work on scales is based on lessons learned in intelligence testing, in which the content of the test items is trivial and the total score is important, psychometricians pay little attention to 'face validity'. . . . For the clinician on the other hand it is the total score which is likely to be uninformative, whereas the scores on individual items may be of great interest. . . . Nonetheless, the most useful scale will be one which is both statistically sound and clinically interesting.

Later he says:

There are scales which are 'valid-by-definition', i.e. scales in which the items themselves are meaningful and informative to the clinician. Many items from the developmental scales are of this kind. There are gaps in our knowledge of developmental scales, but they are already useful.

The gaps in the developmental scales seem to be (i) knowledge of the most essential items which represent either crucial skills or stages in the acquisition of those skills, (ii) knowledge of the interplay of different skills, and (iii) knowledge of the age variation in the acquisition of skills among children. It seems that there is an urgent need for research into these problems.

It does seem possible to make practical use now of the knowledge contained in the developmental scales to help handicapped children, either by using one of the standardised developmental scales or by using an *ad hoc* scale. Among the best known of the standardised developmental scales are those of Gesell (12), Illingworth (17), Sheridan (42) and Griffiths (14). Carr and Stephen, in an unpublished report of a survey of the uses made of developmental scales, found that two out of three of the doctors who replied to their questionnaire used developmental scales in the assessment of babies and young children, and also that a large number used their own *ad hoc* scales. In constructing an *ad hoc* scale it would seem most useful (a) to select items which seem clinically important, and (b) to give these items a general placement by maximising the agreement between different scales in which they occur. In some cases it might only be possible to give a range in time for the achievement of a skill: Dr. Woodward found for instance a large age range for essential stages when developing Piaget's sensori-motor scale. With regard to the selection of items, the suggestion is made here that all the items in the various scales be looked at by a group of experts, who can then select the items. In this way items of interest to one expert only will not be rejected, and moreover the range of items geared approximately to age norms will be as wide as possible, allowing children with a variety of handicaps to be provided with experiences appropriate to their age. For the future perhaps we need a scale which includes activities essential to the achievement of important skills, such as meaningful speech or ambulation, and also a wide range of other items assigned to age levels and pertaining to these scales though not necessarily essential. From this 'master scale' one would hope to derive individual scales tailored to suit the varying handicaps of individual children. At some future time this master scale should be re-standardised, using the available statistical techniques, so that it becomes statistically sound as well as clinically interesting.

Uses of Developmental Scales. (i) Up to now one of the main uses of developmental scales has been in the diagnosis of severe mental subnormality in young children. Illingworth (18) claims that this can be done with a fair degree of accuracy in children under the age of 2 years. So far psychologists have been unsuccessful in attempts to predict later intelligence for normal babies and young children (Hindley (16)).

Further work on the predictive value of early tests in relation to intelligence is needed.

(ii) Another use of developmental scales is in the early detection of special handicaps. In Carr and Stephen's survey almost as many replies indicated the use of the scales for this purpose as for the detection of backwardness. Sheridan, and Illingworth (17), write that developmental assessments are useful in the diagnosis of cerebral palsy and of visual and hearing defects in young children. Both, like Lawson, emphasise that early diagnosis of these conditions is important because it makes early treatment possible.

(iii) A third use of these scales is in assessing the effects of treatment by repeated reassessments at intervals of time. This has been done for children with cerebral palsy and other orthopaedic handicaps by Ingram, Withers and Speltz (19) and by Quibell, Stephen and Whatley (39). Ingram, Withers and Speltz, working in the Crippled Children's Hospital School at Memphis, wanted to select severely involved children with cerebral palsy who would respond to the intensive programme of physical and occupational therapy available; they also wanted an objective assessment of the results of this treatment. They therefore devised a scale, based on Gesell's Developmental Schedules, to give two 'levels' and 'ages', i.e. a motor age and a social age. They publish the scale in their paper. Sixty children, comprising consecutive admissions to the hospital school and those who had been in hospital for one month at least, were assessed on the scale. These were children selected as likely to improve or as doubtful and requiring a trial period. The average age of the children was $3\frac{1}{2}$ years, and after an average stay of 16 months they were reassessed on the same scales. The authors report their results in terms of significant improvement in the children. Improvement was judged to be significant if the change in the child was of practical value to him and the people who cared for him. On the problem of selecting children for the treatment they offered, they found that no child with a Motor Quotient of 15 or less improved significantly. This seems a low cut-off point, which in itself is encouraging; as also is their other finding that 40 out of 60 children improved significantly.

Ingram, Withers and Speltz also used their scales to suggest the level at which treatment should begin. This is another important use because it implies that the clinician responsible for the treatment, in this case physiotherapy and occupational therapy, must have found the scale items clinically interesting, i.e. they gave him the information he needed to initiate and plan treatment. This is a fourth use of developmental scales, which will be referred to again.

Quibell, Stephen and Whatley (39) also used developmental scales to assess results of treatment in young mentally and physically handicapped children. This was a retrospective study of the response to treatment of 40 mentally and physically handicapped children treated in a long-stay orthopaedic children's hospital and school. Their group was made up of all the children with IQs under 70 in the hospital, namely 33 ESN and 7 ineducable children. The children ranged in age from 2–16 years, the main diagnostic groups being children with cerebral palsy and children with spina bifida cystica. The children of 5 years and over were assessed on admission on Quibell's scale of daily living functions, and then reassessed at least one year later; the same procedure was followed with the children under the age of 5 years, except that an *ad hoc* scale of daily living functions derived mainly from Gesell (12) and Griffiths (14) was used, to allow for age. The results were that 30 of the children showed worthwhile improvement in daily living functions, which indicated, as one would expect, that children with IQs under 70 can make worthwhile progress in these skills.

Quibell (39), like Ingram *et al.*, used his scale of items essential for daily living in the initial assessment and treatment plan; this use is described in an earlier paper (Quibell (38)). However the *ad hoc* developmental scale was only used thus in order to assess results; the treatment itself embraced the full range of services available in an orthopaedic hospital. Quibell *et al*, reported their results in terms of improvement in functions essential for daily living because maximum independence in these skills is an essential goal (though not the only one) in the management of severely and chronically handicapped children, for whom the physical handicap dominates the 'clinical picture. Their handicap, as in cerebral palsy, may be ameliorated but it cannot be cured; treatment in its widest sense, however, can best be planned to help the children in every possible way if their abilities and disabilities are known and accepted. Quibell (39) knew that children could only be helped in every possible way if their emotional adjustment, family relationships and educational status were also taken into account. Although they did not report changes in these areas, they did assess emotional adjustment and educational status in a group of the children at the time the study ended. Educational attainment test results were made available by the headmaster of the school, so the assessment of educational status presented no problem. *Emotional adjustment* was assessed by the psychiatrist, one of the authors (Dr. E. Whatley) using the Maudsley descriptive code (Cameron (7)) as an adjunct. The Maudsley code was slightly modified to suit their physically and mentally handicapped population so that the adapted code had 39 items. These items were given equal weight and summed to give a score for each child, and from this an arbitrary rating scale was made on which the children were graded as 'adjusted', 'mildly maladjusted' or 'severely maladjusted'. This method, though crudely used, did provide a complete phenomenological picture of the children's behaviour.

If this assessment of emotional adjustment is looked at from the developmental point of view, there are two matters to be considered. First, no attempt was made to use items from the Child Development Scales to form a sub-scale of emotional development for the assessment of the children under 5 years. It seems probable that, though there are some items in these scales which assess emotional and social development, there are not enough at present to provide an adequate assessment. The second is that emotional adjustment in children is not static. There was some evidence in a follow-up of 17 of the older children in Quibell's group, carried out one year later (unpublished), that some of the children became more maladjusted and that this was not clearly related to physical progress. This is suggestive of the need for further research into the emotional adjustment of handicapped children and into the optimum conditions associated with adjustment. There is evidence from the work of Boles (5) that the attitudes of parents of children with cerebral palsy tend to change with the age of the children, and it therefore seems reasonable to suppose that the attitudes of handicapped children change with age. Meyerson (28) in a review of studies of handicapped children found no acceptable evidence that these children have specific emotional problems; but later work of Wedell (47) indicates that clearly defined diagnostic sub-groups of handicapped children tend to show specific difficulties. However it is probably safe now to say that children with chronic handicaps do have the same kind of emotional problems and are subjected to the same kind of stresses as normal children, but that sometimes these are increased qualitatively and quantitatively by the physical handicap. In the meantime there is no need to wait for research workers to describe the particular difficulties of handicapped children; there is enough knowledge already available of the way in which normal children live and learn that can be, and is being, used in planning the total care of these children. The reality of the handicap may prevent children from living entirely normal lives, but they can be helped to live lives in every way as nearly normal as possible. In working towards this end present findings are practically useful, as well as giving clues for further research. For example Quibell's second follow-up suggested that some dull, physically handicapped children become more maladjusted at adolescence, although they had made adequate progress in independence for daily living activities. Also in this follow-up it seemed that the few young imbecile children who were cared for in small groups on the babies' and toddlers' wards seemed reasonably happy and well adjusted. Both these tentative findings are in line with expectation: adolescents tend to have problems of adjustment, and young children develop most satisfactorily in small family groups. One last comment on the emotional adjustment of handicapped children is that this must be considered in its own right, because one cannot assume it is correlated with any one other specific factor.

To relate the last 3 uses of developmental scales: Ingram's and Quibell's studies suggest that items from Child Development Scales can be grouped into sub-scales which measure meaningful areas of child development, and that in these sub-scales the individual items are meaningful. In work with handicapped children these sub-scales may be used (a) in initial assessment and planning of treatment and (b) in the serial assessments of results. Such scales must be treated with caution; they are imperfect and incomplete, but they can be, and are, useful now, and they will be more useful in the future, provided they are used correctly to assess the development of handicapped children in terms of normal child development. Retardation on a developmental scale may pin-point abnormality, but that is all. Perhaps one advantage of our present imperfect knowledge of child development is that it prevents dogmatism in a difficult and complicated field.

The following report on one baby with gross congenital malformation of arms and legs is presented, to indicate how the information provided by a combination of developmental scales may be used to assess present skills, to make some recommendations and to assess progress.

GIRL V., AGED 14 MONTHS

Assessment 1. Piaget Stages of Sensori-motor Development.

21.12.62: Age 12 months. Piaget Sensori-motor Scale, Stage IV—begins 8–9 months, ends 11–12 months.

27.2.63: Age 14 months. Piaget Sensori-motor Scale, Stage V—begins 12 months, ends 18 months.

Interpretation: V. has made progress in her sensori-motor development over the past few months and it is now appropriate for her chronological age. This would seem to indicate not only cortical development but also hand/eye or hand/foot coordination. She is at the following stages of concept development within this scale:

(i) *Space*—She is interested in learning about size and will put small objects into larger ones. She might be encouraged to do this with meaningful everyday objects as well as toys, such as nesting cups. She has difficulty in grasping objects, so some toys which are easier for her to lift and manipulate might be provided. (In fact this is being done.)

(ii) *Concepts of permanence of objects*—V. is learning that objects have permanence when they are outside her field of vision. She learns this through hiding and finding toys etc.

(iii) *Problem solving at a concrete level*—At this stage babies learn that one object can be affected by another as well as by themselves directly: such activities as e.g. playing a xylophone seems particularly helpful to allow limbless babies to develop this concept, because they need long-handled toys, otherwise they cannot coordinate hand and eye. From her behaviour with toys it may be that V. finds it so difficult to manipulate toys physically that she needs extra encouragement to explore different kinds of activities and materials. Now that she is in the nursery class she will learn from other children provided that she is physically near them, but at this age she still needs to learn mainly from one grown-up.

Assessment 2: Ad hoc Scale. Locomotor Development.

21.12.62: Age 12 months. Locomotor development—9 months approx. omitting stepping reactions.

27.2.63: Age 14 months. Locomotor development—10 months level for trunk control and rolling.

Interpretation: V. has made progress in moving, but she is now at the stage where she would be beginning to walk and of course this is impossible. At this stage a normal child would find out about objects and people for himself by moving up to them; V. can only roll towards objects. It would seem that she is dependent on getting a horizontal vision of her world by being sat up in her 'flower pot' and having things brought to her to play with. It would seem increasingly important within the next six months or so to remember that her experience is limited in this way and to provide her with a variety of everyday objects within touching distance. She does not enjoy her trolley yet, but she is barely old enough for it. One would expect her to make use of it within the next three or four months. She may need encouragement from one adult she knows well as she seems a naturally shy child.

Assessment 3: *Ad hoc Scale. Hearing and Speech.*

21.12.62: Age 12 months. Hearing and speech—9–10 months.
27.2.63: Age 14 months. Hearing and speech—no observed change.

Interpretation: It seems that V. is a little backward in speech. She has moved to a new ward lately and this may have held her up a little. She should be encouraged to make as many sounds as possible; again the other children will help her, but one grown-up will help her more. She should be beginning to understand simple speech and to learn the names of everyday objects. The nursery school class should help her in this.

Assessment: 4: *Ad hoc Scale. Social Development.*

21.12.62: Age 12 months. Social development—about average.
27.2.63: Age 14 months. Social development—she seems average so far.

Interpretation: V.'s development seems about average so far, but this may be because there is very little on which one can judge social behaviour at this age. She may fall behind in the sphere of self-help soon unless she is given extra encouragement to feed herself: dressing and toilet are going to be problems, but there seems to be plenty of time to deal with this, as long as she remains confident and does not get the feeling that she is falling behind the other children. It would not seem this would matter for the next year or two.

V. is making very good progress and does appear to be a happy, well occupied little girl.

Discussion. This report illustrates how achievements affect each other. For example V. cannot grasp easily because her arms and hands are malformed; therefore it is difficult for her to solve the simple problems involved in using one object to move another unless she is helped. However, given appropriate aids she can do it. The Piaget sensori-motor scale suggests what normal children of this age would do, and also what they cannot be expected to do yet but may do next, and the approximate age at which they should move on to the next stage. As a rough guide one can use the *ad hoc* sub-scales of development in this way. The great difficulty is that it is not possible to know exactly how far limitations in one area, due to physical handicap, are going to affect achievements in other areas in the future. The only possible method at present would seem to be to set clearly defined short-term goals in terms of scale items, and provide experiences geared to the achievement of these goals in a total setting beneficial to the child, and then by careful observation to note when and how the child achieves these goals. It would seem necessary to set short time limits and to be guided by the emotional state of the child so that impossible and frustrating goals are abandoned. The observation of V. suggests that children sometimes find their own ways of simulating normal development: she passed objects from her best hand to her best foot at about the time when normal babies would transfer objects from hand to hand. However, although handicapped children can sometimes find their own methods of overcoming their handicap, they need all the intelligent help that can be given. Parents and other people working with handicapped children know a great deal about the development of children, but they also need the kind of systematic and detailed advice on the management of the children which this kind of approach should make possible.

★   ★   ★

To sum up: it seems that knowledge derived from scales of child development provides useful information about the kind of behaviour, or skills, which normal children achieve at stated ages from birth to about five years. This information is based on cross-sectional, not longitudinal, studies of samples of normal children's behaviour in such areas as speech, locomotion, self-care and social behaviour. At present the resultant scales seem most useful in the assessment of locomotor and self-care activities, less adequate in the assessment of speech, and least adequate in social and emotional assessment. Items in the sub-scales are usually placed at one-monthly age intervals up to two or three years, and then at six-monthly or greater intervals up to five years. These scales are therefore most useful with babies and young children. The age ranges between items or skills in the same sub-scales give an approximate idea of the time taken by children to master one skill before moving on to the next. But more research is needed to show how much time is spent by children in practising a skill, and it must be remembered that handicapped children may need more time than normal children in order to achieve skills.

Severely Mentally Handicapped Children

Children with severe mental handicaps and children with severe chronic physical handicaps require long-term care from their parents and professional workers. One aim of such care is to make the lives of both groups of handicapped children as nearly like the lives of normal children as possible.

Although severely mentally handicapped children are a hetero-geneous group, psychologists have shown that some of these children develop like normal children in the areas studied, have the same needs and respond to the same environmental factors. Now psychologists like Lyle (22) and O'Connor and Hermelin (33) are filling in the picture by describing difficulties specific to sub-groups of these children, and methods by which these difficulties may be at least partly overcome.

We do know from the work of Woodward (51), Tizard (44) and Lyle (26) that severely sub-normal children of imbecile level but without associated handicaps, aged 6–13 approximately, develop like normal children of nursery school age, only more slowly in such areas as complex language skills. Tizard (44) and Woodward (53) have shown how knowledge of the normal processes and sequences of development can be used to facilitate progress in mentally handicapped children, because such knowledge makes possible the provision of appropriate experiences and conditions whereby growth is fostered. Dr. Woodward has described intellectual development in her chapter of this book.

Total Care (Family care pattern). The Brooklands experiment (Tizard (44)) proved that 'the methods of child care that are employed in residential nurseries for pre-school children of normal intelligence' can be applied to the care of severely subnormal children of pre-school mental age but of approximately primary school actual age, with good results. As well as the general and specific progress mentioned earlier, the Brooklands children improved clinically in daily life activities such as self-care skills (although this was not actually demonstrated by a statistical comparison with the control group of institution imbeciles). Workers with mentally handicapped children have been interested in developing self-care independence in these children since the time of Itard (20). One well known scale of child development, the Vineland Social Maturity Scale (Doll (10)), was devised as a measure of social competence which should be used as one diagnostic criterion in the ascertainment of mental deficiency.

Speech and language. Lyle in five papers, (22), (23), (24), (25) and (26), describes his findings in relation to the verbal ability, developmental speech patterns and characteristics of 3 groups of imbecile children of nursery school mental age but chronologically 6½–13½ years, and one group of normal children chronologically of nursery school age. All 4 groups were matched for non-verbal IQs. It is not possible to review his findings adequately in this chapter; some have been referred to already. In general Lyle's findings support the hypothesis that trainable imbecile children of nursery school mental age resemble nursery school children of actual nursery school age in certain aspects of speech development. His findings also suggest that level of speech development may be one measure of general progress and adjustment. He demonstrated that, of his three matched groups of imbecile children, the group living at home and attending day centres were most advanced in verbal ability and language skills, followed by the group living at Brooklands, which is run on residential nursery school lines, the least advanced being the institution group. The normal group of children of nursery school age matched for non-verbal IQs were more advanced than any of the imbeciles in the more complex language skills; this is a practically useful finding which applies to imbeciles mentally of nursery school age.

A second aspect of Lyle's work particularly relevant to the use of developmental scales in work with severely mentally handicapped children is that he devised a scale of developmental sequences of early language behaviour from the verbal responses given by the imbeciles and normal children; this scale therefore applies to children of nursery school mental age. In this scale of sequences he distinguished three stages: (i) nil verbal response; (ii) early language responses such as jargon, echolalia and sign language; (iii) meaningful speech. Among his sample of normal children aged $2\frac{1}{2}$–4 years he found none at stages (i) and (ii). This is what one might expect from the standard scales of child development: meaningful speech predominates from $2\frac{1}{2}$ years onwards.

To sum up this section: there is evidence that imbecile children of nursery school mental age go through the same stages of development in speech and social learning as normal younger children, and that they respond to the same patterns of care as normal younger children.

5

Conclusions

We have outlined and illustrated an approach in which knowledge of normal child development is applied to the problems of handicapped children. We have attempted to be systematic, although our coverage is an incomplete one and the assumptions on which our suggestions are based have not always been empirically validated. However we feel that enough is already known about both handicapped children and child development for an attempt to be made to systematise our knowledge. Not only does such an attempt clarify what use we can make of present information, but it is only in this way that it becomes possible to assess the extent of our knowledge, and to indicate in what areas further investigations should be made and what directions these should take.

★   ★   ★

Acknowledgments

We would like to thank Dr. Kenneth Cameron for encouragement to apply this approach to handicapped children, and Dr. David Lawson for permission to quote Case V.

REFERENCES

1. ABERCROMBIE, M. L. J., 1963. Eye movements, perception, and learning. *Little Club Clinics in Developmental Medicine*, No. 9: 52-58.
2. ANTHONY, E. J., 1956. The significance of Jean Piaget for child psychiatry. *Brit. J. Med. Psychol.*, **29**: 20-34.
3. BERKO, M. J., 1954. Some factors in the perceptual deviations of cerebral palsied children. *Cerebral Palsy Rev.*, **15**: 3-4.

4. BIRCH, J. W. and MATTHEWS, J., 1951. The hearing of mental defectives: its measurement and characteristics. *Amer. J. Ment. Defic.*, **55**: 384-393.

5. BOLES, G., 1959. Personality factors in mothers of cerebral palsied children. *Genetic Psychol. Monographs*, **59**: 159-218.

6. BOWLBY, J., 1952. *Maternal Care and Mental Health.* Geneva: W.H.O. Monographs, Series 2.

7. CAMERON, K., 1955. Diagnostic categories in child psychiatry. *Brit. J. Med. Psychol.*, **28**: 67.

8. CLARKE, A. D. B. and CLARKE, A. M., 1959. Recovery from the effects of deprivation. *Acta Psychologica*, **16**: 137-144.

9. CLARKE, A. M. and CLARKE, A. D. B., 1958, (ed.). *Mental Deficiency: the Changing Outlook.* London: Methuen.

10. DOLL, E. A., 1953. *The Measurement of Social Competence.* (A manual for the Vineland Social Maturity Scale.) Washington: United States Educ. Test Bureau.

11. DUNSDON, M. I., 1952. *The Educability of Cerebral Palsied Children.* London: Newnes.

12. GESELL, A. L. and AMATRUDA, C. S., 1949. *Developmental Diagnosis.* London: Cassell.

13. GOLDFARB, W., 1943. The effects of early institutional care on adolescent personality. *J. Exp. Educ.*, **12**: 106-129.

14. GRIFFITHS, R., 1954. *The Abilities of Babies.* London: Univ. of London Press.

15. HILLIARD, L. T. and KIRMAN, B. H., 1957. *Mental Deficiency.* London: Churchill.

16. HINDLEY, C. B., 1960. The Griffiths Scale of infant development: scores and predictions from 3-18 months. *J. Child Psychol. and Psychiat.*, **1**, No. 2: 99-112.

17. ILLINGWORTH, R. S., 1962. An introduction to developmental assessment in the first year. *Little Club Clinics in Developmental Medicine*, No. 3.

18. ILLINGWORTH, R. S. and BIRCH, L. B., 1959. The diagnosis of mental retardation in infancy. *Archs. Disease in Childh.*, **34**, No. 175: 269-273.

19. INGRAM, A. J., WITHERS, E. and SPELTZ, E., 1959. Role of intensive physical and occupational therapy treatment of cerebral palsy; testing and results. *Archs. Phys. Med. and Rehabil.*, **40**: 429.

20. ITARD, J. M. G., 1801. *The Wild Boy of Aveyron.* Trans. by G. and M. Humphrey, 1939. New York: Appleton-Century Co.

21. LAWSON, D., 1958. A cerebral palsy service for children. *Lancet*, 19th April: 840-842.

22. LYLE, J., 1959. The effect of an institution environment upon the verbal development of imbecile children. I. Verbal intelligence. *J. of Ment. Defic. Research*, **3**, Pt. 2, Dec. 1959.

23. —— 1961. The effect of an institution environment upon the verbal development of imbecile children. II. Speech—Language. *J. of Ment. Defic. Research*, Vol. **4**, Part. 1, June 1961.

24. —— 1960. The effect of an institution environment upon the verbal development of imbecile children. III. The Brooklands Experiment. *J. of Ment. Defic. Research*, Vol. **4**, Part. 1, June 1960.

25. —— 1961. Comparison of the language of normal and imbecile children. *J. of Ment. Defic. Research*, **5**, Pt. 1, June 1961.

26. —— 1960. Some factors affecting the speech development of imbecile children in an institution. *Child Psychol. and Psychiat.*, **1**: 121-129.

27. —— 1960. The effect of an institution environment upon the verbal development of imbecile children. *J. of Ment. Defic. Research*, **4**: 14-23

28 MEYERSON, L., 1957. Special disabilities. *Ann. Rev. Psychol.*, **8**: 437-454.

234   CHILD DEVELOPMENT AND HANDICAPPED CHILDREN

29. MUNDAY, L., 1957. Environmental influence on intellectual function as measured by intelligence tests. *Brit. J. Med. Psychol.*, 30: 194.
30. MURPHY, L. B., 1944. In: Hunt, J. McV. (ed.), *Personality and the Behaviour Disorders*, Vol. 2. New York: Ronald Press.
31. NORRIS, M., SPAULDING, P. J. and BRODIE, F. H., 1957. *Blindness in Children*. Chicago: Univ. of Chicago Press.
32. O'CONNOR, N., 1956. The evidence for the permanently disturbing effects of mother-child separation. *Acta Psychol.*, 12: 174-191.
33. O'CONNOR, N. and HERMELIN, B., 1963. *Speech and Thought in Severe Subnormality*. London: Pergamon Press.
34. PARTEN, M. and NEWHALL, S. M., 1943. In: Baker *et al.*, *Child Behaviour and Development*. New York: McGraw-Hill.
35. PIAGET, J., 1932. *The Moral Judgment of the Child*. London: Kegan Paul.
36. —— 1937. Principal factors determining intellectual evolution from childhood to adult life. In: Rapaport, D. (ed.), *Organization and Pathology of Thought* (1951). New York: Columbia University Press.
37. —— 1950. *The Psychology of Intelligence*. London: Routledge and Kegan Paul.
38. QUIBELL, E. P., 1956. The physically handicapped child: functional assessment of the disability as an aid to planning. *Brit. Med. J.*, ii, 991.
39. QUIBELL, E. P., STEPHEN, E. and WHATLEY, E., 1961. A survey of a group of children with mental and physical handicaps treated in an Orthopaedic Hospital. 1959. *Archs. Disease in Childh.*, 36, No. 185: 58-64.
40. RITCHIE RUSSELL, W., 1958. Disturbance of the body image. *Cerebral Palsy Bull.*, No. 4: 7-9.
41. SCHAFFER, H. R., 1958. Objective observations of personality development in early infancy. *Brit. J. Med. Psychol.*, 31: 174-183.
42. SHERIDAN, M. D., 1960. *The Developmental Progress of Infants and Young Children*. London: H.M.S.O.
43. SPIERS, B. W. and SAUNDERS, J., 1962. Aids for congenitally deformed babies. *Physiotherapy*, Dec. 1962: 346-347.
44. TIZARD, J., 1960. Residential care of mentally handicapped children. *Brit. Med. J.*, i, 1041-1046.
45. TIZARD, J. P. M., 1960. In: Report of a discussion on sensory, auditory and speech defects in cerebral palsy. *Cerebral Palsy Bull.*, 2, No. 1: 40-41.
46. TIZARD, J. and GRAD, J. C., 1961. *The Mentally Handicapped and their Families*. London: Oxford Univ. Press.
47. WEDELL, K., 1960. The visual perception of cerebral palsied children. *J. Child Psychol. and Psychiat.*, 1: 215-227.
48. —— 1960. Variations in perceptual ability among types of cerebral palsy. *Cerebral Palsy Bull.*, 2, No. 3: 149-157.
49. —— 1961. Follow-up study of perceptual ability in children with hemiplegia. *Little Club Clinics in Developmental Medicine*, No. 4: 76-85.
50. WOODS, G. E., 1958. The development of body image. *Cerebral Palsy Bull.*, No. 4: 9-17.
51. WOODWARD, M., 1960. Early experience and later social responses of severely subnormal children. *Brit. J. Med. Psychol.*, 33: 123-132.
52. —— Early experience and behaviour disorders in severely subnormal children. *Brit. J. Social and Clinical Psychol.* (In press.)
53. —— 1962. The application of Piaget's theory to the training of the subnormal. *J. of Ment. Subnormality*, Vol. VIII, 1: 3-11.

X

CHILD PSYCHOPATHOLOGY

FREDERICK H. STONE

M.B., CH.B., M.R.C.P. (Glasg.), M.R.C.P. (Lond.)

Consultant in Child Psychiatry, Royal Hospital for Sick Children, Glasgow
Hon. Clinical Lecturer, Glasgow University

1
Introduction

In order to contain the psychopathology of childhood within the confines of a chapter, selection has been necessary, inevitably at the expense of comprehensiveness. A few clinical entities in which the writer is specially interested have been chosen for discussion, but it is hoped that the main controversial issues have been presented without serious omission. The emphasis on ego assessment is in itself a reflection of a current trend, and one which for child psychiatry, far from representing merely a fashion in conceptual thinking, may prove invaluable in the practical tasks of clinical assessment and management.

2
The Psychotic Child

If we consult the texts in clinical psychiatry that were standard at the beginning of this century, we find that reference to childhood psychosis tends to be brief and dogmatic. With the exception of the occasional 'symptomatic psychosis' associated with infections or progressive degenerations of the central nervous system, childhood insanity is practically unknown. A few eponymous entities were recorded, without arousing very much interest, and there the matter rested until in 1943 Kanner (30) described the syndrome of 'early infantile autism'. In addition to delineating a clinical picture Kanner made reference to parents, noting the high incidence of university graduates among the fathers and mothers, who were stated to have a preference for certain professions and skills. Now this was recorded as a statement of fact in a limited series of cases without any inference being drawn. This did not prevent others from doing so, either to question the findings (curiously, no incidence study of sufficient scope to take account of social class, for example, has yet been published), or else to accept them and to draw conclusions. Some regarded these findings as strengthening the case for a hereditary cause, postulating an affinity between aesthetic sensibility and 'vulnerability'. Others invoked the pathogenicity of one or both parents. A type of mother began to emerge from the accumulating clinical descriptions—cold, formal, unspontaneous—and was designated 'schizophrenogenic' (Rank (36)). The child's disorder was considered to be the outcome of a particular variety of maternal deficiency, and intensive psychotherapy, often an attempt at substitute or replacement mothering, was undertaken.

A brief interruption of this history of ideas is required in order to observe that we are involved in an aspect of psychopathology which is inherent in the psychiatry of children, namely the psychopathology of family relationships. It may seem rather quaint to introduce this in a discussion of childhood psychosis, where its relevance may be regarded as peripheral or non-existent. It is our intention, however, to show that it is seldom irrelevant, no matter what the clinical entity displayed by the child, but that the nature of the relevance is readily misconstrued.

Some workers were unimpressed by the 'schizophrenogenic mother' hypothesis, and for interesting, differing reasons. Although some mothers of autistic children were as described, others were not. Even when they were, they had other children who seemed quite normal. This last point arises in many clinical contexts, and it is worth noting here that the counter-argument runs as follows: It is naïve to assume that, because the relationship of a mother to a child is abnormal, it is necessarily so in relation to her other children. Disturbances of parent-child relationship may be specific to a particular child, and may sometimes occur only at a particular time, i.e. there may be a *focal relationship disorder* in contrast to the diffuse variety which involves many or all of the children.

Other clinicians observed that in many families they encountered disturbances of mothering far grosser than that to which infantile autism was being attributed, and yet the children showed relatively minor disorders. To account for this observation it became necessary to introduce an old-new dimension, namely 'predisposition'. Abnormal mothering of the type described, it was claimed, would result in psychotic development only of certain children—those who were constitutionally vulnerable. Bergmann and Escalona (8) view this vulnerability psychophysically as a defect in the 'stimulus barrier'.

Even if a dual-factor hypothesis is accepted, it is capable of a revised interpretation. 'Could it be', some have asked, 'that the disturbed pattern of mothering is a reaction to an abnormally developing child?' (Bender (5)). After all it is not so rare to see marked disorders of mothering and fathering where a child has been born with some congenital handicap. Indeed those who are concerned clinically with the emotional disturbances of such children, whether they are mentally retarded, blind, deaf, paralysed or with physical deformities, lay tremendous emphasis on the part played by 'child-rearing practices' in their aetiology.

This is not an end to the theories about the 'cold' mother and her autistic child. Even if the peculiar and abnormal relationship existing between them is acknowledged, it is possible that both have the same hereditary characteristics and that what we are seeing is the reciprocal interaction of two inherently abnormal personalities. To blur the issue still further, Eisenberg (14) has drawn attention to the high incidence of abnormal personalities among the fathers of autistic children.

It is hardly to be wondered at that some investigators are turning to biochemical research into 'autism', if only to escape from this nightmare of theorising. They would do well to read Jung's monograph *The Psychology of Dementia Praecox* (28), whose concluding paragraphs, in which he acknowledges the qualitative difference from neurosis and speculates about pathogenesis, anticipate much of our current thinking. The notion that certain kinds of stress operating at a certain time might produce organic change is not so far removed from the currently productive hypothesis of auto-immunisation.

Be that as it may, there are already sufficient clinical studies of autistic children to permit at least a glimpse into their inner world and to confirm the existence of *some* psychopathological features qualitatively different from what we observe in the psychoneuroses. Much of their behaviour and developmental retardation begins to be comprehensible when we consider it in relation to ego development. The ego was originally conceptualised by Freud (20) as the part of the personality that is in contact with the outside world, and whose matrix was formed from bodily perceptions. Psychically this was represented by the 'body image'. Ascribed to the ego were such functions as memory, perception, control of motility and reality-testing. The ego also functioned as a barrier against the unconscious. It was postulated that in the early stages of infancy there was a gradual differentiation between the 'self' and the outside world, a laying-down of 'ego boundaries' (cf. Piaget's phases of dualism and a-dualism). Many clinical studies of autistic children (Norman (33); Creak (12)) have stressed these very aspects of personality malfunctioning, namely a failure to achieve a sense of self, distortions of body image, perceptual anomalies, and poor control of motility. Viewed in relation to ego development this implies a hold-up in maturation at a very early level, but does not commit us thereby to a particular aetiological view. Although Freud himself (19) stressed the importance of congenital factors in ego development, and has frequently been so quoted, the how and what of the congenital aspect tended to be ignored till quite recently. In this respect the theoretical contributions of Hartmann (24) are important, and especially the broadening of the view of ego development which he affords in delineating three components: (i) the impact of reality, (ii) instinctual drives, and (iii) hereditary factors.

When a young child shows the clinical features of an overt psychotic disturbance, it is unfortunately true that the prognosis is usually rather poor no matter what treatment is undertaken. The exceptions. to this statement make the professional life of the therapist tolerable, but these cases are few, and we are still inexpert at making accurate predictions. More precise 'ego diagnosis' may help. On the whole, however, it may be felt that in psychosis psychopathological formulation is academic. As far as adult patients are concerned, this is surely contradicted by the work of Freeman (17), for example, who applies psychoanalytic insight to the fostering of good nursing technique, on the basis of comprehending the patient. So it is, we suggest, in the *management* of psychotic children. They are frequently in states of obvious distress whose cause the child can seldom communicate verbally, but which can often be inferred when they are considered in terms of anxiety production and the child's limited resources for its containment.

Moreover the study of psychopathology can serve eminently practical ends, when it leads to the setting up of research projects designed to test experimentally a particular hypothesis. While Anthony (4) has set out with clarity the lines of enquiry relevant to autism, the work remains to be done.

When we come to consider those children and adolescents who are somewhat less deviant, variously described as 'borderline' (Geleerd (21)) or with 'severe ego disturbance' (Weil (43)), the importance of ego assessment cannot be over-stressed. These cases are not rare and their severity is frequently underestimated. Perhaps this is firstly on account of the façade of normality, for they do relate to the interviewer and other people in a sort of way, and speech development may be very good. Secondly they are often initially seized upon as 'interesting cases' because of the rich production of fantasy material. Thirdly the presenting symptomatology is often that commonly associated with quite benign emotional disturbances —nightmares, phobias, tics, or just 'naughtiness'. But if we look more closely at each of these features as an exercise in ego-assessment we discover:

(1) That although these children are not completely out of contact with their environment the capacity for inter-personal relationships is markedly impaired, they lack empathy, and sometimes reveal 'merging' with the other person, i.e. there is evidence of impaired object-relations, and sometimes of defective ego boundaries.

(2) The production of fantasy material in painting, modelling or play, sometimes with vivid symbolism (as if they had been reading Freud), is in fact much too ready. Easy access to primary process (i.e. unconscious) content means inadequate repression, i.e. there is evidence of a defective ego-barrier to the unconscious. Where by contrast ego development, especially early integration, is sound, the clinician has to work hard,

particularly with latency children, for even a glimpse of the unconscious. It is worth reminding ourselves here that the *content* does not help in assessing clinical severity.

(3) The 'ordinariness' of the presenting symptoms is usually a reflection of parental imperception or denial, for a detailed developmental history invariably shows marked deviation in sequence and level. In later life, as Weil points out, some of these children correspond to the 'as if' personality as described by Helen Deutsch, and not a few of them appear in our clinics for the first time as the parents of disturbed children. Here again the psychopathology tends to be underestimated, and such a mother may be taken on as a 'promising case-work assignment', only to reveal herself later, in spite of an attitude of politeness, conformity and respectability, as unable to make use of therapy. Her relationship with the child as with the case-worker and with everyone else is not so much 'disturbed' as 'pseudo'. This in a sense brings the discussion full cycle, since we have already encountered this type of maternal pathology in connection with infantile autism.

Now many of these 'borderline'[1] children can be helped by psychotherapy, but the technique must be modified to afford ego support. This is particularly true at times of crises, whether precipitated by internal or external factors. We suggest moreover that the diagnosis of ego defect, in the present state of our knowledge and therapeutic skill, has prognostic value, for progress will be slow and patchy. This realisation allows parental counselling to be realistically based.

3

The Neurologically Impaired Child

Apart from the researches of Lauretta Bender (6), whose special interest it has been for many years, the psychopathology of children with neurological impairment has been studied relatively little. Particularly valuable are her observations that such cases are not nearly as rare as has been thought among the children attending psychiatric clinics, that the criteria for organic brain disease are very different from those in the adult and are therefore frequently neglected, and that the major problem demanding attention is the concomitant emotional disturbance. Bender attempts to correlate the personality traits of these children with the particular segment of the central nervous system affected, noting, for example, the extreme dependency where there is cerebellar dysfunction causing impairment of balance and the need to cling. Nor does she neglect the parental reactions to this kind of need.

---

[1] The term 'borderline' as here used means that the patient while showing defective reality-testing still maintains some contact. It should not be confused with 'borderline psychosis', increasingly used as a descriptive term for cases showing features of both schizophrenia and affective disorder.

Pond (35) in a major review of the subject places the emphasis somewhat differently, stressing both the social factors and environmental stresses.

In a preliminary study of the psychodynamics, Stone (41), by means of long-term collateral therapeutic contact with a few such children and their parents, has record edsome suggestive findings: (i) The degree of anxiety displayed by these patients was pathologically high. (ii) Rigid defences were maintained by various manoeuvres which apparently served to 'control the environment'. (iii) Characteristic features were the presence of omnipotent fantasies, poor control of motility, and at times impaired hold on reality. (iv) A successful psychotherapeutic technique (in addition to the usual interpretation of defences, and of transference phenomena where appropriate) demanded measures principally aimed at support. It is difficult to convey in words the intensity of the anxiety reactions witnessed in these children (and described spontaneously by the parents). They are of an order said to be encountered only in psychotic and borderline states. 'Catastrophic reactions' as described by Goldstein (22) were frequently observed. Now these anxiety reactions did not appear 'out of the blue' as is said to be typical of brain-damaged cases, but appeared whenever the rigidly organised defences were threatened, for example if the therapist refused the role allocated by the child in his 'identification with the aggressor', or sometimes if the purpose of obsessional rituals was verbalised at an appropriate stage. It was concluded that these various features, the poor control of motility, the tenuous hold on reality and the narcissistic traits, all pointed to *impaired ego functioning*.

The question arises why this should be associated with a neurological lesion. Here again, as in our discussion of the psychotic child, we encounter an aetiological mesh without as yet being able to tease out the crucial strand. We must take account of (*a*) the *matrix* itself, which here is certainly suspect whether the lesion is developmental or acquired (though neurological opinion does not favour a direct correlation between the lesion as such and a particular behaviour pattern); (*b*) *concomitant factors*, e.g. social class, nutrition, prematurity etc.; and (*c*) *genetic factors*, e.g. mode of interaction by parents and others, 'traumatic' episodes etc.

Perhaps it would be more profitable at the present stage to consider pathogenesis rather than aetiology, and it is tentatively suggested that we should examine closely the possibility of distorted perceptual experiences from birth or very early age, and also relevant here is the ethological view of the earliest bond between offspring and mother. In this connection we must take account, in considering perceptual experiences of infants, not only of the special senses, especially tactile, but also of kinaesthetic and balance stimuli.

Yet another feature which seems characteristic of many, if not all, of these neurologically impaired children is a *predisposition to anxiety*. In her monograph with this very title, Greenacre (23), discussing this tendency in adults with severe neuroses or borderline states, reviews a number of researches which indicate the possible relevance of a history of 'severe suffering and frustration occurring in the ante-natal and early post-natal months'. Greenacre is mainly concerned with possible psychological trauma, but longitudinal studies by Pasamanick (34) in the United States and by Drillien (13) in Scotland lend support to the view that hazardous births, and/or prematurity, increase the subsequent vulnerability of the child to emotional disturbance.

So far our focus has been on severe ego disorder, with a number of familiar clinical examples, and before leaving this subject we shall consider the practical and theoretical implications of two common symptom formations. Firstly, 'inexplicable attacks of fear'. These severe anxiety attacks, frequently described with accuracy by the parents, are evidence of disordered affect. It would seem reasonable to assume that *one characteristic of a healthy ego is the ability to tolerate anxiety well*. This is a deceptively simple formulation which raises difficult questions. Do these children experience extreme unease because of the weak 'barrier' to the unconscious, allowing the emergence of terrifying fantasies? Or do quite ordinary external events impinge upon the child in fear-provoking ways because they are distorted in the process or perception? Or is the terror that accompanying the threatened dissolution of the ego boundaries? These questions remain unanswered, but by asking them at all we avoid the risk of over-simplification in considering the aetiological role of parents. If perceptual distortion proves to be important, then all sorts of quite ordinary parental behaviour may well be misinterpreted by the child. Conversely there is a type of parent, often commended as 'insightful', who may be a peculiarly malevolent influence for this type of child, i.e. the parent who meets the child's rage, fear, or grief with something like an interpretation instead of the neglect, reassurance, or comfort which a less 'insightful' but spontaneous parent would supply. Children, and not just ego-impaired children, need parents who represent the real world, who bolster reality-testing.[1] They are ill served by parents who augment fantasy in their misdirected attempt at 'psychological handling'.

Secondly, to turn from anxiety attacks to a different type of symptom which is often described as 'peculiar games or habits': clinically we recognise these to be obsessional or ritualistic, and they can often be seen to appear when anxiety-provoking situations are imminent. We infer that they represent an attempt to ward off anxiety. They are a form of 'defence'. The concept of 'defence' is of course an integral one in a consideration of ego functioning, and in Miss Freud's classic monograph (18) are described the dynamics involved: repression, regression, projection, sublimation etc. What is not yet clear is why a particular individual acquires his own 'defensive style', preferring some manoeuvres rather than others. It has

[1] The reservation should perhaps be made that in the very early stages of infancy there may be a danger in excessive or premature reality enforcement (see Winnicot (44)).

long been realised however that too ready use of defences or exclusive use of one type of defence can result in crippling of the personality, or, more accurately perhaps, reflects a personality which is crippled. It seems that in the ego-impaired child as in the brain-damaged adult (Schilder (40)) there is often a preference for an 'obsessional' defence system.

If in diagnosis the ego pathology is not recognised, such a child may be regarded as having an obsessional neurosis. When we recall that rituals are common in healthy young children (some would describe these as transient neuroses) it is apparent that 'obsessional states' may be symptomatic of all degrees of psychopathology. This of course is true of the great majority of symptom-complexes. Mahler (32) in a masterly review of tics in childhood, and Kahn and Nirsten (29) in a recent paper on 'school phobia', both emphasise this point with many clinical illustrations. It is therefore as absurd to speak of 'the treatment' of tics or school phobia (or any other symptom complex) as it would be for a physician to describe 'the treatment' of loss of weight.

4

The Anti-social Child

Although there is little agreement about the precise meaning of such terms as 'delinquent', 'psychopath' or 'character disorder', the reader will have no difficulty in identifying which children are under consideration. Not that 'anti-social' is a term devoid of complexity or ambiguity. For one thing it is a negative concept, and we shall have to consider why some children are 'pro-social'. Moreover it is not really a clinical category at all but a sociological one, which has to take account of the accepted mores of a given group at a certain time. It is worth recalling before pursuing its psychopathology that it is this group of children which provided the impetus to the development of child psychiatry as a speciality half a century ago. Its implications extend far beyond medicine and take us into the realm of morality and the future of human society. However, the view that psychiatry has the knowledge, let alone the wisdom, to tell people how to lead the good life is not one to which we subscribe.

Our concern here is with the development of the individual conscience, or in psychoanalytic terminology the super-ego. The shift of interest from the neurotic adult to the delinquent youth as the subject of psychoanalytic research was clearly anticipated by Freud in his preface to Aichhorn's *Wayward Youth* (1). As to the theoretical aspects of super-ego development, the present situation may in fairness be described as one of intense reappraisal. There are few satisfactory answers as yet to the problems of the precise mechanisms of introjection and identification, of the necessary preconditions of super-ego development, of the relationship of super-ego to 'ego ideal', and many more (Hartmann and Loewenstein (25)). From the clinical point of view probably no single contribution has made more impact than the monograph prepared for the World Health Organisation by Bowlby, *Maternal Care and Mental Health* (9). This work has tended to highlight three concepts: (i) the clinical entity of the 'affectionless child', (ii) the pathogenic role of early maternal deprivation, and (iii) the transmission theory. The simple sequitur *maternal deprivation produces psychopathy* has long since been modified by Bowlby; he is now concerned with detailed studies of the behaviour of the separated child, which he regards as a mourning reaction (10) and whose possible relation to subsequent psychiatric illness is viewed in the light of ethological considerations.

For all their theoretical differences, few researchers question the importance of the earliest phases of the mother/child relationship for super-ego development. There have been many formulations of the essence of good mothering, few as profound—and incidentally as benevolent to mothers—as Winnicott's. It is curious that, whereas it is the harsh and oppressive parental aspects that are almost invariably associated with super-ego action, it is on tender, loving care that all the emphasis is placed with regard to its precondition of development. There is no doubt that by and large fathers have suffered quite extraordinary neglect both in theoretical formulations and in clinical procedures, but of late consideration has been given to paternal deprivation. Of course not all fathers are harsh, nor all mothers tender, nor for that matter all families patriarchal. Sandler (38) in a recent paper has drawn attention to the pleasant, approving aspects of the super-ego, which some would probably regard as attributes of the ego.

Let us return however to the consideration of the three issues highlighted by Bowlby's work:

The Transmission Theory

If a mother has herself suffered severe emotional deprivation in early childhood, she may have grown to womanhood lacking the ability to give (and receive) affection. Although she may carry out the mechanical tasks of mothering, the essential mother-love component is lacking and her baby is in turn subjected to the same pathogenic experience as herself. From clinical experience we know that this sequence from one generation to the next does sometimes occur, but we also know that there is not a clear-cut cause-and-effect relationship. Not all girls who from their earliest days would be expected to grow into 'affectionless' women do so; nor do all 'affectionless' mothers give a history revealing deprivation. As regards the 'early separation' hypothesis, the present position has been admirably reviewed by Ainsworth in a recent W.H.O. monograph (2).

The principle of the transmission of psychopathology through the generations is one that is generally accepted as an important aspect of the aetiology of childhood emotional disorder. Though numerous publications support this concept by describing 'relationship pathology', often retrospectively from the adult patient, the whole subject lacks precision. It is true that experimental testing of complex hypotheses is very difficult, but this hardly explains the dearth of research studies into childhood psycho-pathology. One method is that of prediction, whose methodological complexity has been considered in detail by Benjamin (7).

Maternal Deprivation

Bowlby has focused on the absence of the mother at a time, roughly between the ages of 12 months and four years, when the child is believed to be maximally susceptible. From his clinical observations he has allocated to separation experience a central position in the theory of the origins of anxiety (11). Working from the hypothesis that the infant is bound to the mother by a number of instinctual response systems, he affirms that conditions of isolation produce the 'elemental experience' of 'primary anxiety'. This view of the infant's basic tie to the mother has similarities with those earlier formulated by Suttie (42), and Fairbairn (16) also places great emphasis on separation anxiety as a precursor of psychopathology. Winnicott (44) too stresses the importance of early deprivation, *or what is experienced as deprivation*, in the genesis of both psychotic defence mechanisms and anti-social character development. His nomenclature is at times formidable, but it should be recognised that he is trying to formulate ideas about the earliest stages of infancy before psychological processes as ordinarily understood even exist. (Some of his main contributions are lucidly summarised in James's (27) recent review of his collected works.) Winnicott's hypotheses about precocious ego development, the 'false self', and the fate of the 'transitional object' could be the starting-point for a host of clinical researches.

The importance of infantile experience for later psychological development has if anything been reinforced by recent contributions from many different vantage-points. Yet there is an extraordinary lack of controlled infant-observation research. An exception is Schaffer's work on the attachment behaviour of infants (39), in which he identifies what would appear to be a crucial developmental milestone at about the age of seven months, marking the onset of specific attachments.

'The Affectionless Character'

Somewhere between the amorality of the affectionless character and the oppressive super-ego of the neurotic patient there is presumably a median zone inhabited by the responsible, internally-directed, mentally-healthy individual. If that is so then whole sections of our communities, being predominantly 'other-directed', are mentally ill even if asymptomatic. This dilemma highlights another aspect of super-ego reappraisal, the question of social norms of morality. Here again while Riesman (37) postulates certain phases in the development of societies, and attempts to correlate them with the group conscience, experimental testing of the hypothesis is in its infancy (Holmes (26)). For child psychiatric practice this is far from an academic matter. Anti-social behaviour is a common symptom, and desperate parents seek help. To the child the clinic is yet another aspect of authority against which rebellion is directed. It is hardly surprising that rapport is not easily established, and if this together with a history of delinquent behaviour be taken as evidence of 'an affectionless character' the child is in danger of being prematurely dismissed to his home or to an institution as 'untreatable'. This raises two issues. Firstly, deprivation even at a critical period can probably result in all degrees of disordered capacity for inter-personal relations. There is no doubt an extreme variety, the pre-psychopath, but it is doubtful if this can be assessed confidently in a short diagnostic contact. Secondly, the untreatability of such children—and the majority of clinical reports are hardly encouraging—may yet prove to have been the result of inappropriate technique, based on the fallacy that if deprivation has been severe psychotherapy must be correspondingly intense. More hopeful results have recently been reported by Alpert (3) from the Child Developmental Centre, New York and by Lavery (31) at the Notre Dame Child Guidance Clinic, Glasgow, using rather similar techniques of management as a preliminary stage to intensive psychotherapy.

5

Ego Weakness

A widely occurring form of personality disturbance which is not gross in its manifestations, even although its ramifications touch on almost every aspect of ego functioning, merits description, for although its recognition is of the greatest prognostic importance it has received little notice in the psychiatric literature. Often the child's disturbance first presents in early latency, and this frequently takes the form of somatic symptoms, of which one of the commonest is recurrent abdominal pain. Anxiety attacks may appear in the form of sleep disturbance, or of 'school phobia' of all grades of severity, which is frequently really a separation anxiety. Other common symptoms are headache or enuresis. All sorts of irrational fears may present, with moments of sudden and extreme distress and equally rapid recovery. This sequence is frequently 'triggered off' in the interview itself, often by the expression of empathy, and the distressed weeping of dramatic onset may easily be mistaken for evidence of depression. It is very striking that when not acutely distressed these children present a deceptive façade of normality, so that for example school reports are singularly void of unusual features. These children, often decidedly immature in appearance, admit to nervousness but are quite unable to be more specific. They may express fear of teachers but cannot say why. They seem aware of a sense of inadequacy, and may declare their unwillingness to grow up—indeed there is a striking lack of emotional investment in the past or the future. No clear picture emerges of their relationships, which seem vague and colourless, and the child does not emerge at all as a well defined person. Their expressed fears are often but the echoes of the fears of adults. There is poor tolerance of anxiety or of conflict. Object-relations are weak, and there is a marked inability to sustain ambivalent relationships. The girl is not very feminine, nor the boy masculine. We cannot yet predict whether in adult life these children will present as intractable neuroses or as inadequate personalities with or without chronic or recurrent psychosomatic disorders. We do know, however, that in childhood they seldom have the resources to benefit from interpretative psychotherapy, although the symptoms can often be alleviated or removed by suggestion or by supportive ego-strengthening techniques. Little can be said with certainty about aetiology, though the relationship with the mother often displays a symbiotic-like attachment, and we can often recognise a failure on the mother's part to differentiate the child's needs from her own.

To describe them as 'ego-weak' is really to beg the question. Perhaps in the present state of our knowledge we should regard their deficiency as one of identity formation.

The concept of *identity*, to which Erikson (15) has contributed so richly in recent years, has wide connotations. The psychosexual stages, oral, anal, genital, each regarded as the determinant of character traits depending on 'fixation points', are given by Erikson a new dimension or 'modality', e.g. 'incorporation' and 'taking' in relation to orality, 'retention' and 'elimination' to anality, etc. It is the interaction of these maturing modalities with environmental experiences which Erikson regards as the essence of psychosocial development. Thus at each stage there are opposing polarities (trust and mistrust, autonomy and shame, etc.), and the conflict between them constitutes successive crises. It is too early to judge how useful this comprehensive scheme of personality development will prove. We have no doubt however of the unique way in which it illuminates many clinical states of adolescents, especially the concept of 'role diffusion' in the identity crises of young adults. There is probably no stage at which the clinical picture may be so deceptively grave as regards prognosis. For example, the reactivation of unresolved oedipal conflicts is common, but the observable turmoil is often the external manifestation of intra-psychic realignment, offering, as it were, a second chance for resolution. Psychotherapeutic intervention can be most rewarding, and here also the 'identity crisis' formulation may prove valuable, highlighting as it does the adolescent's need to make use of the therapist not only as a confidant and interpreter but also as a real person.

6

Postscript

The focus of child psychopathology over the years has been constantly shifting—from id to ego, from neuroses to character disorders, from trauma viewed as life experiences to the pathology of parent/child relationship, from speculation to controlled observation. At last the contributions of experimental psychology, ethology, developmental neurology, sociology, anthropology and psychoanalysis are impinging the one against the other, and all with the clinical psychiatry of childhood.

REFERENCES

1. AICHHORN, A., 1925. *Wayward Youth.* In English, 1951. London: Imago.
2. AINSWORTH, M. D., 1962. In *Deprivation of Maternal Care.* Geneva: W.H.O. Public Health Papers, 14.
3. ALPERT, A., 1963. A special therapeutic technique for prelatency children with a history of deficiency in maternal care. *Amer. J. Orthopsychiat.,* **33,** 1: 161-182.
4. ANTHONY, J., 1958. An experimental approach to the psychopathology of childhood autism. *Brit. J. Med. Psych.,* **31:** 211-225.
5. BENDER, L., 1953. Childhood schizophrenia. *Psych. Quart.,* **27:** 1-19.
6. ———— 1956. *Psychopathology of Children with Organic Brain Disorder.* Springfield, Ill.: Thomas. Oxford: Blackwell.
7. BENJAMIN, J., 1959. In *Dynamic Psychopathology in Childhood.* New York: Grune & Stratton.
8. BERGMAN, P. and ESCALONA, S., 1949. Unusual sensitivities in very young children. *Psychoanal. Study of the Child,* **3-4:** 333-352.
9. BOWLBY, J., 1951. *Maternal Care and Mental Health.* Geneva: W.H.O. Monograph Series No. 2.
10. ———— 1962. Childhood bereavement and psychiatric illness. In *Aspects of Psychiatric Research* (ed. Richter *et al.*). London: Oxford Univ. Press.
11. ———— 1962. Separation anxiety: a critical review of the literature. *J. Child Psychol. and Psychiat.,* **1:** 251-269.
12. CREAK, E. M., 1963. Childhood psychosis. *Brit. J. Psychiat.,* **109:** 84-89.
13. DRILLIEN, C. M., 1963. Obstetric hazard, mental retardation and behaviour disturbance in primary schools. *Dev. Med. and Child Neur.,* **5,** I: 3-13.
14. EISENBERG, L., 1957. Fathers of autistic children. *Amer. J. Orthopsychiat.,* **27:** 715-724.
15. ERIKSON, E., 1958, 1960. *Discussions on Child Development,* Vols. 3 and 4 (ed. Tanner and Inhelder). London: Tavistock Publications.
16. FAIRBAIRN, W. R. D., 1941. *A Revised Psychopathology of the Psychoses and the Neuroses.* Psycho-analytic Studies of the Personality. London: Tavistock 1952.
17. FREEMAN, T., CAMERON, J. L. and McGHIE, A., 1958. *Chronic Schizophrenia.* London: Tavistock.
18. FREUD, A., 1948. *The Ego and the Mechanisms of Defence.* London: Hogarth Press.
19. FREUD, S., 1912. *Dynamics of Transference.* Quoted by Greenacre, *Trauma, Growth and Personality* (1953), Int. Psychoanalytic Lib., p. 28.
20. ———— 1923. *The Ego and the Id.* London: Hogarth Press, 1946.
21. GELEERD, E. R., 1958. Borderline states in childhood and adolescence. *Psychoanal. Study of the Child,* **13:** 279-295.
22. GOLDSTEIN, K., 1939. *The Organism.* New York: American Book Co.

23. GREENACRE, P., 1941. *Psychoanalytic Quarterly*, **10**: 1.
24. HARTMANN, H., 1952. Mutual influences in the developmental of ego and id. *Psychoanal. Study of the Child*, 7: 9-30.
25. HARTMANN, H. and LOEWENSTEIN, R. M., 1962. Notes on the superego. *Psychoanal. Study of the Child*. **17**: 42-81.
26. HOLMES, M. B., 1960. A cross-cultural study of the relationship between values and modal conscience. *In* Muensterberger and Axelrad (ed.), *The Psychoanalytic Study of Society*, Vol. I: 98-181. New York: Internat. Universities Press.
27. JAMES, M., 1962. Infantile narcissistic trauma. Observations on Winnicott's work in infant care and child development. *Intern. J. Psychoanalysis*, **43**, I: 69-79.
28. JUNG, C., 1907. *The Psychology of Dementia Praecox*. New York: Nerv. and Ment. Dis. Pub. Co., 1936.
29. KAHN, J. H. and NIRSTEN, J. P., 1962. School refusal. *Amer. J. Orthopsychiat.*, **32**: 4.
30. KANNER, L., 1943. Autistic disturbance of affective contact. *Nerv. Child*, 2: 217-250.
31. LAVERY, L., 1963. Personal communication.
32. MAHLER, M. S., 1949. A psychoanalytic evaluation of tic. *Psychoanal. Study of the Child*, **3-4**: 279-310.
33. NORMAN, E., 1954. Reality relationship of schizophrenic children. *Brit. J. Med. Psychol.*, **27**: 126.
34. PASAMANICK, B., 1954. The epidemiology of behaviour disorders in childhood. *Neurology and Psychiatry in Childhood*. London: Baillière, Tindall & Cox.
35. POND, D. A., 1961. Psychiatric aspects of epileptic and brain-damaged children. *Brit. Med. J.*, ii: 1377-1382; 1454-1459.
36. RANK, B., 1949. Adaptation of the psychoanalytic technique of the treatment of young children with atypical development. *Amer. J. Orthopsychiat.*,19: 130-139.
37. RIESMAN, D., 1955. *The Lonely Crowd*. Yale University Press.
38. SANDLER, J. et al., 1962. The Classification of Superego Material. *Psychoanal. Study of the Child*, **17**: 107-127.
39. SCHAFFER, H. R., 1963. Some issues for research in the study of attachment behaviour. In *Determinants in Infant Behaviour*, II (ed. Foss). London: Methuen.
40. SCHILDER, P., 1938. Organic background of obsessions and compulsions. *Amer. J. Psychiat.*, **94**: 1397.
41. STONE, F. H., 1961. Psychodynamics of brain-damaged children. *J. Child Psychol. and Psychiat.*, **1**: 203-214.
42. SUTTIE, I. D., 1935. *The Origins of Love and Hate*. London: Kegan Paul.
43. WEIL, A. P., 1953. Certain severe disturbances of ego-development in childhood. *Psychoanal. Study of the Child*, 7: 271.
44. WINNICOTT, D. W., 1951. Transitional objects and transitional phenomena. In *Collected Papers*, 1958. London: Tavistock Press.

PART TWO

CLINICAL ASPECTS OF
CHILD PSYCHIATRY

XI

ORGANISATION OF

CHILD PSYCHIATRIC SERVICES

JOHN G. HOWELLS

M.D., D.P.M.

*Consultant Psychiatrist, Department of Family Psychiatry,
Ipswich and East Suffolk Hospital*

1

Historical

Beginnings

Throughout history there has been a concern for the welfare of the child, but only a dim awareness that some of his disabilities arise from an inner disharmony of his emotional self. Modern child psychiatry owes much to contributions from adult psychiatry, paediatrics, child guidance and educational psychology.

Few attempts were made by psychiatrists to consider the emotional disabilities of children before the beginning of this century. During the nineteenth century psychiatrists ('alienists') were usually concerned with adult psychosis, and in that period some attention was given to psychosis in children. Henry Maudsley in *Physiology and Pathology of Mind* (29) of 1867 had a chapter on 'Insanity of Early Life'. W. W. Ireland published his *Mental Affections of Children* in 1898 (25).

The first clinical attempts to treat emotional disorder in children were made by the psychoanalysts. Freud's discovery that emotional disorder in adults often has its roots in childhood, together with his theory of infantile sexuality in 1905, gave a great impetus to the exploration of the emotional development and disorders of childhood. In 1909 we have the first published account of a child analysis by Freud, *The Case of Little Hans* (12). As time went by psychiatrists sporadically tended to pay attention to children, and when the Tavistock Clinic opened in London in 1920 its first patient was a child; by 1926 it had inaugurated a department for children. Subsequently clinics were associated with general and teaching hospitals. The Royal Victoria and West Hants Hospital at Bournemouth started a clinic for adults and children in 1928, and the Maudsley Hospital, London, opened a children's department in 1930; this latter clinic was greatly influenced by the psychobiological approach of Adolph Meyer and Leo Kanner of the Johns Hopkins Hospital, Baltimore. The British Psychoanalytical Institute displayed an interest in children from its inception; they were influenced by the work of Melanie Klein and later, in 1938, by that of Anna Freud. In the 1930s Henderson and Gillespie's *Textbook of Psychiatry* (13) devoted a section to 'Child Psychiatry'. Today child psychiatric clinics are firmly established in association with adult psychiatric departments in most of the major teaching and non-teaching general hospitals, in paediatric hospitals, and in some mental hospitals.

As may be expected paediatricians, with their day-by-day clinical work with children, have from early times concerned themselves with nervous disorders in children. In the first English book on paediatrics, Thomas Phaire's *The Boke of Chyldren* (38) published in 1545, sections are devoted to the malady of 'Terrible Dreames and Feare in the Slepe' and 'Of Pissing in the Bedde'. Robert Hutchinson in his book *Lectures on Diseases of Children* (24) of 1904 devoted two chapters to 'Functional Diseases of Children', and in 1918 Hector Cameron published his book *The Nervous Child*. Paediatricians were subsequently to devote more attention to nervous disorders, the work of Spence in Newcastle and Winnicott in London being particularly noteworthy. Most modern English textbooks of paediatrics devote some space to the consideration of the emotional or nervous disorders of childhood.

'Child guidance' has been defined by Gertrude Keir (27) as 'giving expert advice or assistance to parents, educationalists, and to the children themselves, in those individual cases where doubt has arisen about the best way of directing or redirecting the child's mental development'. The contribution of 'child guidance' started with Healey's work with delin- quents in the Juvenile Courts of Cook County in 1909, and was continued with the founding of the Judge Baker Clinic by the Judge Baker Foundation in Boston in 1912. This was followed by the experimental clinics of the National Committee for Mental Hygiene set up with aid from the Common- wealth Fund, and led to the importation of the child guidance movement to England in the 1920s. In 1927 the first child guidance clinic was estab- lished in England; it was the East London Child Guidance Clinic, started as a voluntary effort by the Jewish Health Organisation. In 1928 the Child Guidance Council was started, and it is interesting to quote from the words of the chairman at its first meeting: 'Above all, it must be realised that the work of such a clinic will be educational and social more frequently than medical or clinical in strict sense'. The first demonstration clinic was started with the help of the Commonwealth Fund at Islington in 1929 and was known as the London Child Guidance Clinic. By 1932 the movement had spread outside London and a clinic under a Local Education Authority had been established in Birmingham. In 1944 there were 95 Child Guidance Clinics, of which half were organised by Local Authorities, 22 were staffed by Mental Hospitals and 9 were voluntary. These were in addition to University and Hospital clinics of child psychiatry.

A notable contribution was made by child study and educational psychology. In 1884 Francis Galton set up an 'anthropometric laboratory' to measure human form and faculty. In 1896 Sully opened a laboratory devoted to the psychology and assessment of children of different mental abilities. There was much concern with mental and school tests. Deviations were seen by accident, but rarely was anyone equipped to handle them, or to appreciate their significance. In 1907 Burt was appointed Lecturer in Psychology at the Physiology Department of Liverpool, and in 1913 he was the first psychologist to be appointed to an educational department when he took up his post with the London County Council. In the terms of his duties it was understood, among other things, that 'children who present problems of special difficulty' were to be seen individually. Provision was made for neurotic and psychotic children to be seen by a psychiatrist, but even so the work of the educational psychologist and that of the psychiatrist were not very precisely defined. Later, educational psychologists were appointed to education authorities outside London, Leicester being one of the first to employ them.

The Period of Confusion

At first it was thought that the management of the child's welfare in all its aspects was best undertaken by one organisation. The term 'child guidance' was often interpreted to include guidance of the child in every facet. As time went on it became apparent that no one movement was large enough to satisfy within itself the multiple demands made upon it; thus medical, educational, social and ethical functions were undertaken by separate but co-operating bodies. A psychiatric service for the emotional disorders of the child was yet to crystallise. Between 1930 and the end of the last war followed a period of great confusion about the functioning of the various services designed to help the emotionally disturbed child. A number of factors contributed to this confusion.

The most important single cause was no doubt the lack of a reliable body of knowledge in this field. Clinical services were only slowly developing, and research was virtually non-existent.

An additional cause was the lack of appreciation by many of the nature of emotional disorder, and therefore of the role of the child psychiatrist. Deviations in the emotional behaviour of adults are readily recognised as requiring the expert help of specialists in psychiatry. Deviations in the child's emotional life may be less florid but are just as significant in denoting emotional conditions, requiring the same expert care. If these conditions are neglected they may result in the more obvious adult disorders. The treatment of these conditions requires psychiatric experience in the field of adult and child psychopathology. The main work of the child psychiatrist in the children's field will always be with these emotionally disturbed children, rather than with psychotic children. At times it was wrongly supposed that psychosis was the main concern of the child psychiatrist, when in fact psychosis accounts for less than 1% of patients seen at child psychiatric clinics.

Confusion was also caused by the use of the term 'maladjustment' instead of terms denoting clinical conditions. A document by the Royal Medico-Psychological Association (40) comments thus:

'Maladjustment' is a term descriptive of the individual's relationship with the environment, and the 'maladjustment' may be manifested in any one of a series of social situations. One of these situations may be the school, and such children, because of their psychiatric problems, are unable to make the fullest use of the educational facilities offered them. To regard 'maladjustment' in a child as a clinical entity is inaccurate—the obsessional child slow in school work, the child lacking confidence in reading, and the child liable to a psychotic outburst do not represent the same entities.

Further confusion arose from the tendency to base psychiatric services for children on the school. This encouraged an attitude of mind that regarded events at school as the cause of emotional disturbances in children, thus neglecting the influence of the home environment in aetiology. The same attitude also concentrated attention on the symptomatology manifested by the child at school, thus ignoring a much wider range of symptomatology manifested by the child at home. It also led to the obvious disadvantage of a children's psychiatric service being based upon the child of school age, and so excluding the important pre-school age group.

More confusion was caused by the lack of definition of the work of the educational psychologist. The function of the educational psychologist was primarily to make new work from the psychological laboratories available in the schools. The field covered by the school psychological service included such matters as: ascertainment of unusually gifted pupils, ascertainment of dull children needing special educational provision, methods of remedial teaching, vocational guidance, and new learning techniques. With a background of training in education, the educational psychologist could hardly be regarded as an expert in clinical problems and able to diagnose minor from major emotional problems, physical from emotional problems, and to take a clinical history from parents. Despite this the educational psychologist sometimes took on medical functions, such as being a diagnostician responsible for referring children from the schools to the child psychiatrist. This is now properly regarded as the function of the school doctor.

Yet more confusion arose from the 'team concept', which implied that a team-patient relationship rather than a doctor-patient relationship should be encouraged. The team tended, through the case conference, to be the diagnostic agency and to be collectively responsible for treatment.

This concept cut across the clinical responsibility of the psychiatrist for his patient, and indeed the responsibility of each professional worker for his own work. Inevitably it fostered an attitude where the roles of various team members became unclear. The strictures applied by David Levy (28) at the annual meeting of the American Psychiatric Association in 1951 to American child psychiatry applied equally to child psychiatry in Great Britain: 'We have been remiss in studying the delineation of functions and thereby failed to aid in the optimal distribution of the energy of the members of the team.'

To the above was added the confusion springing from the tendency to study the child in isolation. There was an inordinate interest in the intra-psychic phenomena of the child, which was encouraged by the work of some psychoanalysts. The child's emotional environment, in particular the influences of its parents and of the rest of the family, tended to be given little prominence. The links between child and adult psychiatry were ignored, and thus such matters as that the emotionally disturbed child might later become a disturbed parent were insufficiently realised, or that helping the disturbed parent should take account of that parent's child-hood. Child and adult psychiatry are indivisible.

Disentanglement

This can be said to have begun with the Blacker Report (1) of 1946, which divided the children's services into Child Guidance Centres with a largely educational function, and Child Psychiatric Clinics with a clinical function. The matter was made crystal-clear by the National Health Service Act of 1946 (37), in which the Health Service accepted the respon-sibility for psychiatric disorder in children, both emotional disorder and psychosis. A memorandum (33) issued in 1947 stated: 'The Regional Board will be responsible for the provision and development of medical services for children suffering from mental illness and maladjustment.' A complementary circular (30) issued by the Ministry of Education made clear the responsibility of the Local Authority for a purely educational service.

The matter, now clarified, was not long allowed to rest. Reaction set in, with the result that in October 1950 the Ministry of Education set up a committee, the Committee on Maladjusted Children, which reported five years later in 1955 (31). The committee had as its terms of reference: 'To enquire into and report upon the medical, educational and social problems relating to maladjusted children, with reference to their treatment *within the educational system*' (my italics). The fact that its terms of reference confined it to a consideration of the problem within the educational system seriously affected the usefulness of this committee. Unfortunately the committee's findings tended to be regarded as applying to child psychiatry outside the educational system, and this started a further period of confusion.

The principal recommendation of this committee, which became known as the Underwood Committee, was that it advocated the setting up of what it called 'joint' clinics. These were clinics in which the staff (other than the psychiatrist) and the premises were supplied by local authorities (the educational service, the school health service, and the public health service), while the psychiatrist was to be supplied by the hospital service. This meant that in effect four authorities were to be concerned with each 'joint' child guidance clinic.

However, while the Underwood Committee had been sitting, events had taken their own course. Child psychiatric clinics had been established at most of the major teaching and non-teaching general hospitals. The Royal Medico-Psychological Association in its memorandum on the Organisation of Child Psychiatric Services had made clear the medical function in regard to emotionally disturbed children. The report of the Underwood Committee was contrary to clinical developments at that time, and contrary to clinical opinion, which hastened to condemn the report. The British Paediatric Association (5), the Royal Medico-Psychological Association (41) and the British Medical Association (2) all condemned the findings of the Underwood Committee, and advocated a child psychiatric service based on the hospital service. Further opposition by medical authorities was unleashed by the publication of circulars (32) from the Ministry of Education advocating the 'joint clinic'. Very recently the 'Association of Undergraduate Teachers of Psychiatry' has issued a memorandum (8) calling for a child psychiatric service based upon the hospital. A Special Committee of specialists, all members of the British Medical Association (3), published a report which had as its main recommendation: 'The child psychiatric service should in future be centred at a hospital.' This was endorsed by the Porritt Committee (4) (*A Review of the Medical Services in Great Britain*) in 1962.

Today

The position now is that most of the large child psychiatric clinics are within the hospital service. In 1956 there were 64 hospital child psychiatric clinics, which by 1961 had increased to 102 clinics. Of these, 72 clinics were held at general hospitals, 17 at children's hospitals and 13 at psychiatric hospitals. These hospital clinics contain all the in-patient facilities for disturbed children and all the training posts in child psychiatry. There are still many smaller clinics which are the responsibility of the local authorities and not of the Health Service, and of these approximately two-thirds are 'joint' clinics and one-third entirely the responsibility of the local authority. Purely local authority clinics staffed by psychiatrists are likely to disappear, if only because the salary scales for psychiatrists under local authorities are considerably lower than for those within the Health Service. Work in the 'joint' clinics is unpopular with some psychiatrists because of the many administrative difficulties inherent in running a service which is the responsibility of four different authorities. A further handicap is the isolation from medical specialist colleagues within the hospital service.

In 1942 James M. Cunningham (10) in the U.S.A. advised: 'It would seem imperative, if public support is to be obtained for a psychiatric service for children on a State-wide basis, to designate the service by a title which would indicate its psychiatric nature.' In Great Britain the present tendency is to refer to children's psychiatric services at hospitals as 'child psychiatric clinics', and the Royal Medico-Psychological Association (40) has advocated dropping the term 'child guidance'. In future there are likely to be departments of child psychiatry or child psychiatric clinics at hospitals throughout the Health Service, and an educational psychology service maintained by Local Education Authorities which may be called 'school psychological' or 'educational psychology' services.

The child psychiatric clinics will be concerned with supplying a clinical service primarily for the investigation and treatment of emotional illness in children and to a much smaller extent for mentally ill (psychotic) children. Emotional disorder in children manifests itself in changes of mood, such as apathy, anxiety, phobias, obsessions, lack of concentration, sleep disturbances and tension, and also by such psychosomatic signs as restlessness, anorexia, tics, speech anomalies, enuresis, encopresis and indeed signs of dysfunction in any body system, and lastly by deviations of behaviour such as awkwardness, aggression, destructiveness, temper tantrums and many signs of delinquent anti-social attitudes. In addition a very small number, approximately 1% of children accepted at such clinics, manifest signs of mental illness or psychosis.

Future Trends

In recent years there has been a significant trend towards working more with parents. At one time it was thought that the parents merited nothing more than 'advice and reassurance', on the assumption that parents merely lacked knowledge of child care. It is now generally felt that parents often require investigation and treatment in their own right as emotionally ill individuals. This has been long recognised by such clinics as the 'Department of Parents and Children' at the Tavistock Clinic, London.

In one general hospital unit, the Department of Family Psychiatry of the Ipswich and East Suffolk Hospital, practice has been extended to the point at which the family itself is regarded as the functional unit, and the child or indeed a patient of any age group is regarded as an introduction to the family (19). There are four channels of referral from the family: an adult intake clinic, a marital problems intake clinic, an adolescent intake clinic and a children intake clinic. Once a patient is accepted through the intake clinic, the department works towards the involvement of all the family members in investigation and treatment. The family is not regarded as just a background to be modified in order to help the presenting family member; the family itself is the functional unit and the presenting family member is given no more (but no less) attention than the other family members. This development is termed 'Family Psychiatry' (21). A child psychiatric clinic (22) thus becomes an intake clinic with special facilities for the reception and diagnosis of children's problems, and by having it within a department of family psychiatry it is possible to offer assistance to the rest of the family and so attain the desirable aim of a healthy child in a healthy family. Furthermore investigation of a family, initiated by acceptance of an adult, adolescent, or marital partners at their respective intake clinic, often leads to help being given to the children of the family. Thus children of pathological families are not overlooked even if they are not themselves the subject of a referral.

Professional Body

The Royal Medico-Psychological Association, founded in 1841 and thus the oldest psychiatric organisation in the world, is the professional body of psychiatrists in Great Britain. At first the clinical problems of children were not considered apart from general psychiatry. But in 1942 a separate committee was established for child psychiatrists, and by 1946 this became a Section of the Association. The Section's membership has steadily grown and in January 1963 stood at 650 members, approximately half of whom are practising child psychiatrists while the remainder are psychiatrists with an interest in the field. It is unlikely that there is any practising or trainee child psychiatrist who is not a member of this body. It has been deemed essential by thoughtful psychiatrists that there should be a professional body able to foster the legitimate interests of child psychiatrists and child psychiatry, to act as a forum for clinical discussion, and to sponsor research. It is also a body which may be consulted by appropriate authorities. The existence of such a body has already exercised a profound influence upon the standards of practice within child psychiatry in Great Britain.

2

Facilities

Siting of Units

In future the hospital facilities of an area will be concentrated at the district general hospital. Thus the ideal siting for the children's psychiatric department is at such a hospital. There are great advantages in being associated with a general hospital—the children's psychiatric department becomes integrated with the other clinical services of the area, it collaborates with psychiatric and other departments within the hospital, and it is readily accepted by the public. Furthermore referrals from the general practitioner are encouraged, special investigations are easily available, inpatient facilities are adjacent, all members of the staff have the same employing authority, conditions of service are as for other clinical person-

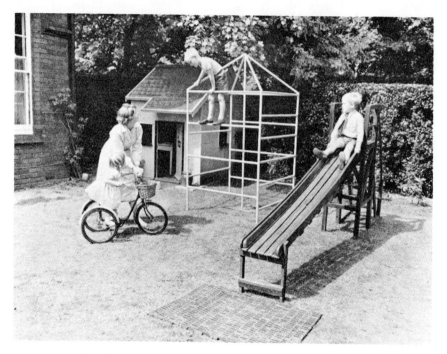

A

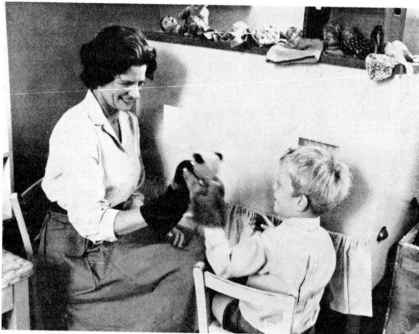

B

PLATE 1. A. A play waiting garden.

B. Puppetry in Play Therapy.

nel, and a contribution is made to the management of the sick child in hospital and to the understanding of psychiatric matters by the nursing, medical and other professional staff.

The children's psychiatric clinic is best attached to the psychiatric department of the general hospital. Such an arrangement allows for collaboration between colleagues, for the pooling of clinical resources and for the integration of the teaching programmes. The management of a child's problems often calls for assistance to the adult members of the family, and vice versa. Child and adult psychiatry are indivisible. In addition the children's psychiatric clinic co-operates with the departments in the hospital which accept child patients, especially paediatric, surgical, orthopaedic, ophthalmologic, ear nose and throat, etc.

In large urban areas, where a separate paediatric hospital exists it may require a child psychiatry department. Departments may also be placed at mental hospitals when these supply the out-patient psychiatric facilities to an area, or in local authority clinics if the psychiatric services are based on them.

Structure

The architecture should be a blend of the domestic and of the functional. This does not necessarily call for a building designed as a house; it is possible to design a hospital building so that it embodies domestic features. In internal decoration special attention should be paid to the use of colour, so that an atmosphere of warmth, welcome and brightness is created. Colours must blend, or otherwise there will be a feeling of restlessness and disharmony. Lighting in the corridors and offices should be bright, but in interview rooms the lighting should be reflected from walls or ceilings, thus giving a more subdued and relaxed atmosphere. Whenever possible, as in waiting, interview and staff rooms, curtains, carpets, wooden furniture, flowers and plants should add to the general feeling of warmth and relaxation.

The waiting room, usually sited on the ground floor, should be in two sections: one for adults and children together, the other for children alone in the form of play room or waiting garden. The main office should contain a switchboard, desks and facilities for storing records, for duplicating and for photocopying. The interview rooms, which should be sufficient in number for all members of the staff, have normally two functions: that of an office and that of an interview room—the latter being more important than the former. It should be possible to arrange the furniture so that interviewing takes place away from the desk, for instance round a small side table on which flowers are placed. Instantaneous recording facilities are very helpful, though they call for attention to sound-proofing and ventilation. The work of the clinical psychologist is greatly aided by having a storage room for test materials.

Play rooms are normally situated on the ground floor. Each room should contain all the facilities required for child psychotherapy. In addition to individual play rooms there should be a large room suitable for group and club activities. One room should cater for adolescent activities. Further features are a two-way screen or short-circuit television for teaching purposes, ample storage facilities for play materials, and a children's library.

A staff room suitable for seminars, for reading and for the departmental library is an essential. A clinical room allows for the storage of drugs, syringe work and routine urine testing. A small kitchen is necessary for staff requirements and also for club and group activities. Amenities for staff include cloakrooms, separate toilet accommodation and parking. Most of the interview rooms should have an outside telephone, and communication between staff is facilitated by an internal telephone system. In addition there should be a telephone booth for the use of patients.

Case notes can be kept in individual filing systems in each interview room, while a master file is maintained in a locked filing system in the general office. At the closure of a case the notes are brought together in one file and remain in a 'temporarily closed' cabinet for twelve months, after which they are removed to the records room. Should a case be re-opened, the notes are broken up into unit notes and held in the locked cabinet of the professional worker concerned.

The utmost care should be taken to guard the confidential nature of case notes, and it is a useful practice for each member of staff on appointment to sign a statement that he has read the warning notice about their confidential nature.

Staff

General. In a document of 1960, *Recruitment and Training of the Child Psychiatrist* (42), the Royal Medico-Psychological Association estimated that one full-time trained consultant child psychiatrist with complementary junior psychiatric staff and allied professional staff were required for 200,000 of the population. It added that future experience would probably show that this was an underestimate of the needs. Thus in Great Britain a total of 230 child psychiatrists would be required. In 1960 there was an equivalent of 160 full-time child psychiatrists. It called for a programme of training to produce the 230 child psychiatrists in the next five years, after which the position should be reviewed. In Sweden one child psychiatric team to 140,000 of the population has already been attained; plans have been made to allow of one team per 50,000 of the population.

The clinical team in child psychiatry usually consists of: psychiatrist, clinical or educational psychologist, social worker, and child therapist. In the past child psychiatrists have been in short supply, and therefore there has been a high ratio of social workers to psychiatrists, even 3 or 4 to 1. Ideal ratios should be as follows: one psychiatrist, one social worker, half-time clinical psychologist, half-time child psychotherapist. In urban areas there is much to be said for the social worker working closely with a particular child psychiatrist. In rural areas it is less time-consuming for social workers to be given geographical areas.

In the recruitment of staff emphasis should be placed upon the emotional stability of the applicants. Natural stability in a staff member is rewarding both to himself and to his patient, and even the best analytical therapy is seldom an adequate substitute for it.

Recruitment and Training. The majority of child psychiatrists come from the field of general psychiatry. Thus all the factors affecting the recruitment of general psychiatrists ultimately impinge upon the recruitment of child psychiatrists. These include the changed attitude of Medicine towards psychiatry, the sounder training in psychiatry for medical students, the availability of posts in general psychiatry, and the equitable distribution of merit awards. There are additional factors appertaining to child psychiatry. These include the opportunity for the medical student to acquire a knowledge of child psychiatry, the availability of training and training posts in child psychiatry for the general psychiatrist, good facilities for clinical work, and opportunities for research.

Child psychiatrists have also come from paediatrics, public health, general practice and general medicine. Trainees from these fields are expected, however, to undertake a comprehensive training in general psychiatry before specialising in child psychiatry.

Trainees in child psychiatry after completing their training in general psychiatry are usually of the Senior Registrar grade. The Royal Medico-Psychological Association (42) estimated that in 1960 there were the equivalent of 16 full-time training posts in child psychiatry. It called for an additional 24 training posts, making a total of 40.

Initially the child psychiatrist undertakes a comprehensive training in general psychiatry. It is an advantage if at this stage he has particular experience of the management and treatment of the neurotic patient. This general training usually takes place at the Senior House Officer and Registrar levels. Specialisation in child psychiatry follows at the Senior Registrar level, this being normally for a period of three years. Particular attention is given to the understanding and management of the psychopathology of the child and adult neurotic patient and their families. Training takes place at clinics orientated towards teaching and research which are able to offer a comprehensive training. Before commencing training in child psychiatry, the trainee will normally hold a diploma or higher qualification in psychological medicine. During his training a child psychiatrist often obtains the M.D. of his university by a thesis on some aspect of his clinical field.

Davies and Stein (11) in 1963 reported the results of a follow-up of doctors who left the junior staff of the Maudsley Hospital between 1st January 1946 and 31st December 1958, a period of 13 years. The follow-up was concerned with the posts held on 1st January 1959. Information was available on 287 of the 299 doctors who left the Maudsley during the years under review, 274 doctors being actually in posts at that time. The second largest group was that of doctors who had specialised in child psychiatry (18% of the doctors); doctors working in the United Kingdom accounted for 22%. Sex influenced the choice of child psychiatry in that 26% of posts were occupied by women, as against 6% in all other sub-groups of psychiatry. Child psychiatry showed a relatively high proportion of grade one (consultants) posts, most of which were in clinics rather than in universities or teaching hospitals; at the fifth year after leaving the Maudsley, of the 18% who were in child psychiatry, 44% were in grade one (consultants), and 41% in grade two (S.M.H.O.).

Psychologists in the Health Service are recruited from Honours Graduates in Psychology of the universities. The clinical psychologist undertakes a training period of three years under a senior clinical psychologist, or joins one of the training courses for clinical psychologists. A number of such courses are available; each Regional Hospital Board is now organising training programmes. A number of psychologists are attracted to the field, but, currently, retention is difficult because of unfavourable salary scales.

Social workers are recruited from the ranks of those who hold a Social Science Diploma or Degree in Social Science at one of the universities. The psychiatric social worker takes an additional one-year postgraduate course for a Mental Health Diploma. In recent years universities have started generic courses for social workers; this may be a step towards the amalgamation of the various groups of social workers into one professional organisation.

Child psychotherapists are recruited from psychology or occupational therapy. The Association of Child Psychotherapists (non-medical) accepts psychologists for training in child psychotherapy. It supervises a number of recognised training courses; each student is required to undergo a personal analysis at a centre approved by the training council. The training period is usually for three years, part-time. Occupational therapists are accepted for training in child psychotherapy at the Department of Family Psychiatry, Ipswich and East Suffolk Hospital. Here, graduate occupational therapists undertake a two years full-time training in play observation, play diagnosis and play therapy. A personal analysis is not required and the training is eclectic.

Functions. The functions of the psychiatrist are outlined in a memorandum by the Royal Medico-Psychological Association (43). The clinical director of a department of child psychiatry is normally a child psychiatrist, who undertakes clinical responsibility for any patient referred to him; he has additional duties in relation to teaching, research, health promotion and advising the hospital authorities on matters appropriate to his field.

The clinical psychologist utilises a large number of psychological procedures for the assessment of children, parents and families. Discussion between the psychiatrist and the psychologist outlines the areas to be assessed. Thereafter the psychologist uses the appropriate procedure and makes his report. A typical psychological report contains room for the test findings, a systematic assessment of the patient in the test situation, a discussion of the results, including an estimate of their probable accuracy, the relation of the findings to any previous test results and to the findings on other members of the family, recommendations for further testing, and it usually concludes with a summary. Further discussion may reveal extra areas for assessment. Care is taken to prepare child or adult for the test situation. Experience has shown that an adequate rapport is essential to produce meaningful results, and in the case of children it may be necessary for the child to attend for a number of occasions before testing commences. Follow-up examination, at completion of treatment, is valuable. In addition, the psychologist has teaching and research functions.

A social history is usually compiled by a social worker on the patient's first attendance. This gives a base-line for further work with the family. The traditional pattern of social history is giving way to a format which takes into account the emotional experiences of the patient. Great importance is attached to obtaining adequate rapport with the patient, even at the cost of not obtaining a complete account during the first interview. To the social history from the patient is added relevant information from other agencies. But the social worker's great contribution comes in management. Many social procedures are available for manipulating the emotional climate of the patient to his advantage. This exacting, but rewarding, task requires not only individual case-work, but also co-operation from a large number of family social agencies. Thus a useful feature of the social work unit is an information cabinet containing particulars of statutory and voluntary agencies, welfare services and other relevant information. All placements of children in hostels, special boarding schools, boarding schools, foster homes, convalescent homes, etc. are arranged by the social worker. A number of social workers have specialised in intensive interview therapy with parents. This method is not always as rewarding as the use of case-work with manipulation of the patient's environment, and carries the danger of neglecting altogether this latter important work. In addition, social workers are engaged in teaching and research.

The child psychotherapist undertakes the investigation and treatment of the child patient under the supervision of the psychiatrist.

Co-ordination of Staff Activities. Various patterns of co-ordinating the activities of staff members have been developed. The traditional practice in child psychiatry is for all staff members to meet together in a large case conference. But this has certain disadvantages for day to day clinical work— it is time-consuming, tends to promote a committee-patient relationship, often undermines the responsibility of each professional worker for his clinical work, and leads to group dependence. As a teaching medium, however, the value of the case conference cannot be denied.

Another pattern employed is that of the small case conference procedure: the psychiatrist, social worker, clinical psychologist and child psychotherapist concerned with an individual child meet together. Close collaboration over a period of time allows for many things to go unsaid. Decisions are rapidly arrived at by the group, whilst each individual worker retains responsibility for his own contribution.

Yet another pattern is that of the psychiatrist meeting each member of the professional expert staff in individual interviews once a week. The advantages of this method are speed, the fact that one aspect of the case can be thrashed out thoroughly, and that there is no wastage of time due to other professional workers standing by when discussion is irrelevant to their contribution. New cases can be quickly explored and decisions taken on treatment. Opportunity can also be taken to discuss matters of common interest between the two professional groups.

Administrative co-ordination is also important, and this can be achieved by the staff meeting together once a week to co-ordinate appointments and to discuss matters of general interest.

Administrative Staff. A department cannot function without an administrative officer and an adequate number of personal secretaries, shorthand typists and clerks. A carefully selected receptionist with charm and poise is invaluable in the reception of patients. In addition, a porter may be required for sundry duties, handy-man work and moving play material in the play rooms. The cleaners complete the staff.

The administrative staff should be responsible for maintaining the waiting list, sending out appointments, maintaining records and card indexes, compiling statistics, requisitioning material, and the day-to-day upkeep of the building. In a hospital department they are responsible to the clinical director of the department and to the hospital secretary.

In-patient Accommodation

General. Under Section 17 of the National Health Service Act, 1946, it is made the duty of the Regional Hospital Boards 'generally to administer, on behalf of the Minister, the hospital and specialised services provided in their area'. The Minister discusses child psychiatry in Section D of the Memorandum to Regional Hospital Boards (47) 13. Para. 38 states the position in regard to in-patient facilities: '38. The Regional Board will be responsible for the provision and development of medical services for children suffering from mental illness and maladjustment. In-patient accommodation will be required in hostels and hospitals for those needing residential treatment.' (33.)

Types of Accommodation. This can be conveniently considered as it applies to children up to the age of 12, and to adolescents up to the age of 18:

> *Children: Short-term units.* These are for diagnosis, short-term therapy, and emergencies. They should be in small family units of

8–12 beds, and be closely attached to the out-patient child psychiatric facilities of the district general hospital. The special means of investigation—psychometric, electroencephalographic, pathological etc.—should be readily available.

Children: Medium-stay units. These units admit for periods of stabilisation those children who are too disturbed for placement in hostels, foster homes etc. The length of stay may vary from six months to two years. They should be in family units of 8–12 beds. There are advantages in having these with or close to the children's out-patient clinics and with the short-term units. It makes for economy of services, and children can pass readily from one unit to the other.

Children: Units for psychotic children. These should be planned on a Regional basis. The optimum size is that of the family group type of 12 beds. Facilities for investigation and research should be readily available. Long-term care is required for most patients.

Adolescents: Units for the medium-stay care of disturbed adolescents. The aim of these units is to give intensive treatment over a period of 6 months to 2 years to emotionally disturbed adolescents who are unfitted for other accommodation. Family care should be supplied in units of 8–12 beds. They should be in the district general hospital in association with the department of psychiatry. Sexes are normally segregated, but there is room for experimentation with mixed units.

Adolescents: Units for psychotic adolescents. These should be in units of 12 beds in mental hospitals alongside the same facilities for adults. In future they will be close to or at the District General Hospital.

Adolescents: Night hospitals or hostels. These should be of the family type with house-parents, and catering for groups of 12 adolescents. They are invaluable for adolescents who still require some skilled help while working locally. They should be under the supervision of the main psychiatric hospital, but need not be located with it.

Supporting Services. Children tend to be kept in the above units for longer than it is necessary, unless a number of supporting services are available. For children there should be hostels or special boarding schools, supplied under the provisions of the 1944 Education Act. Some children may need foster home placement by the Children's Department of the local authorities or by voluntary societies.

Assessment of Need. Shortage of in-patient beds for children and adolescents is reflected in the statistics. In 1956 there were 237 children's beds and 86 adolescents' beds in England and Wales (including those in teaching hospitals). By 1961 these had increased to 412 children's beds and

298 adolescents' beds, either established or proposed. Despite this increase the figures still show that only a quarter of the beds considered necessary by the Royal Medico-Psychological Association have been supplied for children, and only one-fifth for adolescents. The Royal Medico-Psychological Association (39) had recommended 20 beds for half a million of the population for children, and 20 beds for half a million of the population for adolescents. Sweden, where one child in six seen in the out-patient child psychiatric clinic is admitted, has twice as many beds for children as England and Wales on a relative population basis.

The Ministry of Health (36) in 1964 has recommended the development of more in-patient facilities. They consider that their interim objectives involve no risk of over-provision, and have recommended that as an initial aim the number of children's beds should be increased to 20–25 per million of the population for short-term care, with additional provision for long-term treatment on the scale, at first, of 25 beds per Region. They recommended that the provision for adolescents should be increased to 20–25 beds per million.

The catchment areas of most child psychiatric units have half a million rather than a million population. A reasonable initial provision of beds for units serving a population of half a million would be: (1) a short-term diagnostic unit of 8–12 beds; (2) a medium-stay unit for children of 8–12 beds; (3) a Regional unit of 24 beds for psychotic children, in two ward units of 12 beds; (4) a unit for emotionally disturbed adolescents of 24 beds, laid in two family units of 12; (5) a unit for psychotic adolescents at a mental hospital, with provision of one unit of 12 beds; (6) a hostel or night hospital, with provision of two family units of 12 beds.

Staffing. The success of in-patient units depends on staff selection more than on any other single factor. Staff are likely to be successful if kindly, warm-hearted, unsentimental, intelligent and with a good sense of humour. These qualities usually go with stability and good relationships with their own parents in childhood and later. The dedicated, the sentimental and the hypermoral are unlikely to be successful.

Professional staff can be shared with the children's out-patient service. The in-patient units should be in the charge of a responsible nursing officer, trained in both the mental and the general hospital field. The nursing staff should be permanent, and nurses in training should visit for observation only, this being an essential part of their training. Nursing assistants, recruited from the local community, can be invaluable in this work. In medium- and long-stay units additional provision must be made for teachers (34) of formal school subjects, and for instructors in various crafts.

The ratio of staff to patients is high, and sometimes may need to be on a one-to-one basis. There is much to be said for project nursing whereby one member of the staff is responsible for a number of children. Especially in the long-term units, time should be available for staff to keep in touch with discharged patients.

Treatment of children should go hand in hand with treatment of the parents and the family. Children should not be discharged to an unsatisfactory home.

Lay-out. The lay-out should be as domestic as possible, with adequate facilities for indoor and outdoor recreation. Provision will also have to be made for a quiet room for study, interview rooms for professional staff, a library, accommodation for pets and a schoolroom.

Voluntary Help

The work of the professional staff can be supplemented by that of voluntary helpers. They can function as a small group, as a Circle of Friends, or in the case of a large unit as a League of Friends. They are usually affiliated to the National League of Hospital Friends. Such groups can serve as useful links between the department and the voluntary charitable organisations in the community, can provide funds for material aid when this is not available from any other source, and can also initiate projects which are not recognised as coming within the purview of any statutory body. The Friends acquire funds through donations from voluntary bodies, from the Sunday Cinema Fund, and by organising fund-raising activities of their own. Small sums of money readily available at the right moment can be invaluable to patients in urgent need.

Research

Leo Kanner (26) ended his Maudsley lecture to the Royal Medico-Psychological Association in 1958 with a plea for research in child psychiatry. This is only beginning to be answered in Great Britain. There is still a widespread tendency to rely upon anecdote and speculation, while systematic investigations are few. This is illustrated by the fact that there is probably no single valid estimate of the results of therapy in child psychiatry. The position is improving as some psychiatrists begin to apply themselves to fundamental research by drawing upon contributions from ethology, ethnology, experimental psychology, developmental psychology, and neuro-physiology. Follow-up studies (18), despite their difficulties, have a real value in the assessment of procedures, organisation and therapy.

With the pressure of clinical work, research will be put aside unless there is a special allotment of time to it. Some senior clinical posts should be designated as joint clinical-and-research posts; personal research assistants and facilities should then be provided. Research administration should have ample accommodation in a quiet but accessible part of the building. Information about an individual patient can be recorded on item sheets and transferred to punch cards to be available for retrospective research. Adequate library facilities are essential.

Teaching

Professional Staff. Time and facilities are essential if effective teaching is to be done. The best teaching affords experience in the whole range of clinical disorders, at the same time allowing the close study of a small number of selected patients. The apprenticeship system, backed by formal instruction in seminars and case conferences, has much to recommend it. Library facilities are required that include not only books and reprints but also tape recordings selected for their teaching value.

Related Professions. It is also necessary to arouse interest in and give instruction to related professions. The best propaganda is a good clinical service. The professions include the following: general practitioner, school medical officer, health visitor, school nurse, district nurse, midwife, social and welfare worker, staff of Children's Departments, staff of day nurseries, teacher and hospital nurse.

The Public. Experience shows that it is more effective to concentrate teaching on key personnel, i.e. members of the related professions, than upon members of the public: key personnel in their day-to-day work can informally influence public opinion.

3

Clinical Procedures

The Clinical Material

The service covers the age group 0–17, which includes the infant, the pre-school child, the school child and the adolescent. While it would be wrong to neglect the needs of any one age group, the infant and pre-school child, because of their ability to change, are of particular importance.

The following points should be noted:

1. An analysis of case material shows that the great majority of patients are emotionally disturbed children. Their emotional disturbance is a result of emotional stress, usually produced within the family. Psychosis, whether it be organic or functional, is rare in children. An analysis of a thousand cases at the Children's Intake Clinic, Department of Family Psychiatry, Ipswich and East Suffolk Hospital showed that only six patients, i.e. 0·6%, were referred for psychosis. Therefore the children's service must be primarily orientated to the clinical needs of the emotionally disturbed child—99·4% of the intake.

2. The incidence of emotional disorder in children is usually given as 1–2% of all children per year. Variations in this figure will depend upon the standard adopted by the observer. In general, it is the most awkward or attention-attracting symptom that receives the earliest investigation; less obvious but equally serious symptoms can easily be overlooked. Furthermore, the greater the skill of the diagnostician, the more numerous the children referred.

As part of a large survey of psychiatric disorders in the population of Aarhus and its county, a survey financed by the Ford Foundation, a small but very thorough study of psychological disorders in childhood was made on the island of Samsø (Denmark) by Lange, Mogensen and Fenger. They found that 15·5% of all children up to fifteen years of age were in need of psychiatric care. Statisticians estimate this as equivalent to 2–3% of children needing care per year, and suggest that the figure quoted above, on which present planning is often based, may be an underestimate.

3. One of the striking results of a direct link with the home through the general practitioner is the increase in the percentage of under-five children referred. Table 1 shows that by 1959 in the town of Ipswich, where the service is particularly accessible to the general practitioner, the percentage of under-fives stood at 17·5%.

TABLE 1

Referrals by age group in Ipswich 1959

Age	Number	%
Under 5	38	17·5
5–10	105	48·1
11–15	75	34·4

4. Table 2 shows that in each age group there is a preponderance of boys over girls, especially in the groups 5–10 years. This may indicate that boys are more disturbed than girls. On the other hand it may indicate that a selection factor is operating, as for example that disturbed boys are more prone to behaviour which attracts the attention of referral agencies. Should there be such a selection factor, it would seem important to circumvent it, so that future mothers may receive the same help as future fathers.

TABLE 2

Sex distribution among Ipswich children referred 1951–1960

Age	Total	Boys	Girls	Ratio
0–4	266	156	110	3 : 2
5–10	825	519	306	5 : 3
11–15	395	246	149	3 : 2

Crombie and Cross (9) showed that in a year 72% of males between the ages of five and fourteen were seen by the general practitioner for 1·3 episodes of 15·3 minutes' duration, while 85·1% of females of the same range were seen for 1·7 episodes of 17·1 minutes each. This slight preponderance of females over males seen by general practitioners is the reverse of the proportion seen at child psychiatric clinics. It suggests that some selective factor must be at work in the referrals from general practitioners to psychiatric clinics.

5. The distribution of intelligence in emotionally disturbed children referred to a psychiatric clinic closely follows the curve of normal distribution, the mean IQ of children being 97·05. (See Fig. 1).

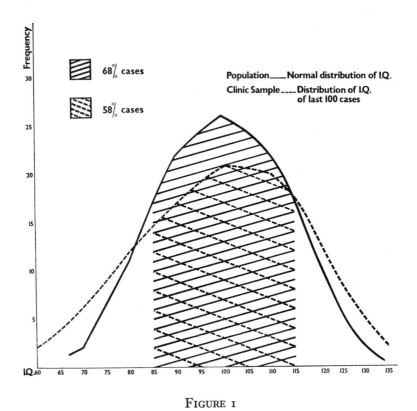

FIGURE I

6. Mentally sub-normal children should be accepted by this service if they manifest emotional problems.

7. Not only should the child who is referred be investigated, but also the other children in the family.

8. It is not possible to separate the child's condition from that of his parents or other adult members of the family. Thus the service should offer help to parents and parent substitutes.

9. When a child becomes emotionally disturbed, the whole of his personality is disturbed. In a particular child a cluster of symptoms, or only one symptom, may predominate. Because it attracts attention it causes concern to the parents or others in contact with the child, and so becomes the reason for referral.

Referral of Patients

General. The aim in referral procedure is to get the patient to the right clinic in the shortest possible time. Success will depend upon taking account of some of the following factors:

1. The attitude of the community towards the service will tend to determine whether patients are referred readily or not. The opinions held about the service by the usual referral agencies are probably much more influential in encouraging acceptance of it than the opinions of the public, which are largely fashioned by those of the agencies. An understanding family or school doctor prepares his patients for a psychiatric interview and fosters rapport between clinic and patient. Unfortunately the problems referred to a new service are likely to be the more severe ones, and success more difficult to obtain.

2. In dealing with children accessibility to the source of the disturbance, the home, is very important, and on this fact largely depends the number of children ascertained as emotionally disturbed. The aetiological importance of the family has sometimes been underestimated and undue emphasis given to the child's school life. In the important pre-school age group, of course, the school cannot be a factor. In the school-age group it would appear that the intensity and length of contact between child and school is much less than is sometimes supposed. Normally, a child in his school years spends approximately one-third of his waking time at school and two-thirds of his time outside the influence of school. It must also be remembered that the intensity of contact between child and adult is very much less at school than it is at home. At home, in a family with two children, he will have a relationship on a one-to-one ratio with an adult: at school he will be fortunate to have a relationship on a one-to-thirty ratio with a teacher. Furthermore, each year contacts made with the school-teacher will be broken; indeed in the later years he will meet a variety of teachers, each of whom he will see for only a short time each week. Thus the school would appear to be less important than the home aetiologically; but naturally it still provides opportunities for the ascertainment of ill children.

Children in care are referred from the Children's Departments of the Local Authorities. One child in every 200 is in care at any one time (14). Some of these children are very disturbed, and since the community is acting as a parent surrogate it has a special responsibility for them.

3. The age of the patient causes him to present more readily to some services than to others.

The infant or toddler is likely to come to the notice of the home doctor or the home nurse. One investigation (9) shows that 93·1% of children under five were seen by a family doctor during a year for the mean number of 2·0 times, for a mean of 9·55 minutes on each occasion. Probably no other agency approaches this degree of contact. A child may also be seen at an infant welfare clinic. Mothers are much more willing to attend welfare centres during the first year of a child's life than they are when the child is older; about 75% of the mothers attend with children under one year, whereas only about 27% of the mothers with children between one and five do so.

When a child is of school age the family doctor and the school health service are important sources of referral. The cases referred from the school are likely to be ascertained by the school teacher, who acts to some degree as a parent surrogate and whose awareness of emotional problems will be a decisive factor in determining whether she refers or not. Additional patients come from the courts and other hospital clinics.

The adolescent at work is likely to come from the home doctor, the factory doctor or the home nurse, while adolescents still at school may come via the school health service. Some adolescents may come through the courts, and others through hospital clinics.

The family doctor is the doctor most in touch with the home, and therefore has certain advantages over all other agencies. He is normally in touch with the family for many years, has a great amount of information available about the family and its social setting, and has knowledge of the family as a whole. An urban general practitioner has analysed his case material, and finds that for 78% of his patients he is doctor to the whole family—truly a 'family doctor' (15). In rural areas the percentage is probably even higher. Cammock et al. (7) have recently confirmed these findings. Referrals from general practitioners have steadily increased over the years as can be seen from the experience of one clinic (see Table 3).

TABLE 3

Year	G.P.s and Hospitals	School Medical Officer	Others
	%	%	%
1950	56	36	8
1951	61	37	2
1952	64	34	2
1953	62	32	5
1954	68	27	5
1955	78	18	3
1956	68	29	3
1957	76	21	3
1958	76	20	4
1959	82	16	2

4. The type of problem or symptom presenting in the patient will to some extent determine which agency ascertains him. General practitioners and infant welfare clinics usually refer patients with physical and emotional

symptoms, while the teacher sends problems of discipline and of failure to make progress in school work. Courts of law may send patients with behaviour disorders—in the first place for a medical report and subsequently with a recommendation for treatment.

Children with psychosomatic problems predominate in referrals from other hospital clinics. Such children are seen at surgical as well as medical and paediatric departments. For example the general surgical department sees patients with obscure abdominal pains, the orthopaedic department accident-prone cases, the obstetric department early disturbances of mother-infant relationship. The ophthalmologist sees emotionally determined squints and headaches; from the ear, nose and throat department come such problems as pseudo-deafness, pseudo-backwardness and chronic rhinitis.

Procedure

General Practitioner. A convenient practice is for each practitioner to be supplied with a number of appointment slips, each having a space for notes. These are sent direct by post to the clinic and are placed in a confidential file until the case is seen.

School Medical Officer. The teacher refers her problems to the school medical officer by personal contact at school health inspections or by telephone or by letter. Others in the educational field have opportunities of observing difficulties in the child, for instance the speech therapist, the educational psychologist and the school nurse. All these agencies refer the children to the school medical officer for referral to the psychiatrist.

The school medical officer should be regarded as being in the same position relative to the teacher and the child as the general practitioner to the parent and child. It is his responsibility to assess the problem, and to exclude non-psychiatric conditions, such as the deaf child, the child with visual difficulties, the subnormal child or the child with physical disabilities. Before referral, the school medical officer can usually discuss the child with the general practitioner. Where the school medical officer can himself manage a problem he is encouraged to do so. When a child is referred from school, it is important to discuss the matter with the parents in order to enlist their co-operation; without this measure great difficulty may arise later.

At this point it may be worth while clarifying the distinction between the school psychology service and the psychiatric service for school children, by an analogy with diabetes in the physical field. Information about a diabetic child's behaviour at school might aid the diagnostic measures of the school medical officer and the hospital paediatrician. An approach is therefore made to the teacher by the medical service to gather information to assist diagnosis. After treatment, it may be helpful to the teacher to receive guidance on the handling of the diabetic child at school from the school medical officer or the paediatrician. Thus a school visit from the medical social worker can be of value. Furthermore the child, because of his disability, may be retarded in school work to such an extent that the teacher may need to use special educational facilities which require the advice of the school psychological service. There is thus no confusion of function between the school psychological service, the school health service and the hospital paediatric service.

Similarly in dealing with an emotionally disturbed child a 'link is needed between the teacher and the psychiatric service through the psychiatric social worker in order to provide information for diagnosis. During and after treatment a similar contact is required between the psychiatric service and the teacher in order to help her in her handling of the child. Furthermore the child, because of his disability, may sometimes be retarded in school work to such an extent that the teacher may require the advice of the school psychological service. Again there is no confusion between the school psychology service, the school health service and the psychiatric service for school children.

Infant Welfare Clinics. The Medical Officer, usually after conferring with the general practitioner, refers the child direct to the clinic, Some have advocated that a child psychiatric clinic should be placed at every Infant Welfare Clinic. Except in special circumstances, such as at a large centre or a teaching unit, that is neither necessary nor practicable; the same request could be advanced by the many hospital and local authority clinics. The real need is for adequate liaison, for advice to be offered immediately by telephone, and for urgent cases to be seen at once.

Direct Referrals. From time to time patients knock at the clinic's door and ask to be seen. This is usually because the matter is immediately urgent, because they are new to the area, or because they have alienated the sympathies of the usual sources of referral. It is a disadvantage if the referring agencies are by-passed and the patient becomes his own diagnostician. Moreover the usual referring agencies lose interest, and many advantages are lost.

Urgent cases should be accepted as a matter of emergency and then referred back to their own doctors. Less urgent cases can be referred back to their own doctors but, should this present any difficulty, the clinic can approach the doctor on their behalf. Administrative convenience should not be allowed to come before the welfare of the patient.

Juvenile Courts. Magistrates usually remand the patient for a medical report and allow the full period of three weeks.

Waiting List. A steady flow of cases keeps the clinical staff at optimum efficiency, and for this a waiting list is required. Urgent cases should be seen at once, fairly urgent cases within five days, and the remainder within two weeks. Such arrangements call for some elasticity in administration. Waiting lists were the subject of an enquiry by the Ministry of Health, 1958 (35).

A psychiatric service should give a rapid diagnostic service or it will hamper the activities of other agencies. If however it accepts for prolonged treatment all the cases requiring it, then, with the staff available, a long waiting list will soon accumulate. Selection of cases for treatment is essential, as it allows the available staff to be used to the best advantage, prevents the accumulation of a long waiting list and lets patients pass straight from diagnosis to treatment, a highly desirable practice.

Other measures which have been found helpful in maintaining a short waiting list are: the omission of routine case conferences and thus saving time, placing one person in charge of the waiting list, and sending a pre-paid-reply postcard with the appointment.

Failure Rate. For first attendances it can be as low as 6% or as high as 75%. The most significant factor in a low failure rate is a short waiting list. Other factors are the co-operation of referring agencies and the acceptance of the service by the community.

Reception. A pleasant letter should invite the patient to attend, and it can be accompanied by a brochure giving information likely to be required before attendance. Most clinics have an appointment system. Patients should be received by a receptionist or voluntary worker in the waiting area.

Evening clinics are popular with fathers who cannot attend during the day and with mothers who require their husbands to look after the children. A special clinic for adolescents allows them, when appropriate, to attend without parents. Once a new patient has attended it is a helpful practice to explain that, should he become acutely distressed for any reason, he has only to telephone the department and an immediate appointment or home visit will be arranged.

Investigation

General. A clinical investigation is based upon the following principles:

1. The first aim is to make a diagnosis. It has to be established whether the presenting patient is sent with an emotional disorder or with some other clinical entity. A diagnosis is made from elucidating positive psychiatric findings and not from negative physical findings.

2. The second aim is to reveal quickly the true emotional condition of the patient by appraising his psychopathology, bearing in mind the dynamic continuum of the past and the present.

3. The focus of the investigation moves from the presenting child to all members of the family as soon as possible. The moment when this is possible varies from family to family.

4. Assessment must be made of the family's assets as well as of its liabilities.

5. The emotional forces bearing on the child from without the family must be taken into account, and include influences from relatives, friends, neighbours, schoolmates, and teachers.

6. The establishment of rapport between the clinical personnel and

the child and its family is of fundamental importance. Given rapport, the relevant information will in time be forthcoming.

Procedure

First Attendance. One practice is as follows. The psychiatrist first sees the parents, who have both been invited to the interview. A history of the complaint is taken from the parents. The child is then seen alone by the psychiatrist, and a systematic appraisal is made of him in either a play or an interview situation, depending on his age. The parents and the child may be seen together. Physical and neurological examination of the child is undertaken at this interview or, more usually, at the subsequent one. Great care is taken to make the physical examination a pleasant and rapport-building experience for the child.

It is important for the psychiatrist to see the problem as it presents in its natural state. The above procedure has advantages in that the first emotional release is an opportunity to establish rapport, and the psychiatrist has a real experience of the situation rather than a condensed or 'second-hand' version.

At the first interview the following *additional information* can be available:

(a) *Hospital records.* They are useful in explaining previous ill health and the reason for hospital admissions.

(b) *School Medical Officer's records.* When children are referred from school, the records are usually sent by the school medical officer with his referring letter. When the general practitioner refers a patient, it is possible to borrow the records from the Health Authority.

(c) *School report.* This is usually forwarded automatically when a child is referred by the school medical officer. When a general practitioner refers a child it can be supplied by the school on request. The school reports may be supplemented later by school visits by the social worker.

(d) *General Practitioner's report.* Should the child be referred by a school doctor, the psychiatrist can ask for a letter to be sent to the general practitioner inviting information about his patient.

At the first attendance one or more of the following special procedures may be required:

(a) *Social history.* The psychiatrist outlines the initial formulation on the child to the social worker, and the policy in regard to the social history is discussed between them. The social history is usually undertaken at the first interview. It may be supplemented by a home visit later.

(b) *Psychometric tests.* The initial formulation on the child is discussed with the clinical psychologist and the problems for solution are defined. Without this definition the procedure is as valueless as sending a patient to an X-ray department without a specific request. The patient is usually seen at the first attendance. Additional appointments if required are arranged between the psychologist and the parents.

(c) *Play diagnosis.* This is not undertaken at the first interview, since the psychiatrist will already have observed the child in a play situation. The initial formulation is discussed between the psychiatrist and the child therapist, who then pursues her investigations in one or more subsequent interviews.

(d) *Pathological investigations.* Urine analysis usually takes place in the psychiatric clinic. More elaborate investigations call for the services of the Pathological Department.

(e) *Radiological examination.*

(f) *Electroencephalographic examination.*

(g) *In-patient observation.*

Second and subsequent attendances. The second attendance usually takes place during the following week, when all the reports are to hand. The psychiatrist now makes his second formulation. Some cases can be closed at this point and sent back to the referring agency. After this attendance, a first report is prepared for the referring doctor.

In most cases, however, further attendances are necessary in order to elucidate the psychopathology. Father, mother, relatives or 'third parties' may need to be seen at day or evening sessions; other children in the family may require investigation. Usually it is not felt that the investigation is complete until a picture of the psychodynamics of the whole family is obtained.

Individual procedures can be supplemented by Family Group Diagnosis (21), whereby all members of the family are interviewed together. Families accept this procedure remarkably easily, and the psychiatrist should never deny himself the opportunity of seeing the interplay of the family dynamics at first hand. Time must be allowed for the true pattern to emerge. The relationships of the family with the community are also readily revealed, and in particular their relationships with the extended family.

Staff Liaison. The clinical responsibility for the patient should be borne throughout by his psychiatrist. The ethical position is that a referring doctor requires an opinion on his patient by a specialist, and also requires that treatment beyond his resources be undertaken by the specialist. The psychiatrist can call on the assistance of a number of expert non-medical colleagues, who, while not taking responsibility for the patient, are responsible for the work they undertake with the patient. Each professional worker is administratively responsible to the senior worker in his unit, and in turn to the clinical director of the department. But each professional clinical worker is solely responsible for his own clinical work, and in this work collaborates directly with the psychiatrist concerned with that case. Each expert worker requires such information as will enable him to carry out his work effectively.

Reports

General. The purpose of a report is to give all who can help a patient as much information as they need for their purpose, *after obtaining the full consent of the patient.* The basis of the work between the psychiatrist and the patient is the ability of the patient to communicate meaningful emotional happenings. This can only occur when the patient knows that the information imparted will not be divulged to others without his consent. At the same time he cannot be helped by other agencies unless they have enough information for their purpose. This information may be the whole, or more usually a part, of the information known to the clinic. It must be passed on to them with the full knowledge of the patient, so that if he wishes he may elect not to seek this further help. Agencies readily accept the position when it is put to them in this way, and difficulties seldom arise in practice.

Reports are usually sent after the second diagnostic attendance. Follow-up reports are sent at intervals if many attendances occur. A final report is sent to the referring doctor at the closure of the case.

General Practitioner and Hospital Reports. The report goes direct to the family doctor when a child patient has been referred by him. If a hospital department is also involved, then a copy of the report goes to the consultant concerned.

With child patients it is often essential to seek the help of the school medical officer. In this event a copy of the report is sent to him, with the consent of the doctor and his patient, so that he can advise his education authority. Sometimes the teacher has been the instigator of the referral, and it is then desirable that her interest should be maintained and her help sought; a non-medical report is therefore sent to the teacher through the school medical officer and the director of education. This may be followed by a school visit, which is more valuable than a written report. Even if the teacher has not played any part in the referral she may still in some cases be able to make a useful contribution. No contact with a school should take place without the awareness and agreement of the parents.

School Medical Officer Referrals. Here the report on a child patient goes direct to the school medical officer, who is responsible for advising the education or health authority. A copy is sent to the general practitioner. Communication is established with the teacher as already described. In those cases where there is a special educational problem a report is sent to the educational psychologist, so that she can arrange for specialist help, and an informal contact invariably follows.

Court Referrals. A medical recommendation is made direct to the Magistrates through the Clerk of the Court.

4

Treatment

General. The following matters are relevant to the planning of a therapeutic service:

1. The ideal aim is the complete cure of the patient and his family.

2. Sometimes it is unrealistic to expect a total cure and a modified aim becomes necessary, as in any other clinical field.

3. The art of medicine must not be overlooked. Every patient and his family is unique, and the constellation of factors which produced the disturbance cannot be covered by any general rule.

4. The patient must show improvement not only within the therapeutic situation but also within the family setting.

5. Individual or group psychotherapy may be required by one or more members of the family, irrespective of the child who was initially referred.

6. Advantages arise from the fact that one clinic attends to both adults and children from the same family. Firstly, most of the knowledge required for the treatment of child and parent is identical. Secondly, the parents' childhood experiences are an important factor in the present child-parent situation. Thirdly, the treatment of child and adult can be synchronised. Fourthly, rapport can be developed with the whole family. Failure to appreciate that the parents of disturbed children are usually themselves also disturbed has sometimes led to advice and reassurance alone being offered to parents. This procedure has a very limited effect.

7. A great deal can be achieved through extra-clinic environmental management.

8. There is a place for an in-patient service for the short-term investigation and the short-term and long-term treatment of children, adults and families.

9. Selected foster homes offer the best form of substitute home care for children.

10. A clinical service should not be obliged to offer all the necessary therapeutic measures to every patient. Other agencies may be able to offer some forms of help just as effectively. The family doctor is in a particularly advantageous position to offer supportive therapy. Supportive work may be done by the home nurse, the teacher, the welfare worker and the clergy. Tasks such as remedial teaching, the ascertainment of educationally backward or bright children who need special school facilities, and vocational guidance, can be undertaken by the School Psychological Service of the local education authority.

Intra-Clinic Therapy

General. At the initial formulation a preliminary plan of therapy is made. The early process of therapy may have begun at the sending of the first appointment. The preliminary plan may need alteration as further information comes to hand. The number of family members under therapy may change or the emphasis of the therapy alter.

In some clinics it is usual for parent therapy to be the prime task of the psychiatrist, while the child psychotherapist treats the child in collaboration with him and the social worker uses case-work in extra-clinic therapy. In others the child therapy is undertaken by the psychiatrist while the social worker undertakes case-work with the parents.

The average British child psychiatrist is not psychoanalytically trained. Psychoanalysis still however contributes significantly to psychopathological concepts. Some maintain that it is possible to manage psychopathology by using different techniques and interpretations from psychoanalysis and still reach the same 'depth'. There is little doubt that we are on the edge of a more questioning attitude towards the scientific basis of psychoanalysis. In some quarters there is a desire to start afresh and to make a new approach based upon systematic research.

The range of treatment for the child and the adult will be briefly described. For the adolescent, according to his maturity, an adult or a child approach is employed.

Child Therapy. The child psychotherapist undertakes the investigation and treatment of the child patient, under the supervision of the psychiatrist. Together psychiatrist and child therapist outline the project for that child. The first aim is usually to establish rapport, for which much play material is utilised. Thereafter systematic observation of the child takes place in the play situation (16); this gives a base-line for comparison later on. Play diagnosis follows. The aim here is to encourage the child to reveal his problems as he knows them, and also to express what he knows about himself and his relationships within the family, the school and the neighbourhood. A young child can only communicate through play; an older child may spontaneously verbalise to the therapist. The play medium appropriate to the child's age, sex and inclination is supplied. It is usual to corroborate information obtained through one medium by that disclosed by another. Play therapy is the final technique, and is employed for one of the following reasons: (a) to support the child while the parents are receiving treatment; (b) to support the child when the environment cannot be changed, or when he cannot be separated from it; (c) to help to separate the child from his parents, for either short or lengthy periods; (d) to make a real change in the child's personality. The relationship between therapist and child is the most potent therapeutic medium. Within the safety of this relationship, the child expresses his fears, guilt, and hate, and, sharing these with the therapist, is encouraged to healthier reactions. With adolescents art therapy is often a useful medium. The child psychotherapist can also organise group activities, either in the form of group therapy with a small number of children, or in the form of supportive clubs for children during the evening and at the week-end. She also has a large part to play in the programme of the day hospital.

Parent Therapy. (a) Advice to parents. This is straightforward work, and includes for example estimating and giving an opinion on intelligence; the differential diagnosis of somatic symptoms; the diagnosis and advice on treatment of acute confusional states.

(b) Supportive therapy. Where there are many material difficulties, the great majority of such problems are usually handled by the social worker. It involves winning the confidence of a family and encouraging and supporting them to take the right measures to help themselves.

Supportive work on patients who may have considerable emotional difficulties may be the task of the psychiatrist or of the social worker. In every case the issues must be weighed up in emotional terms. The aim is to reduce stress, and to mobilise restitution factors through the decisions made possible by the relationship.

Group supportive therapy for adults either in one sex or mixed groups is a valuable supportive measure.

(c) Prolonged therapy. This may last from six months to four years, with daily, weekly or fortnightly sessions, depending on the resources of the clinic. Interviews normally last 60 minutes, but are frequently extended to 90 minutes and sometimes even longer. A close relationship between patient and therapist makes possible the resolution of those adverse situations in the past which are at the root of the present disturbance, and so a reintegration of the personality is effected. Therapy may be on an individual, group or family-group basis.

Family-Group Therapy (21) is a procedure whereby all the members of the family of all ages are treated together. It can be effective in revealing and resolving the attitudes of family members, and their capacity to make up for deficiencies in the family situation is mobilised. According to the demands of the clinical situation, Family-Group Therapy may need to be supplemented by individual therapy; the two forms of therapy should be regarded as complementary to one another.

(d) Drugs. These are utilised as sedatives, hypnotics, tranquillisers, anticonvulsants and as aids to psychotherapy.

Extra-Clinic Therapy

This is the manipulation of the pattern of emotional influences playing upon the family, from within and without, for the betterment of the family. An example of such a manipulation would be to supply 'day foster care' (17, 23, 20) in a foster home or special day nursery for a child deprived of healthy emotional care by a disturbed parent.

The procedures embraces: (a) basing all the measures on a right emotional analysis of the family in the first place; (b) the understanding of the family in emotional terms by all those who have to do with the family, especially the social worker, the family doctor, the health visitor, the mid-wife, the district nurse, and the school welfare officer, so that emotional solutions can be planned for the emotional problems; (c) liaison between the individuals who are dealing with the family; (d) building up new community facilities to help the emotionally ill. Extra-clinic therapy often calls for facilities which may not, at the moment, be available, as community services tend to be geared to meet the physical rather than the emotional needs of the patients.

The effectiveness of extra-clinic therapy has often been underestimated. Poor results may arise from overlooking the importance of the preliminary estimate being in emotional terms, or, if a correct assessment has been made, from the necessary facilities not being available.

Reports

From time to time during treatment a 'progress' report is sent to the referring agency. A final report is sent to them at the closure of the case.

Follow-up

At the end of one year after closure it is a useful procedure to make a 'follow-up' contact by the social worker who undertook casework on that family. This practice has several objectives. Patients derive comfort from the thought that contact with the Department will be renewed in a year's time. Any further help that is required can be arranged. An evaluation of the help given to the family can be made: some patients are able, with the detachment of time, to give a better assessment of the way in which the clinic helped. Follow-up studies can also be used to study the development and natural history of emotional problems (18).

Health Promotion

The personality benefits from positive emotional influences. Every individual should therefore be nourished by such influences. It follows that it is desirable to re-plan all community activities so that the maximum positive emotional influences are brought to bear on everyone, thus creating a health-promoting or salutiferous community (21).

In order to improve the collective influences, there should be an analysis of every activity, standard and institution of the community, leading to an assessment of its emotional value for the individual and for the family, followed by a decision to encourage those situations that promote emotional health and to remedy those that are emotionally unfavourable.

One illustration that may be cited concerns the influence of individuals. Positive emotional influences are received from contact with stable individuals. Therefore these individuals should be deployed at the points where they can exert the greatest beneficial effect upon others. The strong must help the weak. The deployment of stable individuals in this way is one measure likely to produce the optimum conditions for emotional health.

Satisfaction of material needs to a large degree, together with the recognition of emotional phenomena, makes it now within our grasp to enter this new phase of community action. A perceptible improvement may be all that can be achieved by community action in one generation, but this will have a cumulative effect over the generations. Individuals are most susceptible to emotional influences in their early, formative years, and special attention should be paid to this fact when planning community measures.

Thus the psychiatric service for children has a duty to make its findings on the emotional life of the child known to those agencies able to effect improvements in community living.

REFERENCES

1. BLACKER, C. P., 1946. *Neurosis and the Mental Health Service*. London: Oxford University Press.
2. British Medical Association, 1958. *Comments of the Council on the Draft Circular*.
3. 1962a. *Report of Sub-Committee on Child Psychiatric Services*.
4. 1962b. *Review of the Medical Services in Great Britain*.
5. British Paediatric Association, 1957. *Report of Psychology Sub-Committee*.
6. CAMERON, H., 1918. *The Nervous Child*. London: Oxford Univ. Press.
7. CAMMOCK, D. W. *et al.*, 1961. *Lancet*, i: 213.
8. Child Psychiatry, 1961. *Lancet*, ii: 1249.
9. CROMBIE, D. L. and CROSS, K. W., 1956. *Brit. J. Prev. Soc. Med.*, 10: 141.
10. CUNNINGHAM, J. M., 1942. *Amer. J. Psychiat.*, 12: 147.
11. DAVIES, D. L. and STEIN, L., 1963. *Proc. Roy. Soc. Med.*, 56: 115.
12. FREUD, S., 1950. *Collected Papers*, Vol. 3. London: Hogarth Press.
13. HENDERSON, D. K. and GILLESPIE, R. D., 1932. *A Textbook of Psychiatry*. London: Oxford Univ. Press.
14. Home Office, 1959. *Children in Care in England and Wales*. H.M.S.O.
15. HORN, R. Personal communication.
16. HOWELLS, J. G., 1953. A systematic approach to the play observation and play exploration of the neurotic child. *Report 2nd Conf. Occup. Therapists*.
17. 1956. *Lancet*, ii: 1254.
18. 1961. Follow-up studies in child psychiatry. *Proc. 3rd World Congr. Psychiat.*
19. 1962. *J. Ment. Sci.*, 108: 675.
20. 1963a. *Amer. J. Psychiat.*, 119: 922.
21. 1963b. *Family Psychiatry*. Edinburgh: Oliver & Boyd.
22. 1963c. Child psychiatry as an aspect of family psychiatry. *Proc. 2nd European Congr. Pedopsychiat.*, Rome.
23. HOWELLS, J. G. and LAYNG, J., 1955. *Lancet*, ii: 285.
24. HUTCHINSON, R., 1904. *Lectures on Diseases of Children*. London: Arnold.
25. IRELAND, W. W., 1898. *The Mental Affections of Children*. Philadelphia: Blakiston.
26. KANNER, L., 1959. *J. Ment. Sci.*, 105: 581.
27. KEIR, G., 1952. *Brit. J. Educ. Psychol.*, 22: 5.
28. LEVY, D. M., 1951. *Amer. J. Psychiat.*, 108: 481.
29. MAUDSLEY, H., 1867. *Physiology and Pathology of Mind*. London.
30. Ministry of Education, 1948. Circular 179. H.M.S.O.

31.   1955. *Report of the Committee on Maladjusted Children.* H.M.S.O.
32.   1959. Circular 347. H.M.S.O.
33. Ministry of Health, 1947. Memorandum, R.H.B. 47 (13). H.M.S.O.
34.   1956. H.M. (56) 81. H.M.S.O.
35.   1958. SAC (M.H.) (58) 5. H.M.S.O.
36.   1964. H.M. (64) 4. H.M.S.O.
37. National Health Service Act, 1946. H.M.S.O.
38. PHAIRE, T., 1545. *The Boke of Chyldren.* Reprinted by Livingstone, 1955. London.
39. Royal Medico-Psychological Association, 1956. *In-patient Accommodation for Children and Adolescent Patients.*
40.   1957. *Memorandum on the Committee on Maladjusted Children.*
41.   1958. *The Provision of Psychiatric Services for Children and Adolescents.*
42.   1960. *The Recruitment and Training of the Child Psychiatrist.*
43.   1961. *The Functions of the Medical Director of a Child Psychiatry (Child Guidance) Clinic.*

XII

THE PSYCHIATRY OF ADOLESCENTS

Wilfrid Warren

M.A., M.D., D.P.M.

Physician, Children's and Adolescents' Department, Bethlem Royal Hospital and the Maudsley Hospital, London

1

Introduction

Adolescence is defined as the state of growing up, between childhood and manhood or womanhood. The age period covered cannot be exactly delimited, as it depends on the individual's speed of physical development, which is variable, while the processes of psychological maturation are not only inexact but rather obscure. It is not easy to decide when any individual has fully grown up; and it will certainly be later than the teens. However for practical purposes the psychiatry of adolescents can be regarded as referring to those who are in their second decade of life.

2

Psychological Characteristics

While the majority of youngsters no doubt pass through adolescence without particular difficulty, these years, which involve changes and readjustments in relation to family, school, work and social life, are commonly believed to give rise to stresses and sometimes to disturbances of emotion or of behaviour. For how many this may be so is uncertain, but minor upsets can be looked on as part of normal living, and no doubt teenagers themselves, their parents or their teachers usually resolve them. Only when disturbance is more marked or not so resolved can it be regarded as abnormal, and thus it is a small minority of adolescents who reach the psychiatrist. He will then need to be intuitively aware of their characteristic ways of thinking, feeling and behaving, if he is to be *en rapport* with them towards elucidating the psychiatric problems that they present.

A number of facets of adolescent psychological development therefore need to be kept in mind. Briefly, puberty leads to a recrudescence and heightening of the sexual drive, genitality now coming to the fore. In whatever ways sexuality previously was manifest, there is now a concentration on eroticism, and with this an as yet relative lack of self-integration. Pre-genital interests may also recrudesce and so, for instance, habits of cleanliness may for the time being lapse. Expressions of sexuality can now be tumultuous and sometimes appear anomalous. Such behaviour may give rise to complaint and then need to be judged clinically as to whether it is a fleeting anomalous display likely to go on to normal sexuality, or the beginnings of more lasting deviation. At the same time normal sexuality can give rise to stress, leading to manifestations of anxiety that may occasionally require sympathetic help.

Besides sexuality, the adolescent's intellectual life now becomes enriched by an influx of new interests and then attitudes, often highly emotionally toned. They may be of short duration but meanwhile, perhaps running contrary to the parents' viewpoint, give rise to disapproval and so to clashes between them. At the same time introspection and phantasy life in general become intensified, and, unless excessive, such self-interest has a unifying influence in the face of feelings of insecurity. Adolescents commonly are unsure of themselves and are apt to compare themselves unfavourably with others; they may well adopt poses that are self-protective but irritating to an older generation.

Growth of independence is important, as successful emancipation from the family is necessary to achieve maturity. Adolescents strive towards this, although at the same time there may well be a harking back to the security of childhood so that there is ambivalence of feelings; they still need the unobtrusive support of adults. Parents, long used to guide the child, may not find it easy to relinquish their authority, while the child's strivings forward can specifically stir up parental neurotic conflicts; considerable stress then results for either side and the parents can lose control of the situation. The dissensions and anxieties of early years, meanwhile perhaps laid over by the apparent conformity of later childhood, may well reappear on the surface around puberty. In the over-protected child, for example, strivings towards independence can give rise to much anxiety and guilt; for the over-restricted rebellion can become overt; those who have been deprived of parental affection may now become particularly unstable or rebellious. In any case loyalties tend to change to new objects beyond the home. Most adolescents gain security from associating with their peers and this may be turned to constructive use or, on the other hand, sometimes lead to 'gang' activities. These youngsters tend to lean on some interested adult in or outside the family circle rather than on the parents; considerable support may thus be obtained, and such a role seems to be ready cast for the psychotherapist.

In all, the adolescent attitude is typically that of ambivalence (3).

Selfishness is combined with a capacity for self-sacrifice; their loves tend to be passionate, yet cease or change for little reason. Hard work subsides into apathy; enthusiastic sociability is replaced by a desire for solitude. On one occasion they show a submissive attitude, on another rebelliousness with touchy and inconsiderate roughness. These rather bewildering changes of behaviour are the hall-marks of the immature.

3

Physical Development

An appraisal of physical status is an important part of the total assessment of the adolescent patient, and Tanner's (6) comprehensive review of adolescent development supplies much detailed information on this matter. Thus physical examination should take note of the patient's physical habitus, the stage of sexual development reached, and of any physical abnormalities that could be relevant to the patient's well-being.

The normal age range through which children reach puberty is wide, the average age for both sexes now being the thirteenth year; the development of the secondary sex characters both precedes and follows puberty. It is useful to have ready clinical landmarks by which to judge this development, and in girls puberty can be taken as the date on which the first period occurs. The onset of seminal emissions in boys is not easy to determine, so that Crampton's criteria to measure puberty are still useful, although not practical in retrospect: boys with no pubic hair, or with fine unpigmented hair, are pre-pubertal; those with straight pigmented hair are pubertal; while those with the normal 'kinked' pigmented hair are post-pubertal. It is to be noted that the average age at which puberty is attained in both sexes has become progressively lower in the last few decades, and this fact of earlier physical development today compared with that of older generations has important implications for adolescent behaviour.

A spurt in growth precedes puberty that is greater in boys than in girls, but some girls gain a temporary advantage if it comes earlier. For instance a pre-pubertal boy of 13 years may find that his 12-year-old sister has reached puberty and for the time being has grown larger than he, to his disadvantage. Genetical determinants lie behind the age at which the adolescent growth spurt occurs and puberty is reached, while those who are taller and bigger earlier on tend to mature the earlier. Physical illness or malnutrition can delay growth, and there is some evidence that stress can do so; those in whom delay has occurred tend to catch up later.

In practice it will be uncommon for a patient to be found with a developmental status outside the normal range for his or her particular age (see (6) for further details on development), but anxieties on this score, covert in the patient or overt in the parents, sometimes occur and require to be alleviated. It is important for an adolescent to feel the same as his or her peers; to be immature in sexual development compared with them, for instance, puts that boy or girl at a disadvantage and so can be a source of anxiety. Tanner describes how on average those who mature earlier tend not only to be more robust physically, but also temporarily to score more highly in tests of intelligence; this may sometimes be of significance in the competition for secondary school places. With puberty the physiological response to exercise greatly improves, especially in boys—another advantage for those who reach puberty earlier. The unusually tall or small youngster might feel particularly his discrepancy from others, and so do those others who have some physical anomaly such as obesity, gynaecomastia of puberty, or acne vulgaris. It is thus helpful to pay attention to an adolescent's physical well-being, to try and build up his self-regard and so his sense of security.

4

Psychiatric Ill-Health

The clinical psychiatry of adolescents is concerned with those syndromes or illnesses to be found in teenagers, and also in some 12- or even 11-year-olds in these days of earlier physical development; but whatever the problem these patients usually show characteristics that reflect the outlook and behaviour typical of their age. In some the symptoms shown may be similar to those found in younger children, and denote sometimes a prolongation into adolescence of psychiatric disturbance dating back to a much younger age; in others the ill-health now apparent is characterised by the sort of symptoms commonly seen later on in adult patients; and it may be added that some young adults when psychiatrically disturbed show behaviour more appropriate to teenagers. The psychiatric disorders apparent at these different age levels therefore form a continuum; it is a *sine qua non* that for clinical practice with adolescents familiarity with the psychiatry both of childhood and of adulthood is required. In all, these various kinds of psychiatric ill-health in adolescence cover a wide if circumscribed field and, as in younger children, usually come about when any factor or combination of factors interferes with a healthy response to the increasing demands of life, or with the cutting of earlier emotional ties. In the more serious psychotic disorders and in some personality abnormalities the aetiology at present remains obscure, although in all kinds of psychiatric ill-health adolescence itself has become an intrinsic, if indeterminate, factor of varying importance.

For healthy development through childhood and adolescence the constitutional factor is important. Heredity, the presence of physical diseases or imperfections, including brain damage or other abnormalities, perhaps showing on electroencephalography, may all have caused and may continue to cause handicap in individuals. Likewise the level of intelligence and the temperament of the child are of concern and sometimes a handicap, not always appreciated until well into school life. The fact of mental subnormality has not always been diagnosed before the teens, while in any case some retarded children first come to show behaviour disorders or other symptoms around puberty. By the time of adolescence educational retardation may have become marked, whatever the level of intelligence, and so by now comprise another form of handicap.

The environment of the child is equally relevant. Detrimental material conditions deny the youngster stimuli and outlets necessary for physical activity, or for using his imaginative or creative capacities. Socially acceptable outlets for the instinctual needs of youth may also be lacking. More important, the child is wholly dependent on the family for the sort of upbringing that he has had. For some there has been no home background, or one so unstable or detrimental that the effects of emotional deprivation are only too apparent. Some parents have been, for psychiatric or other reasons, unable to give an emotionally secure upbringing; family interrelationships may have been most faulty. The youngster of any age needs stable and secure affection in the home and also consistent but reasonable authority; both may have been lacking. If an only child, the lack of brothers and sisters tends to impede the child's growth towards independence; their presence sometimes gives rise to rivalries which can also be a drawback. In all, the interactions between the emotional life of the growing child and of the family are so fundamentally important that it is often not feasible to consider one without the other; it is only in late adolescence that the family tends to lose its hold.

The causes underlying psychiatric ill-health in adolescence are thus many, so that a broad physical, psychological, psychopathological and sociological approach is needed for their elucidation. The syndromes that present are equally varied, while sometimes the clinical picture shown is polymorphic and not readily fitted into a definite category. Each patient presents a unique problem and it is not possible to describe all the diversities met, although examples can be picked out; it is also only feasible to hint at the psychopathological processes at work in each case.

In general, psychiatrically disturbed adolescents present with clusters of symptoms pointing to various syndromes, and as in younger children there is much overlap between them. Cameron's (2) views on the classification of psychiatric conditions in children are in many respects relevant to adolescents. First, and perhaps most commonly, there are patients reacting to stress by disturbances of behaviour, who merge with others showing the more overt expressions of anxiety; these veer into yet others who are reacting at a more unconscious level and showing a typical neurotic picture. Among these latter are to be found children with examples of the various neuroses ordinarily seen in adult patients. In the other direction, so to speak, those with behaviour disturbances shift into the large group showing the various conduct disorders, and so to those who are definitely anti-social and then confirmed delinquents. Some patients not only show neurotic symptoms but are also anti-social in their behaviour. Any of these kinds of patients may have had increasingly faulty inter-personal relationships with members of their families or outside the home. In any of these there may be features that point to some kind of personality abnormality and whose import time will prove or disprove. Finally, and in a sense somewhat apart, are those who develop a psychotic condition; with these there may be difficulties in diagnosis early on because of associated behaviour disorders or neurotic symptoms.

Behaviour Disturbances

Disturbances in the field of behaviour give rise to diverse symptoms, often similar to those occurring in younger children; frequently they are a continuation of similar symptoms apparent at an earlier age, or have reappeared in adolescence. They include for instance disturbances of eating: overeating, faddiness or anorexia; enuresis or encopresis; sleep disturbances; such habits as nail biting or thumb sucking; over-activity, fidgetiness or tics; disturbances of speech, and so on. There are those who exhibit temper tantrums; cantankerous, attention-seeking or jealous behaviour; showing off, defiance or disobedience. There are others who are very shy, withdrawn or even showing elective mutism. This list is by no means complete; in many patients such disturbed behaviour will have arisen mainly from disturbed inter-personal relationships within the family, and in any case it is likely to give rise to them. How many or how severe these different symptoms are found to be is as variable as in younger children. They may comprise the whole of the complaint, or they may sometimes be expressions of underlying neurotic anxiety or depression, or conceal some personality disorder to be revealed by the subsequent career of the patient.

Anxiety and tension are apt to be expressed particularly by difficult or aggressive behaviour, since adolescents are prone to act out their feelings in these ways. Alternatively they are expressed more directly, as in adults, by hypochondriacal symptoms which sometimes lead to fruitless physical investigation, or through various fears and phantasies. These last may have a barely concealed sexual content and be most prominent for instance when the patient settles down for the night. The father may then well sometimes be an object of fear, while there is a clinging to the mother— the underlying basis perhaps for some cases of so-called 'school phobia'.

Depression may be the outstanding symptom in some patients, though usually it is more labile in quality than in adult patients. Depersonalisation is an occasional accompaniment, while associated tension is common. Because of its lability the depression is not always recognised for what it is, especially when self-damaging activities appear to be attention-seeking and with a 'hysterical' flavour. Such gestures indicate, however, that the patient requires careful assessment to decide what measures are required for his protection, as a serious attempt at suicide does sometimes ensue. Depressed adolescents often show other behaviour disorders too which may well mask the underlying depression. Such a state of depression may be reactive and neurotic in kind; but such cases merge with others where the depression is psychotic in character.

The occurrence of attention-seeking, apparently motivated behaviour, especially in girls, gives a special significance to the term *hysterical*. Furthermore such behaviour in one girl in a group may well be copied by others who have similar propensities. These sorts of patients of either sex can be overtly aggressive or have severe outbursts of temper, thus causing considerable problems of handling. There can again be marked accompanying tension or a tendency to regression to behaviour more appropriate to a much younger child. Such instability is sometimes called *psychopathic* because of the patient's apparent impulsiveness, and perhaps because of associated running away or delinquent acts. The label 'psychopathic personality' is nevertheless very rarely justified at this age, as most settle down with increased maturity. On the other hand an occasional patient with these sorts of behaviour patterns shows evidence of brain damage, or it may be associated with manifestations pointing to an epileptic condition. Such handicaps need to be diagnosed, as appropriate drug therapy may well help towards the amelioration of difficult behaviour.

Neurotic Syndromes

While in many adolescent patients the manifestations of neurotic ill-health have been seen to be indeterminate and their symptoms not pointing to any clear-cut condition, in others a definite neurotic entity, nosologically the same as in older people, is seen to develop, or occasionally is found to have dated back to earlier years. For example a *phobic state*, usually with an inability to travel or to go out, can develop rather insidiously, drag on and lead to severe curtailment of the patient's social or working life during adolescence. Most with this condition seem to improve with increasing age, perhaps leaving behind minor phobic symptoms by early adult life, but an occasional patient continues to be severely crippled. Some adolescents can be seen to be 'punishing' their parents by their phobias or bidding for some other form of 'secondary gain'; this can be equally true of other neurotic conditions such as obsessional neurosis. So-called *school phobia*, with refusal to attend school perhaps for long periods, has become a common condition in children, mostly of eleven years of age or older, and is generally regarded as the presenting symptom of an underlying neurotic condition; Kahn (4) gives a comprehensive list of writers on this condition. The term, however, may sometimes have come to be used too widely to cover truancy or cases where failure to attend school has been connived at by the parents, but most 'school-phobics' do give rise to considerable problems of management and treatment. Such patients first need a careful assessment, and in a small minority there is found to be a well marked depression, or an underlying phobic state for which the outlook is uncertain; some of these latter after leaving school are still unable to go out to work. In general, while those exhibiting 'school phobia' are likely to be treated on an out-patient basis in the first place and with a successful outcome in a proportion of them, others will require treatment away from home in a hospital unit or a hostel, and perhaps later placement as maladjusted in a boarding school.

Hysterical conversion states seem these days to be more commonly found in adolescents than in adults; for example a paralysed limb, loss of memory, pseudodementia, fugue states or repeated hysterical 'swoons'. These last will sometimes have to be distinguished from epileptiform attacks, and the boundaries between the two conditions are not always well defined. Treatment requires careful planning in order to relieve a hysterical condition, with attention paid to the total circumstances of the patient. Short-cut methods involving 'suggestion' seem to be notably unsuccessful. The underlying personality is important: if such a conversion state appears to be mostly reactive to particular stresses in a patient with a reasonably well integrated personality, then it is the more amenable to adequate treatment; on the other hand if the patient proves, as occasionally happens, to have an underlying severe hysterical personality disorder, the prognosis is then more uncertain. A permanent crippling resulting from a hysterical paralysis is not unknown.

Anorexia nervosa may start insidiously in early adolescence, and is more commonly found in girls at this early age than is usually described. While it inevitably gives rise to problems of prolonged care and treatment, the outlook for future adjustment on follow-up generally seems to be better than for older women. It appears typically and for no obvious reason in a girl who is emotionally immature, prim and inhibited, and obsessional features and depression may also be noticeable. Such patients essentially are apt to be most resistive to a psychotherapeutic exploration of the underlying psychopathology, treatment being directed to their general care and well-being over a long period of time.

Obsessional neurosis occurs fairly often in adolescents, a few having shown well marked obsessional symptoms earlier in childhood. More develop compulsive rituals for the first time acutely around puberty, perhaps associated with stresses at that time; less often obsessive ruminative thinking appears at a somewhat older age. As with younger children, it is common to find that the patient has involved the mother in the rituals, so that she may for instance be up for hours trying to get the patient to bed at night. Rituals marked at home are sometimes hardly noticeable at school. With adequate treatment, which may well include admission into hospital, most of these patients appear to settle down in due course, at any rate during adolescence; their later progress in adult life remains to be seen, as it is well known that obsessional neurosis sometimes recurs. The prognosis for those who have a history of it dating back into earlier childhood needs to be more guarded, while occasionally an adolescent is found to have a markedly obsessional personality, which can be a severe handicap since it does not seem to alter much with treatment or with time.

Tics, with or without associated obsessional symptoms, generally seem to occur less commonly than in somewhat younger children. However an adolescent is sometimes seen in whom severe tics have long been developing and have by now become a severe handicap, perhaps with associated compulsive utterances. These tics may improve considerably with treatment, which means relief from all stresses for some time, perhaps away from the home environment; but in others the syndrome becomes indistinguishable from that known after Gilles de la Tourette.

Conduct Disorders

These are symptoms that are anti-social or can easily become so, for example, lying, stealing, truancy or sexual misbehaviour, but they also include behaviour that is generally anti-authoritarian, sometimes amounting to being 'out of control'. Such could have started earlier and then increased, or have first become overt in adolescence. How many with these sorts of disorders reach the Courts and are dealt with there appears to depend to some extent on the circumstances. All can obviously be assessed from the psychiatric point of view, although it is sometimes in practice a debatable point how far some individual delinquent can be regarded as psychiatrically disturbed, or whether social or moral factors may have had more importance in causing the misconduct.

The incidence of conduct disorders and of delinquency in adolescents is high and of general concern, but when adolescents have been charged in Court and then referred, psychiatric factors are usually suspected as being important. This is likely, for instance, when behaviour disorders or neurotic symptoms are also present, when there appear to be handicaps, or when the family appears to be psychiatrically disturbed. How far such delinquent adolescents can benefit from psychiatric treatment depends on a number of factors, including what provision can effectively be made for their care as well as for their treatment, and whether they can so be 'contained'. Some of these patients are apt to 'act out' their difficulties by committing further offences, which may then of necessity lead to further measures by the Court to bring them under control. Until this has been done psychiatric treatment may not always be practicable, whether it be on an out-patient or in-patient basis or in some after committal, perhaps to an approved school (9).

Personality Disorders

It has been pointed out that personality is still developing throughout adolescence, and that there must therefore be caution before inferring that an apparent abnormality of personality will become a settled feature of that patient's make-up. Certain adolescents are most unstable, impulsive, aggressive or repeatedly delinquent, and should this be so in an older patient it might then be taken as indicative of a psychopathic personality. But most adolescents of this kind appear to become more stable with maturation, although should this not happen they would still need, except in rare and severe cases, to be observed over some years before such a diagnosis could be made. Various factors, including the favourableness or otherwise of their further environment and their response to any treatment instituted, may determine future stability. Some such unstable patients are found on electroencephalographic examination to have non-specific dysrhythmias, perhaps pointing to 'immaturity'; these dysrhythmias later may become more normal.

Some patients, especially those presenting with neurotic symptoms such as phobias or hypochondriasis, show inadequate traits in their personalities that seem to be well marked. Should such traits continue they will be a considerable handicap and interfere with effectiveness in the future, but again fairly prolonged observation is required before accepting that this is so. Occasionally an adolescent seems to have become set in what can be called an eccentric mode of life: perhaps very withdrawn, with well marked obsessional traits or a preoccupation with esoteric pursuits of his own. He is a misfit and can cause a considerable problem of handling and disposal; he may well become depressed or develop other symptoms, arising from the stresses that come from his inability to fit in with the world as it is. The term 'schizoid' personality applied to a teenager, however, would usually be premature.

Homosexuality is occasionally found to have become well established in a surprisingly young patient of either sex, in contrast to the much more common minor homosexual upsets that occur. The latter are amenable to treatment, but in the former motivation for treatment, which would presumably need to be intensive and prolonged, is sometimes lacking. Other kinds of sexual perversions in adolescents are rarely seen, apart from cases of boys who repeatedly expose themselves. These also sometimes give rise to problems of treatment, particularly when they deny the symptom and then are backed up in the denial by the parents.

Psychotic Disorders

The child who has developed a psychosis early will in due course reach adolescence; sometimes a less severe case, who for this reason has not been placed for care in some institution, has not been diagnosed earlier and now presents as a diagnostic problem. A detailed history may indicate that the patient was apparently normal very early on, and then developed severe and unusual disturbed behaviour, perhaps at the toddler stage; there may then have been symptoms typical of childhood psychosis recalled for the more recent past; disparities in intelligence tests, perhaps indicating patchily a higher level of intelligence than the overall score allows and not accounted for by brain damage, may be found—these among other findings point to the diagnosis of childhood psychosis. Such a child may well have improved over the years, but still remains clearly handicapped, 'odd' perhaps autistic and with obsessional traits, and may now be giving rise to problems of employment or further care.

The incidence of 'adult type' schizophrenia rises from puberty, but with a steeper rise in the third decade. In most adolescent patients the clinical picture is similar to that seen in adults, and as varied (although 'paranoid schizophrenia', typically encountered later in life, seldom appears to occur in youngsters). The onset may be fairly sudden and present with florid symptoms, or insidious and so difficult to diagnose early on; thus behaviour disorders, anxiety or hypochondriasis, for instance, can remain unexplained until definite schizophrenic symptoms such as delusions, hallucinations, thought disorder, or catatonia appear. Some adolescents who develop schizophrenia have previously been apparently normal, while others have shown varied evidence of disturbed behaviour in earlier childhood. The patient's previous psychiatric history therefore does not help in predicting whether he may later develop a psychosis, since it is so variable.

The possible development of schizophrenia in disturbed adolescents needs to be kept constantly in mind, but it can hardly be diagnosed in the absence of clear-cut pathognomonic symptoms. Nevertheless it seems to be suspected more often than is in fact the case. Adolescents are apt to be shy and rapport on interview can be difficult; their answers to questions may be rather incoherent and their mood seemingly inappropriate, perhaps because of an embarrassed smile; they are inclined to be suggestible and so answer in the affirmative to leading questions about their thoughts and perceptions—questions that have been designed to elicit abnormalities. Experience in dealing with adolescents lessens these difficulties of assessment, but in some cases of doubt a period of observation in hospital may be justified to establish or exclude the diagnosis.

Manic-depressive psychosis occurs much less commonly than does schizophrenia in adolescents. A fairly typical case of mania has been encountered in a boy of 11 years, and a case is seen from time to time over the age of puberty. The symptom of depression has already been described, as it occurs in neurotic conditions, but a depressive state of psychotic intensity, with retardation, delusions, ideas of unworthiness and so on, similar to that found in older people, is occasionally encountered, though usually in those of 16 years of age or older. Depressive states in general tend to be rather atypical in adolescence, and sometimes masked by other symptoms; the diagnosis may sometimes only become quite clear in retrospect after a spontaneous recovery has taken place; or more rarely the patient's condition has swung over into that of hypomania. Cases of recurrent depression or cyclothymia are occasionally met, in some instances coinciding with phases of the menstrual cycle.

A psychosis, perhaps a short-lived episode, can in adolescence give a mixed picture and include both schizophrenic and manic or depressive symptoms. The term 'schizo-affective' is appropriate for this, but if the illness continues or recurs it may become diagnosable definitely as schizophrenia, or less often as manic-depressive psychosis. Occasionally a patient is seen with recurrent schizophrenic episodes, leaving the patient less and less normal between them. Again, occasionally a psychotic episode of dramatic onset and of brief duration is seen, which appears to follow some precipitating trauma or some minor physical illness; schizophrenic, manic, or symptoms pointing to a toxic confusional state, may any of them be present. The term 'reactive psychosis' has been used for this condition (10); the immediate prognosis seems favourable, but such patients need to be followed up, since the episode could well herald a further psychotic breakdown.

A toxic confusional state can occur in adolescents, as in adults, perhaps following some infection. It needs to be kept in mind in the differential diagnosis of any acute psychotic state in the young, as does the possibility of encephalitis. The taking of such drugs as amphetamine or marihuana may be becoming more common and lead to a psychotic condition. Finally, in view of the increasing numbers of people with venereal infections, juvenile 'general paralysis of the insane' may come to be seen again in adolescents.

Psychosomatic Disorders

These occur in adolescence as they do at other ages, and give rise to the same problems of diagnosis and treatment. The list of possible disorders is a long one, but there do not seem to be features in such cases that are especial for adolescents and distinguish them from those occurring in general.

5

Treatment

Provisions for Treatment

The psychiatric techniques that can be used for the care and treatment of adolescent patients depend in the first place on the facilities that are provided. Special clinic or out-patient facilities are very scarce. Younger teenagers can be suitably dealt with in child psychiatric or child guidance clinics, and similarly older patients can be readily coped with in out-patient clinics for adults, but there are patients in between who are apt to be handled rather inadequately in either. They may dislike a children's clinic where the psychological and social worker facilities required for them are readily available, while a psychiatric clinic catering for adults may find it difficult to provide for those who happen to present with essentially childish complaints, educational problems and so on. There is therefore a case to be made out for special clinics for those of adolescent age, with an appropriate set-up and staffing, and 'advertised' as such.

These could be arranged separately in existing children's or perhaps adults' clinic premises; it should be kept in mind that teenagers may need early evening appointments, to avoid missing school at perhaps an important stage in their education or taking time off from their first job.

Separate in-patient units for adolescents who require hospital care are much needed, but are as yet in very short supply. Their siting should be reasonably near to the patients' homes, and they should be backed by the facilities for investigation and treatment of a psychiatric hospital, with the possibility of transferring certain patients when necessary to adult wards. These units should be small enough to be manageable, and with a high staff/patient ratio. A suitable daily programme with the services of a Special School should be arranged. There should be an associated out-patient clinic, for instance for the follow-up care of ex-patients.

Adolescents should not as a rule be housed with younger children, but it is sometimes efficacious to treat certain of them in adult psychiatric wards. Some of the more sophisticated prefer it, the disturbed psychotic or acutely suicidal patient may be more easily looked after, while occasion-ally an adolescent with acutely disturbed behaviour may settle better among older patients. Most, however, are best treated among their own age group; they tend to disturb older patients, and should not witness undesir-able behaviour and conversation by adults. Those adolescents whose illness has become chronic and who need long-term hospital care form a special category. They take up valuable beds in an adolescent unit, but this has to be weighed against the risk of further deterioration in a 'chronic ward'.

Other kinds of provision, besides out-patient and in-patient units, are at times required for adolescents with psychiatric problems. They may present in children's homes or hostels, remand homes, approved schools and so on; a psychiatrist may best be employed there on a sessional basis to deal with them on the spot and to advise the staff. Some patients, whether or not they have had in-patient treatment, may need to be placed away from home. Deeming as maladjusted and placement in a suitable boarding school may provide for those who are younger, but near to or after school-leaving age hostel accommodation may be required—yet it is most difficult to get it for those who have shown psychiatric disturbance or who are not yet earning sufficient to keep themselves. Residential jobs or industrial training are also needed for some who are suitable. For those more handicapped, day hospital care may be called for; or hostel or night hospital accommodation with psychiatric treatment available in the even-ings—for those, that is, who are fit enough to go out to work by day. These are a part of community care in general, and if available could keep some adolescents out of hospital and help to rehabilitate them.

The total management of disturbed adolescents may well require the professional help of other non-psychiatric workers who normally deal with teenagers. They may in fact provide the framework in which psychiatric treatment can take place, or complement it, or provide for after-care. For instance, psychiatric treatment may not be feasible until the patient has been brought under control by those whose role it is to do this when necessary; 'character training' is hardly the responsibility of the psychiatrist, and yet is needed for some patients; educational retardation can hold back the full rehabilitation of a patient who has been psychiatrically disturbed; while practical advice on what work is locally available may be important at some stage of treatment. Again, provision for the care of those adolescents without a home or with a detrimental home background is sometimes an urgent problem. Thus familiarity with the professional roles of the various officers concerned with these matters will lead to a co-ordinated approach to problems of these kinds, to the patients' advantage.

Investigation and Treatment

It is again only possible to remark here on those aspects of investigation and treatment that are of particular concern for adolescent patients; although their scope includes many familiar to the practice of child and adult psychiatry, their choice depends on the particular bent of the psychiatrist. However, as the range of disorders is wide and their aetiology diverse, a broad approach is implied. Any plan of treatment depends on an adequate diagnostic formulation made after weighing up all the contributory factors, and on then using the differing kinds of facilities for furthering treatment that are available at the various stages of the patient's care. To view a problem from too narrow a viewpoint is apt to lead to incomplete diagnosis and then treatment. To take some rather gross examples: some physical abnormality needing treatment may not be discovered; a faulty assessment of the patient's level of intelligence can result from using psychological tests unsuitable for the age level; or psychopathology at work in the family is not fully appreciated, because the other members of the family have not been assessed. It may be added that electroencephalography sometimes reveals a pertinent but unsuspected abnormality.

Out-patient Clinic Treatment

As psychiatric services are at present organised, an adolescent seldom seeks advice or treatment for himself or herself, although some might well do so if they knew how to set about it. Psychiatric experience among young University students points to this. Normally it is the parents or others responsible who make complaints about the patient, particularly in the field of behaviour; and so the referral is initiated, the adolescent patient perhaps being an unwilling, or puzzled and fearful, victim. Should the adolescent refuse to come to the clinic, as sometimes happens, a domiciliary visit may then be justified to assess the situation. It is important to try and gain the patient's co-operation from the beginning, and hence it may be wise to see him or her briefly to explain the situation and the role of the psychiatrist before taking a history from the informants and before psychological testing is undertaken. To point out that anything said by the patient is in confidence and will not be reported to the parents may be helpful in establishing rapport from the start. Some adolescents are notoriously unable to express themselves because of shyness or for other reasons, so that an intuitive and sympathetic appreciation by the psychiatrist of the youngster's way of thinking and likely difficulties may allow the patient's complaints or difficulties to be the more readily clarified. The psychiatrist thus needs to be more active in initiating and keeping up discussion when interviewing an adolescent than is usual with older patients. From all this, however, it is clear that the first interview with patient or parents cannot be hurried, if an adequate diagnostic assessment is to be made and then the co-operation of patient and parents gained for a plan of treatment and disposal.

For those who are considered suitable, out-patient treatment includes a number of general measures. These include attention to the environment and if necessary an attempt to adjust it for the benefit of the patient, whether it be in the home, at school or at work; sometimes help in finding suitable leisure activities, or social assistance towards obtaining clothing or other necessities. To have the right kind of clothes compared with other teenagers promotes self-respect. Some kind of physical or drug treatment may be indicated in certain patients, while in others arrangements for remedial education may be important.

Apart from these general measures, some form of psychotherapy for the patient and the family is also necessary for a majority of teenage patients. How this is to be organised will need an early decision; there may be open hostility between patient and parents or covert differences of attitude, or, on the other hand, morbid over-dependence of the patient on the parents and of them on the patient. Should the psychiatrist himself decide to treat the adolescent patient, then someone else working with the psychiatrist, perhaps the psychiatric social worker, may take on the parents —unless the mother, for instance, is considered more psychiatrically ill than the patient. Joint family interviews are sometimes appropriate.

The form of psychotherapy chosen will obviously depend firstly on the kind of problem, and then on the inclinations of the therapist. Tolerant support by the therapist has a particular value with some adolescents, while superficial exploration of the patient's difficulties and discussion of them with him will suffice for many. For a minority, however, psychotherapy will need to be intensive and prolonged. Group therapy might be organised for some patients, if this is considered suitable and not thought to encourage the 'acting-out' of conflicts. On the other hand the use of projective techniques such as painting may be preferred, or practical occupations such as carpentry, either alone with the therapist or in a group.

Whatever form of out-patient psychotherapy is decided upon, much will depend on the willingness of the patient to partake, and so on the.

development of a dependent relationship of the patient on the therapist. Adolescents may well express their hostility by failing to keep appointments, while the risk of 'acting-out' their tensions by difficult behaviour, suicidal gestures, aggressive acts or committing offences is well known in certain patients, and may be a bar to the more intensive forms of therapy. A point can thus sometimes be reached when out-patient treatment is not feasible; in-patient treatment may then be the answer, or it may sometimes be necessary for the patient to be brought under control, perhaps through the Court. Such unruly adolescents are apt to be brought first to the psychiatrist in a last effort to avoid this and without appreciation that out-patient treatment may not be a practical solution, or that 'training' may be more important than treatment.

Fortunately the majority of adolescent patients do respond to out-patient treatment whatever the diagnosis, although support may sometimes be required for a long time. Once the adolescent has matured further, and feels more independent and able to cope, he or she may no longer feel the need to come. The parental background by then will be a less significant influence on the patient.

Meanwhile the parents may need considerable help, whether it be advice in handling the patient, practical help in bettering conditions in the family, or more intensive therapy in helping them to readjust themselves and to deal with their own emotional difficulties. An occasional parent will require arrangements to be made for formal psychiatric treatment in his or her own right. Again, others concerned with the patient, whether it be the Children's Officer, Probation Officer, teacher and so on, may require advice and support in handling the patient, the permission of the parents having first been obtained.

In-patient Treatment

The indications for the admission of adolescents into a psychiatric hospital for observation, investigation, care and treatment are largely the same as for other ages, but for adolescents there may be further particular reasons requiring their admission. The lack of suitable hospital places, however, gives rise at times to acute difficulty on behalf of some patient, and is apt then to lead to less desirable disposal. Out-patient treatment may have failed to make headway because of adverse influences in the family, so that for this or for other reasons separation from the family may be imperative. The marked quick improvement that sometimes results in some teen-aged patient after separation from the mother makes clear the morbid influence which she had exerted and to which the child was reacting. Once away from her such a patient can quickly mature. In others, for example, phobic symptoms may have confined the patient to the home, or so-called 'school phobia' may have become prolonged and attempts as an out-patient failed to get the child back to school; obsessional rituals may have disrupted the home, although perhaps hardly apparent once in hospital; or behaviour to parents has become so difficult that they have in effect lost control, even when misbehaviour outside the home has not been apparent.

Admission to hospital should be part of a long-term constructive plan, made after first visualising the likely outcome of hospital treatment and what further steps, if any, may be required after discharge; this may mean further placement away from home. To place the patient in hospital may solve some impasse for those outside, but it may not always be in the patient's best interests. For instance a girl of sixteen years may have got out of control and now become promiscuous: placed in hospital she may be prevented from offending for the time being; but unless hospital treatment stops these tendencies, she may relapse again into further promiscuity after discharge; time has passed and being now over seventeen years of age she can no longer be pulled up by a juvenile court. It can be added, in regard to delinquent patients, that a hospital has the facilities to cope with psychiatrically disturbed behaviour, but that should there be repeated absconding or delinquent acts committed on or from the hospital premises, in-patient care can become impossible to maintain.

Below the age of 16 years parents decide admission of a child, but over 16 years it is the patient who has volition. Occasionally an adolescent expresses active dislike of the idea of hospital treatment, although it is considered by the psychiatrist to be in his or her best interest and the parents agree. Planning for the tactful management of admission is then important in order to prevent complete refusal by the patient. However, if moral support of the parents is considered likely to be helpful to ensure it, the referring agents rather than the hospital staff should undertake it, and if necessary supervise the journey to hospital. Most unwilling youngsters settle once in hospital, although a quick absconding home again may have to be faced.

Organisation of Adolescent Unit

It is convenient and usually beneficial to house patients of the same age group together in hospital and with a suitable daily programme. An adolescent unit, however, not only ensures this but also acquires a dynamic quality of its own. The régimes of some of the adolescent units set up have been described elsewhere (1, 5, 7, 8), but certain points can here be stressed.

Placement of adolescents together away from parents and home, but with adult staff to care for them, inevitably creates a continuous group situation in which all, patients and staff, are involved. Though difficult to define, it undoubtedly has therapeutic value by encouraging a number of patients to unbend, to work out their conflicts and to mature, unless they are too ill to take part. Very real and sometimes valuable relationships spring up between patients, although these need supervision to avoid occasional hurt feelings or to control and modify strong hatreds: the situation amongst the patients can sometimes become 'explosive', and if allowed to get out of hand then becomes disruptive. This group situation, particularly valuable for those with neurotic complaints or behaviour disorders, is not quite paralleled among groups of older patients, who do not 'act out' in the same way. It certainly cannot be ignored and it needs constant assessment and guidance. The personalities of the staff are therefore significant and they need to be suitable for handling young people, while the kinds of patients admitted at any one time need to be regulated with an eye on the group situation. For instance, a balance should be kept between possibly withdrawn, aggressive and attention-seeking patients.

While the group situation is important, individual psychotherapy of varying intensity is also required for a number of patients. This is likely to need to take into account the individual patient's current problems in relation to living in the unit, and how they may reflect or repeat past difficulties. In any case the time in the unit is a broadly educational experience, as the patient thus gets to know other young people who also have their problems, and has a chance to develop aptitudes and new interests, while gaps in formal education can be repaired by appropriate remedial teaching. Youngsters of this age are quickly developing and their education can proceed at the same time as their treatment; that is, if they are well enough to benefit from it.

Physical Treatment

The wide range of physical and pharmacological treatments available for such conditions as schizophrenia, depressive states, personality disorders, epilepsy, brain damage and so on may all be applicable to patients of adolescent age in the same way as to those of other ages. But the indications for their use and their effect are sometimes less clear-cut, particularly in depressive or tension states, so that their choice is a matter of experienced judgement. General rules can hardly be laid down for their application to what are variable individual problems. Nevertheless, while sedatives have always had an important place in treatment, since the advent of the tranquillisers an adolescent unit has become a more peaceful community to manage.

Home Background

While the patient is in hospital the family background again usually requires careful attention. Parents, deeply involved in their adolescent child's neurotic disturbance, may react sharply to the separation experience. A mother has been known to break down, perhaps into depression, and require psychiatric treatment in her own right; or parents can become acutely anxious about the treatment of the child, or even occasionally paranoid towards the hospital, and then may remove the child against advice. The child, perhaps at first acutely homesick and maybe repeating a long acquired habit of controlling the parents, can put strong pressure on parents to take him home. On the other hand an occasional patient reacts by refusing to have anything to do with the parents in order to punish them. All these possibilities have to be watched for and the parents' anxieties anticipated and dealt with. They may need further to sort out their faulty attitudes and the part they played in leading to the child's disturbance. They may well receive the patient back in due course in a new guise, more mature and less dependent: they have to be prepared for this. They may sometimes have to learn to cope with what will be a psychiatrically handicapped child. For all these reasons, much time with them is spent by the hospital staff throughout the child's stay in hospital. The psychiatric social worker will be particularly concerned with this.

Discharge from Hospital

Some adolescent patients admitted for observation or investigation only need to remain a fairly short period; most, whatever the diagnosis, seem to gain maximum benefit from treatment by a stay of about three months to a year; a few can benefit from a longer stay. This estimate does not include patients with chronic conditions severe enough to have to remain for a very long time in hospital, who present a separate problem of treatment and disposal. Most patients naturally return home; but for some there is no home background, or it is considered too detrimental or a relapse too likely to happen: a placement elsewhere will be required. It is wise to look ahead and plan it well before the patient is ready for discharge. Difficulties and delays in finding a suitable placement can sometimes be formidable, and meanwhile the patient has become too well to remain in hospital and, by now bored and frustrated, starts mischief-making. In any case there is usually an optimum period for a patient to stay; the neurotic patient may get over-dependent on what is a sheltered community, and this is particularly true for the 'hysteric', who sometimes once more begins to deteriorate; the deprived child will develop roots that will be painful to tear up again. However in most cases a strong relationship will have sprung up with the hospital staff, so that, if distance does not preclude it, out-patient after-care is best carried out by the same people who looked after the patient in hospital.

6

Prognosis

To predict the outcome of psychiatric disorders occurring in adolescence for the distant future and when adult status has been reached, is not easy. By contrast the near future can usually be envisaged with some assurance. The effects of maturation, which may help towards a better integration, are uncertain, while the circumstances of the patient's future environment, and whether they will influence towards good or ill, are mostly unknown. Growing-up involves many changes which can be helpful or the reverse: school-leaving and then a new and expanding working life; emancipation from the home with widening social horizons and the acquisition of new friends; the likelihood of an increasingly active sexual life, ending for many in marriage and parenthood. A patient may manage to get away from seriously detrimental home circumstances, or new difficulties or troubles may arise. For instance a near relative, important to the patient's well-being, may die, or long-lasting illness in the home create a new hazard. The future indeed remains unknown.

There is still a serious lack of knowledge of the subsequent careers of psychiatrically disturbed children and adolescents to guide prognosis. At the same time differing yardsticks for measuring future mental health or ill-health need to be kept in mind. There are degrees of psychiatric sickness: from those who require to remain continuously in hospital, through others who can carry on with psychiatric supervision, to those who, while not receiving any form of treatment, are in varying degree handicapped by symptoms or defects of personality from leading a full life, whether it be in their working career, leisure activities or the achievement of a satisfactory marriage. Another yardstick is freedom or otherwise from anti-social conduct, which in practice can usually only be measured in terms of offences known and Court sentences received. Many adolescents who have been anti-social later settle down to conform; a few become recidivists. It is rare, but not unknown, for patients who early showed behaviour disorders or neurotic symptoms later to turn to anti-social conduct.

It is obvious that the long-term prognosis must remain uncertain for many adolescent patients, although cautious optimism is justified unless there are clear reasons to the contrary. For instance, schizophrenia of insidious onset and which does not clear up has an ominous outlook, while for others who have had a psychotic breakdown the future remains uncertain. Those with severe and long-standing personality disorders will not easily change, but growing-up may well soften less serious quirks. Those with neurotic or behaviour disorders are more likely than not to improve with time, but there are exceptions, notably among some severely phobic patients and those with a severe and continuing obsessional neurosis. In any case obsessional neurosis is apt to be a recurrent disorder and only time will show if it will recur.

It seems that adequately controlled, long-term follow-up studies of children and adolescents who have psychiatric disorders are much needed; the retrospective histories of psychiatrically sick adults can only give a distorted picture. Again, what relationships there are between psychiatric ill-health occurring early and that which may occur later on in life is largely unknown; so is the question which among psychiatrically disturbed children and adolescents grow up into fully mentally healthy adults, or how far they do so and how far some remain handicapped.

REFERENCES

1. CAMERON, K., 1953. *Amer. J. Psychiat.*, **109**: 653.
2.   1955. *Brit. J. Med. Psychol.*, **28**: 67.
3. FREUD, ANNA, 1948. *The Ego and the Mechanisms of Defence*. London: Hogarth Press.
4. KAHN, J. H. and NIRSTEN, J. P., 1962. *Amer. J. Orthopsychiat.*, **32**: 707.
5. SANDS, D. E., 1953. *J. Ment. Sci.*, **99**: 123.
6. TANNER, J. M., 1962. *Growth and Adolescence*, 2nd ed. Oxford: Blackwell Scientific Publications.
7. TURLE, G. C., 1960. *J. Ment. Sci.*, **106**: 1320.
8. WARREN, W., 1952. *Lancet*, i: 147.
9.   1956. *Med. Press*, **235**: No. 6110.
10. WARREN, W. and CAMERON, K., 1950. *J. Ment. Sci.*, **96**: 448.

XIII

THE PSYCHOSOMATIC APPROACH

IN CHILD PSYCHIATRY

Philip Pinkerton
M.B., Ch.B., M.D., D.P.M.

*Physician in Charge, Departments of Psychological Medicine, Royal Liverpool
and Alder Hey Children's Hospitals, Liverpool
Lecturer in Child Psychiatry, University of Liverpool
Consultant to the Liverpool School Health Service and Children's Department*

Il n'y a pas de maladies, seulement des malades.—Trousseau

1

Introduction

The Whole Patient Concept

Increasing lip-service is paid nowadays to the concept of psychosomatic medicine. It is fashionable to speak about the comprehensive study of the whole patient, and to decry the narrower mechanistic approach to clinical problems. In theory this sounds laudable, but in practice old prejudices of medical thought die hard, and it is difficult for doctors trained in the disciplines of organic medicine to embrace the broader principles of psychodynamics.

Moreover in the present state of our knowledge considerable doubt still persists as to what constitutes a psychosomatic disorder. Some authorities claim that, in a sense, all disease is psychosomatic, since both mind and matter are involved. There is wider acceptance for the opposite view, that we should restrict the term to those conditions in which emotional factors can be shown to play a convincing role both in the genesis and in the perpetuation of the disorder, e.g. ulcerative colitis, the periodic syndrome, asthma or migraine.

Almost certainly the diagnostic criteria for each of these particular disorders will require to be modified in the light of future research, but this need not invalidate the whole patient concept. At the present stage it seems wiser to refer to the psychosomatic approach, rather than to focus upon specific psychosomatic disorder.

2

General Considerations

The Either/Or Fallacy

One major obstacle to this comprehensive approach, especially among non-psychiatric colleagues, is the persistence of the 'either/or' theory of aetiology. By tradition a disorder is either organically determined, and therefore 'genuine', or it is 'functionally' determined, and by implication less worthy of our attention; certainly it will appear less serious in import. The fallacy of such reasoning can be illustrated from the example of asthma.

Asthma is not a specific disease entity. On the contrary, it is a non-specific reaction, which can be provoked in susceptible patients by a wide variety of different stresses. Broncho-spasm may be triggered off, for example, by physical irritants, or by upper respiratory tract infection, or by inhaling or ingesting certain allergens; or indeed it may be induced by emotional stress. Different stimuli, it will be noted, may provoke an identical attack in the same child at different times; or the asthma may only develop, say as a sequel to infection, when the patient is emotionally disturbed. When the child is not under stress he may well escape an attack, even if comparable infection is present in the upper respiratory tract. Here, the broncho-spasm is a reaction to the summation of two or more potential stimuli; but once established, the attack holds the same significance whether induced by emotional or by more 'concrete' factors. It is worth remembering that broncho-spasm can proceed to status asthmaticus and may even end fatally, though it is 'only' of psychogenic origin.

In the assessment of any given case, therefore, as in every psycho-somatic disorder, it is wise to review all the aetiological possibilities, emotional as well as physical, rather than try to establish a causal relationship with one factor by the exclusion of the others. The 'either/or' mentality is outmoded in this field: it should be replaced by the 'how much organic, how much functional' approach.

The Meaning of Psychogenesis

At once this raises a further problem: how to equate organic with functional or psychogenic factors, where both are suspected to contribute to a composite aetiology. It is misleading, for example, to list the causal factors in asthma as allergic, infective, and emotional, because the pathological processes governing chest infection and allergy are standard in every case, whereas psychopathological processes are not. On the contrary, they are so profoundly individual in character that no two cases are alike. Thus, in broncho-spasm induced by allergy, the offending foreign protein may vary but the pattern of patient response is the same, and therefore the allergic factor in asthma has a universal connotation. In contrast the 'psychological' factor has no such universal connotation.

It may be that the asthmatic response in one child is a reaction to intense over-possessiveness by the mother, and that the patient is almost literally being smothered. Alternatively the asthma may represent a suppressed aggressive reaction, occurring in response to excessive parental aspirations, or based upon unfair discrimination within the family. In yet a third child asthma may develop as the somatic expression of tension originally generated in the mother but now communicated to the child; the source of such tension could be maternal fear of transmitting her own genetic tendency to asthma, or could be based upon an infinite variety of equally morbid fears, holding significance only for the parents. The term 'psychogenic' has therefore many different individual meanings; in fact it varies with each case.

Non-specificity of Emotional Stress

It is particularly difficult for the doctor trained in the more rigid nosological entities of organic medicine to appreciate the individual nature of psychodynamics. In this field the potential causes are legion, but the actual grouping of emotional factors in any given case is specific for that child, in terms of his make-up, his life experiences and his relationship with his parents and with his immediate environment. It will be seen therefore that the designation 'psychological factor' may only be used in the broadest aetiological sense. It cannot be equated with pathological processes proper. Even when a case formulation sounds convincing objectively, and even when it is known to have formed the basis of similar cases previously, it should not be accepted as valid for the case in question until subjective confirmation is provided, either by the child, through the medium of his play activities, or verbally, as in older children, or from the parents. In organic medicine the clinical course of the disorder is universally recognisable by objective means. In the psychosomatic field stress cannot be judged by its external effects, only by what it signifies to the patient.

Subjective Significance of Stress

Stress in this context represents personal emotional stress, of special significance to the patient but not necessarily to anyone else. Indeed the emotional factor concerned may seem quite trivial (Paulley (24)), and therefore its relationship to the attack (of colitis or asthma or migraine) may not be appreciated, and may be missed. Major events, such as the death of a parent or desertion by father, emerge readily in the history, and of course these may well be aetiologically important. More often however the relevant factors seem objectively unimportant: perhaps a secret fear of ridicule when the child is undressing for gymnastics in school; or a sense of outrage that grannie favours the older grandson and always takes his part; or unfulfilled aspirations to do well in school to meet the unspoken hopes of a proud father. The vital point always is the significance with which these essentially personal factors are imbued by the patient, not the factors in themselves.

This, then, is one of the major paradoxes encountered in psychosomatic medicine. Under the broad heading of psychogenic contribution a large number of potentialities qualify for consideration, e.g. suppressed anger, suppressed resentment, humiliation, jealousy, frustration, emotional smothering, communicated anxiety, emotional deprivation, and reaction to perfectionism or to carping pressure by the parents. But from all the many recognisable formulae of interaction between parents and child, or between siblings and child, or between patient and his personal environment, only one grouping is applicable to the individual case, and that is the interpretation which 'fits'. Psychogenic stress factors, therefore, are specific for particular cases of any given disorder, but non-specific for the syndrome itself. In this sense there is no single psychological cause underlying asthma, or any other psychosomatic disorder. The 'cause' is only case-specific.

Common Misconceptions of Psychogenesis

To accept this paradox and learn successfully to explore the psychopathological hinterland beyond the disorder, some readjustment in outlook and feeling is called for in the doctor—what Balint (5) describes as 'a limited though considerable change in personality'. Nowhere is this reorientation more necessary than in the field of psychosomatic medicine, because here the family doctor, the paediatrician and the child psychiatrist tread common ground, and it is vital they should speak a common language. Yet certain naïve ideas continue to flourish among non-psychiatric physicians regarding psychogenic motivation in children. The most popular of these is the theory that psychosomatic symptoms always represent a device to gain attention, assuming their emotional origin.

There is confusion here between primary psychogenesis, if it exists, and secondary gain. Once a disorder has become established, and especially if it evokes parental concern, with corresponding relaxation of discipline, some children are tempted to take advantage of the situation and 'cash in' upon their own symptoms. In these circumstances perpetuation of the disorder is often engineered by the child himself at very near the conscious level, and the motivation might then be described loosely as attention seeking. This occurs most often however as a secondary elaboration, if it occurs at all. Where psychogenic factors are thought to play a significant role, as for example in ulcerative colitis or cyclical vomiting, it is difficult to conceive how attention seeking could be invoked as a motive. In any case, by implication, this kind of response would be consciously or near-consciously determined, and in such disorders that seems very hard to credit. The mechanism involved is, of course, unconscious motivation, but this is a difficult concept for the organicist to grasp, no doubt because of his closer association with the concrete and objective data of the organic field. Hence the more serious and disabling the condition, the less easy it is for our non-psychiatric colleagues to credit a psychogenic contribution. Yet it is precisely in this group that we should be collaborating most closely with them, because of the potential benefits accruing to the patient.

It is surely a reflection on our medical schools that so many doctors remain unfamiliar with the real significance of emotional factors in cases which come under our joint care. Too often psychogenic stress is equated still with situational or socio-economic stress, so that in taking the history a search is made only for gross factors such as paternal drunkenness, or a broken home, or a mother who goes out to full-time work. This is not to decry the significance of such factors, but to emphasise that their absence does not necessarily mean a contented child in a secure home. Conversely, if there is genuine warmth of relationship between the child and his parents, material hardships are of little account, and children will tolerate the most severe privations if only their basic security and sense of belonging is not destroyed. In short, stress cannot be judged by the outside observer.

On the other hand the child who is under personal emotional duress need not *appear* nervous or restless or distressed. Yet so often the family doctor will comment 'He doesn't look as if he need see a psychiatrist', or 'He looks normal enough to me'. If emotional conflicts are being expressed through somatic channels, it is in fact unlikely that the child will exhibit overt signs of anxiety or tension, i.e. utilise a neurotic channel as well. Therefore our colleagues must learn to relinquish this rather naïve concept of what constitutes 'a case for the child psychiatrist', and adopt a more sophisticated view of psychopathology as it applies in this field.

It is, of course, unrealistic to suggest that the general practitioner or the paediatrician should aim to become skilled in the psychotherapy of psychosomatic disorders. But it will help if they can acquire a better understanding of the dynamics involved, and thereby overcome their prejudices and misgivings. These relate to the days of the alienist and the closed mental hospital, but they continue to bedevil our association. We will make small therapeutic headway with lay parents, and therefore with their children as patients, until we have overcome bias in our own profession, which is subtly conveyed from doubting doctor to misguided mother upon referral to the mysterious psychiatrist. If we are to work together in professional collaboration in a field which is our joint concern, we must acquire a common basis of appreciating the aetiological factors involved. We shall be probing for subtleties of feeling which may not be obvious, which may appear disproportionate in import to the strength of somatic reaction they provoke, and which may not emerge until we have taken time to gain the patient's confidence and trust by a sympathetic and un-hurried approach.

The Doctor-Patient 'Couple'

This factor of consultative time is of central importance. Apley and

MacKeith (3) remind us that 'it is acceptable to go to a doctor with a bodily symptom: but many people are afraid that they will be laughed at if they ask for help merely because they feel anxious.' Repeatedly one can demonstrate a kind of 'collar-stud abscess' effect, in which for the first half-hour history-taking is conducted at a formal and relatively objective level. During this phase the patient (or parent) may present a number of 'offers' or 'propositions' (Balint (4)) concerning his illness, with greater or lesser emphasis upon 'acceptable complaints' depending on the outlook and attitude of the doctor. Then, but only after the patient's confidence has been gained, are we allowed to reach the 'deeper layers of pus' and so uncover the mainsprings of personal fear or frustration in the particular case. If there is insufficient time available or if the doctor is impatient he may never penetrate beyond the superficial presentation, and only the somatic aspect of the problem will emerge, to be dealt with perhaps symptomatically and often therefore unsatisfactorily. 'Diagnosis is sometimes like peeling successive skins off an onion: under each diagnostic solution, another problem may be hidden' (3). Yudkin (34) presents graphic illustrations of the same point. We must always treat the whole patient, and that includes his psyche.

Alleged Dangers of Psychotherapy

Many non-psychiatric physicians, however, are hesitant about this counsel. They adduce twin arguments in favour of non-intervention. On the one hand they express fear of uncovering or releasing more potent emotional forces than they, or the patient, can handle successfully. Such concern is perfectly understandable, and should be met with the assurance that danger signals operate in this sphere, just as they do in organic medicine. If during abdominal palpation the patient winces, we instinctively take note of his reaction, but we do not continue probing the area to make it more tender; our next step, on the basis of our diagnostic suspicions, is to arrange definitive treatment by the appropriate specialist for the suspected lesion. Similarly if his exploration for underlying emotional factors should prove untimely, so that the parent or child shows increasing distress or resistance, the doctor takes note and diplomatically suspends investigation. At that stage no great harm will have been done, and there will now be a diagnostic lead for the psychiatrist to follow when, subsequently, he is called in to offer more expert help.

It is a question of learning to recognise these danger signals, and practice brings with it familiarity and confidence. The risk of doing harm through lack of skill is not great, so long as active probing is minimised. The doctor's role primarily is to listen, with a sympathetic but attentive ear, for significant pointers in the personal history as it unfolds. Emotionally traumatic material, damaging to the patient, or to the mother, is unlikely to emerge while they themselves control the rate of outflow, so to speak; and if one particular aspect of the background is conspicuously avoided despite gently persistent references to it, it will be wiser to postpone further comment. After all, the silence itself will have been significant.

In our culture the doctor still retains a unique position of trust and confidential status, which we should do nothing to undermine. If on the basis of that trust the patient is prepared to ventilate his difficulties because he feels 'safe' to do so, it is our role, surely, not to discourage him by curtailing his overtures (and prescribing drugs only), but rather to justify his confidence by listening. The risks involved are no greater than in any other sphere of therapeutics, provided that we avoid active probing and interpretation.

On the other hand it is argued that the doctor untrained in psychiatry should not 'dabble' in the realms of the unconscious. This argument assumes that all conflicts which give rise to psychosomatic symptoms are unconsciously determined, and therefore require deep exploration to uncover and resolve. But this is applicable only to some, and certainly these must be left to the skilled therapist. A large number of emotional conflicts, however, are generated at the conscious or pre-conscious level, where they are much more readily accessible and amenable to treatment. It is not so widely appreciated that the patient with a psychosomatic disorder is often to some extent aware of his emotional tensions already, and of their sources. His difficulty lies not so much in recognising them as in giving vent to his pent-up feelings, and so dissipating the pathological tension. A common feature of the personality structure in these cases is the child's inability to express his feelings. He tends to be emotionally inarticulate, and therefore outwardly compliant; but thereby he is no less prone to anxieties and frustrations than his more articulate peers. Clearly the therapeutic indication is to help him to unburden his grievances or personal worries, through verbal discussion if he is mature enough, or through acting-out the problem in the case of the younger child. The patient may remain vulnerable, and perhaps always tend to utilise somatic pathways for emotional expression, but by releasing his pent-up feelings we reduce the charge which keeps his symptoms going.

Syndrome Shift

Unfortunately the same patient cannot always be relied upon to 'adopt' the same somatic channel of expression, even when he is under similar stress. For example it is common enough to find asthmatic children who 'exchange' their asthma for migraine, or who alternate perhaps between broncho-spasm and eczema, or, as in one case seen recently, between asthma and obesity. It is tempting to postulate a specific 'type' of personality structure underlying each kind of psychosomatic disorder, and indeed various attempts have been made to do so (e.g. by Alexander (1)). However there is no convincing evidence to this effect. On the contrary, the many illustrations of syndrome shift in the same patient during treatment, or under changing circumstances, point to a non-specific relationship between personality traits and certain syndromes (e.g. Van der Valk and Bastiaans (31)). In terms of psychogenesis, it seems, there is neither a specific cause for any given psychosomatic disorder, nor any single personality type specifically prone to a particular syndrome.

Tentative 'Working' Hypothesis

What we can say, however, is that in our clinical experience certain psychodynamic themes recur regularly in association with psychosomatic disorder. The details of these dynamics, and their significance for the patient, vary from case to case, so that each case must be individually assessed. It is helpful nevertheless to construct a diagnostic framework within which any given set of data may be fitted as it emerges.

Similarly in the personality make-up of the children concerned: we recognise certain features or traits which appear repeatedly, and which help to explain why these patients are less able to discharge suppressed emotion freely, and so tend to express it through psychosomatic channels or 'organ language' (Weiss and English (32)). As yet we cannot explain convincingly why one somatic channel should be adopted in preference to another (11), although various psychoanalytic theories have been put forward, e.g. by Bruch (9) and Sperling (29). Nor can we explain why sometimes there should be a shift of channel, nor indeed why a psychosomatic avenue is to be 'preferred' to a neurotic pathway at all, or to expression via delinquent acting-out. We can only say at this stage that genetic and constitutional factors must play some part in determining which reaction finally emerges.

However it is useful in clinical practice to adopt the working concept of a 'sensitive' or vulnerable personality, in the sense that we regard a child as being sensitive perhaps to foreign protein, or a patient with abdominal migraine as being intolerant to fats. By extending this idea of constitutional sensitivity we evolve the concept of the child who is 'allergic' to emotional stress, in the same way as he may be allergic, say, to pollen. Such a child is not necessarily nervous in the lay sense of the word, i.e. he need not be anxiety-prone or excessively fearful, or even unduly reserved. It is simply that he has a lower than average threshold to emotional stresses, but being emotionally inarticulate he tends to react to such stimuli through one of a number of recognisable somatic channels.

3

Psychodynamic Relationships

Faulty Parental Attitudes

Personal conflict affecting children derives mainly from defects in the parent/child relationship, and these defects, or faulty attitudes, in turn develop from one of two main sources. They may stem from the personality structure of the parent (or responsible relative); or they may be moulded by antecedent circumstances in the life and background of the parent, the so-called 'life situation' (Dunbar (15)). More often both sets of factors contribute, and it may be impracticable to differentiate between them.

Over-valuation. Certain themes appear regularly. They include: (*a*) a prolonged period of sterility in the marriage before the birth of the patient. He is perhaps the only child of the union, or if older siblings are already grown up and independent he has become virtually an only child; (*b*) an adverse obstetric record, e.g. habitual abortion, antenatal bleeding, pregnancy toxaemia, complicated delivery, neonatal asphyxia, or prematurity. The common denominator here is risk to the foetus, perhaps associated with risk to the mother's life; (*c*) in the postnatal history, serious illness or injury affecting the child at an earlier age, not necessarily connected with his present disorder, but serving to arouse persisting anxiety in the parents; (*d*) critical and perhaps fatal illness in an older sibling, with symptoms reminiscent to the parents of the younger child's current condition, so that comparisons are inevitably drawn by them, however unfounded; (*e*) marital unhappiness, with isolation of the mother or father emotionally from the marriage partner, and a tendency to 'live through' the child as a vicarious source of emotional satisfaction; (*f*) conversely, during pregnancy, feelings of hostility and rejection towards an unplanned, unwanted, and perhaps even illegitimate child, with reactionary guilt feeling at its birth, leading to compensatory maternal over-solicitude.

These 'models' of various life situations, however diverse, have one thing in common: the likelihood of augmenting the child's emotional value to his parents, and so increasing their emotional investment in him. Such life circumstances form the basis of parental over-valuation.

Over-indulgence. Alternatively (or perhaps additionally), the childhood memories of a mother or father may have been overshadowed by the premature death or chronic invalidism of their own parent, or they may have experienced harsh treatment from their parents, or suffered gross material hardship. Under such circumstances there is often a compensatory drive to 'make it up' to the patient for what they have themselves suffered or been denied at a comparable age. Thus are laid the foundations of parental over-indulgence.

Over-concern. Particularly prevalent, too, is the cryptic fear harboured by parents about familial tendencies to a certain disease and its potential ravages among their own offspring. The common family 'skeletons' are tuberculosis, cancer and mental illness, and it has been aptly remarked (3) that popular lay conceptions about these scourges tend to lag behind current medical thought by at least a generation. Hence young and inexperienced parents are the more readily influenced by the tales and forebodings of their own parents, should there be any family taint of illness.

Among the less intelligent and more credulous elements of the lay public, therefore, it is easy to understand how, say, a child's chronic bronchitic cough might well evoke covert parental fear of tuberculosis if there is an appropriate family history; or how a head injury, or a pronouncement of educational subnormality, or a recurrent pattern of headache in the child, might be feared to foreshadow mental illness (anything to do with the head being especially suspect if there is a family hint of insanity); or how a functional bowel disorder in a recalcitrant child might crystallise parental fears of bowel carcinoma, e.g. 'My father died of cancer of the back passage—could there be any connection?'

It is important to appreciate that such cryptic disease phobias are not always readily elicited from parents. They may be reticent just because they fear so much the validity of a familial loading, and seek unconsciously to ward off the truth; or their reticence may spring from a sense of shame about this 'skeleton in the family cupboard'; or they may withhold relevant data because they fear ridicule of their naïveté. Often the more irrational the phobia, the more tenaciously it is held, and the less the parent will say about it. His reticence, however, need not signify freedom from anxiety; on the contrary, it is just this kind of family history which gives rise to parental over-concern about the physical welfare of the child. Understandably, if the patient is already over-valued, the combination can be pernicious.

Over-protection. It is not always possible to differentiate between over-valuation, over-indulgence and over-concern. In any given case they tend to shade off into one another in significance, but together they yield the parental attitude of over-protection. The detailed evolution of this attitude is, of course, unique for each case, e.g.:

Alan was a pallid, subdued, catarrhal little boy of six. He was referred to the paediatrician for chronic nocturnal cough, plus cervical adenitis, plus indifferent appetite. No significant organic pathology was incriminated, apart from post-nasal catarrh, thought to be the cause of the cough, and the anorexia. Ephedrine nose drops were prescribed, and the mother was firmly reassured. The cough, however, persisted (though now largely as a nervous 'tickle'), and so did mother's anxiety.

This woman was clearly over-concerned and disproportionately protective in attitude. Why?

It emerged that her oldest child, a girl, had died in hospital nine years previously, at the age of one month, with meningitis which had developed from 'an abscess in the ear'. She had not been considered in any danger at first, but had suddenly deteriorated. Mother was profoundly shocked by her death. Alan was born three years later. His mother made no secret of her compensatory investment in him, to the healthy neglect of the two youngest siblings, now aged four years and one year.

When, at the age of three, Alan's cough first developed, she fancied that it was associated with swelling of the cervical glands, especially on the left side, and the left ear had been the site of the abscess in her daughter's case. She recalled having heard that T.B. could cause 'glands in the neck', and after all her grandfather had had tuberculosis. Suppose Alan was now developing tuberculous cervical adenitis? His cough, she reasoned, might aggravate the infection, especially with 'all that straining in the neck'. Conceivably, as with her daughter, this could lead to abscess formation, and so to fatal meningitis.

Set down baldly in print this case summary may perhaps sound trite, ingenuously conceived, and certainly not of serious import. But that is only because it conveys very little of this mother's intensity of feeling. Yet before our reassurance can prove effective, we must be able to appreciate the significance (to her) of her daughter's loss, the strength of her compensatory feeling towards Alan, her unspoken and ill-understood fears of tuberculosis, and the resulting mixture of over-valuation and over-concern which prompted her to hover over this boy, restrict his activities, listen for every cough, and almost literally breathe for him. If her fears sound absurd to us, they are none the less convincing to her, and must be understood as such before we can hope to uncover the roots of her attitude and set it right. This procedure takes time, patience and skill. It cannot be achieved by brief didactic methods.

Ultimately Alan's mother came to see that 'I was putting all my first baby's troubles on to Alan. My mother always said I should try to forget, but I just couldn't—not up till now—it all leads back to my first baby, and I kept getting all worked up—I expect I would have made Alan very nervy in the end.' Six months after their first attendance, Alan had lost his cough, and his pallor, he had developed a healthy appetite and was playing out freely with his school friends. He is no longer a problem, and his mother now has her values in better perspective. She is also better informed, medically.

This woman was not specially anxious in make-up. Her pathological attitude and corresponding mishandling had arisen mainly through the circumstances of her life situation. Alternatively, however, the basis of an over-protective attitude may lie in the personality structure of the parent. The anxiety-prone mother (for it is usually the mother), the 'born worrier', the woman who is herself 'highly strung and sensitive by nature', may quite unwittingly initiate conflict in her relationship with her child through her constitutional inability to handle him with sensible detachment and consistency. But just as it is important not to belittle the fears and prejudices of credulous lay parents, so it is vital for us to stifle any intolerance we may instinctively feel towards the anxiety-ridden, fussing type of parent. She cannot help her emotional vulnerability, and exhorting her 'to pull herself together for the sake of her child' will merely reinforce her self-image of inadequacy and sense of failure, and so increase her guilt feeling. We do not thereby help the child.

Personality Structure versus Stress

On the other hand, the child may not require our help. If he is sufficiently robust in personality structure to withstand the onslaught of over-protective parents and to ride out the emotional stresses buoyantly, there may be no reactive symptoms for us to treat. Alternatively he may rebel against excessive cosseting, and retaliate with provocative, even delinquent behaviour to emphasise his independence and throw off the parental yoke.

David, an only child aged 11, had been a congenital cardiac case operated upon successfully at the age of seven. His mother continued to hover over him, however, because 'you could never be certain that he might not over-strain himself'. David was referred on account of repeated petty thieving from local shops. He admitted that this was an act of bravado, 'just to show her, fussing and carrying on'. His over-anxious mother commented, 'He can be a very self-willed boy'.

Conversely, the child may reflect parental over-anxiety in his own personality structure, so that he reacts to over-protection not with robust defiance but possibly with phobic symptoms, perhaps echoing those of the parents, or remaining dependent, fearful and lacking in self-confidence. We may be asked to see him on account of nightmares, or hypochondriasis, or perhaps enuresis, or maybe failure to adjust in school, and we recognise a regressive or withdrawal type of response in this particular make-up of child.

In every dynamic equation there are always the two aspects to be considered: the personality make-up of the patient, interacting with his immediate environmental situation. If however we assume that our young patient is neither aggressively nor regressively disposed in pattern of response, but is emotionally inarticulate, i.e. constitutionally incapable of expressing himself vigorously even when he is angry or resentful or upset; if we regard him as by nature superficially conforming and acquiescent under stress because of this inability to ventilate pent-up emotion; then this is the constitutional type of coarctate personality who may eventually erupt with psychosomatic disorder in face of intra-familial conflict, provided that he has some form of diathetic predisposition to discharge through somatic channels. This is the essence of the psychosomatic reaction.

If as an example we take the syndrome of asthma in childhood, and study the background of the asthmatic child, we will commonly encounter the classical pattern of maternal over-protection, i.e. the 'hovering, smothering' mother whose anxious tension stifles her child's emotional development and sensitises him to react with broncho-spasm in any situation of intercurrent stress.

Jeanette was a subdued, sensitive little girl, aged seven. She was highly intelligent, but lacked vivacity. She had a baby brother aged two, whom she politely ignored. Jeanette was referred with 'asthmatic bronchitis', present since the age of five. She was well versed in its pharmaceutical treatment, and seemed altogether too preoccupied with her chest condition. She was invariably well mannered and obedient, if rather prim and formal. She avoided rough play and rarely showed any strong emotions. Jeanette's mother was a tense but emotionally controlled young woman, who had been subject to asthma herself in childhood. She recalled her early background with bitterness. She had been 'banished' to a special open air boarding school, because her home was low-lying and damp. But she had hated being away from home, and vowed that she would never allow any child of hers to be sent away. Her over-riding fear was that she might transmit this asthmatic tendency to one of her own children, so she hovered anxiously over Jeanette, because the little girl had always had 'a weak chest'. Accordingly, winter for Jeanette started in late August, and tapered off cautiously in early June. For most of the year she was almost literally wrapped in cotton wool. Two major developments had taken place around Jeanette's fifth birthday. Her baby brother was born, and seven weeks later she first attended school. Within two weeks of enrolment she had her first attack of asthma, and thereafter she spent more time at home than in school because of recurrent attacks.

If we analyse this case record, various themes, already familiar, can be discerned. It is difficult to convey in words the suppressed tension of Jeanette's mother and the controlled intensity of her protective feelings. But once these are understood, it is not too difficult to appreciate the long-term impact of these emotions upon Jeanette—cooped up in her domestic 'hot-house' and zealously guarded against the elements. Yet on the surface the little girl continued to appear unruffled, if perhaps a shade too deferential and composed. What would emerge, one wondered, if this façade were to crack? And crack it did under the additional strain of two extraneous precipitating stresses: the birth of her baby brother and the sense of rivalry so engendered (a perfectly natural reaction), and the demands of a new situation (school). This forced her to leave the baby, unchallenged, in the ascendency at home, and plunged her into an unprivileged world where she had to learn to fend for herself. But in her dependent state she was ill-equipped to adapt, and within two months she was presenting with asthmatic attacks.

It could be argued that the basis of this reaction is entirely mundane, and that in fact Jeanette was simply exposed for the first time to the risk of infection from the group in school, with asthma supervening on the basis of upper respiratory tract infection. It is perhaps not so simple to explain why, under psychotherapeutic treatment, Jeanette's susceptibility to 'chest colds' still persisted, but these no longer precipitated asthmatic attacks.

The absurdity of labelling this child's asthma as attention seeking may now be appreciated. Natural jealousy of the baby was certainly one factor, but only a precipitating one; and even at that, the cause-and-effect relationships project far beyond the simple proposition of Jeanette trying to retrieve deflected attention. Their roots lie much further back, incorporating the early childhood impressions of the mother, the influence of these memories upon her subsequent attitude, the genetic component of predisposition to asthma, the patient's personality structure, her reactive dependence and immaturity, and the effects of her 'exposure' to the robust environment of school. The evolution of the problem is in fact vastly more complex than can be conveyed adequately by a single label of motivation, and this is true for most cases of psychosomatic disorder. Ironically, the therapeutic indication in this case was towards emancipating Jeanette from the grip of her 'dear octopus' (Smith, D., *Dear Octopus*) and promoting the child's independence and self-reliance—the converse of her alleged motive of regaining maternal limelight through attention seeking.

Over-valuation plus Parental Domination

Rather a different situation unfolds when, coupled with circumstances of over-valuation, the personality structure of the parent proves to be dominating and obsessionally driving in type. Because emotional investment in the child remains high, there is corresponding over-concern for his welfare and his health, but this is expressed through rigid control rather than through anxious fussing. Reared in this way the emotionally inarticulate child tends to assume a compliant, passive role of unimpeachable behaviour. He is earnest, conscientious, well groomed and orderly, but he lacks initiative, spontaneity and zest. Basically he too is dependent and emotionally immature, despite the superficial impression of bookishness and pseudo-sophistication.

John, aged eleven, was such a child—'sober, steadfast and demure'. His father was a self-made man, proud of his senior position with his firm, but wistful about his own lack of formal education. His boy must have the opportunities for academic advancement that he, the father, had been denied. The mother was a genteel woman of more refined stock. For her, a place in Grammar School meant associating with the better class of boys in the neighbourhood. They could not quite afford a fee-paying school for John, so that much depended on his performance in the 11+ examination. In his earlier childhood John had been subject to episodes of diarrhoea, lasting two to three days, perhaps at six-monthly intervals, and unexplained by items in his diet or by infection. Retrospectively, his parents recalled that these attacks might occur if he was upset or particularly worried, but no blood or mucus had ever been noted in the stools. Now, four months before the crucial examination, John was admitted to hospital with diarrhoea of acute onset, this time associated with blood and slime. His haemoglobin was 70%, he was passing 12/15 stools daily, with much colic. Sigmoidoscopy confirmed the diagnosis of early ulcerative colitis.

The obvious deduction here might be to incriminate excessive pressure at school, but John's IQ (WISC Full Scale) proved to be 126 and his position in the A form was invariably among the first six. The 11+ in fact was simply the culminating point in a heavily loaded personal history of deferential conduct, anxiety to please his parents, excessive consideration for others and, significantly, complete disinclination to defend his own rights. Numerous workers have referred to the link between the onset of colitis in these vulnerable children and the loss, threatened, phantasied, or actual, of affection or approval from a key figure in the child's life, usually a parent (Engel (17); Prugh (28); Groen (20)). In this case the threat involved was of disappointing father's academic ambitions for the boy and mother's

social aspirations, with the consequent danger of losing parental appro-
bation. But this of course was merely the precipitant in a constellation of
contributory factors, which included the boy's personality structure, the
presumed vulnerability of his bowel to react to personal stress, and the
dominant personality of the father, rigidly overshadowing the child's life
and suppressing any flicker of independence and self-assertion.

Clearly, therefore, the whole situation has to be taken into account,
not just the precipitating stress. Nor must it be assumed that ulcerative
colitis in children need necessarily be associated with this particular type
of background, or indeed with any psychodynamic conflict situation. For
example, in a twenty-year survey of 62 cases undertaken by Platt, Schlesinger and Benson (27), 'in at least half the cases there were no obvious
predisposing or precipitating psychological causes'. Similarly with 23 cases
of juvenile ulcerative colitis who came to major operation, out of a large
series of 106 cases studied by Ehrenpreis et al. (16), none of the 23 disclosed
'any psychologic factors considered to be of aetiologic importance in the
patient's disease', although the investigation was carried out by a team of
child psychiatrists.

Conversely, and perhaps more confusing still, the parent/child
relationship outlined above may operate in the personal background of
other psychosomatic disorders, e.g. eczema, or the periodic syndrome of
repeated vomiting, headache and abdominal pain. In other words, when
it does operate it need not exclusively evoke the response of ulcerative
colitis, or indeed any psychosomatic condition. This 'choice of organ'
provides an intriguing field for further research.

Parental Domination plus Rejection

Consider now the obverse situation in which a strong-willed, dominant
mother or father entertains negative rather than positive feelings towards
the child, and in effect rejects him emotionally. Certain life situations may
have conspired to bring about such an attitude, exactly as the attitude of
over-valuation was seen to be moulded. For example, there may have been
disruption of the parent/child bond at an early stage of development,
through chronic illness of the parent or through his prolonged absence for
other reasons, or because the child was himself ill and away in hospital.
In many instances (O'Connor (23)) no apparent harm is sustained, but in
other cases the child undoubtedly suffers emotional deprivation (7), (12),
and the bond may never be fully restored. Mutual recriminations tend to
build up between the child and his father, or between mother and child,
and these in turn may contribute to a progressively hardening attitude of
rejection. Twenty years after the second World War we are still encountering cases, now in their late adolescence, in whom the basic defect is a
continuing failure of communication with a father who was isolated too
long from his family on overseas duty (perhaps as a prisoner of war) and
has never really learned to bridge the resulting emotional chasm.

Alternatively, the status of the child may affect the relationships within the home. His statutory status as an adopted child, or as a stepson, may be responsible for subtle changes in parental attitude following the unplanned arrival of a natural offspring at a later stage in the marriage. Or it may be the child's physical status which determines an attitude of rejection. Commonly physical handicaps tend to induce attitudes of parental over-concern and protection, but there are instances of the child attracting negative feelings simply because he is not wholesome; he has, perhaps, some kind of blemish, and in a subtle way the parent (mother or father) interprets this as a reflection on himself, i.e. on his capacity to procreate perfectly healthy specimens. In a similar manner a guilt-ridden mother may link her child's disability (say his spasticity) with her unsuccessful efforts to procure his abortion during pregnancy, and though entirely unrelated the handicap serves as a constant reminder, repeatedly evoking her guilt feelings, and so contributing perhaps to deep-rooted rejection. Such feelings are not readily uncovered, and are very rarely appreciated at a conscious level by the parent. The influence they exert may be none the less potent.

Correspondingly, the patient's intellectual status may induce an unwitting attitude of rejection, if as a mentally subnormal child he brings a sense of stigma upon the parents and makes them feel ashamed rather than protective. Or it may be that his behaviour pattern is unacceptable because he is too flamboyant or unduly mischievous, or uncouth, and unknowingly resurrects, perhaps, the family skeleton of some psychopathic uncle who ended up in prison and whose genetic influence is now fearfully if secretly recalled.

The significance of these various themes, as and when they emerge in history taking, must be evaluated separately for each case. As we have seen, psychopathology is an individual matter, and the very factors which might evoke sympathy and over-valuation in some parents will induce diametrically opposite feelings in others, and in others again yield no pathology of attitude whatever.

However, if we encounter the combination of a determined dominating parent and a rejecting attitude, motivated by any of the above sets of circumstances, and if the child too should prove not inarticulate but equally strong-willed and robust in personality structure, the scene is set for major conflict of yet another kind, which may present psychosomatically. The toddler stage of child development is recognised by all disciplines as the phase of defiance, the age of initial self-assertion and revolt against parental omnipotence. During this phase too efforts are made to train the infant in toilet control, in acceptable feeding patterns, and in acquiring an appropriate sleep rhythm. Against such a backcloth of parent/child friction, and classically in the toddler stage, it requires only that undue pressure be brought to bear by a carping parent to ensure 'bowel cleanliness', or to achieve 'a balanced diet', or a 'proper night's sleep', and the child is liable to react sharply with bowel negativism, or a major feeding problem, or with protracted sleep disturbance.

Characteristically these are fastidious, rigid mothers, who cannot tolerate 'a dirty child'. In any case this may have been an unplanned and unwelcome addition to the family, so that the prospect of renewed burdening with soiled napkins heightens maternal determination to 'train' the child virtually from birth. Continued acceptance within the family is therefore made conditional: he will be loved and approved only if he is 'clean'—and to this righteous end all the energies of the perfectionist parent are directed. To a negativistic child, the challenge is irresistible.

At the other end of the alimentary tract, the focus of conflict may centre upon adequate food intake, i.e. 'adequate' as judged by the parents.

Alison, for example, was a premature baby, weighing 4 lb. at birth. Duration of the pregnancy was eight months. Alison had been conceived pre-maritally, and her mother, aged 24, admitted two unsuccessful attempts to procure abortion. Hurried marriage followed the second failure, but mother's feelings towards the unborn child remained ambivalent. Rejection continued to vie with the maternal instinct all through a stormy first year of life, punctuated by bronchitis, septic vaccination, and poor weight gain. Gossiping neighbours began to comment about the child's 'skinny' appearance and fretful temper. Covertly they hinted about maternal neglect, until Alison's mother became quite paranoid, with mounting determination to 'feed her up'. At the age of three, when first seen, Alison weighed a puny 23 lb., all skin and bone, despite her mother's heroic efforts, literally at forced feeding. Careful and detailed investigation failed to reveal any organic basis for the child's failure to thrive. Equally, Alison's adamant resistance to eating was clearly demonstrable as a gesture of supreme defiance against her coercive mother.

Chronic and serious sleep disorder may be evoked under similar circumstances in a negativistic child, and can play absolute havoc with the entire household.

However, such is the complexity of psychodynamic relationships that behaviour patterns indistinguishable from the above may be established, not so much in response to parental domination as in response to parental anxiety. In these cases the area of parent/child conflict is often determined by antecedent life circumstances. Grandfather, perhaps, had died from colonic carcinoma, and 'he had suffered with chronic constipation for years'. Add to this the layman's irrational fears about the evil effects of constipation, plus a basis for over-valuing a particular child, and we may readily understand how a mother can feel driven to insist upon bowel regularity in her child through anxious over-concern rather than fastidious revulsion. Alternatively, a family history of (say) tuberculosis, with resulting tuberculo-phobia, may prompt the over-anxious mother to make an issue of feeding if her over-valued child remains excessively thin.

In this group of disorders, therefore, the same syndrome may be produced by radically differing parental attitudes, based upon different personality structures, plus a variety of motivations and individually relevant life situations. The one common denominator is the evoking of negativism in the child, expressed in conflict with the parents over a particular physiological function. The cardinal mistake which these parents make is to take issue over a function which they cannot dictate because the child retains its own voluntary control. It follows that, strictly speaking, these conditions should not be classified as psychosomatic, because although the presenting symptoms are somatic there is no primary organic contribution. The aetiology is psychogenic, and what is more, it is volitionally determined in the first instance. Nevertheless they are included here because they illustrate the value of the psychosomatic in contrast to the local or symptomatic approach, which must fail because it takes no account of the underlying dynamics. As one of my medical students so aptly put it, in answer to a question on bowel negativism, 'You must treat the whole child, and not just the hole in the child.'

Psychosomatic or not, it should be borne in mind that resistance to defaecation by the young child can be so determined and so protracted that it may produce major physical repercussions, including radiologically demonstrable megacolon (Pinkerton (25)). Once chronic atonia of colonic musculature has become established it is much more difficult to reverse the syndrome, and treatment may then have to continue for years. In at least one case of 'psychogenic megacolon' in my own series, the ultimate outcome in adolescence was a partial colectomy. This proved necessary before normal bowel function could be restored, in a colon which had become grossly atonic and saccular over a period of years, after parental refusal to co-operate in insight therapy. Histological section of the resected gut revealed no pathology other than loss of elasticity. Psychologically, too, if untreated these children tend to become bland and superficially innured to their condition in its more chronic phases, so that what began as conscious negativism tends to be submerged in time below the level of readily accessible material. Treatment is thereby considerably hampered.

A much more common sequel in childhood to emotionally determined constipation is fissure-in-ano. Surgical opinion often transposes the sequence of development, by claiming that the fissure antedates the constipation. This is an interesting example of the doctor's need to find a concrete cause, if possible, for the disorder he is treating, because the treatment is so much more straightforward in that 'one can actually do something'. In fact a fissure never develops *sui generis*, and must be secondary to established constipation. Nevertheless it represents a very painful secondary development, and admittedly if left untreated it may well preclude successful resolution of the basic psychogenic 'fault'. All the more reason therefore for a joint consultative approach between paediatric surgeon and child psychiatrist, to break the vicious spiral of emotional resistance to defaecation: hard, craggy stool—anal fissure—excruciating pain—greater resistance to defaecation, and fear of it—obstipation—megacolon. In true psychosomatic disorder, organic and emotional factors operate, so to speak, in parallel. In this and allied syndromes they operate, initially, in series, the psychogenic preceding the organic. Ultimately, of course, both contributions play their role in perpetuating the disorder.

Parental Aloofness plus Rejection

Reverting to the concept of the inarticulate or emotionally coarctate child, the prototype of the psychosomatic case: a stressful milieu may be engendered for him not by a dominating parent, but by parental withdrawal and detachment. This is a pattern sometimes observed in supercilious parents who prefer sophisticated adult society to the unspoilt directness of children, or who are preoccupied with their business or professional career to the exclusion of 'sticky-fingered kids'. Enough that they provide financial support for their family, without mortgaging their precious time, interest, and intellect. Father or mother may qualify equally for this haughty role of cold disdain, which is in effect a rejecting attitude, and which so often contributes to a rarified emotional atmosphere within the home. Couple this subtler form of deprivation, inimical to the well-being of marriage partner and children alike, with a vulnerable personality structure in the child exposed to it, and psychosomatic disorder may again result (as, of course, may alternative patterns of reaction).

Roberta, aged 14, was a tall but painfully thin child, weighing 74 lb. on referral. The presenting problem was complete disinclination for food, of nine months' duration. Father was a meek and mild civil servant, the mother a qualified biochemist who lived for her work. An older boy, aged 19, was the mother's favourite. She openly preferred her 'masculine' son, and had hardly bothered to conceal her disappointment over the birth of a daughter (hence the name). 'I dislike syrupy sentiment in girls.' During her childhood Roberta had tried unsuccessfully to establish a filial relationship with this emotional 'iceberg'. The child herself was shy to demonstrate her feelings. Rebuffed by her mother, and with small comfort from father, she felt ashamed of her femininity, and as puberty advanced she embarked upon voluntary dieting 'to keep my figure trim'. Pride in her womanhood was replaced by jealous attempts to emulate her favoured brother. Insidiously, this conscious plan to restrict her intake merged into progressive anorexia, with listlessness, genuine aversion to meals, emotional lability, alarming loss of weight (32 lb. in nine months), and surreptitious concealment of food items when pressed by her (now) anxious mother to eat. The very thought of food now gave her a physical sense of revulsion. This was no longer a response controlled volitionally at conscious level, but a case of anorexia nervosa, potentiated unconsciously, and grave in import because of the hazard of death through inanition. During treatment Roberta actually disclosed her repressed wish to die. This had provided the cryptic mainspring of her resistance to eating, and was clearly, if unconsciously, directed at mother.

A similar theme of intellectual hauteur yielded an entirely different pattern of psychosomatic response in the following case:

Anthony, aged 12, was referred with recurrent attacks of severe central abdominal pain, associated with nausea and sometimes headache. These attacks recurred at intervals of 6–8 weeks, and might last up to 36 hours. No organic cause could be incriminated, but his mother, a tense woman, suffered with regular and crippling attacks of migraine. Anthony was a conscientious and most reliable boy, a pillar of good conduct in school, and extremely attentive to his mother at home. A younger brother, aged 10, was noticeably more impish, outgoing and carefree. He was also symptom-free. Anthony's 'bilious' attacks seemed related to excitement, or alternatively 'to come on when things get beyond me and I snap at the children'. Father was an intelligent but snobbish man, a highly successful sales promoter, whose job took him all over the world. 'He loves us, of course, but he is wrapped up in making money to secure our future.' This man had opted out of the ordinary business of fatherhood, coming home only at week-ends, when he insisted on a quiet atmosphere 'to allow him to relax'. Clearly, he expected his wife to shoulder the routine responsibilities of home and children. 'When we do go out together, neither of us is sufficiently relaxed to enjoy it.' So mother was as neglected emotionally as her children.

It was easy to demonstrate to her how closely her own attacks of migraine were linked with waves of covert resentment, periodically welling up inside her, because, as she said, 'it all seemed so unfair'. She could not ventilate these recriminations with her husband: 'He won't listen; you can't argue with him; he dismisses the topic.' From this point we could more readily trace Anthony's equivalent sense of frustration. He too felt rebuffed by the vacuum created by his father; and this, together with his awareness of mother's suppressed tension, led every so often to his own episodes of so-called 'abdominal migraine' (Farquhar (18)). The trigger might be a bout of mother's irritability, but the loading dynamics pointed to this inaccessible father. Significantly, the more articulate younger child seemed able to find his emotional outlets elsewhere, with school friends and in particular with a favourite maternal uncle. He had escaped his mother's genetic taint of 'migraine susceptibility'.

Parental Inadequacy as a Source of Flux

Finally, in our consideration of pathological attitudes and the reactive disorders which they may evoke, we must study the complementary attitude of parental irresponsibility and emotional inadequacy as a stress-provoking factor. This type of parent tends to be immature and shallow in outlook. Perhaps he is simply a hedonist, but more often he is himself the victim of deprivation in his own childhood, through desertion by his mother or father or through some other tragedy. Now therefore he seeks in his marriage the mother figure denied to him in reality earlier on. To him the arrival of a child represents a competitor for his 'maternal' wife's affection, and there is rejection of the baby in consequence, often presenting as emotional neglect, sometimes associated with actual cruelty. This tragic sequence may apply equally to the mother who has been emotionally deprived in childhood. Inevitably marital friction ensues, and adds to the child's established sense of insecurity and division of loyalties.

Classically this background yields a reactive pattern of delinquency (Glueck and Glueck (19)), based on the abdication of parental authority and interest. It does not usually in my experience give rise to psycho-somatic disorder. Yet, paradoxically, it is just this kind of gross situation which tends to be equated with 'psychological stress' in the mind of the uninitiated physician, and which is seized upon therefore as a potential source of symptomatology, if emotional factors are suspected at all.

On the whole stress factors underlying psychosomatic states tend to be 'more subtle, less obvious, and essentially of personal significance to the patient. Nevertheless from time to time the 'broken home' theme, based on parental defection or character weakness, does emerge as the relevant emotional contribution—the exception, so to speak, which proves the rule. But this paradox is more apparent than real, because the child in these circumstances is reacting, not to the overt cruelty or parental harshness, nor to the marital rows or conditions of neglect, but to the sense of bewilderment and feeling of confused orientation which stem from the father's or mother's unpredictability: the fine words but broken promises, the lack of depth, and the failure to measure up to the child's personal image of parenthood. Children can grow accustomed to the most terrible privations materially, as shown by the appalling records of war-time concentration camps, without disruption of their intimate bonds and loyalties. It is the damage to their sense of personal significance, the covert undermining of fundamental ties, which throws them into emotional imbalance.

Since 'home' has so little to offer these children, the majority, it would seem, are driven to seek vicarious outlets beyond the home, often by associating with other deprived children in gangs and so drifting inevitably into delinquent activities. This is one form of self-expression, however unacceptable to society. But occasionally there is the child who lacks the drive and initiative and capacity to ventilate these pent-up feelings through acting-out, but who instead 'bottles up' his emotions because, as we have seen, he is inarticulate and 'alone'; he feels the same sense of hurt and abandonment, but he cannot give overt expression to it. This is the potential candidate for psychosomatic disorder, but as such he reacts to the element of personal duress in his domestic situation rather than to the gross factor of material deprivation.

Girls, it seems, are more commonly affected in this way than boys. The syndrome with which they may present includes lassitude, anergy, and attacks of acute abdominal pain, as if, in 'organ language' (32), they were no longer able to 'stomach' the doubts and divided allegiances of their difficult family situations.

There is no periodicity about this syndrome; it is not usually associated with vomiting or nausea, nor is there any link with 'rheumatic' limb pains, as often in the 'periodic syndrome' (Apley (2)). Many are referred as suspected mesenteric adenitis, or as cases of 'grumbling appendix', or as renal problems, but no convincing lesion shows up on investigation, and the clinical picture assumes a closer similarity to the old descriptions of neuras-thenia, with which indeed it has much in common.

To sum up: running through these various psychodynamic themes we can trace a single continuous thread. It is the need to evaluate the whole child, as he interacts with his personal environment, within the home, at school, and in his neighbourhood society. For the child psychiatrist this means *including* the child's physical state in our assessment (not excluding physical disorder), and for the paediatrician it means surely that psyche, as well as soma, must be considered.

4

Principles of Treatment

Reorientation of Prevailing Bias

By definition, psychosomatic conditions present with physical disorder in the child. This will lead the parents to consult their family doctor in the first place, and possibly through him a paediatrician or paediatric surgeon. Very few cases will be referred primarily for psychiatric opinion. Four groups of people, therefore, qualify for potential reorientation of their attitudes to the problem before referral to a child psychiatrist can be of much value, if indeed the child is to be referred at all.

Allaying Medical Disquiet. The key figure is the family doctor. Unless we enjoy his full confidence, we are unlikely to gain his co-operation and approval in treating the emotional components of the syndrome. The same applies to the paediatric consultant, of whom Chapman and Loeb (10) have this to say: 'His ability to explain the importance of emotional factors is, itself, an important factor in whether parents will actually follow up the suggestion of psychiatric referral.' This means that we must collaborate as closely as possible with our non-psychiatric colleagues, not only in the management of specific cases, but through arranging clinical meetings and case seminars of joint interest at our base clinic or hospital centre, or better still, if time permits, through organising joint consultations with the family doctor or paediatrician. In this way we present a united medical front which is more likely to impress the parents (and therefore the patient) with the validity of the psychosomatic thesis (Pinkerton (25)). However costly such a programme in professional time, it is vital that we bring child psychiatry out of its former isolation into closer liaison with the general children's hospital. Our colleagues can thereby see us at work, so that they gain a more informed impression of what we have to offer (and of our limitations in treatment), and can then judge for themselves the value or otherwise of our potential contribution to psychosomatic disorder.

Inherent in all this is the challenge to present as lucid and convincing a statement of the principles of our discipline as is possible in the present transitional stage of our knowledge. In this field of collaborative endeavour with the organic physician there is no room on our part for woolly thinking or abstruse terminology, which confuses rather than clarifies, and which often cloaks our own ignorance. Before we exhort our colleagues to abandon their misconceived ideas let us make sure that these really are misconceptions, and that modern psychiatric practice is both soundly based and responsibly self-critical. There is the vital need to inculcate this teaching at the undergraduate level, at an early stage in medical curriculum (6; 8; 13).

Allaying Parental Disquiet. Even when we have overcome medical prejudice, however, we have still to allay parental misgivings, and often the fears of the child himself at 'coming to see a psychiatrist'. Two popular misapprehensions persist among lay parents in this connection: there is the implication that their child may be mentally deranged, or the equally stigmatising suggestion of mental subnormality. Should there be a familial taint in either respect, parental anxiety will be proportionately enhanced. Fortunately in psychosomatic practice both these fears can usually be dismissed at once and with authority.

Not so readily resolved, but just as frequently encountered, is the parental resistance which is based upon purely personal motivation. It is a curious paradox that parents (doctors as well as laymen) find comfort in the firm diagnosis of a 'respectable' organic lesion in their child. It is not simply that the pronouncement of an accredited disease, for which appropriate treatment can be prescribed, brings a sense of relief. It is the reassurance that they, the parents, are not involved in its aetiology and are thereby absolved from any imputation of blame. I can vividly recall the incongruity of one mother's relieved smile when she was told that her little girl's headaches and vomiting attacks were due, not to migraine (like mother's), but to cerebral tumour!

Ventilating Doubts and Misgivings

Therefore, as long as they attend their family doctor or the paediatric clinic with their child, these parents feel secure and, curiously, free from shame. Indeed we find them patronisingly concerned for the child's welfare. If their role is protective, it is also objective. But suggest referral to a psychiatrist, and at once they feel threatened by the unspoken implication that they are at fault, or at the very least that 'people will talk'. In some this evokes a sharp guilt reaction; in others a strong protest of denial. But those who disclaim the loudest are often the most deeply involved. Their anti-psychiatric sentiments mask their underlying uneasiness. 'The lady doth protest too much, methinks.' (*Hamlet*, III. ii. 347.)

If they remain unvoiced, such covert misgivings will continue to fester and so sabotage our therapeutic efforts. But if they are brought to the surface, we can at least assess the nature and strength of parental resistance and plan our therapeutic campaign accordingly. Our first task therefore is to encourage ventilation of these fears and prejudices. We will best achieve this by listening. A sympathetic hearing is often the means of disarming mistrust and gaining the confidence of parents and patient alike.

Realigning the Lay Concept of Disease

Parents (and the patients themselves) are orientated to think of this kind of disorder in physical terms, calling for concrete and tangible measures prescribed with traditional didactic authority. They themselves simply take what is prescribed; their role is passive; they do not expect to make any active contribution. This is the kernel of the matter, the point from which any conceptual realignment must start. Now there are still very few family doctors or paediatricians who will consider psychiatric referral of a suspected psychosomatic disorder at the outset in conjunction with their own standard treatment measures. Almost certainly some form of symptomatic therapy will have been tried first, and presumably by itself will have proved disappointing, to prompt consulting the psychiatrist. Sometimes, regrettably, one 'respectable' measure after another has been persevered with, though each with no greater success than the last, until in desperation the child psychiatrist is called in as a 'last ditch' measure. But by this time the child's condition is so chronic and entrenched that psychotherapeutic intervention is rarely practicable. The case has become inaccessible in the way that a neglected neoplasm becomes inoperable.

Gordon was aged 14½ at the time of psychiatric referral for 'vocational guidance'. He had suffered with asthma since the age of three, and now presented the typical fixed 'barrel-chest' associated with emphysematous changes. Even though protected by steroids, he was not entirely free from attacks especially when reference was made to any plans after leaving his special school. He felt very insecure about his future. In retrospect, the onset of his asthma could be traced to his enrolment in a day nursery, shortly after the death by accident of his father and his devoted mother's enforced return to office work. A convincing relationship could be educed in his case between emotional stress factors, operating at the relevant time, and reactive symptom formation in the child (and incidentally in the mother, who suffered with intractable neuro-dermatitis). But at the time of referral, nearly 12 years later, this formulation was of academic interest only. Gordon was an established 'hospital bird', a firm favourite with the nurses and all too ominously at home in the ward whenever a relapse brought him back. At this stage both he and his mother 'need' the boy's asthma, so to speak, as a justification for their respective life patterns, and each would strenuously resist any attempts at psychotherapeutic reorientation. Apart from this, the irreversible structural changes in the boy's chest now afford the strongest argument against psychiatric intervention, because undeniably he has a physical disability which psychotherapy can no longer alter. He will remain permanently handicapped by it, both physically and emotionally.

Clearly, therefore, it is vital to see the child at an early stage in the development of his disorder if an emotional component is even faintly suspected.

In our approach to the parent, we might begin by indicating that the response to purely physical or pharmaceutical measures had so far been disappointing. For example, as soon as the drug is suspended the child perhaps tends to relapse, or he may continue to have attacks even under treatment, or alternatively the condition may tend to return as soon as he is discharged from hospital. The implication, surely, is that something more is called for: an approach more comprehensive than symptomatic treatment, an approach which takes cognisance of the whole child, interacting with concomitant situations in his personal environment. These suggestions are introduced cautiously, on a broad discussion front. To lay people they represent new and unfamiliar ideas, and therefore we must carefully gauge their effect upon parent and patient alike, judging how far and how fast we may proceed in proportion to the degree of acceptance or resistance we encounter. Slowly, sometimes imperceptibly, there comes a subtle change of emphasis in the description of the illness (Pinkerton (26)), perhaps a shift from its objective signs and symptoms to the significance which these hold for the parent, until, in time and with patience, spontaneous reference may be made to a possible cause-and-effect relationship between parental attitude and the disorder under discussion. Here are the first glimmerings of insight.

Insight Promotion: Spontaneous versus Didactic Approach

I say 'spontaneous reference', because the whole art of promoting insight in the parent, as in the child, lies in guiding him unobtrusively towards a self-acquired realisation of the relevant dynamics. The doctors with whom we shall be working in this conjoint field, trained as they are in authoritarian traditions, are tempted involuntarily to 'tell the patient'. They must learn to suppress this temptation. In practice, you cannot 'tell' the patient anything which he is not yet ready emotionally to hear (i.e. to accept with understanding). In contrast to the organic field, the patient must develop insight if he is to co-operate with us in treatment, and without his insightful contribution no treatment will succeed. This is where dynamically orientated therapy differs so radically from organotherapy. But because the relevant dynamics often seem so obvious to us, objectively, we are irresistibly drawn to explain them didactically to the patient or parent as we would an organic lesion. We tend to forget that, for those who are intimately (subjectively) involved in the situation, those dynamic relationships are by no means so clear or so acceptable. On the contrary, considerable readjustment is necessary before the 'subject' can acquire true understanding. This takes time on his part, patience on our part, and mutual co-operation.

It is frequently argued that the doctor saves clinical time by dogmatic explanation instead of waiting for spontaneous insight to dawn. In fact he wastes time, and he may even impair the therapeutic relationship in one of two ways. By 'telling' the parent, he courts the risk of promoting intellectual ('cortical') insight, i.e. a superficial quasi-appreciation of the problem, at the expense of true ('thalamic') insight, acquired on the emotional plane. Parents so indoctrinated represent a more serious obstacle to successful treatment than those completely devoid of understanding, because they *think* they understand, and their spurious familiarity with the problem may well defeat subsequent attempts to penetrate their unconscious defence mechanisms by promoting *genuine* insight.

Alternatively, didactic statements too often provoke a deep sense of guilt in the parent. If we say that she has contributed to the problem we must mean that she is really to blame, and in this way the doctor's well-intentioned explanation is unwittingly misinterpreted as censure. Our task is to convey an understanding of how parents may be involved and yet not at fault; this can only be achieved by fostering insight from within. If we attempt to impose it, however convincingly, we heighten anxiety or generate resentment, depending on parental reaction to this guilt feeling. Either way we undermine our own therapeutic efforts, and the family may withdraw altogether. There is one potential exception to this principle—the intellectually dull parent. He or she may accept unequivocal counsel, but only because they lack the endowment to appreciate its implications, and do not therefore feel threatened.

The Concrete Demonstration

At the other extreme are those parents who cannot or will not countenance the suggestion that emotional factors may be operating in the case of their child, without a concrete demonstration to convince them. The most effective procedure here (if facilities permit) is to admit the patient to hospital for a period of planned separation, in the appropriate ward setting. If we can engineer a stable routine of detached handling by anxiety-free nursing staff, in a group atmosphere devoid of tension, and if we can emphasise the positive aspects of health by having the child ambulant and fully occupied (inclusive of hospital school), the presenting symptoms are likely to remit without recourse to specific drug treatment or other special measures. It is a universal observation, for example, that asthmatic attacks in children are rarely seen in hospital. Faced with such an illuminating demonstration, even the most recalcitrant parents are likely to be shaken in their negative convictions.

The Follow-through

But this is merely the beginning. We must consolidate the initial breach in parental resistance; otherwise their doubts and misgivings soon return. Yet this elementary principle is still neglected in many children's hospitals, where the standard practice is to discharge the patient upon remission of symptoms, without adequate follow-up. The whole point of a practical demonstration (i.e. handling the case in hospital!) is lost, unless we engineer that the right conclusions are drawn from the exercise. How, for example, was the remission achieved? Could it have been linked with uninvolved management in a consistent, tension-free atmosphere? If so, might not the parents' own tensions and dynamic 'bias' have contributed, conversely, to the disorder in its development and perpetuation?

Consolidating the Advantage

Once this link is conceded, however tenuously, the way is open to further therapeutic exploitation. We may now trace with the parents the origins of their basic attitudes to the child. What factors prompted them to adopt the views they hold, and how have those views come to be moulded and crystallised? By taking the parents back through the years we help them to see for themselves the connection with their own antecedent life circumstances, or with their own personality characteristics, and how their outlook and approach to the child have been influenced accordingly. In short, we promote their deepening insight. In the process, emphasis is steered away from the presenting symptoms and focused upon the motivating dynamics which have generated these symptoms, because realignment of parental attitude ultimately depends upon understanding those dynamics.

Dispelling Specific Fears

We have now reached a point at which parents may be encouraged to ventilate furtively harboured fears or forebodings about a particular disease or 'taint' which has afflicted their family. Brusque dismissal of these fears, because they sound ridiculous to us, will not in itself dispel them. Neither will bluff reassurance which is not specific. Indeed either approach may well increase parental anxiety, and so undermine such confidence as is already established in the doctor. However absurd or unlikely the association with the child's disorder, these lay misgivings must be treated with respect, and we must try to appreciate how a false connection might have come to be built up on the basis of half-understood and misapplied elementary medical data. Only if we do this are we likely to dispense successful reassurance.

Direct Therapy with the Child

Complementary to these procedures there is, of course, the need to undertake concurrent therapy directly with the patient. However this work is of such central importance that a separate chapter is being entirely devoted to it. The principles of direct treatment with children that are valid for other clinical groups apply equally to psychosomatic disorders. For our immediate purpose they may be summarised as follows: (1) to establish sufficient rapport with the child (either as out-patient or in-patient), to win his confidence, and so penetrate his defensive façade; (2) to define, with him, his basic problems, either through the medium of projective play techniques or, with older children, through verbal discussion; (3) to encourage him to work through these difficulties, by expressive play therapy where appropriate, with the aim of releasing pent-up emotion; (4) following this release, to promote or restore the child's stability and sense of perspective. In respect of the 'psychosomatic' case and the inarticulate state which so much contributes to it, we might regard such therapy as a means of 'ungagging' or emancipating the patient from the strangulating restrictions imposed by his own personality structure. We seek to encourage the discharge of emotion through alternative channels, less taxing to the patient himself, and no less acceptable to society, by precluding his tendency to 'take it out' on his own body.

Comprehensive Treatment: the Combined Approach

Winnicott (33) has referred to the need for 'symptom tolerance' in a group of disorders which are at once the purview of the paediatric physician and the child psychiatrist. Among paediatricians there is the understandable tendency to try to resolve presenting symptoms by direct treatment as early as possible in the course of the disorder. They are intolerant, so to speak, of the persistence of symptoms. The discipline of child psychiatry, on the other hand, advocates the frequent need to tolerate symptoms while basic treatment is being directed at the real core of the problem, the primary emotional factors underlying. These differing attitudes are derived from the difference in training between the two disciplines, but they need not preclude a combined approach to therapy, provided certain safeguards are observed. Prescribing bronchodilators to relieve the asthmatic child's spasm, or phenobarbitone to relieve the pain of 'abdominal migraine', are valuable adjuncts to psychotherapy, so long as they are recognised for the symptomatic measures they are and not misrepresented as 'cures'. The danger lies in equating the resolution of symptoms with therapeutic repletion, and thereby neglecting to explore the all-important hinterland of psychodynamics. As a result the doctor, the parent, and the patient are all lulled into false security. Conversely, a truly conjoint approach, wary of such pitfalls, may actually enhance successful treatment by reinforcing parental reassurance, and by promoting continuity of management. The recent introduction of powerful new drugs has added fresh impetus to this theme. Steroid therapy, for example, has been shown to facilitate psychotherapy in the treatment of ulcerative colitis (22; 30), while chlorpromazine has been used with equal success to enhance vital rapport in anorexia nervosa (14; 21). While the trend in the field of medicine as a whole is towards increasing specialisation, this move towards integration of therapy is a welcome counter-measure.

5

Conclusion

The organs and tissues of the human body have only a limited repertoire of responses to a wide variety of noxious stimuli, and nowhere is this more clearly demonstrated than in psychosomatic disorder. If therefore we are to pursue meaningful research into the ultimate aetiology of these conditions. we must promote progressive liaison between the disciplines of paediatrics and child psychiatry, so that each reinforces the contribution of the other. In so doing we subscribe to the fundamental principle of reintegrating psychological medicine with medicine as a whole. There can be no finer aim.

REFERENCES

1. ALEXANDER, F., 1952. *Psychosomatic Medicine, its Principles and Applications.* London: Allen and Unwin.
2. APLEY, J., 1958. A common denominator in the recurrent pains of childhood. *Proc. Roy. Soc. Med.,* **51**: 1023.
3. APLEY, J. and MACKEITH, R., 1962. *The Child and His Symptoms. A Psychosomatic Approach.* Oxford: Blackwell.
4. BALINT, M., 1955. The Doctor, his patient, and the illness. *Lancet,* i: 683-688.
5. ⸺ 1957. *The Doctor, his Patient, and the Illness,* p. 299. London: Pitman Medical Publishing Co.
6. BARTON HALL, S., HEARNSHAW, L. S. and HEATHERINGTON, R. R., 1961. The teaching of psychology in the medical curriculum. *J. Ment. Sci.,* **107**: 451, 1003.
7. BOWLBY, J., 1961. Separation anxiety: a critical review of the literature. *J. Child Psychol. and Psychiat.,* 1: 251.
8. BRITISH MEDICAL STUDENTS' ASSOCIATION, 1959. *Report on Teaching of Psychiatry.*
9. BRUCH, H., 1943. Psychiatric aspects of obesity in children. *Amer. J. Psychiat.,* **99**: 752.
10. CHAPMAN, A. H. and LOEB, D. G., 1955. Psychosomatic gastro-intestinal problems in children. *Amer. J. Dis. Child.,* **89**: 717-724.
11. CHAUDHARY, N. A. and TRUELOVE, S. C., 1961. Human colonic motility: a comparative study of normal subjects, patients with ulcerative colitis, and patients with the irritable colon syndrome. (Effects of emotions.) *Gastroenterology,* **40**: 1: 27.
12. CLARKE, A. D. B. and CLARKE, A. M., 1960. Some recent advances in the study of early deprivation. *J. Child Psychol. and Psychiat.,* 1: 26.
13. COLLEGE OF GENERAL PRACTITIONERS, 1958. *Psychological Medicine in General Practice.*
14. DALLY, P. J., 1962. Pharmacological Aspects of Physical Methods of Treatment, in *Principles of Treatments of Psychosomatic Disorders.* Oxford: Pergamon Press. (In preparation.)
15. DUNBAR, H. F., 1943. *Psychosomatic Diagnosis.* New York: P. B. Hoeber.
16. EHRENPREIS, T. *et al.,* 1960. Surgical treatment of ulcerative colitis in children. *Acta Paediat.,* **49**: 810.
17. ENGEL, G. L., 1955. Studies of ulcerative colitis. *Amer. J. Med.,* **19**: 231.
18. FARQUHAR, H. G., 1956. Abdominal migraine in children. *Brit. Med. J.,* i: 1082.
19. GLUECK, S. and GLUECK, E., 1960. *Predicting Delinquency and Crime.* London. Oxford Univ. Press.
20. GROEN, J. and VAN DER VALK, J. M., 1956. Psychosomatic aspects of ulcerative colitis. *Gastroenterologia,* **86**: 591.
21. HOLZEL, A, 1961. Dept. of Child Health, University of Manchester. Unpublished case data.

22. JAMESON, G. K., 1959. Steroid therapy adjuvant to psychotherapy of childhood ulcerative colitis. *Dis. Nerv. Syst.*, **20**: 130-134.
23. O'CONNOR, N., 1956. The evidence for the permanently disturbing effects of mother-child separation. *Acta Psychol.*, **12**: 174-191.
24. PAULLEY, J. W., 1956. Psychotherapy in ulcerative colitis. *Lancet*, ii, 215-218.
25. PINKERTON, P., 1958. Psychogenic megacolon in children: the implications of bowel negativism. *Archs. Disease in Childh.*, **33**: 170, 371-380.
26. —— 1961. Teaching by tape: a method of undergraduate instruction in child psychiatry. *Lancet*, ii: 308-309.
27. PLATT, J. W., SCHLESINGER, B. E., and BENSON, P. F., 1960. Ulcerative colitis in childhood: a study of its natural history. *Quart. J. Med.*, **29**: 257-277.
28. PRUGH, D. G., 1951. Emotional factors in ulcerative colitis in children. *Gastroenterology*, **18**: 339.
29. SPERLING, M., 1946. Psychoanalytic study of ulcerative colitis in children. *Psychoanal. Quart.*, **15**: 302.
30. VAN DER VALK, J., 1962. Clinical and Physiological Aspects of Physical Methods of Treatment, in *Principles of Treatments of Psychosomatic Disorders*. Oxford: Pergamon Press. (In preparation.)
31. VAN DER VALK, J. and BASTIAANS, J., 1961. *The Role of Psychosomatic Disorder in Adult Life*. Oxford: Pergamon Press. (In preparation.)
32. WEISS, E. and ENGLISH, O. S., 1957. *Psychosomatic Medicine*. Philadelphia: Saunders.
33 WINNICOTT, D. W., 1953. Symptom tolerance in paediatrics. *Proc. Roy. Soc. Med.*, **46**, 8: 675-684.
34. YUDKIN, S., 1961. Six children with coughs: the second diagnosis. *Lancet*, ii: 561-563.

XIV

DISORDERS OF SPEECH IN CHILDHOOD

C. WORSTER-DROUGHT

M.A., M.D., F.R.C.P., HON.F.C.S.T.

*Consulting Physician, West End Hospital for Neurology and Neurosurgery
Hon. Medical Director, Moor House School for Children Suffering from Speech
Disorders, Oxted, Surrey*

1

Introduction

Speech does not consist in the mere uttering of words, as the faculty of 'speaking' is essentially a mental process concerned with the acquisition of language. Each country has its own particular code or language which is learned in childhood by its inhabitants, in the first instance by sound. The normal child at first does not recognise words as such, but distinguishes their implication from the intonation, pitch and rhythm of the speaker's voice in the same way as the more intelligent animals such as the dog and horse. Later the child learns to attach meaning to each word, since by association words eventually stand for the objects or actions to which they refer. When the child reacts in the same way to a word as he would to the situation for which the word stands, he is said to know the 'meaning' of the word. Subsequently, by the process of education, a knowledge of the symbols of written and printed words is acquired. Thus spoken words can be permanently recorded.

By a 'speech disorder' we mean some defect in the faculty of presenting spoken language. It is necessary to distinguish between (1) the primary factor of comprehending and formulating spoken language, which is a function of the brain, and (2) articulation, which depends on the integrity of the nerve and muscular structures governing the utterance of words. These structures include various nerve cells in the cerebrum and medulla, the nerve tracts and the peripheral nerves to which they give rise, and the muscles of the lips, tongue, soft palate, larynx and pharynx which these nerves supply. A disturbance of the higher speech areas or of their connections in the brain results in the disorder of speech known as 'aphasia', or in lesser degree 'dysphasia'. When on the other hand the speech defect is due merely to imperfect articulation, the term 'dysarthria' is used. We therefore recognise two main classes of speech disorder: (1) Aphasia or dysphasia, and (2) Dysarthria. A third disorder in which the voice only is affected is termed 'dysphonia', or 'aphonia' if the voice is completely lost. Dysphonia is often associated with dysarthria.

In patients suffering from aphasia, the higher intellectual processes continue to function, though in some cases imperfectly, but those areas of the brain concerned with the receptive process of comprehending spoken language or those controlling the motor act of speaking are disordered or undeveloped, yet the patient has no paralysis of the muscles concerned with speech, nor is he deaf or blind. In other words 'aphasia' implies a disorder in the comprehension and/or the formulation of words and sentences; this disorder probably depends on a deficiency of memory for the symbols, whether spoken or written, by means of which we exchange ideas with other individuals. An aphasic patient, unless his mental faculties are impaired, can usually communicate quite well by means of gesture and pantomime.

For a perfect interchange of ideas between individuals, two main processes are necessary: (1) Reception, and (2) Execution or Expression. The receptive process includes the hearing and comprehension of spoken language; also the seeing and understanding of written or printed words and figures. The memories of words *heard* and *seen* appear to depend mainly on the integrity of certain specialised areas of the brain, termed respectively the 'auditory word area' and the 'visual word area'. Either of these areas may be relatively undeveloped, injured or diseased. Consequently we can distinguish two varieties of disordered reception or 'receptive aphasia': (1) Auditory aphasia—the inability to understand spoken language although hearing itself is intact, also known as 'word-deafness', and (2) Visual aphasia—the inability to appreciate written or printed language although sight is normal, also termed 'word-blindness', alexia or dyslexia.

The expressive or executive element in speech consists of the motor act of self-expression in words, either vocally by talking or by means of writing. Every voluntary motor act learned by an individual is accompanied by a conscious sensation of muscular movement, and by repetition such sensations become implanted, as it were, in the brain as 'kinaesthetic memories'. These kinaesthetic memories of the motor acts of speech are coordinated by means of a special area situated in the fore-part of the brain, especially in the posterior portion of the inferior frontal convolution. If this area, known as Broca's area, is destroyed or diseased, executive or expressive aphasia results owing to the loss of kinaesthetic memories for the utterance of words. Similarly, if the development of this area is imperfect or delayed, executive speech is only slowly or imperfectly acquired.

The age at which normal children begin to talk varies considerably.

Some children are able to say two or three words at or shortly after the age of twelve months. Many children as a result of imitation will say a few words quite early in their second year, and most normal children can produce short sentences by the age of two years. Admittedly there are exceptions, some otherwise normal children only acquiring adequate speech by the end of their third year. Sometimes such late development of speech is a family characteristic; in general however, if a child does not speak by the age of three years, some defect in the mechanism of speech is usually present. It is seldom that a really satisfactory investigation can be carried out at such an early age, and the mistake is often made of regarding the child as mentally deficient when, in fact, the speech defect is later shown to be due to an entirely different cause. Usually therefore a full investigation has to be postponed until a later age. In practice one finds that most speech-defective children are brought up for examination as they approach school age, between four and five years. The first step then is to ascertain whether an absence of intelligible speech or the presence of faulty speech exhibited by a particular child is due to dysarthria, i.e. inability to articulate properly, or to a lack of normal function of either the brain as a whole or of one or more of the special areas of the brain concerned with speech. Accurate investigation of the cause of a child's speech defect is essential, since on the establishment of an exact diagnosis depend not only the outlook regarding the child's ability to acquire normal or approximately normal speech but also decisions about the necessary type of treatment and appropriate form of education.

For the complete investigation of speech-defective children at or approaching school age, a coordinated team of workers is essential. At Moor House School for Children Suffering from Speech Defects, Oxted, Surrey, the team consists of neurologist, psychiatrist, otologist, plastic surgeon, educational psychologist and speech therapists, while facilities exist for consultations with a neuro-surgeon and paediatrician, as well as for reference to radiological and electroencephalographic departments (3). With most cases it is necessary to admit the child to the in-patient diagnostic section of the School for about a week; out-patient investigation is less satisfactory as affording little or no opportunity for observation, and if the child lives at a distance several visits to the clinic at short intervals are exhausting for the child and often impracticable for the parents.

2

Varieties of Speech Disorder in Children

We find that the children approaching school age referred for investigation fall into one or other of the following seven categories.

(1) *Mental Deficiency*

Children in whom absence or delay in the development of speech is due to mental defect are referred to a department for speech disorders very frequently, and in the investigation of any speech defect this condition is usually the first that must be excluded. The diagnosis is made by means of suitable intelligence tests carried out by an educational psychologist, preferably one with experience in dealing with children suffering from speech disorders. When the child is unable to understand spoken instructions adequately, the assessment must be made entirely on performance (non-verbal) tests, such as non-verbal items from the Collins-Drever Scale, Set A in children below the age of 7 years, or from the Wechsler Scale in children over 5 years. With mentally subnormal children between 4 and 6 years of age, non-verbal tests from the Collins-Drever Scale, Set B may be used. We have found, however, that this scale gives an approximately ten per cent over-estimate in the child's non-verbal IQ, for which allowance has to be made.

(2) Various Forms of Deafness

If a child hears only imperfectly he cannot learn properly to understand spoken language, nor will he attain adequate speech without accurate diagnosis and appropriate treatment. Speech deficiency in children is frequently due to some form of deafness, usually congenital but sometimes acquired in infancy as the result of bilateral middle-ear infection or of meningitis, which in some cases involves the auditory nerves.

In most children whose speech defect is due to deafness, as seen in a department for speech disorders, the deafness is only partial. These cases are of two varieties: (a) Generalised reduction in auditory acuity, i.e. the hearing defect involves the entire range of frequencies, and (b) High-frequency or high-tone deafness, in which the child is deaf only for the higher frequencies, and consequently cannot hear such sounds as S and Sh adequately. Low-frequency or 'bass' deafness also occurs but is comparatively rare.

The diagnosis of hearing defects in children—especially of partial deafness in young children—is often difficult to establish with certainty, and careful observation and investigation are usually necessary. A history of rubella in the mother during the earlier months of pregnancy is very significant, for this disease frequently gives rise to various developmental defects in the offspring. The final diagnosis rests on accurate audiometry and other tests, repeated at intervals for confirmation. At Moor House School we have found that with patience and careful training in the application of an ordinary pure-tone audiometer it is often possible to obtain reliable audiograms even in children of four to five years of age. In some cases, as I indicate later, hearing defects may coexist with a degree of receptive aphasia.

(3) Organic Disorders of the Nervous System

This category comprises a heterogeneous group of cases, and includes the various forms of 'cerebral palsy' which result from incomplete or faulty development of various parts of the brain, as well as destructive lesions caused by head injury at birth, failure to breathe adequately at birth (anoxia) and postnatal disease. Among the various forms of cerebral palsy, we have the following:

Congenital cerebral diplegia. This is also known as 'spastic diplegia' and 'Little's disease'. The muscles, especially those of the lower limbs, are spastic and partially paralysed. Some cases may result from birth injury, but most appear to be due to incomplete development of the motor cells of the brain cortex, and of the nerve tracts—especially the pyramidal tracts—to which these cells give rise. Owing to the relative deficiency of nerve supply, the muscles of articulation may also be affected with slight spasticity. Voluntary movement of the face, lips, tongue and soft palate may be quite good, but the spasticity reveals itself when some executive speech is acquired, the utterance being jerky, staccato and somewhat explosive. Further, many cases show varying degrees of mental defect, which is then the primary factor in the delayed acquisition of speech.

Congenital suprabulbar paresis (4). In this interesting condition the impaired development appears confined to the tract of nerve fibres (the cortico-bulbar tract) proceeding from the motor cells of the lower part of the Rolandic cerebral cortex to the cranial nerve nuclei situated in the medulla or bulb. From these nuclei arise the vagus (10th) and hypoglossal (12th) nerves, fibres from which supply the muscles concerned with articulation and phonation. The result is varying degrees of spasticity and paralysis of the orbicularis oris muscle of the lips, the tongue, soft palate, laryngeal and pharyngeal muscles, either separately or combined. Speech is dysarthric, being slurred and indistinct with deficient lingual and labial sounds.

The extent of the paresis or paralysis varies in different cases. In the form of the disorder which I have termed the 'complete syndrome' the child shows weakness or paralysis of the muscle that 'rounds' the lip (orbicularis oris), other facial movements being normal; weakness or paralysis of the tongue, even protrusion being absent; also paresis of the soft palate, together with impairment of swallowing. The jaw jerk is usually very brisk. In cases showing the 'incomplete syndrome' only portions of the speech musculature are affected. Probably the mildest manifestation of congenital suprabulbar paresis is an isolated paralysis or weakness of the soft palate in association with a brisk jaw jerk. The palatal palsy, as a result of deficient oro-nasal closure, causes the voice to be nasal in character, a condition known as 'hyper-rhinophonia'. Similarly one may meet with an almost isolated paralysis of the orbicularis oris or of the tongue. Quite frequently the tongue is protruded fairly well while lateral and upward movements are entirely absent. Those cases with inability to protrude the tongue are not infrequently mistaken for examples of 'tied tongue', and we have met with several cases in which the frenum linguae has been divided unnecessarily and with no beneficial result.

In severe cases, owing to the weakness of the lips and difficulty in swallowing, the accumulation of saliva is uncontrolled and dribbling is practically continuous. This causes the child considerable anxiety and discomfort, rendering him self-conscious and impairing his social relationships. In order to improve the nasality of speech in these cases of suprabulbar paresis, an operation on the soft palate—a palatoplasty or so-called 'push-back'—can be performed, which gives the palate greater length and so improves the closure of the naso-pharynx (oro-nasal closure) during speech. In severe cases it may be necessary, in addition, to keep the soft palate elevated by means of a flap of tissue from the pharynx (pharyngoplasty) (7). Such operations can usually be performed only in a Plastic Surgical Unit. We have found that these operations not only improve the nasality of voice but also the power of swallowing, thus increasing the control and disposal of saliva with consequent abolition or reduction in dribbling. In order further to improve speech and 'educate' the palate in its new position following operation, speech therapy is advisable in most cases.

In children the diagnosis of congenital suprabulbar paresis has to be made from 'Parkinsonism' resulting from an earlier attack of encephalitis. In these latter cases however, in addition to a history suggesting encephalitis, the condition does not date from birth, and there is usually some muscular hypertonia of the limbs. Also the spasticity or paresis is not confined to the lips, tongue and palate, but affects as well the facial muscles as a whole, with rigidity and poverty of movement. In addition there is frequently some form of conduct disorder.

Double hemiplegia. In this disorder there is a severe spastic paralysis on both sides of the body, affecting the legs, arms, face and tongue. The muscles of articulation, therefore, are affected in the same manner as in congenital suprabulbar paresis, but with the addition of spastic weakness of all the facial muscles and upper neurone paresis of all four limbs. In most cases there is a considerable degree of mental deficiency. The condition differs from the Little type of cerebral or spastic diplegia, as in the latter the lower limbs are mainly affected and the cranial musculature scarcely at all.

Congenital hemiplegia. This is almost invariably associated with faulty or delayed development of the speech areas of the brain, which results in failure of speech to appear at the usual age. The affected hemisphere of the brain—on the opposite side to the hemiplegia—is underdeveloped or atrophied. This can be demonstrated by air-encephalography, which reveals widely dilated ventricles in the hemisphere contralateral to the hemiplegia. The exact cause of the unilateral deficiency is obscure. Injury to the affected side of the brain at birth may account for a few of the cases but not for the majority, since we meet with the condition in cases of breech-presentation birth, when a head injury is unusual, and even in children born by Caesarian section. The probable explanation is that the affected hemisphere fails to develop fully.

If the left cerebral hemisphere is affected, the brain cells subserving motor function as well as those of the potential speech areas fail to develop adequately; consequently the child has a right-sided muscular weakness, is left-handed, and the potential speech areas in the right cerebral hemisphere become functional although their development is almost invariably delayed. Nevertheless, even when the hemiplegia is left-sided and the child of normal intelligence, the appearance of executive speech is ,usually retarded. In other words, whichever cerebral hemisphere is affected, we have found that the acquisition of speech is still delayed, in spite of L. Roberts (1) finding in adults that handedness and cerebral dominance for speech are practically independent variables.

Bilateral athetosis. This is also termed 'congenital athetosis' and Vogts' syndrome. Many of the children suffering from this condition are of normal intelligence, but dysarthria is usually severe. In addition to the involuntary athetoid movements of the limbs and usually of the face and tongue, speech is jerky, explosive and indistinct. Kernicterus may give rise to the same athetoid symptoms. Some cases of bilateral athetosis can be improved by speech therapy, their speech being rendered at least intelligible.

Ataxias of articulation. In some disorders of the nervous system articulation is indistinct, not from paralysis but from incoordination (ataxia) of the muscles of articulation. In affections of the cerebellum in children from injury, from relative underdevelopment, from so-called 'cerebellar encephalitis' (inflammation) and from Friedreich's hereditary ataxia, the articulation is slow, laboured and monotonous together with a jerky irregularity. Phonation is sometimes even more affected than articulation, the utterance being curiously explosive with pronounced separation of the syllables. Occasionally, especially in Friedrich's ataxia, the patient talks as if he had a foreign body in his mouth; this type of speech has been aptly termed 'hot-potato' speech.

In Sydenham's chorea, articulation may be incoordinate owing to sudden jerky movements of the respiratory muscles, tongue and face. Speech is therefore hesitant and jerky.

Nuclear and infranuclear affections. These lesions cause dysarthria, and include disorders of the cranial nerve nuclei in the medulla or bulb, or of the structures below this level, i.e. of the peripheral nerves supplying the muscles of articulation or of the muscles themselves.

Facial paralysis occurs in childhood from injury to the facial nerve or from involvement of the nerve by meningitis at the base of the brain, or from spreading suppuration from acute inflammation of the middle ear. Also the nucleus of the facial nerve may be affected in poliomyelitis. Unilateral facial paralysis causes only a transient dysarthria, as compensation is soon established, but in severe bilateral facial palsy the articulation of labial consonants is much impaired.

Paralysis of the soft palate, especially as a result of diphtheria or of bulbar poliomyelitis, causes dysphonia and dysarthria in the same manner as in congenital cleft-palate, since the naso-pharynx cannot be shut off from the mouth. As a result the voice is nasal and certain consonants are altered (*B* becomes *M*, *D* becomes *N*, and *K* becomes *Ng*), rendering utterance as a whole very indistinct.

The soft palate may also be paralysed as a result of congenital deficiency of its muscular structure. Paralysis of the palate in congenital suprabulbar paresis and double hemiplegia has already been mentioned.

Affections of the motor nerve to the tongue (hypoglossal nerve) cause paralysis and wasting of the tongue, and result from congenital defects of the nerve nucleus, bulbar poliomyelitis and injury to the nerve. If they are bilateral the patient will have difficulty in pronouncing lingual sounds.

Lesions of the recurrent nerve to the larynx, usually unilateral, cause paralysis of one vocal cord and render the voice weak and hoarse; they also impair the pronunciation of vowels, but do not interfere with the articulation of consonants.

(4) *Various Forms of Aphasia*

For practical purposes cases of aphasia in children can be divided into two main groups:

Executive or expressive aphasia. In this the child is unable to express himself in spoken language or is very slow in learning to do so, although understanding all that is said to him. He is almost invariably able to indicate his needs by gesture and mime.

Receptive aphasia. In this the child does not understand spoken language. It follows that in receptive aphasia of congenital origin, being unable to learn to understand what is said to him in the ordinary way although otherwise normal, he cannot acquire adequate speech.

A comparatively rare form of receptive aphasia of congenital or developmental origin is that of so-called 'word-deafness', which for reasons we will give later is probably better termed 'congenital auditory imperception' (5, 2). Diagnosis may be difficult, but the condition is usually distinguishable from deafness by the obtaining of a normal audiogram, or one indicating that the hearing loss is wholly insufficient to account for the child's failure in learning to comprehend spoken language. Owing to the disorganisation of the speech mechanism which inevitably results from this receptive aphasia, the child often develops a method of vocal expression of his own, i.e. an individual language, termed 'idioglossia', consisting in an extreme form of mispronounced and ill-expressed conventional language. When the patient has acquired some speech as a result of treatment, he pronounces his words either as he sees them formed by the speaker's lips or as he hears them uttered, but he remains unable to distinguish between many word-sounds and his speech is different from that of the normal child, being monotonous and often lacking the usual division into syllables.

In cases we have investigated it was found that, although the outstanding defect was failure to understand the meaning of spoken words, there was in some examples an additional inability to appreciate the significance of less specialised sounds, for example to distinguish between different types of bell or between different animal noises (5, 2). In some cases there was also a mild but definite degree of actual deafness, though quite insufficient to account for the child's failure in learning to comprehend spoken language (6). It appeared therefore that the designation 'word-deafness' was too limited in scope to apply to this condition; moreover hearing-loss as such plays no part in many of the cases, and very little if any in other cases, spoken language being heard but not understood. Consequently I. M. Allen and I suggested the term 'congenital auditory imperception', as describing more completely the fundamental defect (5, 2). The pathological basis probably consists in an incomplete development of the auditory word-areas in the temporal lobes of the brain.

Inability to appreciate the significance of symbols such as letters and figures—so-called 'word-blindness', also termed 'alexia' and 'dyslexia'—is another form of receptive aphasia due probably to a developmental defect. Compared with the corresponding condition in the auditory field—congenital auditory imperception—dyslexia is frequent. Again 'word-blindness' is an unsatisfactory designation, in that there is no blindness: the child sees words perfectly but does not understand their meaning. In most cases the child readily learns to recognise and name single letters and single figures and often words of two letters, but he has great difficulty in appreciating the significance of three or more letters and similar groups of figures. In some cases the child has difficulty only with words and not figures, or vice versa. Dyslexia is often associated with mirror-writing. With regular and continued individual tuition, many cases gradually improve and eventually acquire some reading ability.

In other examples of aphasia of developmental origin, the aphasia is purely executive or expressive, so that although the child may be normal in all other respects, understanding everything said to him, the appearance of adequate vocal speech is considerably delayed. Such a condition is best termed 'developmental executive aphasia'. At its first appearance speech is confined to single words, usually reinforced by gesture, but as further speech is acquired articulation is invariably faulty, incorrect letters and syllables being substituted for the correct ones and various syllables and word-endings omitted or mutilated. This disorder of articulation secondary to developmental executive aphasia is best termed 'developmental dysarthria'. Provided the child's intelligence is at least average, these cases gradually improve and respond very well to speech therapy.

Acquired executive aphasia is also met with in children as a result of a lesion on the left side of the brain in right-handed children and on the right side in left-handed children. Such a lesion can follow head injury, brain abscess or brain tumour, or occasionally encephalitis complicating one or other of the common infectious diseases, especially measles. In cases of executive aphasia due to head injury, the response to speech therapy is usually very good; but when the aphasia follows brain abscess the results are not so satisfactory, and in addition to other factors the child frequently suffers from epilepsy. Tumours involving the speech areas that are amenable to total removal by operation are very rare, but in the few examples I have met with the results of speech therapy have been very good.

An executive aphasia may also occur in association with epilepsy, especially following a series of convulsive attacks or, less often, an isolated fit. The aphasia may continue for any period from a few hours to several weeks, but usually improves with adequate control of the fits by anti-epileptic medication.

(5) *Mechanical Defects*

These include such conditions as congenital cleft palate, with or without hare-lip; a congenitally short soft palate; a relatively immobile tongue owing to a short frenum; and, in older children, various dental defects. The child with a cleft palate exhibits a characteristic nasal speech known as 'hyper-rhinophonia'. Provided closure of the naso-pharynx by a mobile and adequate soft palate has been secured as a result of suitable surgical measures, the response to speech therapy in most cases is very good. Tongue-tie, although often diagnosed in infancy, is, in fact, a comparatively rare condition. In no circumstances should the frenum linguae be cut in infancy, since even if short it often stretches with growth. In later child life, division of the frenum should be carried out only when the observer, by endeavouring to lift the tongue upwards and forwards with his fingers, demonstrates a shortened frenum or one reaching too far forwards beneath the tongue. As I have previously mentioned, several of our cases of congenital suprabulbar paresis, elsewhere and at an earlier age, had been mistaken for tongue-tied children owing to the relative immobility of the tongue, and had been subjected to an unnecessary and ineffectual operation.

In some children, although the soft palate is fully mobile and of normal length, the entrance to the naso-pharynx is so large that even the normal mobile palate cannot effect adequate oro-nasal closure. The result is a severe degree of hyper-rhinophonia (nasality) in executive speech. For this condition I would suggest the designation 'pharyngomegaly'. The most appropriate treatment is that of a palato-pharyngoplasty operation, followed by speech therapy.

(6) *Functional Disturbances*

These comprise disorders of speech with no recognisable organic or structural defect either in the central nervous system or in the peripheral organs of speech, and include cases of stammering or stuttering as well as the various forms of imperfect articulation known as 'dyslalia'.

Stammering and stuttering are terms used synonymously to denote a spasmodic type of speech disorder with which we are all familiar. Strictly speaking 'stammer' represents the hesitant utterance and 'stutter' the element of repetition in the defect, but the distinction is of no practical importance. In Great Britain the term 'stammering' is more widely used to describe this type of speech disorder, while 'stuttering' is preferred in America.

Physiological stammering, sometimes termed 'primary stammering', consists in hesitation, repetitions and prolongations in speech; they often occur during the normal development of language between the ages of two and four years as purely transient phenomena. Such disturbances of speech are unaccompanied by awareness or anxiety on the part of the child.

Pathological stammering or 'secondary stammering' is a term applied to the more persistent stammer which usually appears between four and seven years of age, and in some cases occurs as a prolongation of a stage of physiological or primary stammer.

There has for long been considerable controversy concerning the causation of stammering, and several theories have been propounded in the attempt to explain the phenomenon. The subject has been complicated by the fact that many observers who have studied the condition have done so only in adolescents and adults. By this age possible causative factors have become obscured by many secondary manifestations, mainly psychological, such as self-consciousness, fear of ridicule and feelings of inferiority. The observer of these effects has had the inevitable tendency to find psychological explanations for the primary speech defect as well as for the secondary manifestations.

In the majority of cases the child starts to talk quite normally, but begins to stammer between the ages of four and seven years. Stammer is much more common in boys than in girls, fully 80% to 90% of the cases being boys. Left-handed tendencies have been present in 60% of cases and can nearly always be traced in parents or near-relatives. By the time the stammer is established, the boy is right-handed, at least for the purpose of writing. When seen at the onset of stammer the children are usually quite normal in all other respects, and there are seldom any grounds for describing them as more 'nervous', i.e. psychologically disturbed or maladjusted, than other children.

Among the hypotheses that have been advanced in explanation of the causation and mechanism of stammering are the following:

(a) The theory of 'handedness', that is, the attempt to convert an inherently left-handed child into a right-handed one. Such outside interference with the development of a dominant cerebral hemisphere in integrating the mechanism necessary for normal speech may lead to a stammer. From the age of two the child begins to establish his handedness, and also his habits of speech. In most individuals the left hemisphere of the brain becomes dominant, and consequently the higher speech areas are located on this side of the brain in association with right-handedness.

Some delay in the onset of speech and in the preferential use of either hand is not uncommon in the history of children who begin to stammer at the early age of three years. A second critical period is when the child is just beginning to learn to read and write, i.e. to acquire graphic language, and is attempting to correlate these two new unilateral brain functions with speech which itself is still in a somewhat developmental stage. Thus, if an inherently left-handed child is thwarted in the dominant use of his left hand at the time his education begins, he is liable to develop a stammer. The reverse also applies, namely the attempt to convert an innate right-handed child to the dominant use of the left hand.

(b) The theory of lack of symmetry in function, that is, an absence of harmony between the three sets of muscle systems necessary for speech, viz. respiratory, vocal and articulatory, in association with emotional disturbances such as anxiety, apprehension and embarrassment. These two factors—physical and psychological—thus constitute a vicious circle.

(c) The theory that stammering is purely psychological in origin and dependent on emotional disturbance and maladjustment. The psycho-analytical view, based on the observations of Freud, postulates that stammering results from the attempt to repress from consciousness, into the unconscious, various painful memories and disturbing thoughts in order that they may not be betrayed by speech. If stammering were of purely psychological origin, it is difficult to understand why the condition is so much more frequent in boys than in girls.

Although 'handedness' undoubtedly plays some part in the aetiology of stammering, it is probable that the disorder has a multiple origin which space does not allow discussion of in this chapter. Also it must be admitted that the treatment of stammering is, as yet, far from satisfactory. At present the condition is best treated by a combination of psychotherapy and speech therapy.

Some stammerers acquire various tricks, chiefly as a result of their efforts to overcome or mask the stammer. Thus, extra noises may be thrown in, for example sudden inspiratory gruntings or whooping noises, or the patient may produce facial grimaces and even contortions of his limbs.

Various articulative tics or habit-spasms are met with in nervous and emotionally disturbed children, sometimes in conjunction with some degree of stammer. The child's speech may be interrupted by weird pharyngeal barking or grunting noises. Articulation may be monosyllabic, an extra breath being taken between each syllable. Again, speech may be jumbled up in the most extraordinary manner, although the child usually interpolates, now and again, a clearly articulated sentence among other unintelligible phrases.

A purely hysterical stammer is uncommon in children. When present it is more frequent in girls than in boys, and usually appears at about the time of puberty or later. Some cases of hysterical stammer result from the attempted imitation of a true stammerer; as a rule these children are somewhat maladjusted. Appropriate treatment usually yields satisfactory results. Similarly 'hysterical mutism', so common as a manifestation of a war psychoneurosis, is rare in young children, but it is occasionally met with in older girls as a result of emotional disturbance and auto-suggestion.

The condition known as 'lalling' is a normal phase in the development of speech in childhood. The form of words is changed by substituting one sound for another, or by the omission and elision of some of the syllables. There may also be a lack of precision in the pronunciation of certain consonants, for example the substitution of the uvular *R* for the ordinary laryngo-palatal *R*, or *V* for *Th*, *W* for *R*, so that 'broken reed' becomes 'bwoken weed'. When lalling persists beyond the usual age for adjustment, the condition is termed 'dyslalia'. Lisping, also termed 'sigmatism', consists in the substitution of *Th* for *S*.

In exceptional cases of dyslalia, although most of the vowels are pronounced correctly, the consonants are so mutilated, mispronounced and substituted that the child appears to be speaking a language entirely of his own, constituting a form of 'idioglossia'. Although unintelligible to those not acquainted with the child, his language is usually well understood by parents and others continually in contact with him.

With the gradual acquisition of speech in cases of developmental executive aphasia, such speech is at first almost invariably 'dyslalic'. As indicated previously, this form is best termed 'developmental dysarthria'.

(7) *Psychotic Children*

In these cases there is considerable maladjustment to ordinary surroundings, and the speech defect is usually one of retarded and inadequate speech development due to purely psychological causes. Speech, when it appears, almost invariably assumes the form of a severe dyslalia.

3

Conclusion

Any child who is not talking by the age of three years, and any older child who has a speech defect, should be referred to a department for speech disorders. Many of the larger general hospitals now have such a department, as have also the special hospitals for diseases of the nervous system and most hospitals for children. For children with speech disorders who have attained school age, reference is usually made to the Principal School Medical Officer for the county or borough. In conjunction with the Local Educational Authority, he then makes arrangements either for the child to attend a speech clinic for appropriate treatment, or, if the speech disorder is very severe and the cause obscure, for specialist investigation.

REFERENCES

1. ROBERTS, L., 1955. Handedness and cerebral dominance. *Trans. Amer. Neurol. Ass.*, 1955: 143.
2. WORSTER-DROUGHT, C., 1943. Congenital auditory imperception. *Medical Press and Circular*, **210**: 411.
3.   1953. *Residential Speech Therapy*. London: W. Heinemann.
4.   1956. Congenital suprabulbar paresis. *J. Otology and Laryngology*, **70**: 453.
5. WORSTER-DROUGHT, C. and ALLEN, I. M., 1929, 1930. Congenital auditory imperception. *J. Neurol. and Psychopathol.*, 1929, **9**: 193; 1929, **9**: 289; and 1930, **10**: 193.
6. WORSTER-DROUGHT, C., HUDSON-SMITH, S. and MANNING, M., 1959. Further observations on congenital auditory imperception. *Proc. Internat. Assoc. of Logopaedics* 1959: 133. Berne: S. Karger.
7. WYNN-WILLIAMS, D , 1958. The surgical treatment of congenital suprabulbar paresis. *Speech Pathol. and Therapy*, April 1958: 18.

XV

ACCIDENT-PRONENESS

GERARD VAUGHAN

M.B., M.R.C.P., D.P.M.

*Physician in Charge, Department of Child Psychiatry,
Guy's Hospital, London*

1

The Problem

One-third of the total number of children between one and fourteen years of age who die in Britain each year die as the result of accidents. Accidents kill more children at these ages than any single disease—more than the four most fatal diseases of childhood combined. Each year nearly two thousand children are killed in accidents of all kinds (42), and over fifty thousand are injured in road accidents alone (45).

These are disturbing figures, and it is surprising that more is not being done; there is, in fact, so much public and parliamentary complacency towards the whole problem of accident prevention that in 1958 the *British Medical Journal* suggested that this was 'a phenomenon which deserves study in its own right' (8).

One of the difficulties has been that it is a complicated field in which physical, geographical, medical, social and psychological factors all play their part. We have moved out of an era where accidents were thought to be due to *carelessness* alone, to be corrected by simple *safety* measures, into one where it is recognised that further improvements will only come about if all the underlying factors are considered.

This chapter is concerned with accident-proneness, but there are also wider implications for the children's psychiatrist who is interested in preventive medicine. He must, of course, be able to recognise and treat children who are specially vulnerable to accidents, but this is only a part of his job. Together with psychologists, he should also be prepared to advise on training programmes for both children and parents; to see that these are appropriate to the needs of the child; and to advise on children's behaviour at different ages in dangerous situations, as this will largely determine the way in which the child perceives and understands the dangers he has to face.

A 'personality' factor is the main cause of accidents in adults (29, 35, 38, 47). Less than 10% of accidents are due to chance. Mechanical factors account for under 10%, lack of skill for under 8%, and physical and mental defects for some 2% or less of industrial accidents (4, 29). Intelligence is only important to the extent that a minimum level is needed, for example, to drive a car (10). This means that between 80 and 90% of adult accidents are due to a personality factor.

Most accidents in children, especially young children, are preventable; many are due to negligence on the part of adults (33). For example, three-quarters of the parents of one group of children were directly responsible for the accidents in their children (50). The high incidence of poisoning in young children is also clearly related to adult carelessness. Even in quite young children, therefore, a personality factor in the parents may be significant.

It has long been known that certain people have more accidents than others (27)—that is, that the majority of accidents occur to a minority of the population. This is well known in insurance and industrial records. In a group of pilots, for instance, only 31% of the pilots were responsible for all the accidents, and 7·6% of these pilots were responsible for half of them. Similar results were found in a group of truck drivers (43), where it was also noticed that when a driver with a history of accidents moved to a different kind of work he frequently carried his accident record into his new job.

Farmer and Chambers coined the term 'accident-prone' in 1926 to describe such people (20), and in the same year Marbe called the tendency towards multiple accidents the accident habit—suggesting that accidents don't just happen, but occur because certain people have a tendency to make them occur (37).

In the early 1930s, and again in the late 1940s and early 1950s, many attempts were made to define and recognise this condition. There was great enthusiasm at first and detailed criteria were set out for the recognition of accident-prone individuals, but as time went on it was discovered that these criteria did not always fit the people they were intended to describe. The results were disappointing—so much so that the initial enthusiasm gave way to scepticism and some people doubted whether there was really a clinical entity of accident-proneness at all, or suggested its importance had been overrated (2).

So we are left today with the main questions only partly answered. Does accident-proneness really exist? If so, what causes it? How can it be recognised? Can it be prevented? And, perhaps most important of all, does it occur in children as well as adults?

This is of special importance to the children's psychiatrist, as it has been suggested that children can be accident-prone, and also that the characteristic personality of the accident-prone adult is established during childhood in response to parental authority (4, 52).

Unfortunately, so far as the children's specialist is concerned, most of the investigations have been into adult accidents, though results have been applied freely and often uncritically to children.

Early reports were concerned mainly with possible psychodynamic factors, or were surveys of large groups of patients who had suffered accidents, whereas more recent studies have looked at the whole family background as well as the patient. The result has been a clearer understanding of the problems involved.

Recent investigations show that, while it is true that a relatively small group of people suffer most accidents, this group is a constantly changing one, with new individuals moving in as others leave (47). Two other points also emerge. Having accidents is not a fixed trait but a shifting pattern during maturation (53). Adults and children who have previously been accident-free can become accident-prone under certain circumstances (47). In fact it now appears that almost any normal individual may become temporarily accident-prone under emotional stress.

The inference from these studies is that it is the maladjusted individual who is liable to accidents (38).

2

Incidence of Accidents

While the death-rate from accidents in most Western countries is now well known (51) there are still no figures for the total number of accidents, many of which cause severe and crippling handicaps. Nelson mentions two million children incapacitated each year in the U.S.A. and a further 50,000 crippled (40). Smid and Logan say there is one death in every 190 accidents; that for every death 25 children are permanently handicapped; and that one child in every 10 injured needs to be admitted to hospital (50).

Accidents can occur in many different situations: in the home, at school, in the playground or in the streets. The majority occur in the home. In Britain in 1960 the four commonest causes of death among children from accidents in the home were (44):

				0-4 years	5-14 years
Suffocation and choking	.	.	.	471	11
Burns and scalds	.	.	.	103	45
Falls . . .	.	.	.	50	15
Poisoning . . .	.	.	.	38	17
Others .	.	.	.	97	42
Totals . .	.	.	.	759	130

Hospital records may give a more reliable estimate of the overall incidence of home accidents than has been previously realised. MacQueen has recently made a study of these in Aberdeen (36). 4,527 home accidents occurred in a population of 186,190 persons between 1st September 1955 and 31st August 1957; of these 95% came via hospitals, general practitioners and health visitors. No less than 91·6% were known to the hospitals. 55·6% of the accidents occurred in children. In this connection therefore the London Ambulance figures for 1962 throw an interesting light on the overall causes of accidents in the home among children. Ambulances were called to 2,027 children, the reasons for 1,328 of these calls being as follows:

	0-4 years	5-14 years
Poisoning	270	17
Boiling liquids	129	42
Falls from one level to another (e.g. tables)	118	24
Falls over objects on the same level .	56	40
Hit by object	54	38
Falls in the garden	42	45
Falls from a window	41	48
Falls downstairs	39	47
Knife-like wounds (spikes, glass) . .	33	60
Cooking-stove accidents . . .	32	19
Burns from fires	28	22
Gassing	24	15
Suffocation	23	2
Accidents in the bath	4	2
Falls from ladders	3	2
Electric shock	1	2
Trapped by window	1	5

The emphasis on poisoning in young children is to be expected. Other points of interest are the high incidence of knife-like wounds in older children, and the general infrequency of accidents due to electric shock. Whereas ambulances were called to more home accidents for young than older children, as would be expected the opposite was the case for accidents in the streets. In the same year ambulances were called to 2,983 accidents involving children in the streets—552 for children under 4 years, and 2,431 for children aged 5-14 years. (Population in thousands: boys 0–4 yrs., 127; 5–14 yrs., 193; girls 0–4 yrs., 121; 5–14 yrs., 185.)

Road accidents provide the other major cause of death. In 1962, 761 children under 14 were killed on the roads (255 were under 5 years of age) and 52,545 were injured—a decrease of 1,906 on the previous year, and the seventh best year on record (45).

It is not surprising that the greatest incidence of accidents is in infants and pre-school children. Between 2 and 5 years there are twice as many accidents as at all other ages. The peak is reached around 5 years, and there is a sudden decrease around 9 years.

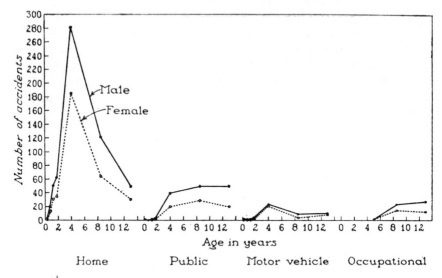

Fig. 1.—Major classification of accidents of children according to sex and age. (From A. C. Smid and G. B. Logan, *Minnesota Medicine*, **39**: 394, 1956.)

Young children are very dependent on their parents and limited in their activities, and accidents are therefore largely due to negligence by the adults looking after them (33, 50). Once they can walk their range of activity increases dramatically, and so do the risks they face.

Certain accidents are more common at one age than another. Burns and falls are common in 2-year-olds, when children are first beginning to walk around the house. An active 2-year-old interested in his surroundings is also particularly liable to be poisoned, to cut and bruise himself and to fall into water and be drowned. Plastic bags are a special danger. When he is 3 he is beginning to run, and to climb; he is then likely to fall, be burnt or be hit in the street. Older children take more responsibility for their own safety, but there is still a high accident rate—by drowning, bicycle and car accidents.

It is interesting to see within one type of accident the effect of age on its form. In falls, for instance, the site is affected—the 2-year-old tends to hit his forehead because he leans forward as he runs; older children hit their noses because they are more upright. 3- and 4-year-olds hit their teeth, the 5-year-old his collar-bone, the 6-year-old his arms, and the 8-year-old his legs (4).

At all ages boys are injured 2 to 3 times as often as girls. It is usually said that this is because boys are more restless, adventurous, aggressive, concentrate less well, and are less mature than girls. However girls receive burns more often than boys (4), perhaps because they are in the home more or more often in the kitchen, and wear clothes which are likely to catch fire easily. Factors such as overcrowding, oil heaters and inflammable clothes all contribute to accidents from burning (11). In areas where steps have been taken to combat these factors, severe burns needing hospital admission either occur equally in both sexes or show a slightly higher incidence amongst boys. Among 200 consecutive admissions to the burns unit at Guy's Hospital there were 123 boys and 77 girls (86 of these children were under 2 years of age) (9).

3

Psychological Factors and Accident-proneness

Current views on accident-proneness need to be considered in the context of the main investigations which have been made into this problem.

The most important and widely known of these is an investigation by Flanders Dunbar into patients with fractures (14, 15, 16, 17, 18). Her conclusions profoundly influenced all subsequent investigations, and marked a transition between individual case reports along psychodynamic lines and the experimental studies on groups of patients which followed. The fracture patients were intended to be the controls for a group of cardiac patients. At the time Dunbar was unaware of the work on accident-proneness in industry. 79% of the fracture patients had had two or more previous accidents, compared with only 11% or less in the other groups. 40% had a history of accidents in the near family. This was more than three times as high as the rates in her other patients.

She divided accidents into true or apparently genuine accidents, and those where a personality factor seemed to be involved, with the following results:

	% of patients having true accidents	% of patients having personality-factor accidents
Cardiacs	10	12
Fractures	10	90

The high rate of personality-factor accidents in the fracture group fits in well with other earlier observations. The fracture patients as a group had abnormal attitudes and reactions towards their environment. They showed a marked tendency to impulsive behaviour under stress, especially when this involved someone in authority—to such an extent that the authors suggested not only that this was something in the make-up of fracture patients which predisposed them to accidents but that this trait was also present in their families.

The fracture patients were characteristically jerky, tense, restless people who were popular, made up their minds quickly, and aimed at immediate rather than long-range goals. They responded to situations by actions rather than thoughts. From early childhood their responses were impulsive. In childhood they were likely to have run away from home, played truant, told lies and been guilty of stealing. Early neurotic traits were common. As adults they were always in a hurry, were tense and often were heavy smokers. Many were intensely interested in sport, body culture and heavy machines. They were boastful, took chances, left school early, and found it difficult to hold a regular job. The outstanding feature in their development was their continual conflict with authority, at first within their families, then at school, later towards social and religious bodies and employers, and finally in their marriages. There was a high incidence of childless marriages, small families and divorce. Accidents tended to occur when strong aggressive feelings were aroused in the patient, and pressure from outside authorities had become too great; aggression showed in a wish to punish themselves in order to punish those whom they regarded as responsible for their frustration. The majority of the patients had at least one over-strict parent.

There were two other interesting features. First, a specific worry in the patient's personal life had preceded the accident in 80–90% of the cases. Second, the injury was usually regarded as a punishment and something 'deserved'; remarks such as 'It serves me right' were common. This aspect was only present immediately after the accident, and was then repressed. It was usually followed by a preoccupation with the details of the injury itself.

Dunbar's findings have been given extensively because, though her patient's ages were from 12 years upwards, and though Dunbar herself did not think accident-proneness was a significant factor in childhood, others have not agreed over this, and there are certainly many similarities between the personality difficulties she describes in adults and what others have found in children.

Dunbar originally said, '80–90% of all accidents are due to a personality factor which can be diagnosed before the habit develops but which cannot be adequately dealt with by education or improvement of machinery.' She also gave an overall profile of the 'accident-prone' person (14). However, her hope that accident-proneness could be diagnosed in advance of the accidents has not been substantiated: she subsequently found that some of the patients had only one accident, or had several accidents in succession and then no more. To explain this she suggested later that, although the patient is prone to accidents, the accident only occurs when the strain in the patient's life becomes too great.

Dunbar's conclusions can be criticised because they were based on retrospective histories only, and the patients were all fracture patients—these are only 7% of all injuries and are more frequent in injured women than injured men. The special selection of cases also led her to conclude, incorrectly, that age and sex play no part. From the standpoint of child psychiatry the most significant observations in this work, apart from the overall profile of the accident-prone individual, were: (*a*) that inner tension of any kind is turned into impulsive action; (*b*) that the home background is usually disturbed; and (*c*) that there is a 'stress situation' immediately preceding the accident.

The inability of the patients to talk about the events leading to the accident has been commented on frequently, and can sometimes make enquiries into accidents specially difficult. A number of people have noticed this in children, and have also commented on an apparent lack of concern in both the children and their parents by comparison with other groups (34).

Personality features similar to those described by Dunbar have been found by many different people investigating a wide range of occupations. There is a general agreement on a history of conflict with authority and of difficulties in childhood which are later carried into adult life. That the majority of accident-prone patients have had a disturbed home background seems certain, whether they are taxi-drivers (52), Air Force personnel (32) or children (19, 38).

It has already been mentioned that physical factors play only a small part. Fabian and Bender discussed the predisposing factors in 86 children admitted to the Bellevue Hospital, New York because of behaviour disorders following head injuries (19). Specific factors—mental subnormality, epilepsy, disease of the central nervous system etc.—were found in only 21 children. Of the remaining 65 children in whom no specific predisposing factor was found, 51% had been involved in two or more major accidents and 15% in three or more. 83% of these children had a disturbed family background in which a large number of the siblings had a history of behaviour disorders and accidents. Fabian and Bender believed that unsettled home conditions create insecurity and aggression in children, which is then acted-out in the environment, i.e. that accidents are aggressive gestures turned against themselves by children, although actually aimed at their parents. They point out that it is common for children when they feel they are being unfairly treated to wish they were ill or dead so that their parents will feel sorry for them. These ideas are not usually acted-out, but some children will act-out their phantasies, and an accident can then occur.

Rawson has suggested a similar process (43). He says:

The majority of accident-prone people seem to have this tendency to act out their hate or guilt feeling. The explanation is not so far-fetched as it might at first appear. Primitive men and children consider all 'accidents' to be purposive. The concept of 'accident' is inculcated in the child by repetition. It becomes a useful way of denying purpose and provides a convenient cloak for hostility. . . . Because of the early taboo against interpersonal hostility the tendency is soon developed in children to hurt themselves in lieu of the person to whom the real hostility is directed. In temper tantrums children stamp their feet, bang their heads, pull their hair, hit, scratch and bite themselves. Older children become more subtle and have repeated accidents usually caused by taking absurd risks, such as jumping down a flight of stairs.

Rawson says that an accident may become 'a useful way of denying purpose':

A mother while scolding her child rocked too energetically on her chair and bumped the child's head. The child started to cry, but the mother soothed it by explaining that the bump was 'just an accident'. An hour later at dinner the child spilled a bowl of hot soup on the mother's lap, and before it could be scolded it volunteered that the occurrence was an 'accident' (1).

A seven-year-old girl was asked, 'What ought you to do if another girl hits you by accident?' She replied, 'Hit her back by accident' (5).

Two types of benefit from accidents are described in the literature (1, 14, 43), but in practice there is often considerable overlap between them:

(a) *Primary gain*—the accident fulfils a self-destructive wish. Freud called this 'the traumatophilic diathesis' (21, 22). Although outwardly unintentional, he suggested that the accident served an inner need which was not recognised by the patient. Menninger made a special study of certain accident patients and came to the same conclusion, saying that the underlying emotion was usually an aggressive one. He also pointed out that sometimes one part of the body can be injured repeatedly as a substitute for the whole (39); Dunbar made a rather similar observation on some of her fracture patients.

(b) *Secondary gain*—the accident helps the person to avoid an unpleasant or dangerous situation. Dunbar tells the story of a Roman Catholic woman who inexplicably broke her hip on the way to confession at which she would have had to admit to using contraceptives (18). This type of accident, however, may be more simply explained by anxiety and tension resulting in altered judgment and inattention. One author gives the example of a boy who, 'forced into the background by his small sister, intentionally hurt himself by letting himself fall from a chair: but then, when caressed by his parents, he admits, while weeping—from pain or for joy, "I did it on purpose." ' (41.) Bakwin says that 'a high percentage of accidents in children occur when they are doing things forbidden by their parents.' (4.)

Sometimes accidents occur in a welter of disorganised tension and anxiety, as part of a series of stress symptoms; abdominal pains, headaches, or nausea and vomiting have usually preceded the accident. The accident then appears to be a desperate call for attention—an unconscious cry for help, not in anger but in need. A pubertal girl had the following symptoms in succession: headaches, then pains in her back, followed by abdominal pains together with headaches and vomiting; she then had an 'accident' in which she caught her hand in a door, and a crush fracture was suspected, but the X-Ray was normal; and finally she developed a rash on her face, which proved to be dermatitis artefacta.

Are accidents in children ever distorted attempts at suicide? Melanie Klein certainly thought that repeated accidents could be (30), and so did Bender and Schilder (6), but most people have not found this (38, 47). More often there is a desire by the patient for adequate integration and adaptation. Super-ego drives push the individual into using destructive behaviour in order to defend himself, i.e. in an attempt to rid himself of guilt (38). In this connection it may be relevant that many accident-prone children have been found to be very poor at adapting to changed situations (3, 25, 31). Gluck examined 83 accident cases aged 7–9 years. These children were less able to adjust promptly to new circumstances than other children. Also they were less able to attend to more than one thing at a time (25). Krall found the same (31), using an interesting doll play technique.

Children do not usually appreciate that they could die in an accident, nor see death as an end to life: 'The idea of death does not enter into the child's fundamental concept of life', say Schilder and Wechsler (46); and as an important corollary to this Bender and Schilder add, 'This attitude plays an important role in their gambles with life.' (6.) Certainly it can enable children to play dangerous games and precipitate situations regardless of possible injury to themselves.

Accident-prone adults are also injury-prone. Are there injury-prone children? Elizabeth Fuller examined the First Aid Charts of 61 nursery school children aged 22–55 months (23). Boys were injured more often than girls (5 to 4). 50% of the boys' injuries occurred in 27% of the boys, whereas 50% of the girls' injuries involved only 14% of them. Injuries became less frequent in the older children and the difference in incidence between boys and girls became more marked.

In a later study (24) she examined 'second grade' children. This time she chose an unusual sample, in that the class chosen was known to have 5 times as many accidents as any other class in the school. The most frequently injured children were socially isolated, unpopular children. She says that 3- and 4-year-olds are more skilled socially—they more often want to hurt each other in their social relationships. She suggests that small children hurt each other indiscriminately, friends as well as enemies, whereas older children only hurt their enemies. The socially isolated children were more individualistic, more aggressive in their general behaviour, and more interested in seeking revenge than other children. This is interesting when one considers the comments already made that some children show their feelings in aggressive acts against objects or other children when they are criticised or scolded by adults. It suggests that criticism from other children may also be a factor.

Accident-prone children, like accident-prone adults, tend to be physically robust and have a better health record than accident-free children. Birnbach found this in a study of the home, health, social and emotional adjustments of 55 accident-repeating and 48 accident-free boys at a junior high school (7). He found, however, on the Bell adjustment inventory that the accident group appeared less well adjusted than the others, with indications that this was particularly the case in their home and general social adjustment. The accident-free group were better adjusted in these respects, as well as having a better knowledge of safety. 20% of the accident group came from broken homes. They tended to be aggressive and to try and control situations by force. Under stress they were impulsive and rebellious. Their teachers said they were less polite, less reliable, less hard working and generally more inadequate than the accident-free group.

Accident children not only tend to be more aggressive than accident-free children, but may also be less realistic in their handling of their environment.

As well as being more aggressive, it seems that they may also be less able to put their feelings into words (31).

In addition to the 'impulsive' child, Langford has suggested that there are at least two other kinds of accident-prone personality. In a well written preliminary report in 1953 (34), which incidentally brings out many of the features already referred to, he and his colleagues examine nine children who had been involved in multiple accidents and compare them with nine accident-free children. They make the point that both groups of children seemed less disturbed than children usually seen by their psychiatric staff. The accident children found it particularly difficult to deal with outside problems; they and their parents also seemed curiously unconcerned over their injuries—a point rather similar to Dunbar's observation of repression of the guilt and self-blame usually seen immediately after an accident and its replacement by unconcern and preoccupation with details of the injury.

In these children, secondary gains from the accident seemed quite unimportant. The home backgrounds were interesting: although if anything the homes were rather pleasanter than those of the accident-free families, the parents seemed significantly less 'in tune' with their children than other parents. The accident-prone children related to the staff rather better than the others, and here the authors suggest that the accident-free child may derive more from his home and so have less need to turn to outsiders.

Although the group he studied was small, Langford suggests there are at least three kinds of accident-prone child:

(1) A child who is over-active and impulsive; who is popular with adults but not other children. He often wants to be older than he is, and therefore tends to over-extend himself in his attempts to meet his ambitions. He reacts poorly to stresses, becoming disorganised and impulsive. Under

stress he is inclined to disregard danger signals or not to recognise them.

(2) A child who is immature emotionally, who lacks supervision from his parents, who insists on autonomy and self-determination, and who therefore tends to compete with older children in dangerous circumstances.

(3) A child who is resentful and hostile towards his parents; whose home is 'bleak and empty'.

While these make three recognisable groups, Langford says of his own survey that the number was too small, and he suspects that if he had examined more children he would have found more types of personality involved. Others have thought the same, and suggested that people of all types of personality may become accident-prone at times of stress (47)— that, in fact, accident-proneness is a feature of maladjustment. This was certainly the view held by Marcus and his colleagues in 1960, after comparing three carefully matched groups of children aged 6 to 10 years: an accident-prone group, an accident-free group, and a group of enuretics (38). Although sceptical of accident-proneness as a special clinical entity, they conclude that accident-prone children do have certain features in common. They found marked difficulties over adjustment in these children, who in this respect resembled the enuretics. Only 7 out of 22 accident-free children had emotional problems, compared with all 23 accident-prone children and all 22 enuretics. The severity or type of emotional problem did not seem significantly different in the accident or the enuretic child. But the accident children were involved in fewer family activities than the other two groups of children, and their parents tended to be anxious, insecure and non-assertive, in marked contrast to the parents of the enuretics, who for the most part were aggressively dominating and over-controlling. They quote, as typical of the parent of an accident-prone child, one who said, 'I would rather have a million friends than one enemy.' They did not find any evidence in these children of 'unconscious suicide' or 'hostility turned inward' or of authoritative, punitive parents; nor did they think that the children were acting-out identifications with accident-prone parents. In fact they make the point that family ties were weaker in the accident group. They conclude that 'accidents would be a response to emotional disturbance, a stimulus which under other circumstances might evoke a different response. The conditions under which this behaviour would occur include a hyperactivity which may be constitutional, a tendency to express tension through physical activity, and disturbed family relationships.' Their point that the same emotional stimulus might under different circumstances have led to a different response seems an important one.

The emphasis here is clearly on emotional maladjustment in these children and on disturbance in the parent-child relationship. In this connection, Backett and Johnston recently looked at the family setting of children involved in road accidents (3). Their investigation showed certain characteristic features in the families of these children. They compare two groups of 101 children for a number of aspects: parental health, maternal preoccupation such as going out to work and size of family, family structure, financial level, play facilities, accommodation, history of accidents in other members of the family, and intelligence. They point out how many studies have been made on individuals and how few (they quote Gordon's work on 'host factors' in roa⅃ accidents (26) as an exception) have sought to define the family and social characteristics of the background from which vulnerable children come. There is a need, they say, for more studies between the 'large social epidemiological survey and the small sociological enquiry'. They find the following factors significant in determining accidents:

(1) Maternal preoccupation of some kind—with work, children, or pregnancy.
(2) Illness in the mother or in a near member of the family.
(3) Vulnerable families are more crowded, have less protection during play, and often an absence of even elementary play facilities.

These factors show little overlap and the authors regard them as significant and independent factors, of which overcrowding is the least important. On school ratings, accidents were more frequent where the standards of the parents were low.

It may seem surprising that more has not been said about psychological tests on children. Batteries of various tests have been used frequently, but apart from confirming levels of intelligence and lending support over clinical impressions of, for example, patient's attitudes, they have so far been of no special value.

It seems therefore that accidents among children are determined by at least three major groups of factors: (1) the dangers to which a child is exposed, (2) his physical development—he is more likely to be injured if he is robust and restless, and (3) his psychological adjustment and level of maturation. One, or all, of these may lead to a particular accident.

In very young children the first is obviously the most frequent cause, with negligence and carelessness on the part of his parents a major contributing factor.

It appears certain that under sufficient emotional stress most normal individuals will become temporarily accident-prone, but that only a small number of people are persistently so. This applies to both adults and children, but is complicated in childhood by the additional aspect of the child's level of maturation which may make him particularly vulnerable to certain dangers.

Accident-proneness is closely related to emotional maladjustment, so that it is the maladjusted, particularly the aggressive socially maladjusted, child who is accident-prone. Children who adapt poorly to new circumstances, children with disturbed homes, children who are robust, physically strong but poorly supervised, are the children who are likely to be injured.

Boys are more likely to be hurt than girls; five- and six-year-olds more than children at other ages.

By contrast, who is least likely to get hurt?

An accident is least likely to occur in a healthy well-adjusted young girl, age thirteen, born and reared in a normal, secure and loving home, in which both parents are well adjusted and if she has not experienced or witnessed major o frequent accidents in the past. (SCHULZINGER, 1956 (47).)

We are left then with the conclusion that accident-proneness does exist in childhood, but that it is usually only one aspect of a more general problem of emotional disturbance. There may also be certain special instances where the accident satisfies an unconscious need. It is not possible, it seems, to predict accident-proneness from any clinical profile or battery of psychological tests, and yet, as a syndrome, it undoubtedly exists and can be recognised in retrospect.

4

Management and Prevention

Recognition of Individual Cases

Accidents which have been psychologically precipitated usually occur in a series, the cycle being triggered off by some emotional crisis. This was shown very clearly recently in South Africa by Shaw and Sichel, who demonstrated a general increase in accidents over a period of several months in a number of towns following the Sharpville massacre (49).

From the preceding section of this chapter it will have been evident that accident-proneness in a child has always to be viewed as a behaviour disorder—as an aspect of 'emotional maladjustment—and therefore requiring investigation and treatment as much as any other comparable psychiatric disorder. Probably any child with a history of more than two major accidents, or a child who has been injured in circumstances which suggest that an underlying psychological problem could have brought about the accident, should be investigated for possible accident-proneness. This should include an enquiry into the part played by any adults involved in the accident—and this is especially important in accidents to young children, as the adult and not the child may be the psychologically significant person.

As was discussed earlier in this chapter, while it is not possible to predict any clear clinical profile for the accident-prone person, multiple accidents tend to occur in children who have a history of social difficulties, who exhibit certain aggressive and non-conforming personality traits, who adapt poorly to new circumstances and who quickly turn psychic tension and anxiety into physical activity. Robust, physically strong, restless, poorly supervised boys from disturbed homes are the children most liable to injury.

The accident-prone adult is essentially similar—a man who is likely to be well known to the social agencies and perhaps rather better known to the police than his fellow citizens, who usually comes from a broken home and has marital difficulties.

Treatment

Treatment needs to follow the same general lines as in other comparable psychiatric disorders. The accident-prone child should be encouraged to talk of the accident, particularly the events leading up to it and any anxieties and misconceptions that may have arisen in his mind as a result of it. Sometimes, especially if there has been a considerable gap between the accident and the time when the child has an opportunity to discuss it with a suitably understanding adult prepared to listen to the child's own account of what happened, this process may be a difficult one, since much of the traumatically important memory of the episode will have been repressed. For example, a girl who had been involved in a car accident denied any memory of it until some months later, when she was able to talk about it indirectly after painting a picture in which a girl was about to be drowned at sea. This particular child had been struck by a car after she had correctly carried out her kerb drill. She had thought that the kerb drill would always protect her, and was very upset that it did not, but more than this: she saw the accident as a 'punishment' because she had not been 'a good girl' at home. This sense of personal blame for an accident, which in this case was not in any way caused by herself, is common in children—especially young children—in the same way that young children will often mistakenly assume personal responsibility if their parents die, or separate, or if there is some other major upheaval in their home.

Similarly parents will also need to discuss their anxieties after a major accident and have advice over how best to handle their child, if they are to give the child the sense of security he will require. They will probably need advice over what to do immediately after the accident: how much to tell him, what to say, and how and when to say it. In general any discussion with the child should take place as soon as possible, as truthfully as possible, and in simple words and concepts which will be appropriate to the child's age and understanding. Explanations should not be forced on to a reluctant, shocked child, but there should be an immediate indication of understanding over what has happened, and an implication that the child is safe, together with a willingness to answer any questions that he may wish to ask. Many children will ask a part of what they wish to know, listen to only part of the answer, and then, because they are anxious change the subject, only to return to it later for a further 'helping' of the answer. This is sometimes very confusing for parents who are accustomed to discussing things more completely at one time. Much of this may seem too obvious to mention, but in practice it is these simple procedures which are so frequently overlooked or misunderstood.

Parents, like children, may also assume an unrealistic responsibility

for what has occurred, or may see the accident as a punishment for previous bad behaviour and neglect.

They may need to discuss their part in the accident. They may also
have severe anxieties about the child's future which they are reluctant to
mention: whether or not he is likely to be permanently handicapped, and
the possible implications for his future schooling, employment and even
marriage. Long-term fears around these subjects can sometimes severely
incapacitate a parent who would otherwise have handled the immediate
problems very effectively. They will all bear discussion fairly early on
with a psychiatrist or psychiatric social worker. In practice, however, it is
often the patient's general practitioner or the hospital resident who will
have the best opportunity for this, as they are in touch with the parents
soon after the accident. Inevitably, as things stand at the moment, patients
tend to come to the psychiatrist some time later, and then only when quite
severe psychiatric complications have become evident.

Prevention

This ranges from measures such as the use of non-inflammable
material for children's clothes to considerations of the human factors
which cause accidents. The first are relatively simple and obvious, the
latter complex and often difficult to define. There is a surprising amount of
public apathy considering the size of the problem, and very little money
has been made available for research. Undoubtedly one of the main reasons
for this has been the multiplicity of the causes of accidents. This means that
many different experts need to be involved: local authorities, road and
building engineers, architects, social agencies, psychologists and doctors.
Even in the medical field there are a number of different types of doctor
who need to work together and understand each other's problems over this:
doctors in industrial medicine, public health, and psychiatry as well as
general medicine. The very complexity of the field has meant that the
general public has tended to regard the prevention of accidents as something to be left in the hands of the experts, while the expert has tended to
work in an ever more watertight compartment, safe from intrusion by
his colleagues in the other related fields. Professor Drew (13) in his
Presidential address to the British Psychological Society has made an
admirable review of the contribution which can be made by Psychologists,
in which he made a plea for a less insular approach on the part of Psychologists when investigating these problems. His remarks could be applied
just as forcibly to other specialities.

Despite a good deal of intensive study, it will be clear from the earlier
part of this chapter that the results have so far been in the main contradictory and somewhat unsatisfactory. This is not surprising; even a
review of the subject quickly tends to become a somewhat disjointed list of
observations or a review of areas in which research would be helpful
rather than a presentation of a firm body of knowledge.

Accident prevention resolves itself into steps directed at (1) improving the individual's emotional adjustment, (2) increasing his level of skill, and (3) reducing the dangers to which he is exposed.

The problems of recognising the accident-prone individual have already been discussed. Ideally we would like to recognise that it is 'a risk', before a serious accident occurs. This was the hope of Dunbar and others who followed her, but it still eludes us. Accident-proneness is always a retrospective diagnosis. Children may show all the general features associated with accident-proneness but never have an accident, while those who have had several accidents may then never have a further accident. At present we do better perhaps if we accept only the more general social challenge of helping at whatever level we can, by both social and medical means, the children and adults who emerge from severely unsettled, disturbed homes.

While it is true that simple reduction of the number of dangers, for example in car accidents better cars on better roads driven by more skilled drivers, will reduce the absolute numbers of accidents, the proportion due to human failure remains fairly consistent at between 80-90%, and it is here that psychiatrists and psychologists have most to offer.

Factors such as lack of skill, low intelligence and physical disabilities play a surprisingly small part. Again and again, whether one is studying the effect of alcohol on driving or the effect of fatigue, one comes back to the individual personality involved. The problem really resolves itself into the observation that two people in apparently identical situations will behave very differently and that this will decide between safety and accident. DiMascio, Rinkel and Leiberman (12) have shown that drugs such as lycergic acid and mescalin have quite different effects on behaviour according to the personality structure of the person taking them. Others have made similar observations after alcohol, and when observing people undergoing specific stresses such as exposure to heat or loud noises.

When it comes to improving individual skill we are on firmer ground. Many studies have shown that road accidents, for example, are more likely to occur in the early months, the first six months, of a driver's career (48).

Training schemes can be highly effective. In a number of American studies, for instance, it has been shown that drivers who have not been trained have twice as many accidents as those who have been. In Delaware 1,100 drivers who were formally trained were compared with a similar number of untrained drivers. The untrained drivers had five times as many arrests for serious traffic offences as those who were trained, and four times the number of accidents. Similar results have been found among police drivers in this country (28). However, even these apparently clear results in support of training are open to question. Furthermore there is no clear argument over what constitutes normal driving, what is to be taught, how it should be taught and to what standard.

Women respond to training schemes very much better than men. Girls respond better than boys to road drill instruction. This raises an interesting speculation as to the social adaptability and conformity of women compared with men. The Road Research Laboratory has shown that a higher proportion of women than men will use a pedestrian crossing, and even those women who do not use the actual crossing will cross nearer to it than the men. If however a policeman is placed at the crossing, even though he does not take any active part, the majority of men will then use the crossing, only to revert to their previous behaviour as soon as the policeman goes away. The presence of a policeman has no effect on the behaviour of the women, who continue crossing as before. This kind of observation is of course open to many different interpretations.

This is not the place to go into the general issues of accident prevention—factors of fatigue, working conditions and alcoholism have all been mentioned already. Investigation of human fatigue as a cause has been surprisingly unhelpful so far. Air crew reports and the histories of long-distance lorry drivers have repeatedly shown that accidents are more likely in the first few hours of a long drive or flight. Accidents are rare after 10 hours. By contrast, loss of sleep will lead to a higher accident rate, and a number of studies show that accidents increase in factories when there are long working hours and short rest periods. Diminishing attention and irritability are well known causes in these situations. Drew has investigated flying performances extensively and has commented on the general restriction on the field of attention which occurs after a long period of flying, until responses are confined to only one interest at a time. This is a form of 'tunnel vision'. It appears to be an aspect of the pilot's response to stress, but Drew has pointed out that it is a misnomer to call it 'tunnel vision', because, although peripheral vision is usually lost, actually vision is reduced to that part of the field from which stimuli are expected, and this may be either central or peripheral. Here again more information is needed, and again the response of the individual is partly determined by his personality structure.

Mention has already been made of the part that psychiatrists, together with psychologists and teachers, should be prepared to make in advising training programmes for both children and parents. These have to be appropriate to the needs of the children and in keeping with the ages of the children. This is a field which has as yet hardly been broached, apart from a general programme of teaching road drill in schools.

These then are some of the problems involved in the prevention of accidents. The enormity of the accident rate itself creates its own urgency. In every highly industrial country the ratio of killed in accidents to deaths from other causes is tending to rise every year. The many factors involved create a specially complex situation, but this itself constitutes an even more worthwhile challenge to our society.

REFERENCES

1. ACKERMAN, N. W., and CHIDESTER, L., 1936. 'Accidental' self-injury in children. *Archs. Pediat.*, **53**: 711-721 (November).
2. ADELSTEIN, A. M., 1952. *J. Roy. Statist. Soc.*, **115**: 354.
3. BACKETT, E. M. and JOHNSTON, A. M., 1959. *Brit. Med. J.*, i: 409.
4. BAKWIN, H. and BAKWIN, R., 1960. *Clinical Management of Behaviour Disorders in Children.* Philadelphia and London: W. B. Saunders.
5. BALINT, E. M., 1949. Address given at National Safety Congress, London.
6. BENDER, LAURETTA and SCHILDER, P., 1935. Suicidal preoccupations and attempts in children. *Amer. J. Orthopsychiat.*, **7**, 225.
7. BIRNBACH, S. B., 1948. *Comparative Study of Accident-Repeater and Accident-Free Pupils.* Centre for Safety Education, New York. New York University.
8. *Brit. Med. J.*, ii, 1958: 377.
9. CLARKSON, P. Personal communication.
10. COBB, P. W., 1940. The limit of usefulness of accident rate as a measure of accident proneness. *J. Appl. Psychol.*, **24**: 154-159.
11. *Designing for Safety in the Home,* 1959. London: H.M.S.O.
12. DIMASCIO, A., RINKEL, M. and LEIBERMAN, J., 1961. Personality and psychotomimetic drugs. *Proc. Third World Congr. Psychiat., Montreal, Canada.*
13. DREW, G. C., 1963. The study of accidents. *Bull. Brit. Psychol. Soc.*, **16**, No. 52.
14. DUNBAR, FLANDERS, 1943. *Psychosomatic Diagnosis.* New York: Hoeber.
15. 1944. Susceptibility to accidents. *Med. Clin. N. Amer.*, **28**: 653-662.
16. 1948. *Synopsis of Psychosomatic Diagnosis and Treatment.* St. Louis: C. V. Mosby.
17. 1954. *Emotion and Body Changes,* (2nd ed.). New York: Columbia Univ. Press.
18. DUNBAR, H. F., WOLFE, T. and RIOCH, J., 1936; 1939. Psychic component in fracture. *Amer. J. Psychiat.*, **93**: 649; Part II. *Ibid.*, **95**.
19. FABIAN, A. A. and BENDER, L., 1947. Head injury in children. *Amer. J. Orthopsychiat.*, **17**: 68-79.
20. FARMER, E. and CHAMBERS, E. G., 1939. A study of accident-proneness among motor drivers. Industr. Hlth. Res. Bd., No. 84.
21. FREUD, S., 1936. *The Problem of Anxiety.* New York: Norton.
22. 1938. The psychopathology of everyday life. In *The Basic Writings of Sigmund Freud,* pp. 33-178. New York: Modern Library.
23. FULLER, ELIZABETH M., 1948. Injury-prone children. *Amer. J. Orthopsychiat.*, **18**: 708-723.
24. FULLER, ELIZABETH M., and BAUNE, HELEN, 1951. Injury-proneness and adjustment in a second grade. *Sociometry*, **14**: 210-225.
25. GLUCK, P., 1955. Psychologische Analyse und Prüfung der Unfallaffinität von sieben- bis neun-jahrigen Kindern. *Arch. ges. Psychol.*, **93**: 1-41.
26. GORDON, J. E., 1949. *Amer. J. Publ. Hlth.*, **39**: 504.
27. GREENWOOD, M. and WOODS, H. M., 1919. *The Incidence of Industrial Accidents with Special Reference to Multiple Accidents.* M.R.C., I.F.R.B., Report No. 4. H.M.S.O.
28. GRIME, G., 1958. Research on human factors in road transport. *Ergonomics*, I.
29. HEYMAN, H., 1943. Significance of accidents and their prevention. *Wien. med. Wschr.* (Aug. 14), **93**: 453-459.

30. KLEIN, M., 1937. *Psycho-Analysis of Children*, p. 218. London: Hogarth Press.
31. KRALL, VITA, 1953. Personality characteristics of accident-repeating children. *J. Abnorm. Psych.*, **48**: 99.
32. KUNKLE, E. G., 1946. The psychological background of 'pilot error' in aircraft accidents. *J. Aviation Med.*, **17**: 533-567.
33. *Lancet*, 1948. Injury in the Home. Lancet, i: 758.
34. LANGFORD, W. S., GILDER, R., JR., WILKING, VIRGINIA N., GENN, MINNIE M. and SHERRILL, HELEN H., 1953. Pilot study of childhood accidents: preliminary report. *Pediatrics*, **11**: 405-413.
35. MACKEITH, R., 1952. Accident-proneness. *Guy's Hospital Gazette*, 1952 (February), **66**: 56-59.
36. MACQUEEN, I. A. G., 1960. *A Study of Home Accidents in Aberdeen, Edinburgh and London*. Edinburgh: E. and S. Livingstone.
37. MARBE, K., 1926. Praktische Psychologie der Unfälle und Betriebschäden. *Munchen med. Wschr.*
38. MARCUS *et al.*, 1960. Society for Research in Child Development, Monograph No. 76. Vol. 25, No. 2.
39. MENNINGER, K. A., 1936. Purposive accidents as an expression of self-destructive tendencies. *Int. J. Psychoanal.*, **17**: 6-16.
40. NELSON, E., 1962. *Textbook of Paediatrics*, (7th ed.). London: Saunders.
41. PUTNAM, J. J. and STEVENS, M., 1918. A study of the mental life of the child. *Psychoanalyt. Rev.*, **5**: 514-515.
42. Registrar-General, 1963. *Statistical Review of England and Wales for the Year 1961*. Part 1: Tables, Medical. London: H.M.S.O.
43. RAWSON, A. J., 1944. Accident proneness. *Psychosom. Med.* (January), **6**: 88-94.
44. Royal Society for the Prevention of Accidents. Stat. E.W./60/JAL.
45. Royal Society for the Prevention of Accidents Report. February 1963. Vol. 2: 83.
46. SCHILDER, P., and WECHSLER, D., 1934. The attitudes of children toward death. *J. Genet. Psychol.*, **45**: 406.
47. SCHULZINGER, M. S., 1956. *The Accident Syndrome*. Springfield, Ill.: Thomas.
48. SCOTT, C. and JACKSON, S., 1960. *England and Wales, the Social Survey*. Central Office of Information. London: H.M.S.O.
49. SHAW, LYNETTE and SICHEL, H. S., 1961. The reduction of accidents in a transport company by the determination of accident liability of individual drivers. *Traffic Safety*, **5**, No. 4.
50. SMID, A. C. and LOGAN, G. B., 1956. *Minn. Med.*, **39**: 394.
51. SWAROOP, S., ALBRECHT, R. M. and GRAB, B., 1956. *Bull. W.H.O.*, **15**: 123.
52. TILLMAN, W. A., 1948. *The Psychiatric and Social Approach to the Detection of Accident-prone Drivers*. London, Ont.: Faculty of Graduate Studies, University of Western Ontario.
53. VERNON, H. M., 1937. *Accidents and their Prevention*. New York: Macmillan.

XVI

DELINQUENCY

P. D. Scott
M.A., M.D., D.P.M.

Consultant Physician, Maudsley Hospital, London

1

Introduction

In 1948, as part of a book marking the achievements in a quarter of a century of the American Orthopsychiatric Association, Ben Karpman (65) wrote a monumental 87-page review of knowledge of delinquency. The reader will not always agree with his pungent criticisms, directed mainly against sociological and statistical studies; Shaw's (103) classical findings concerning the distribution of delinquency are dismissed as an elaboration of the obvious; Carr-Saunders' (15) conclusions concerning the interaction of susceptibility and environment are dubbed a 'bromidic truism', while Ackerson's (1) statistical studies on children's behaviour problems are 'chablonne'.* One feels that it is all in good humour, and without doubt the major milestones of progress are covered so well as to make further summary presumptuous. It is highly recommended as a starting-point for a book list on delinquency.

Two further classical papers will bring the reader fully up to date with progress up to twenty years ago: Walter Reckless (93) on the causation of delinquent behaviour, and Metfessel and Lovell (82) on 'Individual Correlates of Crime'. Bovet's (10) monograph serves as a useful and easily obtained introduction up to 1951, followed ten years later in the W.H.O. series by Gibbens' (37) *Trends in Juvenile Delinquency*, and Friedlander's (33) *Psychoanalytic Approach to Juvenile Delinquency* is still a standard work.

---

* Possibly from the German 'Schablone'—mechanical, routine.

The Magnitude of the Problem

The national crime statistics give us some idea of the overall numbers of crimes known to the police and of the nature of the offences according to age and sex, but there are well-known difficulties in interpreting them. We do not know to what extent changes in police policy and in willingness of the public to charge young people affect the figures, and we do not know the extent of the dark figure of unknown crimes. Among the 'under-privileged' boys of the Cambridge Somerville Youth Study (90) 101 were more or less seriously delinquent, yet against only 40 of these were complaints actually registered, and as regards minor infractions something of the order of 1·6% officially came to light in a five-year period. These figures are from a different country and time, but a rather similar state of affairs may exist here. If so, one wonders about the validity of the control groups of supposedly non-delinquent children which have been used in various studies.

According to the 1961 *Criminal Statistics for England and Wales* (Cmnd. 1779), 120,198 persons aged between 8 and 17 years were found guilty of offences. Except in the case of non-indictable offences in boys up to 14 years of age, there are sizeable increases as compared with the previous year. In boys this is most marked (for both indictable and non-indictable offences) in the 14 to 17-year age group.

A striking feature is the very marked increase in offences committed by girls. The percentage increase over the year for girls committing indictable offences is 22·7% in the 8 to 14 group and 23·8% in the 14 to 17 group, while the non-indictable increase for these age groups is 13·8% and 20·9% respectively. These figures are not corrected for the increase in population at risk, which has been considerable, but even so they are striking. Girls up to 17 still only contribute about one sixth of the indictable crime.

The general picture of indictable crime corrected for population at risk is that the 17 to 20 age group is by far the most serious problem and rising steeply, followed by the 14 to 16 age group. The 21 and over group shows relatively slight increase, and the 8 to 13 is the least delinquent and still below the 1951 peak.

The proportion of the commonest crimes (larceny, and breaking and entering) in young people seems to have remained fairly constant. Sexual offences have not increased appreciably, but violence against the person has risen in both the 14 to 16 and the 17 to 20 age groups, especially the latter.

Leslie Wilkins (118) has a possible explanation for some of these figures. He found that children born between 1935 and 1942 'have been more delinquent over the whole of the post-war period than those born in any other seven-year period. Moreover, the highest delinquency rates have occurred among those children who were four or five years old during some part of the war, and this suggests the possibility that disturbances at such ages may have a particularly harmful effect.' There appears to be something particularly significant in social disturbances occurring in the fourth and fifth years of a child's life. He also found that 'youths aged between 17 and 21 in 1955 and onwards, who would have been expected because of their years of birth to be exceptionally delinquent, have in fact been even more delinquent that could have been foretold by the year of birth analysis.'

This important work of Wilkins illustrates the difficulties of obtaining answers sufficiently firm to serve as a basis for preventive action. Thus we do not know what the operative factors of the 'social disturbance' might be—whether absence of father in the armed services, anxiety or preoccupation of the mother, some mental process in the child such as perception of destructive forces associated with war, or even inadequacies in diet or other physical factors; nor do we know, assuming that the children were in some way sensitised or rendered susceptible in those early years, whether specific precipitating factors are required to release or develop a delinquent tendency. But at least his study enables us to acknowledge, at an early stage of the argument, the importance of the timing of any given factor as well as of its nature and intensity.

Prys Williams (119), using the same statistics together with those relating to 1957 to 1961, shows that the expected 'delinquent bulge' has not in fact continued, and suggests that social circumstances can swamp predisposition; he also shows marked differences in offences as between males and females of different age groups. Wilkins's findings are also criticised on statistical grounds by Walters (115).

2

Classification

It is now fully accepted that delinquents are a heterogeneous collection of persons permitting very little generalisation. Even so it is commonly observed that discussions on delinquency, though started with the good resolution of defining the type under consideration, often end in dangerous generalisation. While eventually we must 'identify, describe and classify most of the various orders of delinquent and criminal behaviour, just as naturalists have identified, described and classified practically all of the plants and trees of the world' (95), we have to accept with Sutherland (111) that it is unlikely that any theory of crime could be 'sufficiently precise or specific to aid greatly in understanding or controlling all types of crime'.

It seems that the difficulties of classification are inherent in the fact that delinquents do not fall neatly within the scope of any scientific discipline. The study of delinquency is a field (some would say a marsh) which has attracted the attention of sociologists, psychologists, anthropologists, psychiatrists and others, each with his own terminology and with consequent difficulties in communication. Secondly, delinquency has never been defined any more precisely than that it is 'what the law says it is' (98); though it may sometimes be the product of mental illness, by no stretch of imagination could all delinquency be regarded as such. This being so, the study of delinquency is to a large extent coextensive with the study of human behaviour and personality; indeed the currently most popular and productive typology—that derived from Erikson and the Grants—is in fact a typology of personality, equally applicable to non-delinquents. On the one hand is the view that crime is an inescapable and necessary quality of human nature, well expressed by Joseph Conrad:

L'homme est un animal méchant. Sa méchanceté doit être organisée. Le crime est une condition nécessaire de l'existence organisée. La société est essentiellement criminelle,—ou elle n'existerait pas. C'est l'égoïsme qui sauve tout,—absolument tout,—tout ce que nous abhorrons, tout ce que nous aimons (21).

Yet on the other hand the clinician daily examines young offenders who are reacting to stresses in a manner which is inconclusive—and often self-damaging—and who need, and sometimes respond to, the adjustments that can be made for them. Indeed 'the doctor is not necessarily acting outside his proper scope if he attends to people who are not ill', and he may learn 'a great deal about normal and abnormal psychology which is relevant to the treatment, or the prevention, of some non-pathological states that are socially deviant' (70).

The number of classifications is vast, and many of them overlap in a confusing manner. What actually happens, as D. C. Gibbons (39) has suggested, is that a worker examines some existing studies and adds a number of hunches, finally emerging with a new theory. If such a scheme can support clinical application and if it can be reduced to a standardised approach capable of validation, then real advance may be possible.

In general, classifications are of three sorts: those which are based upon an offender's specific behaviour, those based on his personal qualities, including his motivation, and those based on his interaction with others. In fact any classification which is to have more than academic interest must involve all three elements. That element which is used for the collection of the sample will depend upon the researcher's opportunities and matters not, so long as the other elements are somewhere involved. Thus a delinquent problem may be primarily classified according to the offence committed (e.g. offenders against property, against the person, mixed, first or repeated), or according to personal characteristics (e.g. Friedlander's strong unmodified instinctual urges, lack of independence of the super-ego, weak ego, (34)), or according to interaction with others (e.g. amenables and non-amenables (2), demanding, complaining, conforming, manipulating, defending, identifying (48), positive, confused, apathetic, psychopathic (41)). Since the objective of all classification is the attainment of effective treatment or prevention, we should take particular notice of the Californian study (46), which consistently demonstrated that it was only the consideration of specified environmental treatment (in terms of type of supervisor and type of treatment programme) in relation to specified types of offender (in terms of level of personality integration) which proved significant in distinguishing results of treatment.

As to qualities which might be used in differentiating delinquents, a great deal of confusion exists. In the first place it is often erroneously supposed that a given characteristic is consistently present; thus Chernukin (17) devised a test to identify absconders, but when this was applied in a large remand home it was found that it did in fact identity the boy who at that moment was contemplating absconding, but that in most boys the intention was so intermittent as to reduce the usefulness of the test as a predictor. We know also from Hartshorne and May (55) that dishonesty does not pervade the whole personality but tends to declare itself in certain circumstances. Wootton (124) makes the point that test findings are too readily assumed to represent inherent qualities rather than the results of penal experience, and that the fact of commission of a criminal offence is itself considered so important that any offender is assumed to be likely to differ significantly from those who have not offended. The work of Johnson (63) suggests that the locus and origin of certain anti-social acting-out behaviour may be in the mind of a parent rather than of the offending child, who may simply respond to the appropriate cue and directive, subtly concealed as it may be. She also supports Hartshorne and May in finding 'personality lacunae' as well as broad personality defects.

The comparison of groups of delinquents with control groups of non-delinquents has been a favourite research field for many years, so that the literature is very large, and the methodology (especially collection of samples) not always very sound. Cressy and his colleague (100) reviewed the literature comparing delinquents and non-delinquents by personality tests, and concluded that there were no significant differences: '. . . as often as not the evidence favoured the view that personality traits are distributed in the criminal population in about the same way as in the general population.' Woodward's (123) review of tests of intelligence in delinquents concludes 'that low intelligence plays little or no part in delinquency', but tests of many other capacities seem to have proved their worth. Notably the Q score of the Porteus Maze Test (36), the M.M.P.I. and the Maudsley Personality Inventory have proved useful, while many workers (S. and E. T. Glueck, I. Nye, R. Andry) have elaborated their own inventories. These and other relevant studies are well reviewed by Argyle (3), who classifies them under four headings: (i) Super-ego Strength—tests of cheating, moral value and extra-punitiveness; (ii) Identification—tests of attitude to parents, to authority, to peer groups, and level of aspiration; (iii) Ego Control and Impulsiveness—tests of motor control, time sense, impulsiveness, emotional maturity; (iv) Sympathy—tests of cruelty and aggression, skill at social perception.

Of the many ways of classifying delinquents, it is reasonable to select for special consideration on the one hand those which have a practical clinical application and which help in understanding, and on the other those which have been utilised by other workers or have proved their worth through successful prediction of outcome.

(1) Classification by Parental Attitude. This is associated with Thurstone (112), who was already attempting to measure attitudes in 1931; with Shoben (105), who held that parental attitudes were measurable and were capable of meaningful association with child adjustment, and that relevant and internally consistent variables could be extracted from a pool of variables by sophisticated judges (claims which have subsequently been vigorously attacked); and also with Champney (16), who devised the famous Fels Parent Behavior Rating Scale. This scale was used by Baldwin and his colleagues (5) to make a somewhat over-elaborate, but nevertheless useful, classification of parental attitudes, which has not been bettered; they further correlated parental attitude with characteristics of the resulting children, noting for instance the hostility, over-dependence or precocious self-sufficiency, the inadequate use of intellectual capacity, low originality and low creativity, of the child of rejectant parents, and the differences between 'actively' and 'nonchalantly' rejected children. Similarly the outcome of casually and indulgently autocratic attitudes are noted, while the democratically raised child reminds one of Sunday's child—'all that is healthy, good and gay'! The observed differences in preschool, school and later adjustment of children from the different backgrounds are particularly of interest.

The emphasis in this work is on the quality of parental discipline and its importance in determining child behaviour. In this respect it supports the most reliable earlier work (for example of Healy (56), Burt (13) and Bagot (4)), as well as the best modern research, especially that of J. and W. McCord (81), Sears and his colleagues (102), and Sheldon and Eleanor Glueck (44), all of whom agree that the quality of discipline, *especially inconsistent discipline*, is crucial. This indeed is one of the few firmly established facts in this field.

(2) Jenkins (58, 61) has approached the problem in the reverse direction, classifying the children and then noting the characteristics of their home backgrounds. Adaptive delinquency is associated with physical vigour and an aggressive attitude towards life; adequate maternal care has permitted the development of social responsiveness, but there has been absence of paternal guidance, or conflict with father, the home tends to be cramped, disorderly, unattractive, overcrowded so that the boy 'lives' with street companions. Maladaptive delinquency is associated with a picture of gross poverty of personality organisation, vengefulness, inability to get along with other children, sullenness, negativism and suspicion; in the strong the world is met by direct aggression, in the weak by loss of control alternating with hostile over-dependence; the background is one of gross

frustration of primary needs, and of rejection by both parents, especially the mother. This concept has been widely used by other workers and has a direct and useful practical application; it has made a lasting contribution to the assessment of delinquents.

(3) Another approach full of promise is that of Kinch (67), who, on a basis of a seven-point self-rating scale, classified his series of delinquents into three categories: Pro-Social delinquents tend to be first-time serious offenders, from stable homes, both natural parents are present and have had a harmonious relationship together, the school record is satisfactory and the boys are well adjusted with their peers; Anti-Social delinquents tend to come from urban areas, are gang members and have had many contacts with law enforcement agents from an early age, the homes are typically lower-class, families large, parents usually lax in discipline, siblings also tend to delinquency, school adjustment is unsatisfactory; Asocial delinquents have experienced early and severe parental rejection, are often illegitimately born to a very young mother, the family is often broken and the mother often harsh and inconsistent, the boy has poor peer relations and tends to aggressive bullying. D. C. Gibbons (40) has utilised similar self-concepts in building up an interesting tentative fourteen-item typology of delinquents. Self-concept links up closely with depression and with the concept of a defective body image (66)—both common findings in rejected children, whether delinquent or not, and possibly giving rise to self-comforting behaviour or attempts to make restitution to the self.

(4) The typology which has had the greatest impact, and which has already proved most fruitful, is that developed by the Grants in California. The scheme is outlined in an important paper by Sullivan, Grant and Grant (110). They develop the views in particular of Piaget (88) and Erikson (27), who visualised the growing child as faced with certain developmental hurdles: at six to nine months the problem is whether to trust or mistrust; starting at about 12 to 15 months the problem is to develop autonomy, failure leading to a lasting sense of doubt and success to self-control without loss of self-esteem; from the fourth or fifth year the child must develop initiative without too much sense of guilt. Sullivan and his colleagues believe that emotional and social development follows a trend towards increasing involvement with people, objects and social institutions, which can be meaningfully described in terms of seven successive integrations. Immaturity is viewed as the handicap resulting from a failure to solve the crucial interpersonal problem at one or other of these stages. Such failure may lead the person to become 'fixed at a particular integration level'; the resulting personality difficulties may be successfully covered but the 'core personality' will be revealed under stress. They predict that persons so handicapped are more likely to become delinquent than others, and they describe, for each stage, the problem facing the developing child, the characteristics of the adult who fails to

solve that problem, and the sort of delinquent who may emerge. Of the seven so-called 'I' (Integration) Levels, numbers 2 to 5 are most commonly met in clinical practice, for the level 1 individual is likely to be so incompetent as to be found 'in mental hospitals and in such fringe groupings in the community as skid rows and hobo camps', while those of the higher 'I' levels are usually sufficiently mature to avoid delinquency. The Grants have developed a Social Maturity Scale with a series of critical questions for the screening interview, and a detailed list of personality qualities for each of which the statistical correlation with 'I' levels 2 to 5 has been determined. In 1961 Mrs. Grant (48) prepared a juvenile 'I' level classification which promises to be of great usefulness, and which is already being applied in this country; the classification is supplemented by a detailed treatment plan for each of the types, including a statement of what treatment goals are indicated, and advice on placement, family handling, community support, job and school recommendations, peer group needs, kind of control and kind of therapist.

The scheme is sometimes difficult to apply in that inevitably cases sometimes seem to fall between levels or to cover several of them, and training of the classifier is clearly necessary, but it represents a great advance. Already work from this school has established certain principles: for example that, in assessing treatment effectiveness, it is not only necessary to assess kinds of subject but also 'kinds of supervisors and kinds of programming' (48), and furthermore that a given treatment method, though effective with certain 'amenable' types, may do actual harm to 'non-amenables' (34).

The Grants do not much concern themselves with aetiology, but make the general statement (110) that, if a stressful or threatening situation is too intense or extreme, 'a real resistance to change is generated and desperate measures may be taken to maintain the *status quo* and a feeling of relative security. If such a need continues over an extended period of time, a characteristic pattern or "style of life" may be established.' This is of course quite consistent with psychoanalytic theory, with the 'frustration-aggression' theory associated with Dollard and his colleagues (23), Marquhart (77) and Maier (75), with 'learning theory' (including the theory of critical or optimum periods of learning of the ethologists and of those who have studied maternal deprivation), and with each of the classifications previously mentioned in this chapter.

3

Aetiology

This very large subject may conveniently be dealt with under the headings of social and precipitating factors, inherited factors, physical and mental illness, and predisposing factors.

Social and Precipitating Factors

Some preliminary points need mention before recent work is considered. Social factors are often considered as having their principal action in the here and now, but they may of course have been acting throughout the individual's life, and they may indeed have had their effect upon the parents and the whole family. Professor Roger Wilson (121) has described the social setting of adolescents living in new housing estates: the youngster is no longer tied to the locality for recreation or courting, and no longer shares common experiences and insecurities with his neighbours, many of whom will work far away from the estate; the parents have no clearly defined and acceptable standards, either high or low, in the training of their children; the mothers care a lot, but have no strong neighbourhood pattern to give them support, and the 'lack of common practice is a very great contribution to stress and strain'; a minority of mothers find 'the stress of taking any consistent line about conduct is more than they can manage' and the resulting ill-discipline of their children heightens the anxieties of all the mothers on the estate. Social factors may thus constitute not only the precipitating factors, but the soil in which delinquency developed.

A second point is that it may be unrealistic to try and study delinquency in isolation, for there is much evidence that at least certain types of delinquency are closely associated with other social inefficiencies. Dr. E. G. Knox (68), writing on family health and welfare, proposes a 'law of conglomeration of impairments'; he finds in a study of Newcastle families that between 10 and 20% (depending upon the arbitrary levels taken) of the families are 'deeply immersed among a large number of defects and disabilities'. In a 30-year follow-up on child guidance cases, Robins and O'Neal (97) conclude:

Although there may be psychiatrically normal criminals who pursue crime as a profession while leading stable, well-organised lives in other areas, it seems probable that criminal activities are more frequently only one expression of a grossly disturbed life pattern of which transiency, violence, and unstable family relations, as well as crime, are typical.

Similarly Fairweather and Illsley (29), studying over a ten-year period all the children born in Aberdeen in 1948 who were mentally handicapped, find a similar nexus between social and psychiatric variables, in that these children's families were characterised by a high frequency of poor education and intelligence, marital and occupational instability, ill-informed attitudes to health, nutrition and child care, and that many members of these families intermarried.

J. B. Mays (79, 80) brilliantly portrays the environmental delinquency which in Merseyside dockland

seems to be part and parcel of that established way of living or sub-culture, to which the majority are obliged to conform. Petty larceny, shop-lifting, lorry-skipping, bunking into cinemas without paying, rowdiness and occasional outbursts of physical violence flourish amongst the children of ill-regulated homes and have become almost acceptable modes of behaviour. The deviant boy in such a neighbourhood is the one who abstains from any form of delinquent act and he is likely to be penalised by ostracism and ridicule.

In Mays's experience the 'vast majority of boys who are brought before the juvenile courts are fundamentally normal personalities'. D. H. Stott (108), working with Glasgow delinquents and using a scale of social adjustment, agrees that delinquency is more prevalent in certain 'black-spot' urban areas, but argues that if this sort of delinquency is solely or mainly due to the sub-cultural influence, then these delinquents should be well-adjusted; in fact he found the levels of maladjustment surprisingly similar in high and low delinquency areas, and that disturbed behaviour in non-delinquents rose consistently with the amount of delinquency in the area; once again, finding that delinquency as well as other forms of social inefficiency is concentrated in the 'black spots', he proposed that delinquency is not the outcome of maladjustment but part of it. His conclusions confirm those of the McCords (40), who state that 'social factors' are not strongly related to criminality: a slum neighbourhood can mould a child's personality but only if other factors make him susceptible (see also Hilda Lewis's (71) findings with children from problem families).

Harriett Wilson (120), in her 'Seaport' study of cases referred to Co-ordinating Committees, found that 'referred families living in relative isolation in low-delinquency areas of the city show a rate of delinquency similar to that of those living in clusters in high-delinquency areas.'

We are left with the impression that there are on the one hand fringe or *formes frustes* delinquents, comprising those who are reacting to the local sub-cultural influences as well as those showing minor degrees of pre-disposition (licked rather than bitten, as one might say), while on the other hand there are the hard-core delinquents who, unlike the first category, will not respond to simple measures, whether instituted by the court or by the sensible provisions of social workers (clubs, football pitches, etc.). The proportion of these two categories may well vary from place to place and from time to time, but both must be reckoned with in treatment and prevention.

Sub-cultural delinquency was recently brought into renewed prominence by Cohen (20) and by Cloward and Ohlin (19): delinquency is linked with the working-class boy who (especially in American culture) experiences 'status frustration'; he is thrust, ill prepared, into a highly competitive situation; when he fails in his aspirations towards middle-class standards he seeks comfort amongst similarly frustrated boys, and, together with them, vents his disappointment and restores his sense of purpose through non-utilitarian, malicious and negativistic values and acts, which perpetuate themselves when counter-action causes a protective drawing together. This 'sour-grapes' motivation of delinquency probably has less application in this country, where organised gangs are very rare among delinquents, and where the drive towards higher class values does not seem so great. The clinician, seeing mainly the more serious delinquents (often unable to identify even with their own sub-culture), may not be in the best situation to know the relative proportion of 'aspirants' and 'statics' in the youthful population; nevertheless the strong impression is gained that the characteristics of wanting things immediately and without effort, and of displaying hostility when frustrated, is an early family-derived, rather than culture-derived, development. There must be truth in the aphorism 'unjust deprivation underlies alienation', but the line between just and unjust is difficult to draw, and it is surely true (and research on suicide confirms it) that intensity of aspiration, with marked reaction to loss of status, are not confined to lower classes.

History continues to show very clearly that social correlates of delinquency are not necessarily causes. Thus it is now widely demonstrated, for example by Jephcott and Carter (62), that it is the home within an area, rather than the conditions of the area, which is significant. The significance of the slum area has diminished since it has been shown that 'some of the new housing estates show a considerably higher incidence of juvenile delinquency than the town as a whole' (Mannheim (76)). A further, previously firm, finding, upon which many theories have been based, was the correlation between delinquency and low social class; but Little and Ntsekhe (73), using unusually representative and satisfactory sampling, show that in London the shift is now towards the middle social class of the Registrar General's classification.

The traditional subdivision of causative theories into sociological and psychological is increasingly unsatisfactory; social, like any other, factors must be considered in their quality, intensity, timing and impact on specific types of individual.

Inherited Factors

The well known twin studies (Lange, Kallmann, Healy, Rosanoff, Kranz) have been supplemented by Slater (106), though he was not working specifically with criminals. He points to a striking contrast between the psychoses on the one hand and the psychopathic and neurotic states on the other; in the latter uniovular pairs of twins are less frequently concordant, and some binovular pairs develop very similar troubles despite big differences in intelligence and personality. 'The dividing line between adjustment and maladjustment is not so wide as that between sanity and insanity and more easily over-stepped, so that chance, whether favourable or unfavourable, is more important. Once maladjustment has begun, it may contribute to its own continuance.'

Certain measurable qualities supposed to have a genetical basis and to correlate with delinquency are relevant here. The firmly established link between mesomorphic body build and delinquency (104, 45, 38) illustrates how a particular choice of reaction is facilitated by inherited potentialities.

Rate of development may also in part be genetically determined and seems to correlate with delinquency, though, like so many measurable factors, it does so at both ends of the scale—too much and too little. 70% of Chicago delinquent girls (57) were physically over-developed compared with the norms for their age. Confirming this, MacFarlane (74) states that 'the late maturers tend to have fewer problems at all ages, and show no trends in relation to menarche.' At the other end of the scale 'under-developed children, especially if frail and sickly, may indulge in mis-conduct, partly as compensation for their physical weakness and the unfair treatment that they sometimes receive.' (Neumeyer (83).)

There is also the well known correlation between aggressiveness and electroencephalogram abnormalities (59). But non-specific abnormalities do not necessarily indicate an unfavourable outcome and do not indicate any specific medication.

Birch (9, 18) emphasises the complexity of the interaction between inherited and environmental influences. He studied organismic variability in a series of 105 infants from middle-class American families, isolating nine separate behaviour characteristics. Despite great variation from child to child, the formal characteristics for any one individual remained remark-ably constant. After two years some 90% retained their original position on the scale, and in some cases the stability persisted after five years. Little effect on these characteristics was produced by stresses such as parental death, separation, or birth of siblings; 'although the *form* of activity may have altered, the *style* remains unchanged.' According to these workers the primary patterns of reactivity appear in infancy and persist into childhood. This initial primary reactivity, together with environmental factors, determines the personality structure and temperament, and this throws doubt upon categorical formulations about the dangers of certain happen-ings in the life of the child.

Indirectly confirming such views are the studies (e.g. West (117)) of adult offenders whose criminality develops late in life and for whom careful enquiry fails to reveal the usual psychodynamics in the family background.

Yet if we take a factor such as intelligence which is accepted as primarily controlled by many genes of small effect, we find the opposite tendency—under-estimation of the influence of environment. This is illustrated by animal experiments. Forgus has shown that the environment in which rats were reared substantially affects their problem-solving capacity. Cooper and his colleagues bred two strains of rats:

The bright rats were not made more intelligent by rearing in an enriched environment; but dull rats were improved by this more stimulating upbringing and they reached the level of the bright rats. Similarly, dull rats reared in excep-tionally restricted environments were not made more stupid, but bright rats so reared were made to resemble dull rats.

Barnett (7), from whom these references are taken, continues:

The stimulation derived from variety of experience, resulting from investigation, manipulation, and play, promotes a kind of learning—the kind that makes possible a rapid acquirement of useful habits and particular skills in later life.... The stimulation that a baby monkey gets from a model mother (or an infant from his attachment to a particular person) is more enigmatic; but it probably helps in the development of both intelligence and social behaviour.

Eysenck (28) links anti-social behaviour with extrovert personalities possessing 'greater innate tendencies to inhibition' and with the resulting tendency to learn lessons of socialisation less readily and to retain them less well. Franks (32) expected a second and opposite type: those who learned the lessons of an anti-social environment too well. Further studies have not confirmed these hypotheses. Robin (96), working with approved school boys, argued that if there are these two types of recidivists then their environments should be different. Further, he expected Franks's second type, the introverts, to respond more readily to the training of the school than the extroverts. Using only one test (Maudsley Personality Inventory) for introversion-extroversion, and assessing response to training by speed of licence from the school, he was unable to confirm either of these hypotheses. Tong and Murphy (113) comment on Franks's and Eysenck's theories: 'This sort of explanation will not bear clinical analysis, of course. The description fits the imbecile, not the psychopath, and completely misses the point that the psychopath knows the rules of society but fails to observe a select few.' Field (30, 31) also was unable to confirm these hypotheses, but did find that adult criminals score highly on 'neuroticism' and 'rigidity' (high need for achievement, high and unrealistic aspirations, low capacity to adapt or to assess their opportunities realistically against objective social conditions) as compared with control groups.

The major studies on the importance of inherited factors are handicapped by not knowing what to measure, and by the difficulty of distinguishing very early environmental from truly inherited factors, so that the subject is still wide open. The probability that inherited factors are significant does not in any way diminish the importance of social and psychodynamic factors, nor does it necessarily indicate a nihilistic attitude to treatment or prevention, for it seems quite clear that inherited factors need a specific soil in which to develop.

Physical and Mental Illness

Nearly everyone would agree with Neumeyer (83) that 'any disease or physical weakness may be a factor leading to social failure, and failure may lead to delinquency', and it is equally clear that 'it ought to be generally realised, in all common sense, that any physical peculiarities, defects, or disease of the offender which stand in the way of social success should be as efficiently treated as possible.' Hence the approach of Ogden (84) in arranging surgical treatment (including plastic surgery for cosmetic disabilities) for his Borstal lads; hence also Banay's report (6): 'The Court verdict laid the blame for the delinquency on the crossed eyes and sentenced the defendant to wear glasses'! Certain physiological states, especially fatigue, menstruation (22) and intoxications, may lower the threshold of crime.

Earlier studies uniformly reported a high correlation of defects of physique, malnutrition and physical disease with delinquency; yet recent work suggests that these defects were not causative, for the modern delinquent does not show this picture but is just as numerous. Thus Eilenberg (25) compared 1930 and 1955 samples of London delinquents; he confirmed the quicker physical development and reported a virtual eradication of gross physical disease and malnutrition; the 1955 boys were in fact rather heavier than their non-delinquent schoolfellows; he did note, however, a high incidence of minor physical disease despite improved standards of available medical care. The Gluecks (44) found that 'very little, if any, difference exists between the physical condition of the two groups [delinquent and non-delinquent] as a whole.'

As regards mental illness and organic damage to the central nervous system, the position is less clear. In their further analysis of the Cambridge-Somerville material, the McCords (81) found that, apart from acne, only 'distinct neurological disorder' correlated significantly with delinquency. In an earlier study, Norwood East (24) found 'a record of encephalitis lethargica was present in about 6 per 1,000 of the lads, and of other forms of encephalitis about 11 per 1,000. There was no evidence of significant variation in the proportion according to the nature of the offences committed, nor of any association with the number of previous offences.' Papers such as Levy's (69) and Pygott and Street's (92) on the effects, including delinquency production, of unsuspected organic dementias should serve to keep psychiatrists diagnostically alert. In particular they should look for: changes in personality, whether there is a history of trauma or encephalitis or not; a combination of irritability and explosive or exaggerated reaction to slight provocation; distractibility, educational backwardness; lability of emotions with sudden and unexplained variability of mood and behaviour. These findings, despite absence of grosser symptoms such as headache, vomiting or fits, and despite the absence of clear physical signs, should lead to a more careful investigation.

Prechtl (91) describes a common syndrome in schoolchildren (characterised by choreiform movements affecting mainly the proximal and facial muscles, behaviour and learning difficulties, and hyperkinesis) which he attributes to minimal brain lesions acquired in the perinatal period. He makes the point that such children are difficult to handle, and that disturbances of the mother-child relationship may be secondary rather than causative.

There is much to support Lauretta Bender's (8) aphorism: 'Even an organic brain lesion does not create fundamentally new trends but it merely underscores specific psychological problems.' Grunberg and Pond (52) showed conclusively that the environments of epileptic children with behaviour disorders, and of behaviour-disordered children without epilepsy, are equally disturbed, whereas stable children with epilepsy have a much lower incidence of disturbed or broken homes. Similarly Harrington and Letemendia (54) showed that neither severity of head injury (as judged by duration of unconsciousness), nor its localisation, is always the major factor in determining the nature and persistence of subsequent behaviour disorders in children. The relation of brain damage and epilepsy to constitutional and environmental modifying factors is admirably reviewed by Pond (89).

Despite several careful investigations (12, 85) it is difficult to know what the relationship between mental disorder and delinquency might be, and even more difficult to establish a causative link. The 'law of conglomeration of impairments' (68) has already been mentioned; florid mental illness often prevents inclusion of such cases in samples, and indeed may protect them from prosecution. In Gibbens's (38) study of Borstal boys 27% were mentally abnormal, most of them showing a severe degree of personality disorder; only one was psychotic and one epileptic. However studies of psychiatric patients (Pippard in an observation ward, Curran in a large private practice and Lennox in an epileptic colony) to determine how many have been delinquent suggest that the correlation is a small one, not higher than 10% to 20%, and even so there may be no demonstrable causal link between the mental abnormality and the offence; sometimes, indeed, the two may be observed to alternate.

The clinical conclusion is that mental abnormality, with certain rare exceptions, helps to release delinquency rather than to cause it.

Interesting work has been done with animals and man suggesting that certain rhinencephalic lesions may result in sexually abnormal behaviour which may sometimes be regarded as delinquency, so that there may be rare exceptions to Bender's generalisation.

Space permits only a mention of Pasamanick's (86) theory of the 'continuum of reproductive casualty': abortion, stillbirth, cerebral palsy, epilepsy, mental defect, behaviour disorders, reading and learning difficulties, and tics. This continuum is related to prenatal complications, prematurity and history of previous infant loss; mechanical factors at delivery were found to be less damaging than the toxaemias, ante-partum haemorrhage, placenta praevia, and dystocia. The theory is strongly supported in the delinquency field by D. H. Stott (109), but contrary evidence is also plentiful. The McCords (81) find no significant relationship between delinquency and either prematurity, difficult birth, Caesarean section, the child's general health, or even prolonged enuresis. Brandon (11), utilising the data from the Newcastle 1,000-family study, considered all these factors, finding only psychological stress in pregnancy (a factor which might continue) to be significantly related to 'maladjustment' of the child.

The effect upon the parents of the child's physical or mental disability must be taken into account. Even minor factors may affect an unstable, intolerant parent and lead to cumulative difficulties in the relationship. A parent may have a dread of some particular disfigurement or illness in the child; the highly narcissistic mother may communicate her disappointment or disgust; the father, hoping for vicarious satisfaction through the attainments of a son, may reject the incompetent one; and certain children may have unpleasant associations, having caused pain or embarrassment. The timing of the child's illness may be significant in determining personality, especially increased aggressiveness or dependency: 'But once a child starts to be over-dependent—or is perceived as being so by his mother—he becomes a stimulus to the mother and influences her behaviour to him.' (102.)

In summary, we should agree with Norwood East (24) that it is easy to attach undue significance to disease once an offence has been committed, and that we should be cautious in assuming any causative relationship. In favour of this outlook is the increasingly well supported fact (for example Grunhut (53)) that, where mental disorder and crime have coexisted, the course and prognosis of the two conditions may be quite different and independent.

Predisposing Factors

The most that can be done in brief compass under this heading is to suggest a framework which may unify the many contributions within a single theory, albeit at the risk—or certainty—of over-simplification.

Similar content can be found in the minds of delinquents, of non-delinquents, and indeed of poets, playwrights and novelists. Of prime importance therefore is the ability to control the frontier between thought and action. Control may give way if the impulse or appetite is overwhelmingly strong, whether it be for hunger, sex or recognition, or for a goal less realistic and less easily recognised, such as the reduction of intolerable anxiety or fear. Alternatively the defences or resistance may be weak, whether inherently, as in the mental defective or the small child, or by disease, as in the demented, though here we should note that in children and defectives the only difference may be in the speed of building up resistance rather than in any real incapacity. Finally, the control may not be brought into action owing to failure in communication; orders to the competent guard, as it were, may have been incomprehensible, misinterpreted, conflicting, absent or rejected.

It is reasonable, from what we know of child development, to assume that controls are not ready-made but have to be built up or learnt. And from this certain broad patterns of predisposition, often in palimpsest, may be discerned.

The individual, whether in the peer-group or family, may learn responses which are not acceptable to wider society. Perhaps all must learn different sets of rules for different groups. Where differences are great, confusions may arise, especially in the young. But essentially such individuals will not feel guilty, and should with re-education be able to readjust themselves. Within this group will fall those not uncommon delinquents, well described by Johnson (63), who are faithfully responding to the hidden anti-social suggestions of a parent. The surest way of finding an example of such is to search the files of girls who have illegitimate babies: the common finding is that the girl's mother had problems with her own sexual adjustment, left her antagonistic parents, formed a temporary and unsatisfactory liaison, and when her child arrived soon began both to expect and to dread a similar pattern; through often repeated warnings the girl has constantly before her the expected pattern of behaviour, which ultimately, in a setting of adolescent rebelliousness, is acted-out. Similar mechanisms occur in acquisitive and violent offences: a boy of 16 whose brother had recently been sentenced to a long term of imprisonment and who daily shared in the family resentment, shot a policeman; a young man who had spent most of his life in approved schools, Borstals and prisons had been actively and openly encouraged to resist authority, and had witnessed father's assault upon his school-teacher. Such individuals often appear friendly and entirely 'normal' to the examiner, and are notably lacking in regret or guilt; they are much more likely to be angry at the failure of others to understand them. A variant, described by Greenacre (51), is the situation in which the child is taught only to gratify the parents' narcissism, to behave 'as if' he had accomplished something and thus to evade reality; the indulgent, pleasure-loving mother, contemptuous of her husband's importance and respectability, may inculcate such a pattern in her son. Trouble arises in all these mechanisms if the behaviour of the 'pupil' ultimately embarrasses the 'teacher', who then recants and is likely to be the target for the very behaviour which was taught. Such reversals are common in adolescence: the seductive mother who has fostered an incestuously tinged relationship with her son ultimately finds herself in the position of the sorcerer's apprentice, and her evident alarm only adds fuel to the adolescent's anger and frustration, leading to pathetic court apprearances as 'beyond control'. Three situations infuriate the adolescent more than anything else: a parent who begins to countermand a well learned and previously approved set of responses, one who tries to break up his or her attempts to find a new solution (e.g. belittling him in front of his friends), and one who blames him for something he has not done. A previously amenable boy was run to earth in a café by his mother, who led him out by his ear; he broke every window and readily available article in her flat, to the great joy of his friends on the pavement outside; this was a highly adaptive piece of behaviour which relieved his feelings, checked his mother, and enabled him to rejoin his friends as a hero— very well worth an appearance in court. Perhaps this explains why angry and rebellious responses when they lead to delinquency, as they very frequently do, have such a good prognosis: they represent adaptive behaviour which is often successful and therefore self-limiting, and rebellion implies an initial confidence and courage which may in themselves exclude the more serious personality disorders.

Not all adaptive delinquency, of course, has been directly taught by parents, family or other members of the 'sub-culture'. Much of it is a personally evolved and carefully worked out pattern or behaviour role which permits adjustment to the difficulties and stresses of the situation. Such a role can only be understood by careful enquiry into the capacities of the individual and into the circumstances, particularly the family interrelationships, which obtained during the critical periods when the pattern was emerging. Such patterns have been called 'reparative behaviour'. They commonly occur when a negative lesson which involves the blocking of an important satisfaction has been learnt and accepted, so that an alternative or substitute satisfaction must be found. An obvious example involves sexual perversion. As with any other pattern of behaviour, the paths by which it is acquired are protean. Homosexuality, for example, cannot always be regarded in the Freudian sense as a means of sexual expression despite a phobia of heterosexual genital contact, or as a phobia of being overwhelmed by a relationship with a woman; it may also follow secondarily upon the adoption of a passive and general repudiation of aggression in one who has learnt that to be aggressive is too dangerous. In delinquency practice a third type of homosexual behaviour is more commonly observed: the lonely and affection-deprived youngster, who has perhaps run away from an emotionally unsatisfying home but is as yet too immature to make his own way in the world, is readily seduced into the service of older homosexuals, who are ever on the look-out for such boys; girls are similarly led into heterosexual relationships; both are gratified by being recognised, valued and cared for rather than by sexual activity, which they are readily able to renounce if they are legitimately cared for.

Reparative behaviour is really coextensive with what the learning theorists call the conditioned avoidance reaction, well described by Gwynne Jones (64) and by Trasler (114), in which the individual learns some behavioural trick or some policy which effectively diminishes anxiety and which is utilised *in anticipation* of the unpleasant unconditioned stimulus; for this reason it is very difficult to eradicate. Obviously many factors, including chance environmental circumstances, may determine whether the choice of role or of avoidance reaction proves to be social or anti-social; it is a tragic truth that the two may be separated, as it were, by a hair's breadth. However it is clear that the individual is likely to cling to his reparative behaviour or to his avoidance reaction in a way not to be found in the 'sub-cultural' offender. The latter requires straightforward re-training, which should if possible include the whole family or group, while the former requires a more intricate process involving the winning of the patient's confidence and co-operation (insight helps this process) in order that a legitimate activity may be substituted.

Different again are those very numerous delinquents who have not learnt any firm patterns of response or code of behaviour, because none has been taught. Such delinquents are to be found in the disorganised family in which gross inconsistencies of discipline prevail and in which the parents themselves are unable to demonstrate self-control or firm standards of behaviour. The resulting delinquency is typically early in onset, varied in kind, not usually very destructive nor aggressive, and largely a matter of evasions of anything unpleasant and of unstereotyped acquisitive offences. Long-term residential training is required for the well established delinquent of this sort.

If delinquency could be sufficiently described under these three broad categories (well trained to the wrong standards, reparative and avoidance patterns, and the untrained), the problem would be a great deal easier. Selection of treatment according to motivation, for example, would be practicable; we could sort our cases into the classical headings of those who seek to escape, to find a substitutive or compensatory satisfaction, to strengthen their self-regard or status, directly or indirectly to seek revenge, to obtain maximum self-gratification, to assuage a sense of guilt, to secure their place in the anti-social group by conforming. Yet we know from hard experience that such an approach is not sufficient, and that there are in fact the unadaptive, apparently self-destructive recidivists for whom these relatively simple learning-theory explanations are insufficient.

So many neat classifications and systems of explanation are as it were adultomorphic, assuming a completeness and maturity of the personality structure which is often in fact lacking.

Progress towards understanding repetitive, unadaptive, 'fixated' or 'regressive' behaviour seems to have started independently and at about the same time in the psychoanalytic and experimental psychology camps. The task is not to explain repetitive behaviour (which is a quality of all appetites), nor stereotyped behaviour (a form of mental economy which Buhler showed long ago to have physiological satisfactions of its own), but to explain why these sorts of behaviour sometimes signally fail to respond to the best that we can offer in correction and therapy. It is not that individuals showing this sort of behaviour are unable to learn or forecast what penalties will follow, but that they are unable to act on that knowledge; Maier's rats showed by their manner of jumping that they knew when punishment would follow the stereotyped behaviour, just as our psychopathic offenders can tell us exactly the consequences of their next crime; that psychopaths are unable to 'look ahead' is a great fallacy. In 1908 Yerkes and Dodson, studying speed of habit formation, found that too strong a stimulus or too difficult a discrimination slowed the process, while Cole in 1911 found that strongly punished chicks abandoned all further attempts at learning, and similar results have repeatedly been obtained with mammals. Anderson and Lidell in 1935, however, found that unconfined animals were not so affected. Three possibly important elements (excessive stimulus, difficult discrimination, and confinement) were therefore early established. Meanwhile the psychoanalysts elaborated an explanation of regressive, stereotyped behaviour in terms of identification and frustration. Freud wrote of conscience formation proceeding by repeated partial identification due to temporary frustration by the parent, and described the tendency of frustrated individuals to repeat earlier situations even when painful. Fenichel later stated that frustration is followed by a tendency to regress from object love to identification, and that 'children in general tend to identify themselves more with the parent from whom they have experienced the more impressive frustrations', observations which, in linking frustration and identification, have been amply confirmed for example by Lifton's (72) account of politically directed brain-washing. Other analysts, notably Minna Emch (26), have linked frustration due to an insoluble discrimination with regression and repetitive behaviour.

Previously quoted experimental studies (77, 75, 35, 87) upon animals and man confirm the triad of excessive punishment, insoluble discrimination and confinement as the likely source of maladaptive, stereotyped behaviour. Such circumstances are particularly likely to arise in early childhood, when dependency and identification prevent escape (perhaps aided by modern flat life, smaller numbers of siblings and absence of the extended family). Faults in the parent such as punitiveness, inconsistency, and a capricious inability to take a firm line on the behaviour requirements of the children will in such conditions have their full and 'undiluted' effect.

These considerations go some way also in offering an explanation of what is often, but wrongly, referred to as masochistic delinquency or as 'punishment seeking'. Certainly much, especially maladaptive, crime superficially appears to be bent upon seeking punishment, yet on analysis this is not confirmed and the offender tries all he knows to avoid it. What in reality is sought may be either to be controlled or to be looked after: many adolescents positively insist on being sent to an approved school or Borstal because they fear their own murderous or destructive impulses, and many 'defeated' persons who are afraid, and desperately alone, force society to care for them. The individual who is plagued by fear of passivity or of homosexual attack sometimes compels himself to tilt at every windmill, to accept every challenge: the more hopeless the odds, the greater his impulsion; his life becomes a series of battles—but he does not want to be punished. Sometimes the anti-social act to be satisfying must be actually in the presence or of directed against a figure of authority, which is risking punishment but not directed towards it; the motive may be to seduce or to show superiority by deceiving; a young man derived satisfaction from painstakingly altering the date on his season ticket and 'getting away with it', although he had bought and carried with him a current ticket. Where punishment actually is sought it would seem that it is only in order to avoid a greater disaster or anxiety. This is very fully discussed in a symposium on masochism edited by Jules Masserman (78), in which the following origin of masochism is suggested: the child lives in an aura of inescapable punishment (the triad mentioned above); sooner or later he perceives the temporary liberating effect which follows punishment, and therefore seeks to precipitate it in order to experience temporary relief from anxiety— the makings of a masochistic conditioned avoidance reaction.

Some doubt must be cast upon the classical association between self-punishment, sadism and kleptomania on the one hand and sexual grati-fication on the other. It is not sufficiently realised that certain individuals, or individuals in a certain state of tension, may respond to massive stimul-ation with orgasm or with sexual excitement. It is sometimes assumed that boys who set fire to buildings and linger, masturbating, to watch, or persons who have an orgasm in the act of stealing, are motivated sexually, rather than that the sexual excitation is incidental. Thus observant school-masters know that boys faced with very difficult scholastic problems some-times masturbate; Stekel described a medical student who experienced sexual excitation when feeling 'great anxiety' due to a difficult arith-metical problem; a shoplifting patient experienced orgasm on being challenged outside the shop; a homosexual had an orgasm when threatened and robbed by a soldier whom he was trying to seduce; an R.A.F. rear-gunner had an orgasm when he saw the enemy fighter open fire in his direction; a group of boys discovered that they were sexually stimulated by diving into very cold water and repeated the process for this reason; Gantt's 'neurotic' dog 'Nick' showed an erection when he slipped on a linoleum floor, and had an ejaculation when he sighted his master. Evidently a wide variety of stimuli, especially fear, may in certain circum-stances produce this effect, so that we should not too readily regard these arsonist and stealing children as masochistic or sadistic sexual perverts.

4

Treatment

How to set about treating this fourth, maladaptive, type of delinquency is not known. It can be alleviated and contained by reducing the precipitating frustrating situation in the (somewhat pious) hope that the condition will extinguish itself. It has been suggested (77) that, experimentally, punish-ment eliminates a habit, but that an abnormal fixation requires manual guidance. In the human subject, as opposed to the rat in a Lashley jumping-box, the nearest approach to 'manual guidance' is presumably for a worker to be present with the subject in his hour-by-hour living and to show him what to do when the frustrating situation crops up. The difficulty here is the fact that the frustrating situations for delinquents of this type, as for adult chronic recidivists, so often involve such fundamental and primitive questions as: Am I an individual in my own right who can exist independently? Can I dare to make a relationship or to trust anyone at all? Will all women inevitably reject me? Does all loving involve attacking or being attacked? Being as I am, how can I avoid hating myself? I know what I want to be like, but how can I start towards anything so distant and unattainable? Nearly all of them are problems of relationships. In some persons the incapacities are so great that one nihilistically feels that any attempt at cure, rather than containment in a permanently sheltered environment, might be worse than the 'disease'.

At least we should appreciate *primum non nocere*, for it is so easy to add to the burden of these children's frustrations and to be forced into the situation of repeating the very process which gave rise to the condition —confining them within an institution in which punishments are heavy and not making it clear what is expected of them. It may not necessarily be the supposedly out-of-date institution which is most likely to make this error. Consider the residential school run on so-called permissive principles and its effect on the maladaptive type here described: the confinement may be supplied by not having anywhere else to go; the threat of punishment may really be the child's dread of further failure and 'moving on'; while the permissive attitude and the requirement to take responsibility in group decision, group discussions and even in psychotherapy may be totally incomprehensible and alarming to these particular children, excellent though it might be for others (for example, the timid, overconforming and inhibited child).

Lay people have been led to believe, and now not unnaturally push psychiatrists into fulfilling the principle, that the more 'disturbed' (socially deviant) the child, the more psychiatric treatment must be applied, and that if only sufficient were available all problems would be solved. This is manifestly not true. The indiscriminate 'taking on' for treatment of delinquents in out-patient departments produces appallingly poor results, even though many ultimately do well after token attendance or totally failing to co-operate. The satisfactory results (usually obtaining by providing a relationship, preventing unsuitable treatment methods and heroic reprisals, and interrupting a vicious circle of family tensions through reducing parental anxiety) could equally well have been accomplished by a skilful probation officer.

The psychiatrist's effective sphere is limited as follows. He has an extremely important function of diagnosis. Now diagnosis cannot always be made in an afternoon; it is necessary to keep in contact with the case and to observe response to suggested measures, and to know something of the personalities of the social workers involved, who may need guidance and support. The psychiatrist therefore has also a duty to collect, apply and pass on the results of research.

He is most likely to be effective while the condition is *in statu nascendi*, and he will not be able to do this unless there is an effective means, as described in the Ingleby report (94), for ascertainment and referral of potential problems. Mother-and-baby, well-baby clinics and school medical examinations may be important areas of operation.

As to the treatment of established delinquency, he should concentrate on those problems in which there is a definite psychiatric symptomatology, though even here he will soon discover that if a character disorder exists with a psychiatric condition the two must be tackled together. Character disorders do not do well in ordinary psychiatric hospital wards while their psychiatric condition is being treated. Psychiatric registrars experienced in treating in-patient children for depression, anxiety, phobias, hysteria and obsessional states are often surprised to find similar cases responding as well, or better, in an approved school in which there is psychiatric surveillance.

His particular approach is most requisite in the reparative and conditioned avoidance delinquencies, and in elucidating some of the more complex and subconsciously operated problems of family psychodynamics; he will find however that bestowing of insight is only a preliminary requirement, and that, in general, nearly all success in this field ends in improved communication and relationships.

In trying to help conditioned avoidance delinquency, not too much attention should be paid to the actual offences. More important is the anxiety behind it, and this is likely to be discovered by exploring the phantasy life. The phantasy will be present every day for much of the day and during the night in dreams, while the offences will be occasional and distorted products of it. Once the nature of the anxiety is clear it may be possible to plan an alternative means of avoiding it. The following case may make this clear. A sixteen-year-old apprentice repeatedly stole money and clothes in a manner which made detection certain; he did not understand his behaviour and feared the loss of his job, and that he would be regarded as mad; during one session he was offered a cigarette* at a time when he was particularly unproductive and silent; he was so obviously gratified by this action that the significance of being given things was discussed; he then revealed that he had a frequent phantasy of being given things by his mother (who died during his childhood); when he felt lonely and after his father had restricted his activities or he had quarrelled with his sister, whom father favoured, these phantasies were very active, particularly before a stealing episode; he thought that his difficulty might be related to wishing that he could still be given things by his mother, but this knowledge did not diminish the phantasy or the desire to steal; nor did an attempt to modify father's attitude; he was asked to substitute the thought of being given a cigarette and, to make it more immediately potent, at the significant time to take out his appointment card and to draw

---

* This was before the publication of the Royal College of Physicians' Report on Smoking and Cancer!

a cigarette upon it, knowing that it would be converted into reality at his next meeting, and to say to himself 'I'm all right now' and to concentrate on thoughts of smoking a cigarette; he reported that this reduced his anxiety and relieved the desire to steal; he has not stolen in six months and had no difficulty in leaving treatment (not dependent on the therapist), nor is he a cigarette addict! It will readily be appreciated that this sort of approach to any other sort of delinquent would be ineffective or make the problem worse.

Many authorities have remarked upon the inadequacy of orthodox psychotherapy with the character disorders: 'The psychotherapist who treats the adolescent character-disordered delinquent using orthodox directive or non-directive technique is invariably disappointed.' (Schulman (101).) 'I have watched analysts of all kinds fail in the psychoanalysis of antisocial children . . .' (Winnicott (122).)

It is not surprising, therefore, that some reaction has set in and that alternative modes of treatment have been sought. The danger of course is that the swing will be back to retributive punishment.

Prominent among what might be called reality therapists is Melitta Schmideberg (99), who has for a long time and from a basis of very great experience been expounding a pragmatic and realistic approach to offenders. Recognising the weakness in some parents which prevents them from taking a firm stance with their children, she does not hesitate to face the offender with the stark realities of his situation and with the community's point of view. She accepts initial compulsion to attend for treatment, and through her genuine concern and interest and, one suspects, through her personality, demands and often gets co-operation. Working in close co-operation with the probation officer, and utilising the authoritarian setting, she makes the offender recognise his responsibilities, and is constantly alert to head off any self-excusatory or projective mechanisms.

This approach is elaborated by Glasser (43), who also insists on a forward-looking acceptance by the offender of responsibility for himself, an attitude which must be uniformly pressed by everyone who has anything to do with the offender, from the policeman who arrests him and leaves him locked up to cogitate, to the judge, the psychiatrist and the entire correctional staff. 'Since we'll accept no excuses we never need to ask why'; excuse-finding, expression of antagonism and hostility are all strongly discouraged, not least by the interested, warm, capable attitude of everyone concerned—never returning hostility, never pressing help or lightening guilt, never sympathetic or condescending, never looking for causes but only results.

This is well worth detailed study; but of course the key, as ever, is choosing the right delinquent for the process, a point which neither author sufficiently stresses. The technique is presumably appropriate for the lad in the third group of this chapter who has not been sufficiently trained by weak parents lacking confidence about where to draw limits of behaviour, and who emerges self-centred, undisciplined, having no strong loyalties either social or anti-social, and yet not severely damaged in his capacity to relate to people. To apply the technique to maladaptive delinquency would be hazardous, and for conditioned avoidance reactions and those with a strong anti-social group loyalty, probably ineffective.

Treatment in Corrective Establishments

Two facts are very apparent in this field. Firstly, techniques of handling delinquent children in a residential setting are constantly learnt, forgotten and rediscovered. Well over a hundred years ago the Royal Philanthropic Society of London reorganised its school by splitting it up into cottage groups, each managed by a craftsman and his wife. In 1911 Helenefriderike Stelzner (107) had already established certain principles for the moral education of young psychopaths: the group consisted of 24 children; doors and dormitories were open; the staff included a teacher, a house-mother and helper, a psychiatrist attending at least three times a week; the Head where possible was to be doubly qualified as pedagogue and psychiatrist (rightly implying that a psychiatric training is not necessarily sufficient), and all staff were to work in close co-operation; the regime was in 'family style' with the children taking some responsibility for running the place and for the chores; finally a treatment plan was made individually to suit the mental and physical needs of each child. It would be difficult to improve on these principles today, and it is apparent that they are not often attained. Secondly, it is only very recently that there has been any attempt to assess the effects of treatment scientifically. As Marguerite Grant (49) has written, rules of thumb are still prevalent:

He's illiterate; put him in a school. He's emotionally deprived; love him. He manipulates; surround him with controls. He's hostile and aggressive; give him tranquillisers. He's a homosexual; keep him segregated. There's nothing the matter with him; give him trade training. He's sick; don't stir up anything because we won't be able to handle it. Or simply—he's a delinquent, therefore must have problems; give him group counselling.

J. D. Grant (47) has said that 'Any correctional agency not using a prediction procedure to study the effectiveness of its decisions and operations is perpetuating a crime against the taxpayer'.

One of the first real attempts to assess the effects of residential treatment methods was that by Weeks (116), who attempted to allocate delinquents alternately to two very different schools. On the one hand Highfields was small, short-term, lavishly supplied with staff, relatively permissive in its discipline, and including such methods as 'group guided interaction'. On the other Annandale was a large, long established and long-term school, relatively authoritarian, and lacking the additional advantages of the newer school. Subjects were assessed in standardised fashion before and after. As with subsequent studies upon treatment methods, the results are disconcerting in that there was little difference in outcome between the two schools.

A possible explanation of this is suggested by the series of studies undertaken by the Grants and their colleagues under the State of California Board of Correction, already quoted in this chapter. At least it is now accepted that the effects of treatment can be masked by failure to consider the typology of the offender, the programme to which he is submitted, and the kind of worker who carries it out.

Jenkins (61) suggests that the treatment needs for his adaptive and maladaptive groups are entirely different. An individual of the former needs to have his delinquent activities thwarted and, through a sincere emotional exchange, to have his loyalty group enlarged to include socialised persons. The problem with the maladaptive delinquent however is to reduce his frustrations, and to apply simple social training through warm interpersonal relations despite unacceptable behaviour. Argyle (3) suggests that for those with 'weak ego control' counselling and group therapy should be avoided, and the Grants found that this group did best with the predicted worst level of supervisor. Those with an 'inadequate super-ego' need a warm relationship and intensive contact with at least one authority figure upon whom they can depend for support, but at the same time firm demands and withdrawal of approval when they fail to conform. Those with 'deviant identification' (elsewhere called 'socialised aggressive', 'normal delinquents' and 'sub-cultural types') should be kept out of institutions but separated from the peer group and re-established in a non-delinquent environment; with older offenders the army is suggested, but with younger offenders these indications are difficult to implement; presumably particular attention could be paid to the balancing of the group. The 'lacking sympathy' group (elsewhere called 'love seekers', 'emotionally disturbed delinquents' and ' "I" level 4') comprises those who need group and milieu therapy.

This kind of approach reaches its most impressive and clinically helpful peak in Grant's 'I' level classification for juvenile offenders (48), in which six types are described in detail and linked up with the most appropriate treatment, including the goals of treatment and means of attaining them through work in the community, the institution, the home, what sort of therapist should be chosen, and what sort of support the therapist will need. At 'I' 2 (unsocialised aggressive and passive individuals) therapy, as opposed to reviewing their day-to-day problems, is out of place; emphasis here must be placed on creating a setting which is as little frustrating as possible, clear, unambiguous, simple and gradual, with no great penalties for failure, and a constant attempt to anticipate mounting tension.

'I' 3 (conformists and manipulators) also cannot tolerate psychotherapy but may respond to group guided interaction; the régime must be strict but fair, with sincere and manipulative responses in the subject carefully distinguished from a utilisation of crises when they occur.

At the higher levels of personality integration, persons capable of identification need individual and group therapy to reduce their unconscious conflicts and to solve their personal and social problems; furthermore at these levels their families can usually be involved in group activities. A study of this work would surely help the psychiatrist working in approved schools or other remedial or penal establishments to direct his efforts, especially his individual psychotherapy, as effectively as possible. With over three-quarters of our 117 approved schools involved to some extent with psychiatrists, often working in rather isolated circumstances, some guidance is needed. A paper by Cameron (14) shows how the psychiatrist must work through the staff, supporting them and increasing their confidence and understanding. Horsley (60) also has produced a highly practical outline of the psychiatrist's role in 'staff therapy'; aiming at attitudes of positive acceptance by the staff, better communication, and creative participation by every individual, he describes four essential elements: general staff meetings, 'natter-groups' for the subjects, observer units, and community meetings, as means of unifying staff effort yet keeping it flexible to the needs of individuals.

In brief, the psychiatrist must first gain the confidence of the staff as a whole and create means of communication with them. His further activities can be divided into two. First he must accept or share responsibility for the most difficult cases; he must be at hand at times of crisis to relieve overwhelming anxiety in the staff, and he must be manifestly successful at this; he must be able to make an immediate and practicable decision which will either enable the staff to carry on with a modified plan or else remove the child, perhaps temporarily, to the sick bay, to another institution or to hospital. He should not seek such responsibility, but once it is offered he must be prepared to take it confidently. His success in emergencies, especially his capacity to see what the trouble is and resolve the immediate crisis (whether it be a boy in fear of homosexual assault, exasperation with a letter from home, a building up of frustration in one of whom too much is expected, an epileptic outburst or a psychotic episode), will greatly affect his impact in other spheres. And further, with the individual, the psychiatrist may often play the important part of dealing with immediate conflicts and symptoms and thus keeping the individual girl or boy in the wider treatment situation of the school. The treatment of the delinquent tendency is nearly always the school's task, not the psychiatrist's, but he can act as catalyst in that process, and there is the point that if the subject retreats into medical symptoms, if he absconds or gets himself transferred, the school cannot act. In a sense the subject must become a reasonably good approved school inmate before he can become a good citizen.

In the second place, the psychiatrist should take part, mainly indirectly, in the various treatment processes of the school, being available for consultation informally and taking part in staff meetings and case conferences, integrating and supporting those who are constantly in touch with the inmates; not expecting finally to solve every problem, but rather helping the staff to improve their understanding and to find their own solutions.

Next to the staff, the other inmates are the most important features of the approved school environment, and in this respect the school is largely at the mercy of those who allocate. Too great a proportion of disruptive problems will spoil the therapeutic process, however good the staff, but something may be done by splitting the school into 'houses' or smaller units, balancing the types of problem according to the preference and capability of the house-mother or father and according to the qualities of the other inmates. The capacities of delinquents to help one another is often underestimated, and appeals to a group to treat one of their members with tolerance are often very successful. Whether or not it be called 'group guided interaction' or 'group counselling', if the group is small enough for one man's span of attention and if they spend much time together at meals or for recreation, then something of this sort is likely to happen in an informal manner.

While the staff and other inmates are by far the most significant features of the environment, the physical features and amenities of the place are also important. Pleasant surroundings, enjoyable recreation and games, constructive work, and especially good food, must reduce bickering and dissatisfaction and thus relieve the staff of strain. Furthermore if the boys or girls enjoy themselves they have something to lose, and thus punishments other than withdrawal from activities can be minimised. If staff are engaged in activities which they enjoy and feel to be worth while, then the chances of the inmates identifying with them and sharing enthusiasms is obviously much enhanced.

Competitive sport, such developments as the Duke of Edinburgh's Award, and activities of the 'Outward Bound' type (described by Gittins (42)), may be of value for those who need to gain confidence and initiative, and for the 'self-proving' type of delinquent. But to organise the whole school on these competitive and challenging lines would be a mistake and hindrance.

Contact with the child's home is essential; a great deal of disappointment and wastage of social workers' time, however, might be avoided by grading the degree of involvement, and this necessitates accurate diagnosis. Homes in which the parents have no gross distortion of personality and who have been able to supply affection and security at least in the early years nearly always appreciate and respond to the social worker; absence of the child usually brings out the more positive sides of the relationship, aided by a degree of healthy regret and guilt on both sides. The parents can be helped to identify with the aims of the school and to back up the efforts of the staff, especially at times of crisis (abscondings, initial home-sickness, loss of privileges), and to prepare for the child's homecoming.

The not uncommon anti-socially inclined parent who derives satisfaction from opposing the staff (writing disturbing letters, encouraging absconding, harbouring the child when 'on the run', passing contraband articles and money) can be neutralised. Some parents cannot be worked with, but even so it is rarely wise to endeavour to make the child cut his ties. Some children and adolescents spontaneously try, but to succeed requires a high level of maturity and self-sufficiency which they never seem to possess.

The problem of returning a child to the very environment which provoked the delinquency is a difficult one; it can only partially be answered by overburdened welfare or after-care officers, and a small proportion (perhaps a tenth) are likely to require a permanently sheltered environment (41), while another section will require an escape from home, at least until they have left school and are established in working life. The need for hostels of all kinds is very great.

REFERENCES

1. ACKERSON, L., 1945. *Children's Behavior Problems*, Vol. 2. Univ. of Chicago Press.
2. ADAMS, S., 1961. Interaction between individual interview therapy and treatment amenability in older youth authority wards. Monograph 2, *Inquiries concerning Kinds of Treatment for Kinds of Delinquents*, Paper 3. Board of Correction, State of California, July 1961.
3. ARGYLE, M., 1961. A new approach to the classification of delinquents. *Inquiries concerning Kinds of Treatment for Kinds of Delinquents*. Monograph 2, Board of Correction, State of California, July 1961.
4. BAGOT, J., 1941. *Juvenile Delinquency*. London.
5. BALDWIN, A. L., KALHORN, J. and BREESE, F. H., 1945. Patterns of parent behavior. *Psychol. Monogr.*, **58**, 3: 1-75.
6. BANAY, R. S., 1943. Physical disfigurement as a factor in delinquency and crime. *Federal Probation*, **7**: 20-24.
7. BARNETT, J. A., 1961. The behaviour and needs of infant mammals. *Lancet*, i: 7186.
8. BENDER, L., 1953. *Aggression, Hostility and Anxiety in Children*. Springfield, Illinois: Thomas.
9. BIRCH, H. G., 1960. *Lancet*, ii, October 1960: 967.
10. BOVET, L., 1951. *Psychiatric Aspects of Juvenile Delinquency*. Geneva: W.H.O.
11. BRANDON, S., 1960. *An Epidemiological Study of Maladjustment in Childhood*. M.D. Thesis, University of Durham.
12. BROMBERG, W. and THOMPSON, C. B., 1937. The relation of psychosis, mental deficiency, and personality types to crime. *J. Criminal Law and Criminology*, **28**: 70.
13. BURT, C., 1925. *The Young Delinquent*. London.
14. CAMERON, K., 1960. The role of the psychiatrist in an Approved School. *J. Child. Psychol. and Psychiat.*, **1**: 306-312.
15. CARR-SAUNDERS, A. M. and NETAL, A., 1942. *Young Offenders*. New York: Macmillan.

16. CHAMPNEY, H., 1941. The measurement of parent behavior. *Child Developm.*, 12: 131.
17. CHERNUKIN, PAUL, 1957. Ph.D. Thesis, London University.
18. CHESS, S., THOMAS, A., BIRCH, H. G. and HERTZIG, M., 1960. Implications of a longitudinal study of child development for child psychiatry. *Amer. J. Psychiat.*, 117: 434.
19. CLOWARD, R. A. and OHLIN, L. E., 1961. *Delinquency and Opportunity: A Theory of Delinquent Gangs.* London: Routledge & Kegan Paul.
20. COHEN, A. K., 1956. *Delinquent Boys: The Culture of the Gang.* London: Routledge.
21. CONRAD, J. From a letter written by Conrad to R. B. Cunninghame Graham. G. Jean-Aubry, *Joseph Conrad: Life and Letters*, Vol. I, p. 269. London, 1927.
22. DALTON, K., 1961. Menstruation and crime. *Brit. Med. J.*, ii: 1752.
23. DOLLARD, J., DOOB, L. W., MILLER, N. E., MOWRER, O. H. and SEARS, R. R., 1939. *Frustration and Aggression.* New Haven: Yale Univ. Press.
24. EAST, NORWOOD, 1942. *The Adolescent Criminal: A Medico-sociological Study of 4,000 Male Adolescents.* London: Churchill.
25. EILENBERG, M. D., 1961. Remand home boys: 1930-1955. *Brit. J. Criminol.*, 2, 2: 111.
26. EMCH, M., 1944. On the need to know as related to identification and acting out. *Internat. J. Psychoanal.*, 25: 13.
27. ERIKSON, E. H., 1950. *Childhood and Society.* New York: Norton.
28. EYSENCK, H. J., 1952. *The Scientific Study of Personality.* London: Routledge & Kegan Paul.
29. FAIRWEATHER, D. V. I. and ILLSLEY, R., 1960. *Brit. J. Prev. Soc. Med.*, 14: 149.
30. FIELD, J. G., 1960. *Report to the Prison Commission of an Investigation into the Personality of Recidivists*, July 1960. See also No. 31.
31. FIELD, J. G. and BRENGLEMAN, J. C., 1961. Eyelid conditioning and 3 personality parameters. *J. Abnorm. Soc. Psychol.*, 63: 517-523.
32. FRANKS, C. M., 1956. *Brit. J. Delinq.*, 6, 3: 192.
33. FRIEDLANDER, K., 1947. *The Psychoanalytic Approach to Juvenile Delinquency.* London: Kegan Paul, Trench and Trubner.
34. ———— 1945. The formation of the antisocial character. *Psychoanalytic Study of the Child*, 1.
35. GANTT, W. H., 1944. Experimental basis of neurotic behavior. *Psychosom. Med. Monogr.*, 3: Nos. 3 and 4.
36. GIBBENS, T. C. N. 1958. The Porteus Maze Test and delinquency. *Brit. J. Educ. Psychol.*, 28: 3: 209-216.
37. ———— 1961. *Trends in Juvenile Delinquency.* Geneva: W.H.O.
38. ———— 1963. *Psychiatric Studies of Borstal Boys.* London: Oxford Univ. Press.
39. GIBBONS, D. C. *Prospects and Problems of Delinquent Typology.* Mimeograph in the Dept. of Sociology Library, San Francisco State College.
40. ———— 1962. Prospects and problems of delinquent typology. *Sociol. Inquiry*, 1962: 235-244.
41. GITTINS, J., 1952. *Approved School Boys.* London: H.M.S.O.
42. ———— 1958. *Proc. 5th Internat. Congress on Social Defence, Stockholm*, Aug. 1958.
43. GLASSER, W., 1962. Reality Therapy: A Realistic Approach to the Young Offender. Mimeo. Address at Fall Institute of the British Columbia Corrections Association, Nov. 1962.
44. GLUECK, S. and E. T., 1950. *Unravelling Juvenile Delinquency.* The Commonwealth Fund. New York.
45. ———— 1956. *Physique and Delinquency.* New York: Harper Bros.
46. GRANT, J. D. and GRANT, M. Q., 1959. A group dynamic approach to the

treatment of nonconformists in the navy. *Annals of the American Academy of Political and Social Science*, Vol. 322: 126-135.

47. GRANT, J. D., 1963. Quoted by Maxwell Jones, Briggs and Tuxford, *Brit. J. Criminol.*, **4**, 227.

48. GRANT, M. Q., 1961. *Interpersonal Maturity Level Classification: Juvenile.* Community Treatment Project, State of California Dept. of Youth Authority, March 1961.

49. ——— 1961. *Interaction between Kinds of Treatment and Kinds of Delinquents.* Monograph 2, Board of Correction, State of California, July 1961.

50. GRANT, M.Q. *et al.*, 1957. See No. 110 below.

51. GREENACRE, P., 1945. Conscience in the psychopath. *Amer. J. Orthopsychiat.*, **15**: 495.

52. GRUNBERG, F. and POND, D. A., 1957. *J. Neurol. and Psychiat.*, **20**: 65.

53. GRUNHUT, M., 1961. *Probation and Mental Treatment.* University of Oxford.

54. HARRINGTON, J. A. and LETEMENDIA, F. J. J., 1958. Persistent psychiatric disorders after head injuries in children. *J. Ment. Sci.*, **104**: 1205.

55. HARTSHORNE, H. and MAY, M. A., 1928. *Studies in Deceit.* London: Macmillan.

56. HEALY, W., 1915. *The Individual Delinquent.* London: Heinemann.

57. HEALY, W. and BRONNER, A., 1936. *New Light on Delinquency.* New Haven: Yale Univ. Press.

58. HEWITT, L. E. and JENKINS, R. L., 1946. *Fundamental Patterns of Maladjustment.* Springfield, Ill.: Michigan Child Guidance Institute.

59. HILL, D. and WATTERSON, D., 1942. E.E.G. studies of psychopathic personalities. *J. Neurol. and Psychiat.*, **5**: 47.

60. HORSLEY, S., 1962. Neoteric staff therapy. *J. Ment. Subnorm.*, **7**: 1.

61. JENKINS, R. L., 1955. Adaptive and maladaptive delinquency. *The Nervous Child*, 2: 9.

62. JEPHCOTT, A. P. and CARTER, M. P., 1955. The Social Background of Delinquents. University of Nottingham. Quoted by Harriett Wilson (No. 120).

63. JOHNSON, A. M. and SZUREK, S. A., 1952. The genesis of antisocial acting-out in children and adults. *Psychoanal. Quart.*, **21**: 323.

64. JONES, G., 1958. Neurosis and experimental psychology. *J. Ment. Sci.*, **104**: 55.

65. KARPMAN, B., 1948. Milestones in the advancement of knowledge of the psychopathology of delinquency and crime. In *Orthopsychiatry Retrospect and Prospect* (ed. Lowrey and Sloane). American Orthopsychiatric Association.

66. KAUFMAN, I. and HEIMS, L., 1958. The body image of the juvenile delinquent. *Amer. J. Orthopsychiat.*, **28**: 146-159.

67. KINCH, J. W., 1962. Self conceptions of types of delinquents. *Sociol. Inquiry*, 1962: 228-234.

68. KNOX, E. G., 1962. *Proc. 69th Health Congress, Scarborough*, 1962, p. 14. Royal Society of Health, 90 Buckingham Palace Road, London, S.W. 1.

69. LEVY, S., 1959. Post-encephalitic behavior disorder—a forgotten entity. *Amer. J. Psychiat.*, **115**: 1062.

70. LEWIS, AUBREY, 1953. Health as a Social Concept. *Brit. J. Sociol.*, **4**, 119.

71. LEWIS, H., 1954. *Deprived Children*, p. 84. London: Oxford Univ. Press.

72. LIFTON, R. J., 1961. *Thought Reform and the Psychology of Totalism.* New York: Norton.

73. LITTLE, W. R. and NTSEKHE, 1959. Social class background of young offenders from London. *Brit. J. Delinq.*, **10**: 130.

74. MacFARLANE, J. W., ALLEN, L. and HONZIK, M. P., 1954. *A Developmental Study of the Behavior Problems of Normal Children.* Univ. of California Press.

75. MAIER, M. R. F., 1949. *Frustration: The Study of Behavior without a Goal.* New York: McGraw-Hill.
76. MANNHEIM, H., 1948. *Juvenile Delinquency in an English Middletown,* p. 101. London: Routledge & Kegan Paul.
77. MARQUHART, D. I., 1948. The pattern of punishment and its relation to abnormal fixation in human subjects. *J. Genet. Psychol.,* **39**: 107.
78. MASSERMAN, J., 1959, (ed.). Individual and Family Dynamics. *Science and Psychoanalysis,* Vol. 7. London.
79. MAYS, J. B., 1954. *Growing Up in the City.* Liverpool Univ. Press.
80. 1962. In *Delinquency and Discipline,* pp. 12-14. Councils and Education Press.
81. McCORD, J. and W., 1959. *The Origins of Crime.* New York: Columbia Univ. Press.
82. METFESSEL, M. and LOVELL, C., 1942. Individual correlates of crime. *Psychol. Bull.,* **39**, No. 3.
83. NEUMEYER, M. H., 1949. *Juvenile Delinquency in Modern Society.* New York: Van Nostrand.
84. OGDEN, D. A., 1959. Use of Surgical rehabilitation in young delinquents. *Brit. Med. J.,* i: 432.
85. OLTON, J. E. and FRIEDMAN, S., 1941. A psychiatric study of 100 criminals. *J. Nerv. Ment. Dis.,* **93**: 16.
86. PASAMANICK, B., ROGERS, M. E. and LILIENFELD, A. M., 1956. *Amer. J. Psychiat.,* **112**: 513.
87. PATRICK, J. R., 1934. *J. Comp. Psychol.,* **1811**; 153.
88. PIAGET, J., 1929. *The Child's Conception of the World.* New York: Harcourt Brace.
89. POND, D. A., 1961. Psychiatric aspects of epileptic and brain-damaged children. *Brit. Med. J.,* ii: 1377-1382 and 1454-1459.
90. POWERS, E. and WITMER, H., 1951. *An Experiment in the Prevention of Delinquency.* New York: Columbia Univ. Press.
91. PRECHTL, H. F. R., 1961. Children with Minimal Brain Damage. Address to the Association for Child Psychology and Psychiatry, London, 14th June 1961.
92. PYGOTT, F. and STREET, D. F., 1960. Unsuspected, treatable organic dementia. *Lancet,* i: 1371.
93. RECKLESS, W. C., 1943. Etiology of delinquent and criminal behavior. *Social Science Research Council Bull.,* **50**: New York.
94. 1961. *The Crime Problem.* New York: Appleton-Century-Crofts.
95. *Report of the Committee on Children and Young Persons,* Cmnd. 1191, 1960. London: H.M.S.O. See also *Prevention of Neglect of Children,* Cmnd. 1966, 1963. Edinburgh: H.M.S.O.
96. ROBIN, A. A., 1957. *Brit. J. Delinq.,* **8**: 139.
97. ROBINS, L. N. and O'NEAL, P., 1958. Mortality, mobility and crime: problem children 30 years later. *Amer. Sociol. Rev.,* **23**: 162.
98. RUBIN, S., 1961. *Crime and Juvenile Delinquency.* London: Stevens.
99. SCHMIDEBERG, M., 1960. Making the Patient Aware. *Crime and Delinquency,* July 1960: 255-261. See also *Lancet,* ii, 2nd August 1958.
100. SCHUESSLER, K. F. and CRESSY, D. R., 1950. Personality Characteristics of Criminals. *Amer. J. Sociol.,* **55**: 483-484.
101. SCHULMAN, IRVING, 1955. Dynamics and treatment of antisocial psychopathology in adolescents. *The Nervous Child,* **11**: 35.
102. SEARS, R. R., MACCOBY, E. E. and LEVIN, H., 1957. *Patterns of Child Rearing.* New York: Row Patterson.
103. SHAW, C. R., 1929. *Delinquency Areas.* Univ. of Chicago Press.

104. SHELDON, W. H., 1949. *Varieties of Delinquent Youth.* New York: Harper Bros.
105. SHOBEN, E. J., 1949. Assessment of parental attitudes in relation to child adjustment. *Genet. Psychol. Monogr.*, **39**: 101-148.
106. SLATER, E. T. O., 1953. *Psychotic and Neurotic Illnesses in Twins.* Spec. Rept. Series, No. 278. London: Medical Research Council.
107. STELZNER, H., 1911. *The Psychopathic Constitution and its Sociological Meanings.* Berlin: Karger.
108. STOTT, D. H., 1958. *Interim Report on the Glasgow Survey of Boys put on Probation during 1957.* Univ. of Glasgow, July 1958. (2nd and 3rd reports have followed.)
109. 1959, 1962. *J. Genet. Psychol.*, 1959, **94**: 233. Also *Amer. J. Psychiat.*, 1962, **118**: 781.
110. SULLIVAN, C., GRANT, M. Q. and GRANT, J. D., 1957. The development of interpersonal maturity: applications to delinquency. *Psychiatry*, **20**: 4.
111. SUTHERLAND, E. H. and CRESSY, D. R., 1955. *Principles of Criminology.* Chicago: Lippincott.
112. THURSTONE, L. L., 1931. The measurement of social attitudes. *J. Abnorm. and Soc. Psychol.*, **26**: 249-269.
113. TONG, J. E. and MURPHY, I. C., 1960. A review of stress reactivity research in relation to psychopathology and psychopathic behaviour disorders. *J. Ment. Sci.*, **106**, 1960: 1273-1293.
114. TRASLER, G., 1962. *The Explanation of Criminality.* London: Routledge & Kegan Paul.
115. WALTERS, A. A., 1963. Delinquent Generations. *Brit. J. Criminol.*, **3**: 391.
116. WEEKS, A., 1958. *Youthful Offenders at Highfields.* Ann Arbor: Univ. of Michigan Press.
117. WEST, D. J., 1963. *The Habitual Prisoner.* London: Macmillan.
118. WILKINS, L. T., 1960. *Delinquent Generations.* London: H.M.S.O.
119. WILLIAMS, P., 1962. *Patterns of Teenage Delinquency.* London: Christian, Economic and Social Research Foundation.
120. WILSON, H., 1962. *Delinquency and Child Neglect.* London: George Allen & Unwin.
121. WILSON, Prof. R., Chairman of the Bristol Social Project. Address delivered on 20.2.61. See also *Relieving Stresses of Living on Council Estates.* Bristol Social Project, The Council House, Bristol.
122. WINNICOTT, D. W., 1958. The antisocial tendency. See *Collected Papers*, Ch. 15. London: Tavistock Publications.
123. WOODWARD, M., 1955. The Role of Low Intelligence in Delinquency. *Brit. J. Delinq.*, **5**, 4: 281-303.
124. WOOTTON, B., 1959. *Social Science and Social Pathology.* London: George Allen & Unwin.

XVII

SUICIDAL ATTEMPTS IN

CHILDHOOD AND ADOLESCENCE

P. H. CONNELL*

M.D., D.P.M.

Physician, Bethlem Royal Hospital and the Maudsley Hospital, London

1

Introduction

Although there is a voluminous literature concerning suicide and suicidal attempts in adults, there is very little literature concerning suicide or suicidal attempts in children. Successful suicide is said to be very rare in children, and only recently has the topic of suicidal attempts been brought to the fore, notably in the United States of America and in Sweden.

Suicide can be studied by a number of methods, which include the sociological approach, the anthropological approach, the ecological approach and the psychiatric approach. All these are as important in investigations into suicide and attempted suicide in children and adolescents as they are in relation to adults.

It is the purpose of this chapter to present a short description of the field of suicidal attempts and suicidal threats in children and adolescents, and to pay particular attention to the clinical aspects of diagnosis, precipitating factors and management.

For the purpose of this presentation the following definition of a suicide will be used:

One who dies by his own hand; one who commits self-murder. Also one who attempts or has a tendency to commit suicide. (SHORTER OXFORD DICTIONARY.)

Children are often introduced to the concept of death when they are very young, and the term 'passing away', 'gone to Heaven' or some such

* Formerly Physician in Charge, Child Psychiatry Unit, Newcastle General Hospital, in association with the University of Newcastle.

404 SUICIDAL ATTEMPTS IN CHILDHOOD AND ADOLESCENCE

phrase is used. The concept of life after death, which is pleasant and satisfying, is therefore often the child's first concept of death. Nevertheless if a child tries to kill himself or succeeds, even if this is to go to the pleasant and rewarding 'after life', he is attempting or succeeding in committing suicide. Whenever an individual plans his own self-destruction he is, for the purposes of this presentation, a suicidal individual.

2

Incidence

There are few studies of the incidence of suicidal threats and suicidal attempts in children and adolescents.

Kanner (21) notes that the data furnished by the United States Mortality Statistics, gathered by the Department of Commerce, Bureau of Census, show that in the years 1926–1929 inclusive between 33 and 53 children under the age of 14 years lost their lives annually through self-inflicted deaths. More recent statistics in that country (1942–1946) showed a range of 46–67 deaths from suicide; and of the total number of infantile suicides in the U.S.A. between 1933 and 1946 (74·5% males, 25·5% females), 2·5% were between 5 and 9 years old and the rest ranged from 10–14 years.

Jacobziner (20), writing on attempted suicides in children, noted that there were 299 cases of attempted suicide in children between the ages of 8 and 19, though most of the attempts were at the age of 18, and that the ratio of attempted suicide to suicide was 50 : 1, which would give a figure of 6 successful suicides between these ages. These individuals did not vary from the average population in physical, mental and emotional status. One-third attempted suicide between April and June.

Bergstrand and Otto (7) studied the incidence of suicidal attempts in Swedish children and adolescents for the period 1955–1959 inclusive, and examined the case notes on patients under 21 years of age who had been treated because of suicidal attempts from all hospitals in Sweden, with the exception of some special clinics to which patients of this type were not usually admitted. Of 471 relevant hospitals and advisory institutions, 465 (99%) furnished information. In all, details of 1,727 patients from all parts of Sweden were studied.

The sex distribution was 20% boys and 80% girls. The youngest patient was 10 years old. Incidence increased with age, particularly at the 14-year age level. The number of cases of 16 years and under was about 517. Only some 80 cases were boys. The highest frequency of attempts was in November and the lowest in June and July. Information was obtained from 512 patients concerning the time of day at which the attempt was made: the majority occurred late in the afternoon or during the night before 12 p.m.; only 6% of the attempts were made in the morning. During the period 1955–1958 there were 245 successful suicides (164 males, 81 females) within the age group 0–24 years. Five of these were under 15 years of age (4 males, 1 female), 73 were 15–19 years of age (48 males, 25 females), and 167 were 20–24 years of age (112 males, 55 females).

Bergstrand and Otto (7) also refer to the tendency to conceal suicidal attempts, and note the possibility of registering them as attempts at abortion. They also draw attention to the fact that a large proportion of those who attempt suicide in the age groups investigated take tablets at bedtime, and that it is probable that many of these awake in the morning and the environment does not interpret these as suicidal attempts; they may not even be seen by a doctor.

Toolan (34), writing on 'Suicide and Suicidal Attempts in Children and Adolescents', states that 'contrary to popular opinion, suicide and suicidal attempts are not rare in childhood and adolescence.' Referring to the vital statistics of the country (U.S.A., 1959), he notes that successful suicides were infrequent under 10 years of age and that in fact only 3 such cases were listed. In the 10–14 year old group, however, suicide was encountered more frequently, and there was a distinct increase in the 15–19 year group. He observes that although these figures may appear low, they are in fact higher than the deaths from nephritis and nephrosis, leukemia, all forms of pneumonia, tuberculosis and poliomyelitis in the 15–19 year group. He also stressed that the figures quoted are undoubtedly all under-estimated and that many cases of suicide are concealed by parents and well-meaning physicians under the guise of accidents, and that many accidents are themselves at best thinly disguised attempts at self-destructive activity. Having made this point, Toolan observes that accidents vastly outnumber all other causes of death in childhood and adolescence.

Toolan also notes that in the statistics quoted successful suicides were much commoner in males than females, and that unsuccessful suicidal attempts were very much more common in females than in males. Suicide was especially common among university students, ranking second only to accidents as a cause of death.

Toolan then reviews the statistics from Bellevue Hospital, New York for the year 1960, and notes that of approximately 900 admissions to the child and adolescent services, 102 were for suicidal attempts and threats. Of these, 18 were under 12 years of age, and 84 from 12 to 17 years of age. Toolan's figures therefore also demonstrated the increased incidence with age, particularly at the 14-year-old level.

The range of intellectual functioning was about the usual in the Bellevue patient population, except that fewer mental defectives were encountered among the suicidal population.

It would seem therefore, from the study of these three papers, that the writers agree that there is an increase with age in suicidal attempts among the child and adolescent population, but that there may well be factors which lead to the suppression of suicidal attempts in diagnosis, so that in the younger age group the figures must be particularly suspect.

3

Incidence in Great Britain

In Great Britain there are no available survey figures of suicide or suicidal attempts among children. The writer has had occasion to enquire from colleagues in different parts of Great Britain who are working in the child psychiatric field concerning the number of suicidal attempts they have seen, and has often been met with a blank stare, followed by remarks that none had been seen, or perhaps an isolated case or two, the details of which had been forgotten.

Kenyon (23) studied 43 cases of emergencies among children of 12 years and under seen at the Maudsley Hospital during the year 1958–1959, and noted that only 5 cases (11·6%) were referred on account of threatened or attempted suicide, whereas 22 cases (51·5%) were referred on account of threatened or attempted violence.

The question is posed, therefore, whether Great Britain is in fact different from the U.S.A., Sweden and other countries in that suicidal attempts in children and adolescents are much rarer, or whether there is some mechanism at work which obscures the real incidence of such events in the British population.

Knowledge of the organisation and practice of medicine in Great Britain may supply some theoretical reasons for this apparent dearth of attempted suicides in children and adolescents.

Firstly, most cases of suicidal attempt in children and adolescents may, if the attempt is severe enough to warrant it, attend the casualty department of a general hospital, but if the effect of the attempt is not serious may receive emergency treatment and be discharged back to the care of the family doctor. If the patient requires medical treatment of a more prolonged nature, he will be admitted either to an emergency bed in a general medical ward or to the paediatric ward. After medical treatment has been effective in saving life, the patient may or may not be referred to a psychiatrist, according to the gravity with which the attempt is regarded by the physician, and to the physician's orientation towards psychiatry. A number of cases will be discharged without psychiatric referral (though the recent Ministry of Health recommendation that all cases of attempted suicide be referred for psychiatric examination may cut down the numbers) to the family doctor.

Secondly, the regrettable dichotomy between adult psychiatry and child psychiatry, and the fact that the adolescent age group comprises a kind of 'no man's land', together with the organisational fact that many child psychiatric units have no contact with the local general hospitals, may well lead to the referral of such cases to a psychiatrist from the adult department. He may or may not have an interest in the adolescent age group, and may or may not have had any experience with children or with the particular problems raised by suicidal attempts in children or adolescents.

Thirdly, it must be recognised that in many hospitals in this country there is still inadequate psychiatric cover, the Child Psychiatric Services in particular being grossly inadequate, so that in many instances in which physicians would like to refer for psychiatric help they are forced to deal with the problem themselves as best they can.

Fourthly, it must be recognised that there may well be a tendency to cover up the fact of a suicidal attempt in children because of the social stigma of the use of such a word as 'suicide', as well as a tendency to regard such events as being due to 'silliness' or 'hysterical behaviour'. These labels are used frequently and tend to imply that there was no real intent to commit suicide and that therefore the word suicide may conveniently be avoided.

Fifthly, many cases which show little physical disturbance because of the attempt may be dealt with by the family doctor, or may not even be referred to him.

Finally, it may be that the child, when accessible, appreciates society's disapproval, or finds that the attempt has led to an alleviation of the factors which drove him to make the attempt, so that when interrogated he denies any suicidal intention.

In the Newcastle area there is only one full-time child psychiatric unit, and this has been functioning for only five and a half years. This unit, the University Teaching Unit, though centred at a non-teaching general hospital, has developed close links with the teaching hospital and the child health departments of the general hospitals in the area. The effective total population represented by the number of 41 definite suicidal attempts in children aged 16 or under can be estimated at about 500,000. If the total population of Great Britain is taken to be 47 million, at the same level of incidence the number of suicidal attempts in children of 16 and under for the whole country would be 771 per year. If the total of 64 suicidal attempts and threats in the Newcastle area is taken, this would represent an incidence for the whole country of 1,204 per year.

Taking into account the fact that the Newcastle unit has been functioning for only five years and that there is a long waiting list, these estimates must be regarded as minimal. If the figure of 16 suicidal attempts seen in 1962 alone is used, the incidence for the whole country per year would be 1,600 and this again must be considered a gross underestimate, unless there are social or cultural factors which make Tyneside a unique area.

The facts referred to above clearly demonstrate that the real incidence of suicidal attempts and threats in children and adolescents is still unknown, but that there is good reason to believe it is sufficiently high in this country, as in others, to present a formidable problem to society. If evidence can be produced to demonstrate that such individuals are in fact in need of psychiatric treatment, and that such treatment is of value, then the implications for the provision of psychiatric services will be considerable.

4

Aetiology and Psychopathology

There have been many suggestions and comments concerning the aetiology and psychopathology of suicidal attempts in adults, but on suicidal attempts in children the literature is sparse, and there are very few well documented case reports.

Kanner (21), in his brief chapter on suicide among children, considers that full-fledged mental illness in the form of schizophrenic or depressive psychosis is responsible for children's suicides only in a very small minority of cases. Nevertheless he goes on to recommend that any profound unhappiness in a child, whether it is a symptom of genuine depression or not, calls for a thorough investigation and for remedial measures. He goes on to mention 'the dread of failure in school with the ensuing punishment by strict and unrelenting parents, the fear of the brutalities of an alcoholic and tyrannical father, and misconceptions about the prophesied ill results of masturbation' as aetiological factors. He also mentions spite reactions in emotionally unstable, feeble-minded children, and intelligent, solitary and educationally misguided children, as well as other factors such as 'obsessions and compulsions which render the patient so unhappy that he entertains suicidal ideas'.

Kanner then refers to Bender and Schilder (6), who studied eighteen children under 13 years of age who entertained suicidal preoccupations. The variety of conscious motives all had in common the desire of the child to escape a situation which seemed unbearable. He also quoted Dublin and Bunzel (17), who reported a case of a 12-year-old boy who hanged himself because he had made no friend in his new school, and a 14-year-old boy who wrote a note before he turned on the gas:

To die will be a glorious adventure. It is my belief that my spirit will some day enter into the body of a playwright and will call forth a story of a boy who loved to dream, the story of a boy who was so disillusioned that he couldn't stand it any more. The play will make the man famous and yet it will be my story, so my ambition will not be unfulfilled.

Kanner also refers to Zilboorg (35), who referred to homosexuality and feminine strivings in boys playing a paramount role in the problem; to Bender and Schilder (6), who stress the motive of spite; and to Schachter and Cotte (30), who mention parental death, divorce or desertion, rebellion against the parents, affection hunger, protest against the curtailment of liberty, fear of imprisonment after an anti-social act, an unhappy love affair, and wounded pride.

Finally, Kanner mentions 'suicidal attempts' of children being only staged without the real goal of death, and hysterical children who alarm the family by some means of self-mutilation, with the aim of attracting attention and being talked about.

Chess (13) notes that threats of suicide are made by children of all ages, although they are usually hostile gestures designed to hurt someone in the environment. 'The older the patient,' says Chess, 'the more his acting-out may find expression in anti-social behaviour, nuisance activities, self-destructive trends and even suicidal attempts.' Later Chess notes that among those requiring in-patient care are 'children who respond to anxiety by suicidal attempts'.

Jacobziner (20) suggests, as have others, that the reason for the higher incidence of attempted suicides among girls and among adolescents is probably due to the greater impulsiveness of the young female, who does not premeditate the act, nor actually desire to die. It is, he says, 'in the main a precipitous, impulsive act, a sudden reaction to a stressful situation'. He then suggests that it is possible that many accidents, particularly among children with a history of repeatism or accident-proneness, are subconscious attempts at suicide.

Among the causes of suicide and suicidal attempts among adolescents Jacobziner mentions 'unresolved conflicts, frustrations, disappointments, guilt feelings, loss of self-esteem, fear of punishment and the real or imaginary loss of a love object'. He states that the motivating force is aggression, usually directed towards the love object and serving as a means of punishing the parents. 'It is an act of hostility against a restraining figure. Children get feelings of rage towards frustrating objects, as well as feelings of helplessness, and they become depressed and use a number of defensive mechanisms. When the defensive mechanism breaks down, an attempt at suicide may be made.'

Bergstrand and Otto (7) mention that among the immediate reasons for the suicide attempts in nearly 1,300 cases were love problems (30%) and family problems (25%), girls being in the majority in these two groups. Boys constituted a relatively large part of the group having school problems (4·8% of total), and dominated the group suffering from mental illness (13·5% of total); in these two groups 19% were boys and 8% girls.

In Bergstrand and Otto's material, 83% of the patients belonged to the low income group, and 5% were of foreign origin, chiefly refugee youths. In only 4% were the family conditions of the patients considered entirely normal. Alcoholism in one or both parents was recorded in 15%, and in 28% the parents were mentally ill or revealed neurotic disorders to such a degree that the physician in charge of the case recorded them. A broken home (because of divorce, death of one parent, unmarried mother etc.) was reported in nearly half the cases (44%).

Toolan (34) observes that less than one-third of his cases resided with both parents, and that many of the 'intact' homes were emotionally disorganised. He notes however that few foster children were included in his population. The absence of fathers from the lives of the children studied is specially mentioned.

Toolan provides a diagnostic list, as follows:

Childhood schizophrenia	12
Schizophrenic reaction	33
Personality pattern disorder	10
Personality trait disorder	25
Transient situation reaction	2
Mental deficiency	4
Neurotic reaction	16.

He then goes on to stress that

suicidal attempts have been overlooked in children and adolescents . . . [because of] the erroneous concept that youngsters do not experience depression. It is true that they do not exhibit the signs and symptoms of adult depressive reactions but rather other symptoms. In the latency child behavioural problems (temper tantrums, disobedience, truancy, feeling that no one cares for him, running away from home, accident-proneness, masochistic actions, self-destructive behaviour) often indicate depressive feelings. The youngster is convinced that he is bad, evil, unacceptable. Such feelings lead him into anti-social behaviour which in turn only further reinforces his belief that he is no good. The youngster will often feel inferior to other children; that he is ugly and stupid. Boys, especially, have a need to hide soft, tender, weak sentiments. Denial is often used to ward off depressive feelings.

Toolan observes that the adolescent may exhibit his depression by boredom, restlessness, preoccupation with trivia, loss of interest in things, acting-out by delinquency, sexual promiscuity, alcohol and drugs, excessive fatigue, hypochondriacal preoccupation, and difficulty in concentration. Analysing the causes for the suicidal attempts, Toolan suggests the following categories:

(1) Anger at another which is internalised in the form of guilt and depression;
(2) Attempts to manipulate another to gain love and affection, or to punish another;
(3) A signal of distress;
(4) Reactions to feelings of inner disintegration, as a response to hallucinatory commands etc.;
(5) A desire to join a dead relative.

The common denominator in all depressive reactions, suggests Toolan, is loss of the love object, and he goes on to elaborate this hypothesis in psychoanalytical terms.

Shneidman and Farberow (31) also state that from the psychoanalytical viewpoint the primary dynamic reason for the suicidal attempt is the real or threatened loss of a love object, and refer to Bibring (9), who emphasised that, whenever children feel the threat of the loss of a love object, they not only develop feelings of rage towards the frustrating object but feelings of helplessness and worthlessness as well.

These writers give a few short case histories of suicidal children, in which they quote instances of dying to punish the parents, self-destructive tendencies in a child (one attempt following the use of Dennis Browne Splints for congenital club feet), depressive reaction following the death of a parent, suicidal attempt in a hysterical reaction, suicidal thoughts and actions in anxiety states and compulsion neuroses, character neuroses, perversions and psychoses.

Meerloo (25), writing on suicide at all ages, discusses the concept of death, and notes that the child's concept of death and departure starts early in life, although hidden in the magic thinking of early childhood. He mentions that it usually stems from a loving and caring elderly person's 'passing away'—a phrase which is a denial of the reality of death—this denial mechanism being taught very early to children, who are supposed to look upon death as a pleasant trip to a far away country. 'The ego cannot conceive of its own disappearance, but under the surface is the fear of not being any more, the fear that the body will be a passive prey to fate,' says Meerloo; and again, 'Unconsciously there is always the biological aware-ness and even wisdom of the narrow path of life and that once it will all end.'

'The parents' withdrawal into mourning', notes Meerloo, 'becomes an additional loss for the child who has not received any acceptable clarification of the life-death concept. He gets evasion and subterfuge instead of the double attention needed at the moment.' This may lead to the child identifying with the dead relative, and to the thought that he can get mother's affection only if he is dead. 'Suicide may represent the preco-cious victory of the inner drive toward death. Man's inner destructivity is, like every instinctual tendency (Freud (19)), rooted in both the primary drive to live and in its opposite tendency to return to the inorganic matrix.'

Returning to the special instance of children's motivations, Meerloo states that the child, usually an adolescent, has a different relation to death from that of older people in the decline of life. Death for the young person does not mean an irrevocable fate, but is a getting away from something.

Fear of punishment, loss of self-esteem, and revenge on the punishing parent, are common motives. Thus suicide may be a pathetic complaint against a world without love and mercy. The suicidal act affords at the same time a passive, non-violent revenge on people who want to punish and seemingly annihilate the victim. In his fantasy the individual who commits suicide thinks that as a last triumph he leaves a lonely, sad and mournful world behind him. . . . Especi-ally in suicide by children we realise how much rejection, teasing and vituperation have to do with loss of self-esteem, and how these humiliations can drive the young person to suicide.

Stengel (32) comments upon the fact that the psychoanalytic literature on suicide is surprisingly small, and that the fundamental psychoanalytical propositions have not changed in essentials since Bernfeld (8) formulated them. Referring to Bernfeld, Stengel summarises the psychoanalytic formulations as follows:

(1) A person committing suicide harbours strong unconscious murder impulses against another person. Suicide is an act of revenge.
(2) The murderous impulse will lead to suicide only if the individual unconsciously identifies himself with the hated, previously loved, object so that he kills it in killing himself.
(3) A tendency to self-punishment is usually important. The individual feels guilty on account of his murderous impulses.
(4) Occasionally, the choice of method of suicide has symbolic significance.

Stengel and Cook (33) stress the importance of regarding the successful and the unsuccessful suicide populations as different, and of studying the latter population, and also of recognising the suicidal threat and attempt as an alarm signal (which is an appeal for help from the environment); of recognising the risk to life; and of studying the reaction of the environment to the threat or attempt, and thus obtaining a full understanding of the complex inter-reactions between the individual and his life situation. Suicidal attempts, say Stengel and Cook, can no longer be regarded purely as manifestations of destructive urges.

The question of suicide and depression in children is clearly important, and the reader is referred to Anthony and Scott (3), who note that a depressive reaction of the manic-depressive type is exceedingly rare in childhood; to Kenyon (23), who (among others) suggests that children cannot tolerate a depressive affect and 'act out' instead; to an annotation in the *British Medical Journal* (2) quoting Campbell (12), who discusses in descriptive terms the question of manic-depressive disease in children, and who claims to have seen a large number of such cases even more difficult to diagnose than the endogenous depression of adults; and to Olsen (27), who followed up for a period from 1–14 years 28 manic-depressive patients whose first attack occurred before the age of 19. The frequency of attacks reached its peak at the age of 17 and the attacks were then mainly of mania, whereas mania and depression were equally common from the age of 23.

The question of depression in adults who suffered childhood bereavement is also of interest, and the reader is referred to the papers of Brown (10) and Batchelor and Napier (5).

Bruhn (11), studying adult patients, compared a group of 91 attempted suicides with a control group of 91 psychiatric out-patients who had not attempted suicide, matching the groups for sex, age and occupation. He concluded that the factors of household instability, loss of employment status of breadwinner, residential mobility and marital disharmony, were more prevalent among attempted suicides from broken homes than among non-suicidal psychiatric out-patients also from broken homes.

Balser and Masterson (4) noted that two-thirds of their suicide cases in the adolescent group studied were schizophrenics.

Kaufman (22), writing on crimes of violence and delinquency in schizophrenic children, refers to Reichard and Tillman (28), who in a paper on 'Murder and Suicide as Defences Against Schizophrenic Psychosis' had made the comment: 'Inasmuch as murder and suicide have in common with schizophrenia the factor of unassuageable anger, they may on occasion serve as alternate channels of discharge and thereby preserve the ego from the disintegrating effects of undischarged rage, as manifested in a schizophrenic psychosis.'

Connell (15) examined a group of 100 delinquents committed to an approved school who had been sent to a classifying school for assessment and allocation to a training school. This group was selected at random, apart from being matched for age and intelligence with the total population entering the classifying school during the time of the survey. Twenty-seven of these boys, whose ages ranged from 8 to 17 years, had had suicidal ideas. Of these, seventeen had had vague suicidal ideas of the kind in which the thoughts that life is not worth living, that it would be possible to lie down and go to sleep and not wake up, and the wish to be dead, were prominent, but in which there was no wish actually to take life. Two boys had had vague thoughts that life was not worth living, coupled with the idea of killing themselves, but had not elaborated any particular ideas of method or even considered any method. Eight boys had had definite suicidal ideas, involving not only thoughts of killing themselves but also consideration of method. The latter included jumping in the river, throwing themselves under a bus, putting their head in the gas oven, stabbing themselves with a knife, poisoning themselves, cutting themselves with a razor blade or knife, hanging themselves, and falling downstairs on purpose. At least eleven boys had had these thoughts before being committed to an approved school and at least ten boys had only had these thoughts and feelings after their committal. In the group who had had the thoughts before committal, the thoughts were noted to be associated with the following kinds of stresses: getting into trouble; death of a pet; disturbance in the relationship with an aunt; placement in a boarding school; mother and brother 'getting at him'; having a hard job to do.

The foregoing selections from the many writings concerning suicide, and the few writings on suicide in children and adolescents, have been chosen in order to demonstrate the various methods of approach and thinking on this subject, together with some of the facts which have been published. The reader is referred to the monographs of Durkheim (18), Sainsbury (29), Meerloo (25), Dahlgren (16), Stengel and Cook (33), Dublin and Bunzel (17), Morselli (26) and von Andics (1), which will form a basis for a wider exploration of the subject.

The writings quoted demonstrate the complexity of the problem of suicide and suicidal threats and attempts, and show that views upon aetiology, classification, and association with recognised clinical psychiatric conditions are far from being uniform. As with most subjects about which there is little concrete fact and considerable methodological difficulty in obtaining incidence figures and control groups, speculation and complex and wordy writing abound. Confusion, dogma and enthusiasm sometimes outweigh clinical acumen and objective appraisal.

There are, however, a number of practical clinical issues which those interested in the diagnosis and treatment of suicidal threats and attempts in children and adolescents will have to face. Among these are:

(1) Two opposing views—that full-fledged mental illness in the form of schizophrenic or depressive psychosis is rarely responsible for children's suicides, and that suicidal attempts have been overlooked in children and adolescents because of the erroneous concept that youngsters do not experience depression. This raises the question whether the precipitating causes are themselves directly responsible for suicidal attempts, whether the precipitating cause acts through causing a depressive reaction which then leads to a suicidal attempt, or whether in fact there may be no precipitating cause and the patient becomes depressed and then suicidal.

(2) The observations that a very wide range of stresses may result in suicidal attempts, but that these must be non-specific since they can be experienced by a large number of children without resulting in the suicidal attempt. Thus the question is raised of individual differences between the children who make the attempt and others who, under similar stresses, find other methods of solution.

(3) The possible differences in import and individuality in those who have suicidal thoughts (such as, 'I wish I were dead'), those who have thoughts of actually killing themselves, those who actually make an attempt to kill themselves, those who threaten to do so, and those who actually do kill themselves. Are these a continuum of individuals in which the thought or manifestation is merely a matter of degree, or are they different entities with different psychopathology and different prognosis?

(4) How can the suicide-prone individuals be ascertained before matters become so drastic that suicidal thoughts and attempts occur?

(5) What, if any, are the main features of the clinical examination, diagnosis and treatment of children and adolescents who do make suicidal attempts?

5

Clinical Examination

Those who have had any continuing experience at all with children who have attempted or threatened suicide would agree that no child or adolescent who has thought about killing himself, threatened to kill himself, or attempted to kill himself should be examined or treated with other than all the resources of the psychiatric approach. Only those children, of whom there are many, who when a bit bored or after frustration or punishment say 'I wish I were dead' should be excluded from the above generalisation; and even of these some may show features, such as a disturbed home background, which might indicate full psychiatric, psychometric, educational and social exploration.

There are a number of special points about the examination of children who have made or are suspected of having made suicidal attempts, which the examining psychiatrist should understand if he is to obtain a real picture of the patient and the events under enquiry.

The first of these is the fact that children and adolescents are much more responsive to the environment and to the attitudes and opinions of adult individuals in the environment than are most adults. Thus the actual event of the attempt, the reactions of the parents and family towards it, the attitude of the parents towards the child who has made the attempt, the attitude of the family doctor called in, as well as that of the casualty doctor and the ward doctor if the patient is admitted, may have a very potent effect upon the general and verbal impressions the child may give later at a psychiatric interview. For this reason and for ordinary psychiatric reasons a direct and authoritative approach which goes straight into questions about the full details of the suicidal attempt, how it was done, etc. is very likely to be met with denials that suicide was in fact intended, and by excuses and rationalisation to explain the behaviour. Furthermore, since many children and adolescents attempt suicide because of the reaction to rejection by the parent or parents, and since anxiety and concern about the possible death of the child often lead to overt expressions of concern and of love for him, the immediate stress of the rejection is removed and the child's ability to repress unpleasant memories comes into action. This again may encourage a denial or a much watered down version of what actually happened before and during the suicidal attempt. Alternatively, an unsuccessful attempt which does not require hospital admission may result in scorn, derision and increased expressions of hostility from the parents, who bring the child up to the out-patient psychiatric unit in a state which leads him to believe that removal from home or some dire action may take place, so that he is, at first, unwilling to talk about the stresses at home and the suicidal attempt itself.

A further difficulty arises from the fact that, if the examining psychiatrist uses words such as 'depression', the child may not know what he means, since sophistication of this kind is often lacking and he may deny or admit to 'depression' without really understanding the question.

All the above factors make it imperative that a gentle, non-demanding technique be used in examining the child or adolescent referred, and the examiner's anxiety to discover the true facts should be tempered with caution and patience.

The length of time elapsing between the suicidal attempt and examination by the psychiatrist is also important, in that defensive covering up and repression of the facts and antecedents of the suicide are much more firmly established if the examination is delayed too long, when the real feelings and experiences of the child may be very difficult to elicit and may never be brought to light. One girl, seen personally by the writer in a general hospital about ten days after admission for barbiturate intoxication, repeatedly denied that she had taken any drugs at all, and it was only one year later at follow-up examination that she related what she had done. This, in spite of the fact that there was a significantly high blood barbiturate level and that she was told about this when first examined. In this particular instance the child's denial was fostered and encouraged by parental denial that she had taken tablets or attempted suicide.

For the above reasons it is important that there should be the minimum of questioning by family doctors, casualty officers, paediatric housemen or other persons concerning the full details of the suicidal attempt, and that the fuller enquiry should be left to the psychiatrist. He should have the special techniques and understanding of this kind of interview, and be prepared and able to take the time needed to elicit the facts, even if it requires several interviews with the patient.

One other feature of the examination must be stressed. It is most important that the examining psychiatrist should avoid any suggestion of condemning the act, and that a warm, accepting and friendly approach should be used.

Special enquiry into various aspects of the suicidal attempt will be necessary if the common mistake of classifying these attempts as 'hysterical gestures' or 'silliness' is to be avoided. Thus it may be necessary to find out the following if the full clinical picture is to be assessed:

(a) Was anyone present when the child made the attempt?
(b) Was anyone in the house when the child made the attempt?
(c) Did the child come into the room immediately afterwards and tell a parent that he or she had made the attempt?
(d) Did the child or adolescent tell any friend about the attempt, and did the child leave any instructions either with the friend or in a suicide note?
(e) Where did the child get the tablets from?
(f) Did the child know what the tablets were for?
(g) Did the child take all the tablets, or only some? If the latter, why did the child not take them all?
(h) Had the child made previous attempts?
(i) Had the child made previous suicidal threats?
(j) Had any other member of the family made a suicidal attempt?
(k) Had there been any stress, scene, disagreement, or happening before the attempt?

Only if the answers to the above questions, or most of them, are found is it possible to classify the suicidal attempt in terms of seriousness, dangerousness, goal motivation and so on.

The above full enquiry will need to be made not only with the child, as and when he is able to answer such questions, but also with the parent or others who were present.

The above specific enquiry should be backed up by a comprehensive psychiatric history which will cover the development of the child physically and mentally, the reaction of the child to stresses, and full details of any recent stresses—in particular the death of a relative, death of a close friend, or events leading to a reorientation of family emotional dynamics such as the birth of a sibling, the divorce of the parents, or grandmother coming to stay, as well as any steadily increasing or sudden stresses at school or in the neighbourhood.

The examination of the parent will also need caution and circumspection, as it is common for parents to be unable to face up to the implications of the suicidal attempt without help. In this respect it is important that the examining psychiatrist does show concern about the child—though avoiding condemnation of the suicidal act; and it is often useful, after getting to know the parent, to explore the situation with questions such as 'When did your child first begin to show that she was unhappy?' or similar phrases which assume that the child was unhappy and that it might have been a continuing process. This kind of enquiry will often 'unlock' the parents' feelings and make possible the production of a history of events prior to the actual suicidal attempt.

It will be apparent, from the tenor of these remarks about clinical examination, that one of the dangers of the suicidal attempt situation is that medical measures of resuscitation may be used, the child returned home and the whole episode relegated to the limbo of unpleasant incidents which must be forgotten. The basic cause may therefore never reach the light of day, with the consequent risk of further and possibly successful suicidal attempts, assuming that the first attempt did not produce a permanent reorientation of emotional attitudes in the home which would allow the child a more settled and happy existence.

In all cases where the patient has been referred direct to the psychiatric out-patient clinic, a full and thorough physical examination is necessary.

6

Observations Based upon the Newcastle Population Studied

Case histories demonstrate many of the clinical findings in children and adolescents who have made suicidal threats or attempts, provided these events have been taken seriously enough for a full investigation to be carried out. Cases of depression in childhood or adolescence which have led to suicidal thoughts, but not to overt expression of them nor to suicidal attempts, have not been included in these observations, though children and adolescents of this category have been seen from time to time.

The writer's personal approach to the problem of suicidal threats and attempts can now be stated.

Theoretically there are a number of levels at which children may raise the question of suicide. They can be tabulated as follows, though in practice there may be a degree of overlap:

(1) Non-specific Suicidal Thoughts—'I wish I were dead', 'Life is not worth living', etc. These are common in children and are usually a response to some frustration, boredom or lack of attention, but are short-lived. These thoughts may be voiced aloud in the height of the disappointments or frustration, but do not reach the level of 'I shall kill myself', 'I shall commit suicide', etc. At this level the suicidal idea need not be considered as a serious manifestation unless the idea is expressed often and there is evidence of failure to achieve normality in the interim period.

(2) Specific Suicidal Thoughts—'I wish I were dead', 'I am going to kill myself', 'I shall throw myself under a bus', 'I shall take my mother's tablets', etc. At this level the thoughts, whether expressed verbally in the form of threats or comments, or whether elicited as part of a general examination by the family doctor or hospital doctor in departments other than psychological medicine, must be regarded as indicating a severe emotional disturbance with a definite risk to life. Similarly these thoughts must also be taken very seriously when elicited by psychiatrists.

(3) Suicidal Attempts. Definite attempts on the part of a child or adolescent to take his own life, whatever the concept of death, must always be regarded as being very serious indeed and indicative of a severe breakdown in the emotional homeostasis of the child's life. This applies to all such attempts, whether made in the presence of others or not, and whether the attempt has been dangerous to life or apparently only half-hearted and trivial.

The above statements are made categorically because of the writer's experience that there is in fact a strong tendency for doctors and others to take suicidal threats and attempts in children and adolescents lightly and to call them 'silliness', 'childishness', 'impulsiveness', 'just a gesture', 'hysterical' and so on. This viewpoint has often released the doctor from the responsibility of seeing that full investigations are made and from the responsibility of referring for psychiatric advice. The writer has seen cases of suicidal attempts in children and adolescents who have been seen by adult psychiatrists and have been labelled as 'hysterical', or 'gesture', or 'hyperiridic' (24) (morbid state of hostile tension leading to suicide), when there has been a clear history of tablet taking when alone, a persistent attempt to hide the fact of the tablet taking, no display of 'histrionics', no hostile tension state, and no clear attempt to manipulate the adults in the environment and achieve positive gain from the situation. Although the concept of the 'hyperiridic' suicide appears to be a valid one, it again tends to lead to a failure to elicit previous and continued depression or disturbance in the child, and it encourages concentration upon one aspect of the attempt itself and its antecedents rather than a wider investigation.

Experience demonstrates the extent of the family disturbance and the disturbance in the relationships between the patient and other members of his family.

Certain other important features are also demonstrated:

(1) The clearly reactive nature of the suicidal threat or attempt, so far as the actual event itself is concerned. The stresses these children have to undergo are often very severe, and it is understandable that they feel life is really not worth living. The event immediately preceding the actual threat or attempt at suicide can be regarded as the final insupportable load which, together with previous stresses, leads to the imperative need to consider or attempt suicide as a solution.

(2) The frequent history of 'depression' for some time before the suicidal threat or attempt, which was not understood or taken seriously by the parents but which may, on occasion, be noticed at school and reported.

(3) The frequent history of poor health and depression in the mother, the depression being often of a reactive nature. Such stresses on the parent as marital disharmony, death of the husband, desertion by the husband with the consequent financial strain and total responsibility for the children, as well as situational stresses such as the grandmother coming to live in the home, are often intense.

(4) The finding that many of the children who make suicidal attempts do so 'out of the blue' and had been considered to be sensitive, conscientious, trustworthy, stable and sometimes 'model' children.

(5) The frequent finding that there is in fact a strong motivation for suppression of the details of family tensions by the parents of 'suicidal' children, so that a picture of a stable harmonious family background, with parental harmony, may be presented at first contact with the parents. Only later do the real facts emerge and the picture of a family rent asunder by tensions, jealousies and hostilities becomes manifest.

(6) The observation that in fact the child, by the time the psychiatrist is called in, may have learnt that society's response to the attempt or threat is hostile, or may by then have received enough care, attention and protestations of love and affection from the parents to make the causative stresses at home appear much less severe, so that the whole 'suicide' situation may be either denied or played down.

(7) The observation that some children who are admitted to hospital following a suicidal attempt may in fact settle down fairly quickly and lose their depression, this being likely to be due to the removal from the 'stress' situation and not indicative of a radical change, nor warranting discharge home without psychiatric referral.

(8) The finding that in fact a number of children remain depressed

and need to be transferred to a psychiatric unit, because they require hospital care and treatment for a longer period than is possible in a medical ward which may not itself be entirely suited to their needs.

(9) The high incidence of school anxieties, including those associated with academic work itself, as well as those associated with difficulties in inter-personal relationships with the peer group, with older children and with teachers.

(10) The finding of occasional cases of depressive illness, particularly in the early adolescent years, which do not appear to be mainly reactive in nature, and which in some instances appear to be of the kind often described as 'endogenous depression'.

(11) The finding, on follow-up, of repeated suicidal attempts in some cases, and the use of a suicidal threat later on as a means of manipulating the environment by some children who had previously made a suicidal attempt.

(12) The finding that the suicidal attempt and the suicidal threat do not appear to be separate categories but in the light of the evidence should both be considered as of equal psychiatric seriousness.

7

Treatment and Management

It follows from the foregoing that investigation of cases of suicidal threat or attempt in children and adolescents will indicate that the majority will require treatment, and that those who do not at first investigation appear to be severely disturbed should be followed up for a time because of the tendency to withhold relevant facts at first interview. These measures are indicated not only because of the possible danger to life if the child is not adequately treated, but also, where there is family disturbance, to help the child and the family to more normal mental health in order that the child may, in the few years remaining, be helped to develop into a more stable and adjusted adult.

Treatment can be divided into two main aspects: the immediate emergency treatment, and the long-term treatment.

Immediate Emergency Treatment

In those instances where medical treatment for an acute emergency is called for, attendance at the casualty department and admission to hospital may be required. It may even be politic to admit children to hospital who have taken drugs, even though their medical state does not really warrant such admission, so that investigation of the immediate situation can be arranged from the ward and to avoid the danger of their return home without any future psychiatric help being arranged. Since there is often a long waiting list at many child psychiatric units, it may be possible to obtain more urgent child psychiatric examination while the child is in the ward than if he is referred through the usual channels, thus gaining the advantage of investigation as soon as possible after the attempt.

In those instances where the referral is through the family doctor, it may be necessary to arrange urgent help even if this falls short of the full psychiatric investigation, since it may be imperative for the child to be placed for much of his day in a situation where he is away from stresses that have led to the suicidal attempt.

In some instances urgent admission to a child or adolescent psychiatric unit would be the method of choice, but unfortunately such facilities are few and far between, so that it is rarely possible for such emergency admission to be made, and the child may have to be admitted to an adult psychiatric unit which will provide shelter and care but which will be unsuitable in many other ways.

Where placement in an in-patient unit or a paediatric or medical ward of a general hospital is not available or not warranted, and where separation from home would be deleterious but there is still a need for removal from stress, the Child Psychiatric Day Hospital can be an invaluable method of approach. In this Day Hospital (14) the child can attend five days a week or less, according to the clinical need, and return home in the evenings. In some cases the method of choice may be for the local authority to take the child into temporary care.

The main features of the emergency psychiatric approach can be summarised as follows: (a) the lessening of immediate stresses; (b) the establishment of good rapport with the child, who needs to feel that he is accepted and understood and that there are kindly people who want to, and can, help; (c) the establishment of good rapport with the parent, whose present and later co-operation will be essential; (d) treatment of the depression, if this does not resolve in a few days after (a) has been effected; (e) full evaluation of the individual child and family psychiatric disturbance.

Treatment of the Depression

In those cases where there is a clear history of a depressive reaction—which in the writer's opinion can be equated with the 'reactive depression' of adult life—there is a place for the use of the anti-depressant group of drugs if the depression fails to begin to improve a few days after the other emergency psychiatric measures have been taken.

Nardil, the drug most commonly used by the writer, is of the mono-amine oxidase inhibitor group, and a dose regime of 15 mg. in the morning for three days, then 15 mg. twice a day for two weeks, and then, if there are no untoward side-effects, 15 mg. three times a day, can be recommended. It is important that the reason for giving this drug, its possible side-effects, and the fact that it may take some time before any definite improvement is felt, be discussed with the child and his parents. The drug may need to be continued for several months before it is safe for it to be withdrawn, and withdrawal should be gradual: reduction of the dose to

15 mg. twice a day for three weeks, to 15 mg. in the morning for three weeks, and only then complete withdrawal, is the regime that can be recommended. During this period there should be regular assessments of the patient.

In those much more rare cases where the depression appears to be similar to the 'endogenous depression' of adults (though the symptomatology may be modified in the case of children), Tofranil, 25 mg. once a day for three days, then 25 mg. twice a day for two weeks, and then 25 mg. three times a day, can be recommended. In some instances the dose may need to be increased up to 50 mg. or more three times a day, particularly in the later adolescent age group. Here again the drug may need to be continued for several months, withdrawal should be gradual, and the reason for the drug being prescribed and the possible beneficial and side-effects should be explained to the patient and the parents.

Long-term Treatment

Since most cases of suicidal attempts or threats come from very disturbed family backgrounds, it is often necessary for psychiatric treatment and supervision to be maintained for long periods of time. Only when the child is settled, reasonably happy, showing no depression or excessive or frequent emotional outbursts, where the mother is more confident and assured and where there appears to be a more settled and harmonious relationship between the parents and the patient, is it safe to discharge the child from the clinic.

It has transpired on a number of occasions in cases treated at Newcastle that the relationship with the father may be the vital one, not only in psychodynamic terms but also because of his often vital role in accepting the psychiatric referral, psychiatric treatment and follow-up. A number of children seen in the paediatric or medical wards where no parent, or only the mother, was seen have failed to continue attendance at the psychiatric unit after discharge from the ward.

Ideally, therefore, the ward consultation should be a consultation with both mother and father as well as an examination of the child, so that good contact can be established early when the immediacy of the situation is more likely to result in the parents accepting the need for continued help after discharge from hospital. In a few cases where there has been a second suicidal attempt, this has been due to the failure to get to grips with the family problems, either because of early non-attendance through failure to establish contact with father, or because intensive work with the family has been unfruitful and the basic psychopathological picture has remained unchanged. In the latter situation, long-term placement away from home should always be considered.

The treatment of the family situation may be long and difficult. In many instances the mother requires treatment in her own right on account of an anxiety state or a depressive illness, and since the family dynamics and the concern over the child will be brought up for discussion by whoever treats the mother, this treatment can be advantageously carried out by the psychiatrists of the child psychiatric unit. This means, of course, that the somewhat rigid traditional 'child guidance' approach has to be modified and a much greater flexibility of approach secured to enable the child psychiatrist to treat the mother's or father's psychiatric disorder.

A useful way of providing for this contingency is for two psychiatrists to work together on a case—one treating the child and one treating the mother. In some instances it is possible for one psychiatrist to treat both parent and child. In Newcastle the child psychiatry unit staff run an evening clinic in the adult department once a week for the treatment of adult and adolescent patients, as well as a morning clinic at the Teaching Hospital for the examination of new cases (either adolescents over 16 years of age, or adults) and for treatment of these age groups. In this way fathers and mothers can be seen and treated when it might be inappropriate to carry this out in the children's unit, and the evening clinic in particular is invaluable for seeing fathers, who would resent losing time off work during the day, and adolescents who are at work or at school, for whom it would be unreasonable and possibly deleterious to treatment to insist on daytime attendance.

This kind of organisation, which allows of flexible treatment of child, adolescent and adult, is extremely valuable in dealing with these cases of suicidal attempt or threat, and can be generally recommended for the psychiatric treatment of families.

Individual treatment of the child—apart from pharmacotherapy—does not involve any special measures, and the usual psychotherapeutic methods can be employed. It is important however that the whole topic of the wish to take life be fully discussed at some stage of treatment, and that the child receive reassurance, fairly early in treatment, that there is no condemnation by the therapist, and that the thought or wish or attempt at suicide is understandable and is the experience of other children. Guilt feelings, which are commonly present in the patients who have threatened or attempted suicide, need to be dealt with in psychotherapy.

In many instances when the emergency treatment has been carried out it is clear that the child will benefit from a longer period away from home and away from the stresses. In these instances placement in a children's convalescent hospital in the country where there is normal schooling, such as the one in Northumberland which the writer visits once a month, can be most helpful. Experience has shown however that this placement, to be effective, should in most cases be for a period of at least two months. Return home before this period has elapsed is often followed by relapse.

8

Special Investigations

In cases where there is a school problem it is clearly necessary for full psychometric investigations to be carried out, and it is often advisable for school visits to be made, both to evaluate the school problem itself and also to help to re-establish the child back at school and to help the teachers with their own problems concerning a 'suicidal' child in their midst.

Other special investigations, such as electroencephalography, pathology, X-ray etc., will be carried out where the clinical state indicates the need.

9

Prognosis

In general terms, the prognosis will depend upon the success or failure in re-establishing the child in the family circle and at school, or upon the success or failure in providing suitable alternative long-term placement.

Nevertheless there are certain problems of prognosis and of aetiology which remain unsolved. Why, for instance, do the patients who attempt suicide under the very wide variety of stresses use this method to solve the problem? Is the 'depression' really a reaction to the stress, or is it partly an autonomous condition? Why is it that very many other children under apparently similar severe stresses do not attempt suicide? Why do some children attempt suicide under comparatively mild stresses?

It seems likely that the reason lies in the individual differences of personality and make-up of the children concerned, and that the finding in those who do attempt suicide of a previous personality of sensitiveness, model or conforming adjustment, a too well developed sense of responsibility and a tendency to depressive mood-swings, may point to the important features of these individual differences.

Only when it is possible to examine fully every case of suicidal thoughts, threats or attempts, and when methodologically sound research design can be employed, will the answers to these questions become clearer. Long-term follow-up studies of these children will be essential for assessing the full implications of the suicidal thought, threat and attempt in children and adolescents. It is unfortunate that there is a dearth of academic child psychiatric units, and that the majority of child psychiatric units are either so heavily pressed for clinical service, or so inadequately organised for follow-up into adult life, that such important researches are unlikely to be carried out for a long time to come.

10

Prophylaxis

Little needs to be said about prophylaxis. Since the great majority of cases of suicidal threats and attempts come from disturbed family backgrounds, and since the disturbance of family background has often been present for many years, prophylaxis will be in the field of family mental health from earliest childhood, continuing into adult life. Thus the social 'mental health' services will have a big part to play, and the development of close links between them and the child psychiatric units, with extension of the latter so that cases are seen earlier in the life history of the untoward development, will be important.

At the educational level, wider dissemination of the fact that the 'model', conformist child may be psychiatrically disturbed will be important.

11

Conclusions

The writer has attempted to present the problem of suicidal threats and attempts in children in a general way, as well as giving his personal views based upon a wide experience of such cases. In the interests of space the subject has not been dealt with exhaustively, but certain features of the clinical diagnosis, methods of examination and treatment have been stressed. It is hoped that better understanding and handling of such children will therefore be encouraged.

The main conclusions can be summarised as follows:

(1) Every case of suicidal threat or attempt in childhood and adolescence should be taken seriously and full investigations made. There is likely to be a severe disturbance of the child's relationships with the members of the family.

(2) Most cases will require long and difficult treatment of the child and the family situation. The role of the father is important and should not be overlooked.

(3) The incidence of suicidal threats and attempts in childhood and adolescence is likely to be very much higher than is generally thought, and is considered to comprise a substantial social problem.

(4) The relationship between 'depression' and suicidal threats and attempts is emphasised.

(5) The advantage of the child psychiatric unit operating in the adult field as a part of its work is mentioned.

(6) The need for research and, in particular, follow-up studies of such cases is stressed.

REFERENCES

1. ANDICS, VON, M., 1947. *Suicide and the Meaning of Life*. London: William Hodge.
2. ANON., 1955. Endogenous depression in children. (An annotation.) *Brit. Med. J.*, ii: 425.
3. ANTHONY, J. and SCOTT, P., 1960. Manic-depressive psychosis in childhood. *J. Child Psychol. and Psychiat.*, 1: 53.
4. BALSER, R. and MASTERSON, J., 1959. Suicide in adolescents. *Amer. J. Psychiat.*, 116: 400.
5. BATCHELOR, I. R. C. and NAPIER, M. B., 1953. Broken homes and attempted suicide. *Brit. J. Delinq.*, 4: 99.
6. BENDER, L. and SCHILDER, P., 1937. Suicidal preoccupations and attempts in children. *Amer. J. Orthopsychiat.*, 7: 225.
7. BERGSTRAND, C. G. and OTTO, U., 1962. Suicidal attempts in adolescence and childhood. *Acta Paediat., Stockh.*, 51: 17.
8. BERNFELD, S., 1933. Selbstmord. *Z. Psychoan. Pädag.*, p. 355.
9. BIBRING, E., 1953. The mechanism of depression. *In* Greenacre, P. (ed.), *Affective Disorders*. New York: International Universities Press.
10. BROWN, F., 1961. Depression and childhood bereavement. *J. Ment. Sci.*, 107: 754.
11. BRUHN, G. G., 1962. Broken homes among attempted suicides and psychiatric out-patients. *J. Ment. Sci.*, 108: 772.
12. CAMPBELL, J. D., 1955. Manic-depressive disease in children. *J. Amer. Med. Ass.*, 158: 154.
13. CHESS, S., 1959. *An Introduction to Child Psychiatry*. New York: Grune & Stratton.
14. CONNELL, P. H., 1961. The day hospital approach in child psychiatry. *J. Ment. Sci.*, 107: 969.
15. CONNELL, P. H., 1962. Not yet published.
16. DAHLGREN, K. G., 1945. *On Suicide and Attempted Suicide*. A.-B. Ph. Lund. Lindstedts Univ.-Bokhandel.
17. DUBLIN, L. I. and BUNZEL, B., 1933. *To Be or Not to Be. A Study of Suicide*. New York: Smith &Haas.
18. DURKHEIM, E., 1951. *Suicide*. (Transl.). London: Routledge & Kegan Paul.
19. FREUD, S., 1920. *Jenseits des Lustprinzips*. Vienna: Psycho-analytischer Verlag.
20. JACOBZINER, H., 1960. Attempted suicide in children. *J. Pediat.*, 56: 519.
21. KANNER, L., 1957. *Child Psychiatry*. Springfield, Ill.: Charles C. Thomas.
22. KAUFMAN, I., 1962. Crimes of violence and delinquency in schizophrenic children. *J. Amer. Acad. of Child Psychiat.*, 1: 269.
23. KENYON, F. E., 1962. Emergencies in child psychiatry. *J. Ment. Sci.*, 108: 419.
24. LINDEMANN, E., GORDON, J. E., VAUGHAN, W. T., JR. and IPSEN, J., 1950. Minor disorders. *Proc. Ann. Conf. Milbank Mem. Fund.*, New York.
25. MEERLOO, J. A. M., 1962. *Suicide and Mass Suicide*. New York: Grune & Stratton.
26. MORSELLI, H., 1881. *Suicide*. London: C. Kegan Paul.
27. OLSEN, T. ,1961. Depression. *Acta Psychiat. Scand.*, Suppl. 162, 37: 45.

28. REICHARD, S. and TILLMAN, C., 1950. Murder and suicide as defences against schizophrenic psychosis. *J. Clin. Psychopath.*, **11**: 149.
29. SAINSBURY, P., 1955. *Suicide in London—an Ecological Study.* Maudsley Monograph No. 1. London: Chapman and Hall.
30. SCHACHTER, M. and COTTE, S., 1951. Tentatives, chantages et velléités de suicide chez les jeunes. A. *Criança Portuguesa*, **10**: 109.
31. SCHNEIDMAN, E. S. and FARBEROW, N. L., 1957. *Clues to Suicide.* New York: McGraw-Hill.
32. STENGEL, E., 1960. Old and new trends in suicide research. *Brit. J. Med. Psychol.*, **33**: 283.
33. STENGEL, E. and COOK, N. G., 1958. *Attempted Suicide.* Maudsley Monograph No. 4. London: Oxford University Press.
34. TOOLAN, J. M., 1962. Suicide and suicidal attempts in children and adolescents. *Amer. J. Psychiat.*, **118**: 719-724.
35. ZILBOORG, G., 1937. Considerations on suicide, with particular reference to that of the young. *Amer. J. Orthopsychiat.*, **7**: 15.

XVIII

THE PSYCHIATRIC ASPECTS

OF ADOPTION

HILDA LEWIS

M.D., M.R.C.P.

Consultant Psychiatrist to the Children's Society, London

1

Adoption

Adoption, which from one point of view is a legal and social procedure, is also a decisive act which has a complex psychological setting and momentous psychological consequences. This is particularly so when a child is cut off from his progenitors and blood relations and placed with strangers.

In this country, however, the mother or father of an illegitimate child often uses the device of adoption to remove from the child the legal and social disadvantages of his birth. Legitimately born children also are sometimes 'adopted' after the remarriage of one of their parents who has been widowed or divorced. There are, for example, strong grounds for doing this when a woman after a divorce marries the co-respondent by whom she had had a child who was registered as her former husband's (legitimate) child. These adoptions by one or both natural parents have their inherent psychological problems. The same applies to the many adoptions of children by relatives of the mother or father. In this chapter it is chiefly the problems of the adoption of a child by unrelated persons which will receive consideration.

2

The Legal Aspects

Adoption Statistics

The Registrar General's annual Statistical Reviews show that between 13,000 and 17,000 adoption orders are granted each year. In 1960, for example, there were 15,099. 3,139 (20%) of these were legitimately born children, of whom 1,576 were adopted by one or both parents (as a rule by the mother and her spouse acting as joint adopters after a new marriage). Of the 11,960 illegitimately born children of the 1960 group of adoptions, 2,896 went to one or both parents.

The age at adoption varies very much according to the type of placement. For example in 1960, 48% of the children were adopted in their first year and a further 25% during their next three years. These were predominantly adoptions of illegitimate children by couples neither of whom was the natural parent. Natural parents mostly begin to adopt the child as he approaches school age, as well as later in his childhood, even until he is 15–20 years old (673 in 1960). Children may similarly be adopted by foster-parents in later childhood or adolescence.

Adoption Laws and Regulations*

The custom of adopting children has grown so rapidly that it is hard to believe that the first adoption act regularising the process in this country dates only from 1926, following a private member's bill. Since then there have been a number of revisions and amendments, culminating in the Adoption Act, 1958 (1), which aimed at placing foremost the welfare of the adopted child and at giving him a legal position in the family equal to that of a child born in the ordinary way to the adoptive parents.

The rights of the natural mother to withhold her consent to other people adopting her child are safeguarded until the day of the court hearing. The court hearing at which the adoption is authorised cannot take place until the child has been with the prospective adopters for three months, no period during the child's first six weeks of life counting towards this three months. Although the magistrate may dispense with the mother's final consent if he thinks it is unreasonably withheld, only a few courts have so far ventured to override her wishes expressed at the last stage of the procedure. A further uncertainty for adopters and agencies has been added by a clause in the 1958 Act which permits a natural father to object to the adoption of his illegitimate child, and if the adoption order is refused to make formal application for the child's custody.

Registered Adoption Agencies

The legal procedure by which a parent or both parents apply to adopt their own child is simple, but the regulations laid down for the conduct of Registered Adoption Agencies, and for Local Authorities who supervise the child during the probationary period, are demanding. Adoption Agencies must (a) ascertain that the mother has read and understood an explanatory statement about adoption and given her provisional consent, (b) receive a report on the health, history and background of the infant,

* The proportion of adoptions arranged by registered agencies and local authorities cannot be given precisely. The Hurst Report (1954) estimated it as 25%; a recent study of a large area (to be reported shortly) made it nearly 50%.

(c) review data about the character and suitability of the applicants as ascertained by personal interviews and public and private references, (d) receive a report on the premises of the applicants, and (e) visit the child in his new home before the adoption is put forward to the court.

Direct and Third-party Placings

The Law permits a mother to place her child directly with adopters, or to do so through the intervention of a private third party. It is illegal for payment to be made to the mother or to any third party for this transfer, but it is common knowledge that private arrangements are sometimes made which do not openly contravene the Law, but which provide indirect gain for some of those concerned. In such arrangements the welfare of the child and the suitability of the adopters receive little attention.

In these direct or third-party placings there are other inherent weaknesses: for a full discussion see *Brit. Med. J.*, i, 1960: 1197-1200. Duties to investigate and obtain medical or other reports on the baby and to ascertain the suitability and health of the adopters before placement are not imposed on private third parties. They have only to notify the Children's Department of the Local Authority two weeks beforehand that the child (as a protected person) is being placed. Two weeks' notification is too short a period for making a full social investigation; even this preliminary notice is by-passed if the infant is placed 'as an emergency' with the proposed adopters immediately after it is born. Children's Departments therefore have to act swiftly upon receiving third-party notifications if they are not to be faced with a *fait accompli*, which they could not easily reverse since the baby if removed would be rendered immediately homeless. By the time the case comes before the Court, three months or so later, a Magistrate will be very reluctant to uproot the infant from a placement, even though it is not satisfactory in certain respects. He may refuse an adoption order, but this does not mean that the child will be removed from the home unless moral danger or gross neglect has been proved; as a rule in such a case *de facto* adoption is the outcome. Children's Officers who lodge objections to adoption orders in such cases are sometimes overruled. In this way neurotic or unstable couples will nevertheless, if they are sufficiently determined, manage to secure a child to adopt even after they have been turned down by adoption societies.

If third-party placings were always carried out by responsible and kindly individuals who knew a great deal about the infant and his family and about the adopters, little harm would be done; excellent adoptions are occasionally made in this way, and they have the advantage of minimum delay in satisfying the infant's instinctual needs. It is unfortunately the case, however, that doctors and nurses in contact with unmarried mothers and childless couples not infrequently make hasty and quite unsuitable arrangements, which would have been avoided if they had promptly called in professional social workers familiar with this work.

3

The Social Aspects

Ideals in Placement

Adoption serves two ideals:

1. To give the homeless or unwanted child at the right moment a permanent home with affectionate parents, where his relationships will be emotionally, not less than legally, as nearly as possible the same as if he had been born into this family;
2. To enable a suitable married couple with a satisfactory expectation of life to fulfil their natural desire for parenthood.

Leaving aside adoptions by relatives and the many haphazard third-party arrangements still permitted by our legal system, how often are these ideals realised? Adoption societies believe that the majority of the adoptions they arrange turn out happily. Salzberger (20) estimated as 'successful' 87% of a series of such placings. Further follow-up studies are needed. Success depends in part on the quantity and quality of the information on which the adoptive home is selected, the soundness of the criteria for selection, and the skill of the social worker in introducing the baby to the new home. Introducing a baby is an art depending not only on training but also on sympathetic understanding of the inexperience, hopes, fears, weaknesses and strengths of the prospective parents.

There are grounds for believing that adoption societies which accept only those applicants who have well developed parental attitudes (having, for example, shown a lively interest in the children of friends and relatives), and who are happily married, cheerful and emotionally stable, effect more satisfactory adoptions than those which pay less attention to these criteria.

The Balance of Supply and Demand

The adoptive home that can be found for a child depends obviously on the number and quality of potential homes available. The wider the choice of approved homes, the better for him. Unless there are more parents wanting babies than there are babies to be adopted, agencies find it difficult to find the right home at the right moment, and have to relax some of their standards as regards non-essentials. Exaggerated and incorrect statements in the Press about the large number of couples waiting for each baby (still sometimes quoted as 10 to 1) are to be deplored, because they lead childless couples to assume that it is futile to approach the adoption societies and they therefore seek and obtain a baby through private channels.

It is true that a few adoption societies, troubled by an excess of would-be adoptive parents, adopt a policy of 'rationing' one child to a couple; but this too is to be deplored: adopters who have proved successful with one child should be helped to build up a larger family if they wish.

The Needs of the Children

The problem of adoption was often thought of twenty or thirty years ago as primarily one of satisfying the wishes of childless parents; now it is properly regarded as the problem of meeting a child's needs. The child may be of modest intelligence, not appealing in form or behaviour to many people, of coloured or mixed race, or he may have a more serious handicap, but he still has his rightful claims to a home. Every homeless child is adoptable if suitable parents can be found to adopt him and he is ready to accept them in that role. Unfortunately for those who have become anti-social through deprivation, this may be only a pious hope.

The normal infant. In this country today the great majority of infants are born healthy, thanks to the good physique of their usually young mothers and to the National Health Services. Those offered for adoption come from all classes of society. For these healthy very young babies there is no dearth of would-be adopters who have been unable to produce the children they so much desire to have. Such couples usually want to adopt a child who can measure up as far as possible to one they might have produced themselves: in practice this means a child like one or other of the adopting parents, making the adoption seem more natural and possibly helping to create firmer bonds between child and parents. For example an unusually big child with tiny parents, a brilliantly intellectual child in an isolated farm labourer's cottage, or a simple child in a professor's family, may not feel quite at ease even if he is much loved.

The extraordinary resemblances often noted between adopted children and one or other adoptive parent show that physical 'matching' is often achieved (largely through recording of the height, weight, colouring and other physical features of both sets of parents). Of course many difficulties stand in the way of matching where intellectual capacity is concerned, because most children are placed as infants, before their potential can be judged other than by the roundabout and very uncertain criteria of the occupational and educational achievements of their natural parents.

Matching can be over-stressed. Some experienced workers consider it unimportant.

Another difficulty is that adopters have come disproportionately from the professional and managerial social classes 1 and 2, in which the IQ level is often above average. Thanks to the greater appeal of adoption generally, however, more homes are being offered by people of the skilled manual and technical classes. Children from a very poor social background benefit from being placed in an adoptive home of rather superior status to that of their own families, as Skodak and Skeels (23) have shown so clearly, but problems in adjustment tend to arise more often if there is too large a discrepancy between the social status of the two families (Salzberger (20)).

The character of the home in which the child will develop (and not its economic class) strongly influences his ultimate intellectual functioning, whatever his genetic endowment. A sound adoption society looks for qualities in the adopters which will make them good parents in the fullest sense. In addition it wants to be assured that the home will meet two other basic needs of the child:

1. A warm welcome from other members of the adopter's family, in particular their own parents and their own children if any.

2. Membership of a wider community which will also welcome the child. For adoption societies this means a religious group in which the child will receive spiritual and moral guidance. Adoption societies which have been founded by religious groups insist that adopting parents must be active members of a religious denomination, and that they will bring up the child in it. Local authorities usually take the same view. But in modern society, in which so many citizens do not believe in or observe any religious affiliation, it might be considered unjust to deny them the right to adopt a child except by private arrangement when the child's natural mother would concur. The child may also need protection against a narrow moralistic or over-restrictive upbringing. Some more thinking is required about the means of assessing the spiritual and moral values of a home in relation to the child's happiness within it and to his welfare in the larger community that lies outside his home.

Older infants and children requiring adoption may have experienced many changes of environment, or they may have remained with their mothers neglected and unwanted. Others, perhaps because they were frail in the early months of life, or had a poor family history, could not be placed until their physical and mental normality had been assured after some months of treatment or observation. Skilled social work is needed in placing these children, and thereafter in supervising them to ensure that all goes well.

Older infants who are placed after they have spent months in a nursery are not necessarily abnormal in their emotional responses to foster-parents and adopters who understand and are prepared to cope with the possible difficulties. The belief, widespread of late, that after a period of institutional life a child is likely to be emotionally crippled has very regrettably led to couples being dissuaded from adopting such a child. Provided that the adoptive parents understand the situation, and are introduced gradually, there is no good reason why they should not adopt the child if they wish, after he has had an initial period as a foster-child in their home under the guidance of a social worker who knows the child well. This works especially well with infants who have had consistent and kindly care in a modern nursery or with experienced temporary foster-mothers. Even a baby will take to one particular substitute mother (or father) more readily than to another, and knowledge of his personal reactions may ease the initial stage of adjustment.

Similarly there is a great need to determine and understand an older child's preferences. It is most unwise to proceed with adoption unless the child as well as the foster-parents desire it, and until a sufficient period has been allowed for the child to work through his initial insecurity, which may show itself in deceptively 'good' conforming behaviour, often followed by a period of naughtiness or moodiness. Reference to a psychiatrist is desirable in cases of doubt. However, children's departments and voluntary children's societies arrange many successful adoptions of older infants and children, including handicapped ones.

For example, the Church of England Children's Society in 1961 reported that 84% of all their children in foster-homes were placed with a view to adoption. Many were very simple homes, but in each case the mental and physical health and life expectation of the couple had been reasonably assured, and the child was wanted for his own sake and was sure of a welcome. The immediate result is shown in this Society's annual figures. In 1960 only 7 of 119, and in 1961 only 4 of 143, under 5 years at the time of 'foster-placement with a view to adoption', were returned to the Society and the steps towards adoption stopped. This was sometimes because of complications in the foster-parents' family such as ill health rather than because the child was no longer acceptable. The other (112 + 139) children were legally adopted. After 5 years of age or long periods of institutional care or parental rejection, the outlook for successful adoption is of course poorer (Theis (24)).

Handicapped children, and some older children, do best with middle-aged but robust couples whose own children have grown up and who have a special enjoyment and skill in caring for children, especially for those with some physical or mental limitation.

Children of mixed or coloured races who require adoptive homes present a growing problem in this country because their numbers are increasing, yet applicants to adopt are mostly unwilling to take a child of Eurasian or Euro-African origin. This may spring from the desire of the infertile couple to have a child who will resemble themselves. Racial prejudice may also operate, though it is not the whole story.

Problems connected with adoption about which a psychiatrist may be consulted will be discussed as follows:—Problems arising shortly before adoption placement; those arising during the probationary period; those arising at various points in the child's life after he has been adopted.

4

Problems arising Before Placement

Conflicts over Consent to Adoption

The Natural Mother. No adoption arrangements can take place without the mother of the child coming to a decision in which her deepest emotions are involved. The rule that 6 weeks must elapse before she can officially agree to the placement for adoption aims at giving her time to recover emotionally, and after this there is at least a three months probationary period before an adoption order can be made. A decision for adoption arrived at too hastily because of pressure upon the mother even before the child is born, and perhaps imposed by her parents or by her husband who is not the father of the child, may cause her at some stage of the probationary period suddenly to change her mind. She may snatch her child back from the adopters even at the last moment, i.e. on the day of the legal hearing. She may become mentally ill under the stress, and a psychiatrist will have to explore her conflicts and give her psychotherapy, while at the same time directing a good deal of social work through the psychiatric social worker's department or through a moral welfare worker. He may also have the exacting and responsible task of deciding whether the mother's medical history indicates enough risk of transmissible mental illness in the child to prevent adopters being willing to take him.

Unsuitable and maladjusted mothers. The psychiatrist may also be called in to help unstable women or girls who repeatedly change their minds about giving consent to an adoption though it seems the only satisfactory means of ensuring their child's future care. Such women include in undue proportions those who have themselves experienced life in a broken home, or an unhappy fostering, adoption or institutional care (White Franklin (6)); there are also some older lonely spinsters. These women and girls often need psychiatric help and social support, but once the pregnancy is over and the baby on the scene, they often neither want or accept such help. If the conflict about parting with the child remains though the child has been adopted, such mothers may deliberately run the risk of another illegitimate pregnancy, and the dilemma is repeated. These women need to be spotted as soon as possible in pregnancy by moral welfare officers or maternity clinic staff and referred for psychiatric treatment and help, which can continue after the child's birth, at least until its future is settled. This is now being done in several hospitals which have psychiatric and obstetric departments working closely together.

Breast feeding and weaning of the child. Almost all mothers who cannot keep their infants carry a considerable load of guilt. Breast feeding during the first month, if handled properly, is a therapeutic measure which helps the mother to reduce her guilt, because she feels that she is giving the infant the best help she can before he leaves her. Maternity Homes in which this principle is applied with sympathy and insight seem to have fewer infants snatched back by mothers who change their minds after the child has been placed in an adoptive home (White Franklin (6); Winner (26)). On the other hand prolonged breast feeding and close contact with the baby after she has decided that adoption is inevitable is cruel to an affectionate mother, or harmful to the child if the mother rejects it. Gough (7) gives an illuminating picture of unmarried mothers in a mother-and-baby home awaiting the departure of their babies.

In the hope of saving the mother suffering, some obstetricians and psychiatrists arrange for her not to see the child at all. This is a grave decision to make, and should never be a routine procedure. Statements made by some of these mothers afterwards indicate that their sufferings were far greater than they would have been had they had the satisfaction of seeing their child, nursing it and handing it over to people who seemed likely to give it a good upbringing and who themselves gain from doing so. Except in certain cases of rape or incest, removing the child at its birth should be done only after careful consideration of the psychological aspects of the case (e.g. incipient psychosis or mental subnormality in the mother).

The Child

The psychiatrist may be called on in various ways. He may be assessor for an adoption committee or for adopters, who have before them reports on the child's family, medical history and physical condition* and want an expert opinion on the prognostic significance of certain data; he may be needed to carry out further investigations to appraise the child.

Heredity and Family Background. Mental disease: In giving any advice about genetics and the risk of abnormal heredity, the psychiatrist is very often handicapped by lack of data about the baby's father and his family. However, more detailed social and medical reports, even if obtainable only on the mother's side, may make it clear that the mental illness or other condition is one (such as a neurotic illness) in which the definite genetic component is negligible. Today adopters on the whole are great believers in the importance of environment, and they seldom decide against taking such an infant if the general social competence of the families is reasonably satisfactory.

Children who have a strong family history of schizophrenia or manic-depressive psychosis are not often offered for direct adoption as infants, though advice is often sought when they are older and their foster-parents wish to adopt them. In such cases the foster-parents who are fond of the child are usually prepared to accept the risks, about which however they should be properly informed.

Some applicants to adopt are frightened of taking a young child when socially unsatisfactory conduct is reported in one or both parents. Their fears on hereditary grounds can usually be dispelled, unless the family history reveals such long-standing social inadequacy as to suggest poor basic intelligence. Cases of incest often belong to this last category. Decisions about adoption are then best deferred until a period of at least 6 to 12 months of careful observation in a good foster-home or nursery has revealed what the child is like. Boarding out with a view to adoption can then be arranged, after systematic psychological and physical examination to determine his level of development and health.

Epilepsy and mental defect: When there is a history of definite mental defect or epilepsy in several members or generations of a family, the child's

---

* For discussion of the general medical problems at this stage, see Black and Stone (3), and Lewis (14).

condition at birth and of course his later development have to be reviewed. However, the severe forms of epilepsy are more often due to brain damage or acquired disease than to heredity: 'The forms of epilepsy in which genetic or hereditary factors play a major part are among the most benign and most easily controlled, and the ones that have in many ways the best outlook for the future.' (Pond (19).) Often it is only a matter of obtaining accurate records and reports about a single individual in the family affected to dispel anxiety about the infant being adopted right away.

The position is closely similar in regard to defect. Most children of mental defectives prove to be within the normal range of intelligence (Skeels and Harms (22)), and are usually adoptable through preliminary fostering with the prospective adopters, if not by direct adoption: 'A label of mental deficiency on the parent need not necessarily be a serious thing from the point of view of the potentialities of the child; we have to consider, not only the effects of the mother's environment on her own mental development, but also the special circumstances which caused her to acquire the label.' (Penrose (18).)

Forecasts about what any child's intelligence will be when he is grown up cannot be made from the family history. It is reasonable, however, in placing a very young infant to assume that the chances of average or good mental capacity will be greater if the child has two parents of superior intelligence, than if his parents are both dull or low-average (other things being equal). The risks run by parents who adopt a child of known family background are similar to those of parents with a new-born baby of their own. Applicants who insist that they must have a child of superior intelligence should be kept at arm's length—or, if considered, should be helped to adopt only an older child of known ability.

Measurement of the Child's Present Level of Mental Development and Assessment of Future Capacity. Opinions about the infant's mental normality are unfortunately often sought in the early weeks of life when a firm judgement cannot be made: at most it is possible to say that, if the infant's birth weight and its physical condition and behaviour observed in the first three weeks of life are normal, the chances of a serious mental disability are small. The mother's condition during pregnancy, and the occupations, achievements and mental stability of the near relatives, should also be taken into account. Children who are judged to be premature because of low birth weight, or who show signs of cerebral damage, have a poorer outlook and need repeated paediatric and psychological examination before a firm opinion can be given (Knoblock and Pasamanick (9); Douglas and Blomfield (5)).

In early infancy: The examination of a young infant to discover especially any mental, neurological or sense organ defects usually falls to the paediatrician, who needs to be well trained in giving developmental tests such as Gesell's or Griffiths'. (The reader is referred to Knoblock and Pasamanick (9) and Illingworth (8) for fuller discussion of these matters.)

By the end of 16 weeks (about the time when the adoption of a child may be legalised) an expert can satisfy himself after careful neurological and developmental examination that a child is not grossly mentally defective; by six months an examination in such competent hands should detect retardation or subnormality of less degree, though its significance for the final mental status of the child might need to be reconsidered at 40 weeks or later. It must be emphasised that no authority—paediatric or psychological—has produced evidence that mental superiority can be recognised in infants during the first few months of their lives. Later socio-cultural factors contribute to a considerable degree to the IQ results and, of course, to their intellectual achievements.

In later infancy and childhood: In these matters of assessment in late infancy the child psychiatrist, like his paediatric colleague, needs to be well trained for the particular task. He will often have to assess both emotionally and intellectually older deprived infants and toddlers at Child Guidance Clinics or for a Local Authority before they are placed.

In any case, as regards developmental assessment, there are many areas, especially in rural districts, where expert paediatric or psychiatric examination and assessment of these children is very hard to come by; and if a child is brought to a clinic from a considerable distance he will be fatigued and frightened and give a poor and misleading impression of his abilities. In such circumstances considerable help can be derived from getting the nurses who live with the infant to complete a modified Gesell Questionnaire at 40 weeks (validated for use by nurses by Knoblock and Pasamanick (9) and further improved by them);* the answers given are then compared by the psychiatrist with the paediatric or other medical reports on the child's physical (and neurological) status. Discrepancies between the levels of motor, adaptive, personal-social and language development can be easily picked out. For example, if language behaviour is backward, as it often is in deprived children, and the child is normal in other respects, immediate fostering with a view to adoption can be urged, or if he has to stay longer in the nursery special attention must be paid to speech stimulation. Nurses who have contributed to assessment of a child's capacity by filling out the Gesell forms take a more intelligent interest in their charges, and the results are beneficial all round.

Age at Placement. Cautious preliminaries of the kind here advocated may be hampered or prevented by those doctors (and especially psychiatrists) who hold the view that infants should be placed at all costs with adopters in the early weeks of life, if they are not to run the risks of serious emotional upset and a less secure relationship with their adoptive mother-substitute. It cannot be overlooked, in opposition to this rather sentimental belief, that there is much evidence of highly successful adoptions of many older children, and that Wittenborn (28) could not detect in his exhaustive

---

* Mary Sheridan's Developmental Progress Schedules (21) might be similarly used.

follow-up significant differences in his group of children between those placed in the early weeks and those placed later during the first year of life. Early placement has some advantages for both adopters and infants, but the risks of entrusting a possibly handicapped child to unsuitable adopters are incomparably more serious than those entailed by leaving a child with his natural mother until she has made a firm decision, or by leaving him in a good temporary foster-home or residential nursery until his physical and mental condition is more definable.

Applicants to Adopt a Child

Over the question of applicants to adopt, the psychiatrist may have several tasks:

He may again act as an adviser to an adoption committee, so that he sees case papers and medical reports, perhaps collects further information, and then gives an opinion.

He may be treating a patient who would like to adopt a child and seeks his guidance.

He may be called in to advise and help when an applicant has been turned down for psychiatric reasons by an adoption committee. Adoptive societies have no facilities for helping rejected applicants to cope with the disappointment and distress the adverse decision evokes; delay and uncertainty have often caused such applicants much anxiety while awaiting the outcome of their request. They may need support from a psychiatrist. The unstable resentful applicant who has been rejected by an adoption society is a potential danger to another infant offered privately for adoption without sufficient regard to the suitability of the adopters.

The psychiatrist may find some conflict between his wish to see his childless patient's emotional needs supplied, and his sense of obligation towards a child debarred from a natural upbringing with his blood relations. A neurotic or otherwise unstable patient should be helped to realise that adopting a child may lead to difficulties with which he (or she) is ill-equipped to contend with or to avert. A shaky marriage; non-consummation; impotence; strong emotional reactions caused by infertility; morbid fear of pregnancy; perverted psychosexual relationships in childhood or later—all these point to the need for investigation and other psychiatric help, but not, as a rule, to the fallacious short cut of adopting a child.

Criteria for Accepting Adopters in Doubtful Cases. On the other hand he may be able to give valuable advice to an adoption committee to the effect that they can safely place a child in an adoptive home, where its fundamental needs (security, affection, welcome from the whole family and by religious and other local groups in the community) will be met even though one or other of the adoptive parents has had a mild disability such as well controlled epilepsy, a mild anxiety state associated with miscarriages, post-traumatic neurological disability etc. He must however take account of the couple's general personality, cheerfulness, resourcefulness and their relationship to each other.

Impotence (of psychological as well as of physical origin) is a common reason for a couple seeking to adopt a child. Whether their wish should be gratified is a complex question, certainly not one to be answered with an immediate negative. In some such cases psychiatric treatment has been given without response; AIH (a more suitable solution than adoption) has been tried, but failed; the personality of the man seems good, and the marriage, apart from copulation, is successful and happy. Such a couple may have much to offer a child in need, and the writer has watched some very happy families (with several adopted children) built up in this way. Caution and careful investigation are of course indispensable in deciding this issue.

5

Problems of the Probationary Period

Temporary Adjustment Problems

The process that leads to adopting a child is an endurance test which tends to bring out anxiety, if not morbid tendencies, in the applicants. It is during the probationary period especially that the social workers, and perhaps the psychiatrist, have occasion to detect emotional problems in the adopters as well as possible defects in the child which need further consideration. Most of these are temporary problems of adjustment common to the average (natural) parent; they call for no more than the sympathetic guidance from the social worker or the doctor. There may be doubts about the child's health or mentality, or fears that the natural mother may withdraw her consent before the final step is taken in the court. If it is the child's mental development that is the subject of concern, help should be readily available at Child Guidance Clinics and paediatric departments without subjecting them to the delay of a waiting list, for these adoptive parents have good reason to be more concerned than ordinary parents.

Threatened Breakdown of Placement and Rejection of the Infant

Occasionally the adoptive mother gets into a panic about her capacity to love the child, or has unwarranted fears that the natural mother will take it away. These may be warnings that she is too unstable to adopt a child, and they should be taken seriously; occasionally she is covering up her husband's unwillingness to adopt any child. The unjustified complaints sometimes made about the child itself by one or other partner may have a similar covert motivation. They need to be referred to a psychiatrist to help decide whether the child should be removed or whether help in adjustment should be given. When removing the child seems desirable, action should be taken promptly so far as is legally practicable. If the case drifts on and the adoption is legalised, then if subsequent removal of the child becomes necessary it is incomparably more difficult.

6
Problems arising After Legal Adoption

General Aspects

Adoption societies believe that the majority of adoptions arranged for the right motives turn out happily. When problems arise they may be indistinguishable from those of ordinary parents and children. The special problems in adoption arise because the child has had other parents, and in the majority of cases has been born illegitimate. The child often has some feeling of shame or inferiority about its origins, and the adopters may unfortunately add to this by criticising the natural mother adversely. A recent follow-up of adopted persons when adult showed that it had been particularly difficult for them to accept the fact of their illegitimate birth without suffering.

Telling the Child about his Adoption

Some adopters are able to discuss the facts of the child's background with him frankly and easily in successive stages from his earliest years, without either side being upset. This is the ideal; but adopters are often inhibited and embarrassed by diffidence in handling a very difficult job, or by emotions centring on their inability to produce a child of their own. They may need psychiatric help to overcome these obstacles. On the other hand children are able to accept even painful facts without lasting trauma if they are told them tactfully by loving parents. All follow-up studies of adoption point to the need for the child to know from his infant years that he was adopted, and for him to be able to come back easily to the subject and learn more from his adopters as he matures. Adopters should be supplied with enough information to be able to give the child as real a picture of his natural parents as possible, e.g. if they can describe the physical appearance of the natural parents, or have met the natural mother even briefly, so much the better: children want a tangible picture of their parents. If they have not been told enough or have only suspected that they were adopted, they will weave fantasies about their forebears and may become dreamy and inaccessible—particularly in adolescence, or they may be openly resentful at having been kept in the dark (Kornitzer (11)).

Insecurity and Emotional Rejection

It is tempting to call an adoption successful only if the adopters feel toward the child exactly as if he were their own flesh and blood, and the child feels reciprocally. But this would be to over-simplify the situation. An affectionate and sensible adopter who is bringing up the adopted child very happily may admit to feeling strongly the lack of the intimate physical bond that normally exists between parent and child. This may have obvious causes: the child may resemble neither parent physically or in temperament.

Concealed conflicts—need for treatment. Apart from this, there are varying degrees of reaction to the lack of blood ties, sometimes concealing conflicts in the adoptive parents about parenthood and infertility. This may call for psychiatric treatment, as in the case described by Winnicott (27) in which the adopted mother had guilt about a premarital abortion that had made her sterile; she could not take to the adopted child at first, and it consequently became insecure and developed a head-banging compulsion. Even in a fairly secure adoption, in moments of tension and anger the adopter or the child (especially during adolescence) may throw up the lack of blood relationship to annoy the other, and later deeply regret having done so. Where there is real insecurity or inadequacy of affection between the adopters and the child, strong resentment alternating with guilt may lead to violent emotional scenes and other regrettable behaviour.

Children's attitudes. A young adopted child may show signs of emotional deprivation, e.g. attention-seeking behaviour, petty pilfering, aggressive outbursts, compulsive disorders and food fads. In adolescence he may be delinquent, moody and unhappy. Disturbed behaviour of this kind may represent the child's rejection of his adopters which had occurred from the start because he had had traumatic experiences in early childhood before he came to the adopters. In these cases careful and sometimes prolonged psychiatric help may be required both for adopters and adoptee.

Children adopted at an age when they can even faintly recall their natural parents may get into conflict with their adopters if their attitudes to being adopted had not been sufficiently gone into with them at the time the arrangements for adoption were being made. Such children may run away or try to find their natural parents. Similar difficulties occur when an illegitimate child, who has been brought up to believe that his grandmother is his real mother and his natural mother a sister, suddenly realises the true relationship. Another situation arises when an illegitimate child is adopted by his mother and is brought up as the eldest child in a new family after his mother's marriage to another man. Many children troubled in these ways make a better adjustment when they are helped to recall some of their earlier emotions and to understand better what happened at their birth and to their parents.

Complete emotional rejection of the child by one or both adopters may occur, and the sooner this is recognised the better for the child. Such distressing cases require that, after suitable treatment in a reception centre or with temporary foster-parents, new parents should be found for the child. Complete rejection is usually the result either of the child's being adopted by relatives impulsively or from a sense of duty, or of a haphazard privately arranged adoption by strangers who are not qualified to care for any child. A common instance is that of an adoptive mother who is severely neurotic and immature, as in the following case:

A youngish couple had had their application to adopt refused by a Local Authority on the grounds that the woman appeared neurotic. A few months later they acquired through private channels two-week-old premature illegitimate twin girls. The same Local Authority had to supervise during the probationary period, and as they found the infants well cared for and the woman reasonably well after 9 months, the adoption order was granted. Eight months later a health visitor reported that the mother was emotionally upset and incapable of caring properly for the infants. She was given various short periods of rest away from them, but after another year, when the children were in their third year, one child was found badly bruised from blows by the mother and the other child was in a frightened condition, so that they were removed from her permanently. At this time a psychiatric report on the mother showed that because of her phobias she had slept with her parents until she was 15, her first marriage had ended in divorce, she had married her second husband knowing he was sterile, the marriage was unhappy and, although the husband had wanted to adopt a child, she had been opposed to doing so.

Such a case underlines the importance of close attention being paid to the sexual development and marital history of the couples who apply to adopt, so that the misfortunes due to rejection can be prevented in good time.

Follow-up and Other Investigations

Brief Comments on Previous Studies. A survey of the results of planned research into the problems of adoption show that no controlled observations have been made, longitudinal cohort studies are few, and generalisations premature (Lewis (15)). Particular value attaches to the studies of Skodak and Skeels in Iowa, Wittenborn in New Haven, and the Charities Association of New York State.*

In the Iowa Study (Skodak and Skeels (23)), 100 white children, who had been placed in a rather superior adoptive or unpaid foster-home between 1935 and 1937 when they were under the age of 6 months, and whose mental development was tested on four occasions at roughly three-year intervals, received their final survey in 1946. From the first examination until the end of the ten-year period, the children showed above-average mental development as indicated by IQ scores; their intellectual level was, moreover, consistently higher than would have been predicted from the intellectual, educational and socio-economic level of their natural parents, and was as good as that of children brought up by their natural parents in circumstances comparable to those of the foster or adoptive parents. The most favourable influences seemed to be in the emotional and personal characteristics of the adopters.

* See also the References for a list of more recent works, 1963-64.

The Yale Study (Wittenborn (28)) took adopted children who had been psychologically examined before they were 14 months of age, and reviewed and re-examined them when they were between 4 and 8 years of age. Very small relationships were found between scores on infant examination (by the Gesell tests) and scores on later intelligence tests. Much closer correlations were found between the child's emotional development and the warmth and quality of the relation between the child and adoptive mother. Aggressive children and timid children both tended to be living with adoptive parents who were at odds with one another and rejected the child, or who were over-anxious about the inheritance of undesirable traits. Children told about their adoption in infancy and not worried about it tended to be less clumsy, to speak better, and to have a higher IQ than those not so told. (This finding may reflect the general good qualities of the parents who told them early.) As regards age at placement, there was no evidence that early commitment before adoption to one residential nursery, or on the other hand numerous changes of temporary placement during the first year of life, affected the child's later development, except that the latter children tended to be more independent (rather resembling Kibbutz children). This could be an advantage, although the imputation of such a trait for the child's subsequent relationships with single individuals when adult is not certain.

Wittenborn emphasised that, while he would not make wide generalisations as a result of this follow-up of a small group, he had to conclude that 'much of the effort commonly devoted to an exact evaluation of infants for adoption could more properly be devoted to a study of the applicants who desire to be adoptive parents.'

So far the only large-scale survey which throws light on what happens to adopted children in adult life is the neglected study of nearly 1000 foster-children made by the New York State Charities Association (Sophie Theis (24)). It, too, clearly demonstrated the importance of regarding the qualities of the foster or adoptive parents. The 235 children who had been adopted (more than half of them foundlings) and traced to adult life were superior in social adjustment and educational achievement to the non-adopted. Placement in a secure foster-home before 5 years was generally favourable to a good outcome. Only 14 of the adopted children were 'incapable' by reason of mental or physical handicap, and only 14 because of mild delinquent traits.

There was no significant difference in outcome between children placed in their future homes before the age of 2 and those placed between 2 and 5 years.

Margaret Kornitzer (12) has published a preliminary report on a serial group of some 300 adopters who had been supervised during the probationary period by one Local Authority; many were third-party arrangements or placings with relatives. She also interviewed about 150 adult or adolescent adopted persons. The findings constituted a warning against generalisations, however widely accepted. Many of the happiest placements seemed to run counter to expectations. The presence of own children or other adopted children in an adopted family did not seem to be a disadvantage to an adopted child. One-child adoptions seemed to be the least satisfactory.

A third of the adoptees had not been informed of their adoption until they were old enough to be shocked by it. Feelings of inadequacy, and resentment because they were illegitimately born, were common among the adult adopted children.

Further Need for Research. There is clearly need for well planned research into adoption, but there are many difficulties in sampling and in getting suitable controls, especially if a long-term prospective study is envisaged. Definition of terms, fixing criteria of 'success' or 'failure', and obtaining access to the propositi and their records, also present great technical and practical difficulties. However there is a vast collection of material now in the hands of adoption agencies and Local Authorities, from which useful answers might be obtained if the right questions were asked and the work planned and directed by experienced investigators (Parker (17)).

Need for Better Statistics and Records. The Registrar General's Annual Returns about adoption orders do not state how many resulted from third-party or private placings as distinct from adoption agency placings, nor (since 1960) how many children were adopted by their relatives other than a parent.

Local Authorities might maintain a special register of adopted children who subsequently come into Public Care or pass into the care of persons other than their original adopters. This would reveal the extent, and possibly the causes, of the most serious failures in placement. The Children's Officers of Local Authorities, who are in a strong position for conducting follow-up inquiries, might be given more power to find out what happens to all illegitimate children who do not remain with their mothers. Already some Health Departments do so, by following up until the 5th year of age illegitimate children in their areas through the statutory visits of health workers (Thompson (25); Macdonald (16)).

Adoption agencies might also keep a record of mothers who withdraw their consent after their child has been placed with adopters, and of those who bring successive illegitimate children for adoption.

The keeping of sufficiently detailed and uniform records by Children's Departments and adoption agencies is of course of fundamental importance for any follow-up investigations. Confidentiality and safeguards to prevent identification and interference with adopted families must be fully preserved, but need not prevent the use of the records by bona fide and competent investigators. Most adopters, if approached in the right way when adopting a child, would be glad to promise their co-operation in an inquiry which would be of benefit to adopters and adopted children in the future.

Public Mental Health Aspects

Information of the Public. There is no lack of public interest in adoption. Some statements and letters in the Press are misleading; others draw attention helpfully to salutary principles or abuses. There is a manifest need for articles on special aspects from authoritative sources. There are already several very useful books of general information for adoption workers and adopters (Kornitzer (30); Rowe (30)).

Special Services. The S.C.S.R.A. Information should be readily available in the form not only of literature but also of personal advice to those who are immediately concerned. Mothers wishing to place an illegitimate child can obtain much help, early in their pregnancy and later, from the Moral Welfare Associations and from the Council for the Unmarried Mother and her Child.

The various National Children's Societies and National Adoption Societies have of course always been readily available to would-be adopters, but the rapid increase in legalised adoptions after the second World War showed a need for a central body to serve wider purposes, namely:

1. To provide information (leaflets etc.) about adoption generally and about special aspects;
2. To study how adoption is working, and to take measures to improve its standards.

The Standing Conference of Societies Registered for Adoption was therefore formed with the support of the National Council of Social Service in 1949, and has carried out these central functions ever since. It provides a forum for discussion through its Annual Conferences, and publishes a useful and informative quarterly journal, *Child Adoption*. Current problems are also referred to a central executive committee elected in rotation from the member societies and enlarged by persons with special knowledge. Through its Honorary Secretary postal inquiries are dealt with in consultation with various advisers, and a close liaison is maintained with the Home Office and Health Departments. It has an active Honorary Press Relations Officer. It publishes reports of Conference discussions as well as leaflets for adopters (29). Though keenly alive to the need for follow-up and research, the Standing Conference unfortunately has no funds for organising or conducting such investigations.

7

General Reflections

It has been the aim of this chapter to present a broadly based, though inevitably compressed, review of adoption in this country today, and to indicate the points at which psychiatric help should be sought. Something remains to be said about shortcomings in the practice of adoption agencies and adoption committees, and about improvements which might be made.

Social Work

Some social workers, from inexperience or lack of training, fail to provide as full information as is required about the adoptive home, the motives of the couple who apply to adopt, their childhood and early family relationships, their marriage, their reaction to their infertility, and their capacity to satisfy the child's needs and to help him accept his adopted status. Brenner (4) in a follow-up study of adoptive homes describes the problems of the initial assessment, and discusses how far the worker's appraisal of each home before adoption had provided a correct picture of what it proved to be. Gaps in the information collected in the early case records, due either to lack of experience or to haste from pressure of work, led to less correct prediction of the success of the adoption. Better evaluation of the marital relationship, as judged by the worker's observations of the couple's behaviour towards each other and of the way in which they spoke about and to each other, seemed particularly needed, as well as more systematic recording of their joint attitude to parenthood from the start of their marriage, and of the details of their emotional experience of growing up. Workers occasionally in their interviews mistook the cautious reserve of a good 'parent' for coldness or, conversely but less often, judged a half-hearted and ambivalent applicant to be laudably non-committal. Sometimes the worker made superficial judgements when the couple were not interviewed separately as well as together. Some responded favourably to certain extroverted, mentally alert clients who did not prove successful parents. They sometimes supposed that an affectionate and self-reliant husband would compensate for a rather immature dependent wife—but this was not borne out by success in the adoption.

Untrained or voluntary workers are used by certain small adoption societies to carry out these difficult assignments, and in some cases they work on a rigid set of rules and do not know when to call in expert medical or psychological help. Local Authorities with their wider resources and better qualified personnel can avoid these defects, but something can be lost if no use is made of the sympathy and understanding of human relationships which many mature voluntary workers bring to adoption work. Too much professionalism and deliberate committee procedure can slow things down excessively.

Adoption Committees

It is extremely difficult to determine when a firm 'No' must be given to applicants. In an adoption committee which has to take the decision on this there may be different points of view, varying according to the members' personal bias, their qualifications to make a judgement and the adequacy of the case report, with its special medical details, which is placed before them. It is easy for a wrong decision to be taken by a committee even when, as is usually the case now, detailed medical reports have been made on the adopters and the child. The decision is facilitated when a professional group—social worker, psychiatrist and paediatrician—is available to report on appropriate aspects of a difficult case. Ultimate responsibility must still rest with the committee, who are less directly involved with the clients. It would be profitable, however, if each member of an adoption committee would read Brenner's (4) sober findings regarding the study of the adoption home as a means of diagnosing its suitability.

The Psychiatrist

The psychiatrist who works with children and young people is deeply involved in the problems and consequences of adoption. He becomes a strong advocate of using it to prevent the serious consequences of a child's homelessness or its rejection by its parents. He sees the pregnant school girl or unmarried woman too immature, too isolated or too maladjusted to be able to provide a home for her child; he witnesses the distressing spectacle of a rejected older child in an institution without outside friends, and, most disturbing of all, the anti-social adolescent or young adult who has reacted to his lack of parental support by rejecting any parental figures in his life and turning towards others like himself in an underworld of crime.

When the homeless child grows up unhappy or anti-social, the psychiatrist's thoughts must inevitably turn toward the practical measures of adoption which might have averted such an outcome. A home with some defects, or a home leading to only a partially successful adoption, might have saved the child from such a fate if it had been forthcoming when he needed it and was able to accept it. This must be taken into consideration when the success of adoption is reviewed as a whole.

Towards Better Adoptions

The available resources for investigating the emotional and social problems of the unmarried pregnant woman and for helping her to deal with them are woefully inadequate. In many places the maternity and antenatal services are unequal to the task. Too heavy a burden is at present laid on voluntary bodies such as the Moral Welfare Associations and the Council for the Unmarried Mother and her Child.

Because of the hazards they involve, the number of direct and third-party placements, especially of newly born babies, must be reduced, either by forbidding them by legal enactment or by giving to the Local Authority Children's Departments wider powers to control them. Even with the Law as it stands, Children's Departments can do much to lessen considerably the chances of third-party placement by developing their own adoption work, as the 1958 Act encouraged them to do; they can more safely place a very young baby of uncertain potentialities provisionally with foster-parents with a view to adoption, because of their wider resources of residential care or foster-homes if a breakdown occurs, and of skilled social workers to supervise the foster-homes. They can collect a pool of prospective and carefully vetted adopters which they can draw on in emergencies.

An area which calls for more action and more thought is the preparation of adopters for their exacting job. We know little about this, and as Wittenborn (28) concluded in summing up the Yale Child Development Study, 'additional research might provide the basis for some training of adoptive applicants. . . .'

Undoubtedly adopters need help, information, and guidance or support in dealing with their unfamiliar task and responsibilities. These should be given as fully as possible before they take a child. Classes in ordinary child rearing should be as available for prospective adopters as they are for expectant natural parents. The maternity and child welfare clinics might provide these services for both. Such didactic help and guidance should reinforce the individual parent's healthy instinctual feelings in this direction.

A film entitled 'A Baby Named X' (31), in the U.N. Social Welfare Film Loan Service, showed how an attempt was made to deal with the very difficult problem of unsuitable would-be adopters. When shown at the Annual Conference of Societies Registered for Adoption in 1961 it had a most disturbing effect on most of those who saw it, and was rather adversely criticised. In it a small group of couples who were applying to adopt a child met a number of times in a psychiatrically directed discussion circle; they were also visited in their homes by the social worker, and their backgrounds and earlier history were presented to the onlooker. In the discussion each pair looked at the situation of the other and thereby learned what they would have to offer an adopted child brought into their home. In the end, all but one came to the conclusion that they should not adopt a child.

To enable unsuitable would-be adopters to recognise their shortcomings as prospective parents, and thereby to deflect them from further efforts in that direction, is obviously desirable but hard to bring about. Group discussions, perhaps therapeutically oriented, might serve this purpose in some favourable situated centres.

The psychiatrist, unless he serves on an adoption committee, is likely to have his attention drawn mainly to the difficulties and failures of adoption. But these are few in proportion to the successes. Adopted children not only bring much happiness into the lives of their second parents, but develop as a whole more healthily than anyone who knew the family history and antecedents of the natural parents would have expected.

REFERENCES

1. Adoption Act, 1958. London: H.M.S.O.
2. Adoption Agencies Regulations, 1959. London: H.M.S.O.
3. BLACK, J. A. and STONE, F. H., 1958. *Lancet*, ii: 1272.
4. BRENNER, R. F., 1951. *A Follow-up of Adoptive Families*. Child Ad. Research Com., New York.
5. DOUGLAS, J. W. B. and BLOMFIELD, J. M., 1958. *Children Under Five*, p. 138. London: Allen & Unwin.
6. FRANKLIN, A. WHITE, 1954. *Proc. Roy. Soc. Med.*, **47**: 1044.
7. GOUGH, D., 1961. *Report Conf. S.C.S.R.A.*: 36-41.
8. ILLINGWORTH, R. S., 1963. *The Development of the Infant and Young Child*. Edinburgh and London: E. & S. Livingstone.
9. KNOBLOCK, H. and PASAMANICK, B., 1959. *J. Amer. Med. Assoc.*, **170**: 1384.
10. — 1955. A developmental questionnaire for infants 40 weeks of age. An evaluation. *Monogr. Soc. Res. Child Developm.*, **20**, No. 61, 2.
11. KORNITZER, M., 1962. *New Society*, 18 Oct.: 27-29.
12.   1955. *Report Conf. S.C.S.R.A.*: 21-31.
13. Legitimacy Act, 1959. London: H.M.S.O.
14. LEWIS, H., 1960. *Brit. Med. J.*, i: 1197-1200.
15.   1963. Adoption follow-up in the U.S.A. *Child Adoption*, **42**: 21-27.
16. MACDONALD, E. K., 1956. *Medical Officer*, **96**: 361-365.
17. PARKER, R. A., 1962. *Report Conf. S.C.S.R.A.*: 13-23.
18. PENROSE, L., 1953. *Report Conf. S.C.S.R.A.*: 81.
19. POND, D., 1956. *Report Conf. S.C.S.R.A.*: 31.
20. SALZBERGER, F., 1955. *Survey Based on Adoption Society Case Records*. London: N.A.M.H.
21. SHERIDAN, M., 1960. *The Developmental Progress of Infants and Young Children*. M.O.H. Report No. 102. London: H.M.S.O.
22. SKEELS, H. M. and HARMS, I., 1948. *J. Genet. Psych.*, **72**: 283.
23. SKODAK, M. and SKEELS, H. M., 1949. *Ibid.*, **75**: 85.
24. THEIS, S., 1924. *How Foster Children Turn Out*. New York State Charities Association.
25. THOMPSON, B., 1956. *Brit. J. Prev. and Soc. Med.*, **10**: 75-87.
26. WINNER, A., 1954. Report of Conference. In *Child Adoption*, **13**: 15-24.
27. WINNICOTT, D. W., 1957. *The Child and the Outside World*, pp. 47-51.
28. WITTENBORN, J. R., 1957. *The Placement of Adoptive Children*. Springfield, Ill.: Thomas.
29. *Publications of Standing Conference of Societies Registered for Adoption (S.C.S.R.A.)* (obtainable from Hon. Sec., A. Rampton, Gort Lodge, Petersham, Surrey):—
    Reports of Annual Conferences.
    Journal—*Child Adoption* (published quarterly).
    Leaflets for adopters—'*Adopting a Child*'. '*Adopting the Older Child*'. '*What Shall We Tell our Adopted Child?*'. '*If You Are Adopted*'.
30. *Books of general information:*—
    KORNITZER, M., 1952. *Child Adoption in the Modern World*. London: Putnam.
      1959. *Adoption*. London: Putnam.
    ROWE, JANE, 1959. *Yours by Choice*. London: Mills & Boon.
31. *Film*, 1959. '*A Baby named X*'. The Work of a Private Agency in New York. In United Nations Social Welfare Film Loan Service.

MORE RECENT WORKS

GOODACRE, I., 1963-4. Adoption agencies and their clients. *Child Adoption*, **43**.

HUMPHREY, M., 1963-4. Factors associated with maladjustment in adoptive families. *Child Adoption*, **43**: 25.

KIRK, H. D., 1963a. From Empirical Investigation to Theory and Return. *Annual Meeting of Canadian Political Science Association, Quebec*, 6th June.

1963b. Non-fecund people as parents: some social and psychological considerations. *Fertility and Sterility*, **14**, (3) (May-June). Amer. Soc. for Study of Sterility.

LEWIS, H., 1964. Some recent studies of adoption. *Child Adoption*, **44**: 17-23.

McWHINNIE, A. M., 1964. Adoption work of a Scottish Society. *Child Adoption*, **45**: 9-25.

OUNSTED, C. and HUMPHREY, M., 1963. Adoptive families referred for psychiatric advice. Part I, The children. *Brit. J. Psychiat.*, **109**: 462 (September).

1964. Part II, The Parents. *Ibid.*, **110**: 549.

WITMER, HERZOG, WEINSTEIN and SULLIVAN, 1963. *Independent Adoptions in the State of Florida: a Follow-up Study*. The Russell Sage Foundation, U.S.A.

XIX

THE NEUROPSYCHIATRY OF CHILDHOOD

D. A. POND

M.D., F.R.C.P., D.P.M.

Consultant Physician, University College and Maudsley Hospitals, London

---

1

The Brain-damaged Child

Almost all child psychiatrists recognise a clinical picture that appears to result from damage to a child's brain. Damage may occur at any time in development, but is probably more common at birth or after birth than *in utero*. The damage may be caused in a variety of ways—by infections, vascular disorders, physical trauma, or metabolically. The psychiatric pictures said to be commonly seen (which will be described in detail below) may occur with or without various epileptic disturbances, and with or without frank neurological signs and symptoms. Nothing will be said here of the pure neurology of childhood, which would of course require a volume of its own (such as Ford's (11)), particularly now that more is being discovered about the postnatal functional and anatomical development of the brain and the way in which these changes modify the classical neurological signs and symptoms of adults. This chapter will be mainly concerned with the psychiatric symptoms, and with the special problems of epilepsy.

A child may show an acute, but usually temporary, disturbance of behaviour after a severe head injury, brain infection, vascular accident, or other cerebral insult. Neurosurgeons and paediatricians are familiar with this regression, which most often lasts days rather than weeks but which may be more prolonged and even semi-permanent. The symptoms shown in this phase of regression, of course, very much depend upon the age of the child at the time, but they are usually recognised for what they are and are handled without any special psychiatric assistance. The child psychiatrist is not generally called in until the child's behaviour has been difficult for weeks or months. The clinical picture said to be commonly seen then is that of a very disturbed child with irritability, hyperkinesis, unpredictability, mood-swings and erratic educational performance. However, in a survey of such children seen at the Maudsley Children's Department (see Pond (24)), the symptoms seen were much more varied, and an assessment of the contribution of the brain damage itself to the clinical picture is more difficult to make than appears at first sight.

The Assessment of Brain Damage

Although some of the above mentioned symptoms are commonly found in brain-damaged children, none of them is invariably seen only in such children and never in non-brain-damaged children, so that the evidence for brain damage must be from facts other than the clinical psychiatric symptoms; otherwise the argument will become circular. Such a circular argument has often been made in relation to certain psychological tests, particularly those concerned with perceptual anomalies. It is false logic to argue that, because anomalous results are found in these tests in some children with brain damage, then these anomalous results indicate brain damage in children who only show these changes and no other clinical evidence.

The three main sources of evidence for brain damage are:

(1) History;
(2) Signs and symptoms in the central nervous system;
(3) Special tests—(*a*) physiological, (*b*) psychological.

(1) A history of trauma at birth or subsequently, for example in a car accident, is of course unequivocal evidence of damage at that time; but it is well known that the child's brain shows great powers of recovery from such physical damage. Follow-up studies of unselected head injuries in childhood by neurosurgeons show many fewer sequelae than in comparable series of adult head injuries. In assessing the late effects of such an injury it is easy to commit the fallacy of *post hoc ergo propter hoc*, particularly if the physical symptoms subsequently seen are ascribed to physical damage rather than to the emotional effects of a severe injury. These same arguments apply also to sequelae of infections and vascular accidents. As with adult injuries, the length of the period of unconsciousness at the time of the original trauma is the most reliable single guide to the severity of the damage at that time.

(2) The majority of children with gross motor and reflex disturbances get lumped together as spastics or cerebral palsies (some of whose special problems will be considered below). On the other hand minor asymmetries of power, tone and reflexes have often been described in behaviour problem children, but their significance is uncertain. They imply, if anything, only damage to those parts of the brain concerned with locomotion. It is another

question whether damage in those areas of the brain can be related to psychological disturbances. Also such damage does not imply that there must be damage that may be more significant for psychological disturbance in other areas of the brain. In the clinical population—that is to say in patients with psychological disturbances—left-handedness may be regarded as slight evidence in favour of damage to the dominant left side of the brain, but on the whole too much is made of so-called crossed laterality as a cause of stammering and all sorts of other language disturbances. Left-handedness should imply no more than it says, namely that the control of limb movements is being better done by the right hemisphere than the left. It does not mean that speech or any other functions have also been transferred to the other side or elsewhere.

(3) Electroencephalography (EEG) is such a simple, safe and not unpleasant test that it is probably ordered far more often than it need be. Unfortunately in the field of psychiatry it has turned out to be a rather disappointing technique of investigation. A single random EEG taken months or years after a cerebral trauma is unlikely to give any evidence for or against existing physiological disturbances unless the patient also has epilepsy. Serial EEGs taken at about monthly intervals following trauma may show interesting progressive changes, but any one single record of such a series is of less value. One of the reasons for this is the very wide range of EEG appearances in children. As is well known, the EEG shows striking changes in maturation from birth to the teens. Very little is known about this process of maturation apart from bald description of the actual appearances of the record. The wide differences between EEGs of children in the same age group cannot be correlated with any psychological or physiological process of maturation. Moreover the EEG itself is a very coarse measure of cerebral function, so that widely different conditions can produce very similar EEG tracings. If, for example, a child's EEG months or years after head injury shows an excess of generalised slow activity, this is just as likely to be a constitutional maturational defect present before the injury as it is to be the result of injury. Although there have been various attempts to correlate different kinds of EEG anomaly with particular clinical symptoms, none has so far been clearly proven (see Pond in Hill and Parr (26)). As will be discussed below in more detail, the EEG has for all practical purposes only one useful function in the clinic, namely the sorting out of different forms of epilepsy; but for that it is absolutely indispensable.

The air encephalogram is of course a much more difficult procedure, since for most children it requires a short general anaesthetic and cannot be done except in a properly equipped neurosurgical unit. Like the EEG it is a fairly coarse test, quite large areas of tumour, cyst or cerebral atrophy having to be present before ventricular enlargement or distortion or pooling of air over the cerebral cortex is seen. With children suspected of focal brain damage and epilepsy it is sometimes justified to arrange for their admission to a neurosurgical unit, where not only can an air encephalo-gram be done under a short general anaesthetic but also a satisfactory sleep EEG, with or without special sphenoidal leads, can be obtained. The outcome of these special investigations, however successful, is likely to do no more than prove the existence of past trauma and make likely the presence of persisting anatomical damage, which may or may not be of functional significance. Such tests can do no more than that because of the absence of a proven physiological basis to most psychiatric phenomena.

Psychological tests are frequently administered to children suspected of brain damage, but the results are more equivocal than in adults suspected of dementia or focal disorders. Differences between verbal and performance scores are more inconstant than in adults, and it is probable that a generally low score compared with the score that might be expected from the intelligence level of parents and siblings is more suggestive of brain damage than any sub-test discrepancies. Several tests of visuomotor functions (e.g. the Bender-Gestalt) have been tried, but they have been inadequately standardised, and critical reviews such as Benton's (1) and Graham and Berman's (13) show their limited value. The psychologist's function with brain-damaged children is to help the individual case as regards special educational needs; his contribution to the diagnostic problem is more dubious.

In the assessment of the significance of a brain injury, two very important factors in addition to the site and size of the injury have to be taken into consideration: (a) the previous personality of the child before the trauma occurred, and (b) the handling of the child subsequent to the injury by its family and others in contact with it.

Influence of Previous Personality. Although clinicians have long thought that unstable personalities tended to react badly to cerebral trauma, clear evidence for this has only recently become apparent. The best papers are by Dencker (6) and by Dencker and Löfving (7), who used a twin series in whom one member of each pair had had a head injury. Dencker was mainly interested in the so-called post-traumatic syndrome as seen in adults, but there is no reason why his work should not apply equally to children. The conditions seen in the injured twin were for the most part an exaggeration of symptoms and personality traits seen in the non-injured identical twin. There were also no *significant* differences in various psycho-logical tests, though the injured twin tended to be in general a little slower than the non-injured one.

Pond (24) has found that the commonest causes of brain damage in the child psychiatric population are the events around the time of birth, whether by anoxia or by physical damage with forceps etc. There is a certain amount of evidence that abnormal births are not distributed at random in the population but are seen more often in the lower social classes and families with less satisfactory social standards. Fairweather and Illsley (9), for example, investigating the children in the special schools for subnormality in Aberdeen, found that the majority of such children came from poor homes, and did not think that any extra factors of birth trauma were needed to explain their low intelligence. This is perhaps an extreme view, but their general argument is sound and suggests that heredity, and environmental factors other than just the birth history, have to be taken into account as well. For example, in a further paper entitled 'The Social Aetiology of Foetal Damage', Illsley (21) points out that social class as measured by the husband's occupation can imply differences in the premarital physique and intelligence of the mother, and these factors are known to be related to birth difficulties. In this field correlations abound and causal connections are only too easily assumed.

Effect of Environmental Handling. This refers to the social milieu of the child after the injury, as opposed to the child's state before the injury which was referred to in the preceding paragraph. With both factors, of course, environment and constitution enter into the changes seen in the child, but the disturbances of environmental handling subsequent to the injury can usually be seen going on when the child is referred to a psychiatric clinic, whereas in most cases past history can be established only by inference. Harrington and Letemendia's (16) study of the psychiatric sequelae of head injury in children provides the clearest evidence of the importance of parental handling in relation to psychiatric symptoms in injured children. They followed up a series of cases seen only in neurosurgical units, and cases seen in the Maudsley Child Psychiatric Unit. The papers of Pasamanick and his colleagues (Rogers *et al.* (28)) purport to show the importance of minor brain injury in the production of a wide range of neuropsychiatric disturbances, but much of their work does not seem to be controlled adequately for social factors and, paradoxically, seems to provide good evidence for the significance of the latter rather than the former factors. The paramount importance of the usual causes of disturbance in the child psychiatric population for producing psychiatric symptoms in brain-injured children was clearly brought out by Pond (24) from the Maudsley Child Psychiatric Unit. In his series the symptoms seen and the age at which they occurred in children with brain injury were similar to those in non-injured children, with a highly significant exception of differences of intelligence (Tables I and II).

The tables show a preponderance of boys, as is found in the non-brain-damaged population. Though most of them were damaged at or around the time of birth they did not present at the clinic till late years, and then with symptoms similar to those seen in children without brain damage. Table II lists only hyperkinesis, aggression and neurotic symptoms as these were the only ones seen sufficiently often for analysis, but gross obsessive-compulsive symptoms were sometimes seen, and very rarely a typical autistic psychosis. The proportions of these various symptom groups are probably similar to those seen in the non-brain-damaged child guidance population. Also the great majority of brain-injured children seen in a psychiatric clinic came from the same sort of broken and disturbed homes as the non-injured children.

TABLE I

Brain-damaged Children without Epilepsy (Males, 40; Females, 18)

EVIDENCE FOR BRAIN DAMAGE		AGE WHEN BRAIN DAMAGE SUFFERED	
History only	30	0–1 year	35
Physical signs	21	2–4 years	8
AEG	4	5–9 ,,	7
EEG	3	10+ ,,	2
		Not known	6

INTELLIGENCE LEVEL		AGE WHEN FIRST SEEN AT CLINIC			
Less than 50	8				Expectation
50–79	21				from total
80+	29				clinic cases
Significant discrepancies	11	2–4 years	3	(5%)	6%
		5–9 ,,	21	(36%)	23%
		10–14 ,,	28	(49%)	45%
		15+ ,,	6	(10%)	26%

TABLE II

Brain-damaged Children without Epilepsy (58 Cases)

SOCIAL CLASS	TOTAL	EXPECTED	ENVIRONMENT	
I	8 (14%)	4·7%	Normal home	13
II	9 (16%)	16·2%	Broken	13
III	18 (31%)	55·1%	Institution	4
IV	13 (22%)	10·7%	Other relatives mentally ill	16
V	8 (14%)	13·3%	Abnormal parental attitudes	30
Not known	2 —	—		

	AGE OF BRAIN DAMAGE					AGE WHEN SEEN AT CLINIC			
	0–1	2–4	5–9	10+	N.K.	2–4	5–9	10–14	15+
Hyperkinesis	8	2	1	0	2	2	8	3	0
Aggression	11	4	2	0	2	2	7	10	0
Neurotic symptoms	15	4	5	0	5	0	10	16	3

The apparent syndrome of brain damage would therefore appear to be the effect of unstable previous personality and/or subsequent environmental handling upon a child who, as a result of brain injury, is retarded in the general field of learning, memory and intelligence. The handicap is probably not fundamentally dissimilar to that of dementia in adults, though of course with the basic difference that the demented adult's inability to learn new material is to a greater or lesser extent compensated by the persistence of previously well-learned patterns of behaviour which are not yet present in the young child. It is still an open question whether there are any specific defects in the fields of emotion and volition, as would be suggested by the common symptoms of irritability and hyperkinesis. It is probable that these symptoms are in fact simply those that are appropriate to the child's mental age, so that the disturbances can be included under the general heading of lack or slowness of development.

In addition to these general psychiatric disturbances, there may of course be also focal disorders, such as aphasia, not to mention the special problems of cerebral palsy to be discussed below. However, as is well known, focal disturbances such as aphasia are much less common in children than in adults, and Pond has found at the Maudsley Clinic that in brain-damaged children secondary psychogenic mutism is much commoner than an aphasic disorder. (See also the chapter by Worster-Drought, 'Disorders of Speech in Childhood'.)

In addition to the question of focal psychological disturbances, there is also the question whether there are any focal anatomical lesions such as might even underly the general psychiatric picture of brain damage. Clinico-pathological evidence on this important topic is unfortunately lacking, though it has long been suspected from the clinical material, and is partially confirmed by animal experiments, that the so-called rhinencephalon or deep temporal structures may be of particular importance as the anatomical substrate to emotion and personality generally. On the other hand consciousness and memory are more closely connected with the midbrain and thalamic regions; but the whole subject of the anatomical basis to psychiatric disturbances is too vast to be dealt with here, and is largely without practical clinical application.

Treatment of the Brain-damaged Child

The general principles for handling these children may be deduced from what has been said about the probable nature of their disturbances. The general approach of a child psychiatric clinic to a disturbed child in the family setting is appropriate also to the brain-damaged child, It is essential that the parents, teachers and others accept the child not as one irrevocably damaged, but as one who is slowed down in learning—not merely learning in the narrow educational sense, but generally as regards the usual behaviour that would be appropriate to his chronological age. Endless time and patience are often needed in the process of re-education, but everyone can take comfort from the fact that time is on the side of the parents, teachers and doctors, since the normal processes of ageing appear to cause the worst of the symptoms to subside, particularly the hyperkinesis. On the other hand parents must be prepared for a possible exacerbation at adolescence, especially with boys, who may often appear to become more aggressive at that age, though in fact much of the difference is probably due to the fact that they are bigger and stronger and can therefore knock down parents who were formerly able to control their tantrums.

Many of these children appear to have special educational difficulties. Some are very clumsy in all movements, others may have difficulties in all forms of number work, and still others have reading problems. As has already been stressed, the apparent focal disabilities are probably not evidence of focal cerebral damage, but they do sometimes warrant special investigation by educational psychologists and the designing of specific teaching methods. In general all such handicapped children do better in small groups with distracting stimuli avoided as far as possible. Tizard's (33) work has shown very strikingly how much of the learning difficulties of some retarded children is environmentally determined and can respond to better general handling.

The indications for individual psychotherapy or psychoanalysis in these children are the same as in the non-brain-damaged child, though naturally the frequent low intelligence of the handicapped child means that psychotherapy is comparatively rarely possible. Not uncommonly these children are too disturbed for their own parents to manage, particularly when, as usually happens, the parents have their own problems for whose solution the handicapped child may have become a convenient scapegoat. Under these circumstances a period in an in-patient psychiatric unit or in a special school for maladjusted children is needed. Periods of months rather than weeks away are usually required, but more or less permanent institutionalisation is not usually called for unless the child is a severe mental defective (the special problems of defectives are discussed in the chapter by B. Kirman). The handling of the rest of them probably more closely approximates to what goes on in child psychiatric units than to what goes on within the purely educational orbit.

Many drugs have been tried for controlling the more troublesome symptoms of the brain-damaged child, particularly the irritability and hyperkinesis. Phenobarbitone nearly always makes such children worse rather than better, particularly the younger ones. Amphetamine sometimes has a startling quietening influence, though large doses (up to 30 mg. a day) may be needed; occasionally irritable and hyperkinetic children are not only slowed by it, but also made acutely miserable with the turning in of the aggression to produce a depressive picture. The new tranquillisers may also be given a trial—there is no convincing evidence that one is any better than another—and usually the dosage can be reduced or stopped after a few weeks or months when a new equilibrium between the child and its environment has been established.

Sally, aged 10, illustrates most of the diagnostic difficulties already discussed. Four months before being seen in the clinic she had a severe meningitis, with coma and convulsions. After the illness the parents described a personality change with an increase in irritability and untidiness and, most prominently, a loss of some scholastic abilities already acquired, together with an apparent loss of recent memory. No abnormal physical signs were found, and serial EEGs showed at first only a doubtful excess of slow activity, which improved over 6 months. Extensive psychological tests showed average intelligence, but an apparent impairment of new learning, especially for retention over 24 hours, though learning under stress was if anything better than in unstressed conditions. School reports gave a consistently better picture of behaviour and learning ability than that given by the parents. Psychiatric explorations of parents and child over ensuing months gave evidence of a disturbed mother-child relationship from the beginning, when Sally had been unwanted, having come too early in the marriage; then the mother had returned early to part-time work, and was only at home fully when the second daughter came a few years later. The mother remarked on Sally's apparently enjoying her daily visiting while in hospital, thereby actually getting more of mother's undivided attention than at any other time. Both parents are intelligent, educated and ambitious, especially father, and Sally's early school career suggested that the average IQ scores probably reflected her pre-illness level. The apparent learning difficulty cannot be simply ascribed to brain damage, as the child is and always has been under considerable parental pressure. It is just as likely to be part and parcel of a long-standing psychiatric problem, exacerbated by hospitalisation for a serious physical illness. No clinical observations or special investigations show unequivocal evidence of persistent cerebral disturbance. In the handling of the child drugs were of no value, and her school progress went back to her previous level without special coaching. Mother and child continue attending the clinic for the general psychological difficulties.

Cerebral Palsy

This is of course a heterogeneous group of brain-damaged children with various degrees and types of *motor disorders*, often together with other defects, sensory, intellectual or characterological. Many of the problems of these children (e.g. the surgical treatment of distorted limbs) are outside the scope of this book. Of psychiatric importance are the facts that about half of those reported in various series have IQs below 80 (Hansen (15)) and that disturbances of personality occur in about the same proportion (Floyer (10); Dunsdon (8)).

In general, the more severe the motor defect, the lower is likely to be the intelligence level and the more disturbed the personality. The evidence for differences in intelligence between patients with right- and left-sided palsies is conflicting, and the differences are not therefore likely to be significant. Low intelligence is, of course, a very important factor limiting the rehabilitation of cerebral palsied children, since there is unfortunately no prosthesis for the brain. The behaviour disorders seen do not seem to be in any way specific, but result from the complex interaction of environmental pressures and misunderstandings and the child's own limitations.

Epilepsy complicates the picture in about half the spastics and in a smaller proportion of athetoids (Illingworth (19)). The intelligence is usually lower in those with than in those without epilepsy (Hansen (15)). The fits are sometimes very disabling, but Holt (18) has shown that in many they occur only in the earlier years and then spontaneously die out. It is for intractable cases of epilepsy and behaviour disorder that hemispherectomy may be seriously considered. The operation does not usually increase the motor defect, but a hemianopia may result, if not already present (frequently unsuspected). Of course such surgery can only be contemplated if the pathology is essentially unilateral, and in any case this applies to only a few of those cases disabled enough for surgery to be considered at all.

2

The Epileptic Child

General Introduction

Much has been discovered about epilepsy in the last twenty years, and for general discussion reference should be made to standard texts such as Lennox's two volumes (21), Hill and Driver (17) etc. The particular problems of epilepsy in childhood have been discussed by Pond in Holzel and Tizard (23) and in Pond (24). Epilepsy is a common complication of brain injury, particularly in childhood, and it appears to cause its own additional psychiatric problems, to be described below. The benign and uncomplicated forms of epilepsy, such as the common febrile convulsions or teething fits, do not produce any particular psychological disturbance and are therefore rarely seen by child psychiatrists, who thus get the impression that epileptic convulsions can be of much more serious import than in fact they usually are.

There are three ways in which epileptic attacks may cause additional disturbances: (1) by physiological disturbances produced by the epileptic discharges, as seen (a) in overt clinical attacks and (b) possibly in other ways; (2) through the social handicaps of epilepsy; (3) through the side-effects of anti-convulsant drugs.

Types of Epileptic Attack

The major seizure or *grand mal* attack is the commonest form of fit and the one best known to everyone. Socially such fits can create a good deal of disturbance, but there is no very convincing evidence that the fits themselves cause any damage to the brain unless the sufferer becomes severely anoxic or else goes into *status epilepticus*. This last is, of course, a medical emergency which usually needs hospitalisation. Major fits can be divided into two main types: those that begin suddenly without any aura or focal onset—the centrencephalic type in the accompanying table, and those which begin a focal cortical onset with movements in a limb or an aura which spreads more or less rapidly to involve the whole brain. The details of the major fit pattern itself are of less importance than the details of the onset of the attack, since the latter information usually points to the site of origin of the attacks; the various forms of minor epilepsy are usually even more informative in this connection. There are two main groups of such attacks, corresponding to the two main types of major seizure. The centrencephalic forms of minor attacks are the typical *petit mal* or *absence*, and the generalised myoclonic jerks. The former are usually

TABLE III

*Classification of Epilepsy**

	GROUP 1 GENERALISED EPILEPSIES		GROUP 2 PARTIAL EPILEPSIES	
	(A) Primary subcortical (centrencephalic)	(B) Secondary subcortical	(A) Rhinencephalic (or temporal lobe)	(B) Isocortex
Fit pattern	*Petit mal* ±*grand mal*	*Petit mal* ±generalised myoclonic ± *grand mal*	'Psychomotor' ± *grand mal*	Focal cortical (Jacksonian) ±*grand mal*
EEG (a) Inter-seizure	Symmetrical spike and wave transients	Irregular spike and wave or focal temporal	Temporal lobe spikes (often only in sleep)	Normal or focal spikes
(b) Ictal	Three per second spike and wave	Variable but generalised and irregular spikes and spike and wave complexes	Complex, progressive, usually symmetrical patterns of slow activity	Various, often focal only
Aetiology	Predominantly genetic. Sometimes febrile precipitation of *grand mal*	Various, predominantly diffuse brain damage (e.g. anoxia)	Various, mainly trauma and infections	As above
Age of onset	*Petit mal* from 4–10	From birth	From 4 years	Any age
IQ	Normal	Often subnormal	Normal or subnormal	Normal
Personality	Normal or minor neurotic traits	No specific changes	Severe behaviour disorders	No specific changes, usually normal
Treatment	Diones±amphetamine and phenytoin. Succinimides	All drugs in combination	Primidone, amphetamine. Surgery	Phenobarbitone, phenytoin

* The classification of epileptic attacks has recently been reviewed by an International Committee. The review is to be published in a forthcoming number of *Epilepsia*, to which reference should be made.

seen at school age; the latter are commoner in younger children. Of the minor seizures of focal cortical onset the commonest is the complex type of attack that begins in the deep temporal structures. Children, especially young ones, cannot usually describe their aura in any detail, but it may sometimes be inferred from a child's actions, for example by the way he will suddenly clutch his stomach and run to a parent with obvious signs of fear or distress. In these attacks consciousness may only be partially lost and periods of disturbed behaviour are common post-ictal, so that the whole attack may be dismissed as something entirely psychogenic. Again it is the events at the very onset of the attack which are of the most importance in the differential diagnosis. As far as possible the clinician must decide whether the child has epilepsy or not, and vague formulations such as hystero-epilepsy, epileptic equivalents and so on should be avoided. The child may of course show psychogenic disturbances of consciousness and other episodes of curious behaviour as well, but the presence of undoubted epilepsy carries with it quite different implications for treatment and prognosis from those implied by purely psychogenic disturbances. Furthermore it is important to know as far as possible what sort of epilepsy the child has, since there are again great differences in treatment and prognosis and in the implications for psychological disturbances between one form of epilepsy and another. As has already been mentioned, the EEG is indispensable in sorting out the various forms of epilepsy, a function which it does much better than it answers the question whether a patient has epilepsy or not. Sometimes more than one EEG may be needed, and sleep records can be more informative than waking records. On the other hand the use of convulsant drugs such as metrazol in graduated doses is of much less value in children than in adults. Nevertheless, a small proportion of attacks may be still undiagnosed, and in those circumstances (particularly if the patient has a 'non-specific abnormal' EEG) it may be justifiable to try the therapeutic test of a small dose of an anticonvulsant, using one such as phenytoin which has no significant hypnotic effect and is therefore unlikely to benefit purely psychogenic attacks.

The clinical correlations of the various forms of epilepsy in children are discussed by Pond (24). The physiological disturbances produced by the minor centrencephalic form of attack (Fig. 1) are quite different from those produced by the minor temporal lobe form of attack. In the former there is instantaneous loss of consciousness, with an instantaneous return to full consciousness at the end of the seizure. The patient thus has no knowledge whatever of the attack until it is over, when he becomes aware that the time has moved on a little bit since he last noticed anything. On the other hand the latter form of seizure is often very disturbing, as the aura may be a terrifying experience and the partial disturbance of consciousness like a bad nightmare. These differences are probably related to the different parts of the brain that are mainly involved in the two types of attacks. However, in addition to the disturbances produced in overt clinical attacks, there is some evidence of interference with cerebral activity with even the briefest bursts of generalised spike and wave in the EEG (see Tizard and Margerison (32), and Tizard and Margerison (31A)). It might be expected that even such transient losses of consciousness would have a serious effect on the patient's performance, but paradoxically the intelligence level of most children with *petit mal* is average. This effect may however be in some way related to the curious passivity of personality that patients with *petit mal* often show. In addition to the disturbances associated with spike and wave, Goldie and Green (12) describe more complicated and longer episodes of partial disturbance of concentration seen during psychotherapeutic interviews with patients suffering from *petit mal*. These episodes are not accompanied by any obvious change in the EEG and their physiological status is uncertain. These episodes are different from *petit mal* status as illustrated in Fig. 2.

The timing and frequency of occurrence of all forms of epileptic attack are to some extent affected by the psychological state of the patient, but this applies particularly to the *petit mal* type and generalised spike and wave, as Tizard and Margerison's paper shows. An extreme and bizarre example of the influence of the psyche on seizures is, of course, the rare case of self-induced epilepsy; the largest series of cases of this has been collected by Sherwood and his colleagues (29). Most, if not all, of these children have psychological disturbances, and many of them are of low intelligence. So far no one has been able to explain how and why those patients discover for themselves the epileptogenic effect of intermittent photic stimulation.

Compared with the generalised epilepsies, there is much less certain evidence of interferences of cerebral activity (other than in overt attacks) in patients suffering from temporal lobe and other forms of partial epilepsy. This is probably because the epileptic activity recordable in the EEG from such deep foci is only a very small sample, and probably an unimportant sample, of what is actually going on. From the clinical point of view these attacks are associated with a great deal more psychological intellectual disturbance than *petit mal* seizures; naturally this is partly due to the fact that focal cortical seizures are associated with acquired brain damage, which may be quite extensive even when the patient has no usual clinical neurological signs. This is in contrast to the *petit mal* child, whose epilepsy is usually of mainly genetic origin without evidence of acquired brain damage. However this cannot be the sole cause for the difference, because, for example, in adults even extensive tumours involving the temporal regions do not produce the changes seen in temporal lobe epilepsy (Bingley (2)).

Intelligence and Epilepsy

In general children with fits beginning in the first year of life have low intelligence, since they usually have severe brain damage from birth or even *in utero*. The child who has had so-called hypsarhythmia also is of low intelligence in most cases. This is of course a clinical EEG syndrome, not an aetiological entity, as a variety of causes have been suspected although few proven by autopsy (Millichap *et al.* (22)). In contrast the next chronological groups—febrile convulsions and then *petit mal*—usually have normal intelligence, but the focal epilepsies, especially temporal lobe epilepsy, may be associated with impaired ability. In general patients with many seizures (especially *grand mal*) have lower IQs than those with few seizures, presumably because more fits implies more brain damage in the first place, but also because major fits with anoxia can in some cases produce further brain damage. The fit patterns of mental defectives are often atypical, presumably because the associated severe brain damage modifies

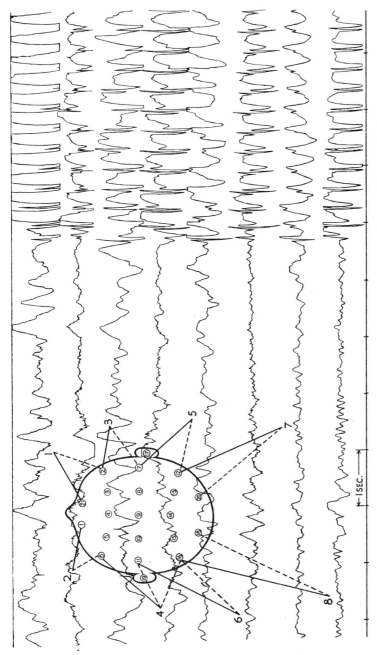

FIG. 1. Girl, aged 8, with R-sided vascular lesion (note the slow activity on the R side (channels 1, 3, 5 and 7) compared with the left before the onset of a *petit mal* attack. The spike and wave complexes are asymmetrical, being of lower amplitude on the injured R side compared with the left. This is an example of secondary centrencephalic minor epilepsy.

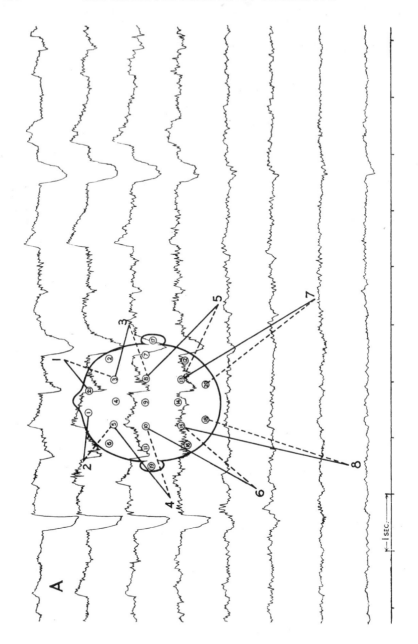

Fig. 2A

FIG. 2B

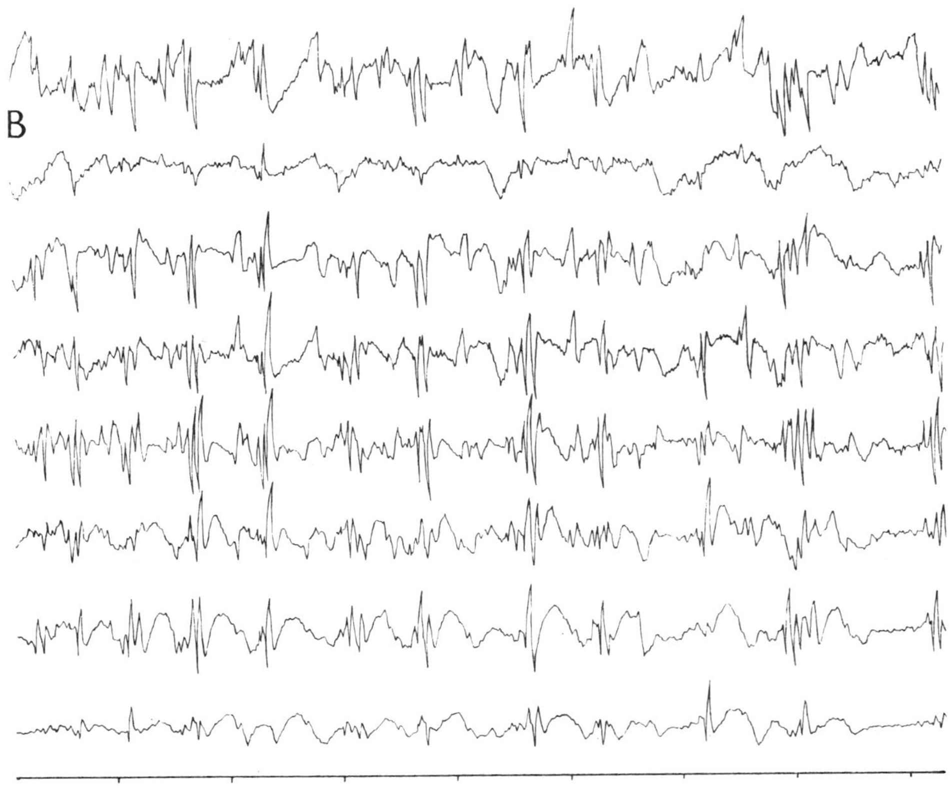

FIGS. 2A and B

Taken at the same gains and speed, in the same recording positions. The E.E.G. of a high grade mental defective girl aged 13 who suffered from long spells of confusion. The first tracing shows her normal interictal record. The second tracing, taken during the confusional spell, shows continuous polyspike and slow wave complexes (petit mal status).

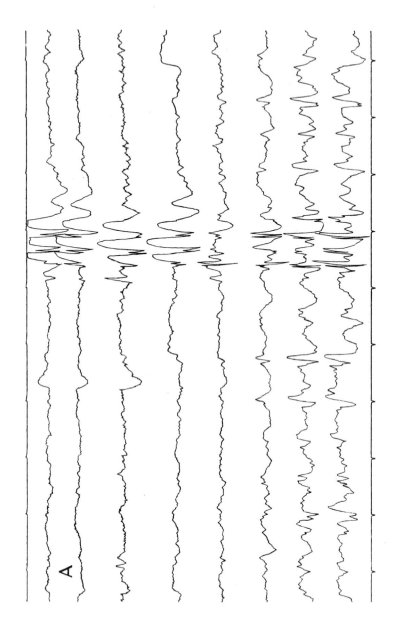

FIG. 3A

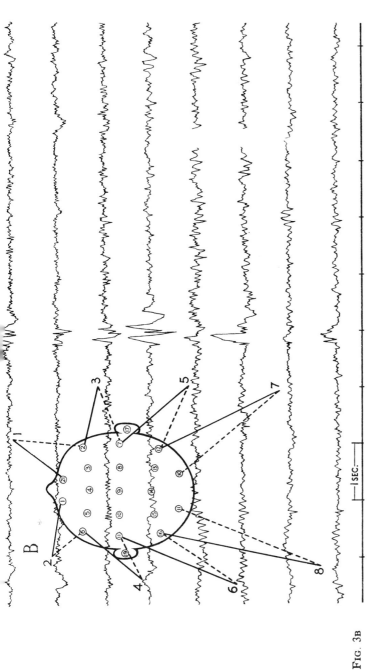

FIG. 3B

FIGS. 3A and B. These two records were taken in 1954 and 1963 respectively, in the same recording positions, to show maturation with the increasing dominance of regular alpha rhythm in the posterior channels. In 1954, when the boy was aged 9, the epileptic activity is mostly in the posterior regions (Channels 7 and 8) but one generalised burst of spike and wave is seen. 9 years later the occipital foci have disappeared and only a left mid-temporal focus is seen (between channels 4 and 6). The boy's epilepsy has diminished in the duration and frequency of fits, but whereas when young he was typically hyperkinetic, he now shows the more adult picture of slowness, bad temper and paranoid tendencies.

the spread of abnormal discharge. Fits are increasingly common the lower the intelligence, rising to over 50% in idiots. Mongols and cretins rarely have epilsepy, but patients with other metabolic and all traumatic conditions have epilepsy commonly (Pond (25)).

Although the majority of children with epilepsy show the normal expected or a slightly slower rate of intellectual development, a few children actually deteriorate intellectually, with a loss of previously acquired functions. There are two common forms of this deterioration: the first is the now well recognised syndrome of infantile spasms or hypsarhythmia already mentioned, which nearly always starts before the first year and runs a stormy course with numerous major and minor seizures. These tend to die out after a few years, but the patient usually remains mentally defective. This appears to be a clinical syndrome with a variety of causes. The second form of deterioration is less well recognised, but Chaudhry and Pond (3) found that drugs were not responsible for epileptic deterioration. Even quite small children tolerate doses up to adult level and combinations of several drugs may be needed, especially if the patient has several different forms of attack (see Table III). Among the most recent advances may be mentioned the substitution of the succinimides (such as Zarontin) for the diones (such as tridione) as the first drugs of choice for *petit mal* and generalised myoclonic epilepsies.

Temporal lobectomy for intractable epilepsy complicated by behaviour disorders is only very rarely needed in childhood, probably because children with such a severe disorder not improving with drugs etc. nearly always have such extensive brain damage that a unilateral lobectomy is of limited value.

Social Problems of Epileptic Children

Although the physiological disturbances described above are of great importance in understanding the limitations of the epileptic child, particularly as regards intelligence rather than personality, the social problems posed by having attacks are in practice far more important in producing the sort of symptoms that bring a child to a psychiatric clinic. This was shown clearly by Grunberg and Pond (14) some years ago. As with brain-damaged children generally, the most important contribution of the Child Psychiatric Clinic to the understanding of the epileptic child lies in the application of its own social and psychological methods of investigation to him. The epileptic has, of course, many real difficulties to face. He must usually adhere rigidly to regular medication, and may have to eschew certain activities that might be dangerous for him, such as swimming or cycling. However he suffers more often from the frustrating effect of over-restriction than from the supposed danger of many activities. Taking slight risks is better than boredom, and an interesting life undoubtedly reduces the tendency to fits. Frequent attacks may lead to slowing up of scholastic progress, though in practice this is far more often due to innate dullness unrelated to attacks, as is shown by the fact that, if and when the attacks can be brought under control by anticonvulsants, no great increase in school progress occurs. In addition to these real handicaps, the epileptic child may suffer from more serious problems as a result of the prejudices and the misunderstandings of those looking after him. Epilepsy is still a dread disease in the popular mind, associated with deterioration in personality and dangerous proclivities to violence or sexual malpractices— all of which, of course, is largely untrue, and when such do occur they result precisely from the over-restriction and over-protectiveness that these fears have engendered. The parents of epileptics benefit greatly from simple explanations of what goes on in their children in such terms as 'scars in the brain' causing over-activity and the 'dampening' thereof by drugs. It is particularly important to stress that it is a physical disease for which neither the child nor themselves can be blamed.

In most parts of the country the educational facilities for epileptics have greatly improved since the war, mainly as a result of programmes of education by school medical officers and others, so that the epileptic child is for the most part accepted in schools appropriate to his intellectual level. Placement in residential schools for epileptic or backward or mal-adjusted children is now necessary in most cases only because of associated behaviour disorders, or because of parental inability to cope with difficult handicapped children. Significantly such residential schools are now called Hospital Schools rather than Colonies, implying that they are places for relatively long-term medical supervision and stabilisation rather than institutions in which people were expected to stay for all their school years or longer. The sort of services that are needed for such handicapped children are well discussed in the World Health Organisation Technical Bulletin No. 130 (34) and in the Cohen Committee Report (4). All child psychiatric services should have an in-patient unit fully able to cope with these problems. According to Pond and Bidwell's Survey (27), children who have had problems during their school age are likely to go on being difficult in employment and other social relationships; hence particular care is needed with this group, especially during the awkward transition from school to work and to greater independence from surveillance by parents and school medical officer. Adolescence brings problems to most children, but especially to those with a social handicap. For epileptics there is the additional problem that many change their pattern of attacks (over half those with *petit mal* develop *grand mal*, for example), and a change of medication is therefore also needed.

REFERENCES

1. BENTON, A. L., 1962. *Child Development*, **33**: 199.
2. BINGLEY, T., 1958. *Acta Psychiat. Scand.*, Suppl. 120.
3. CHAUDHRY, M. R., and POND, D. A., 1961. *J. Neurol. Neurosurg. Psychiat.*, **24**, 213.
4. Cohen Committee Report, 1956. *Cohen Committee Report on the Medical Care of Epileptics.* London: H.M.S.O.
5. CRUICKSHANK, W. M. and BICE, H. V., 1955. In *Cerebral Palsy* (ed. W. M. Cruickshank and G. M. Raus), Chap. IV. Syracuse Univ. Press.
6. DENCKER, S. J., 1958. *Acta Psychiat. Scand.*, Suppl. 123.
7. DENCKER, S. J. and LÖFVING, B., 1958. *Ibid.*, Suppl. 122.
8. DUNSDON, M. L., 1952. *The Educability of Cerebral Palsied Children.* London: Newnes.
9. FAIRWEATHER, D. V. I. and ILLSLEY, R., 1960. *Brit. J. Prev. Soc. Med.*, **14**: 149.
10. FLOYER, E. B., 1955. *A Psychological Study of a City's Cerebral Palsied Children.* London: Brit. Council for Welfare of Spastics.
11. FORD, F. R., 1952. *Diseases of the Nervous System in Infancy, Childhood and Adolescence*, 3rd. ed. C. C. Thomas.
12. GOLDIE, L. and GREEN, J. M., 1961. *Epilepsia* (Amsterdam), 2: 306.
13. GRAHAM, F. K. and BERMAN, P. W., 1961. *Amer. J. Orthopsychiat.*, **31**: 713.
14. GRUNBERG, F. and POND, D. A., 1957. *J. Neurol. Neurosurg. Psychiat.*, **20**: 65.
15. HANSEN, E., 1960. *Acta Psychiat. et Neurol. Scand.*, Suppl. 146.
16. HARRINGTON, J. A. and LETEMENDIA, F. J. J. ,1958. *J. Ment. Sci.*, **104**: 1205.
17. HILL, D. and DRIVER, M., 1962. *Recent Advances in Neurology and Neuropsychiatry*, 7th ed. (ed. R. Brain and E. B. Strauss). London: Churchill.
18. HOLT, K. S., 1961. Little Club Clinics in Developmental Medicine, No. 4. *Hemiplegic Cerebral Palsy in Children and Adults.* Bristol.
19. ILLINGWORTH, R. S., 1958. (ed.), *Recent Advances in Cerebral Palsy.* London: Churchill.
20. ILLSLEY, R., 1961. *J. Ment. Subnorm.*, 7: 86.
21. LENNOX, W. G., 1960. *Epilepsy and Related Disorders* (2 vols.).
22. MILLICHAP, J. G. *et al.*, 1962. *Epilepsia*, 3: 188.
23. POND, D. A., 1958. *Modern Trends in Paediatrics* (ed. A. Holzel and J. P. M. Tizard), Chap. 12. London: Butterworth.
24. —— 1961. *Brit. Med. J.*, ii: 1377 and 1454.
25. —— 1962. *Proc. London Conf. on the Scientific Study of Ment. Def.*, 1: 207.
26. —— 1963. In *Electroencephalography*, 2nd Edition (ed. D. Hill and G. Parr).
27. POND, D. A. and BIDWELL, B. H., 1960. *Epilepsia*, 1: 285.
28. ROGERS, M. E., LILIENFELD, A. M. and PASAMANICK, B., 1955. *Acta Psychiat. Scand.*, Suppl. 102.
29. SHERWOOD, S. L. *et al.*, 1962. *Arch. Neurol. Chicago*, 6: 49.
30. STEPHEN, E., 1958. In *Mental Deficiency* (ed. A. M. Clarke and A. D. B. Clarke).
31. STRAUSS, A. A. and LEHTINEN, L. E., 1947. *Psychopathology of the Brain-injured Child.* New York.
32. TIZARD, B. and MARGERISON, J., 1963. *J. Neurol. Neurosurg. Psychiat.*, **26**: 308.
31A. TIZARD, B. and MARGERISON, J., 1963. *Brit. J. Soc. Clin. Psychol.*, **3**: 6.
33. TIZARD J., 1960. *Brit. Med. J.*, i: 1041.
34. W.H.O., 1957. Technical Report Series, No. 130, *Juvenile Epilepsy.* Geneva.

XX

THE PSYCHOSES OF CHILDHOOD

GERALD O'GORMAN

M.R.C.P., D.P.M.

Physician Superintendent, Borocourt and Smith's Hospitals,
Henley on Thames

1

Introduction

Psychotic illness in childhood, which until about two decades ago was thought to be a rare condition, is now diagnosed with increasing frequency and is recognised as being comparatively common. This recognition is due partly to the writings of psychiatrists like Bender and Kanner in the United States and Creak in this country, and partly to the renewed interest in the writings of older authors, including de Sanctis (42) and Kraepelin (30), who had pointed out that dementia praecox occurring in children or adolescents could lead to a state resembling mental defect, and Earle (13), who described catatonic psychosis in severely defective patients. Following on the work of these authors it was found that a surprisingly high proportion of patients in hospitals for the subnormal were suffering from a schizophrenic type of illness (O'Gorman (38)). This work has suggested not only that schizophrenic reactions are comparatively common in severely subnormal patients, but also that minor degrees of mental subnormality, and even of backwardness or poor academic performance, could be attributed to milder degrees of schizophrenic deviation. Recognition of the comparative commonness of psychosis in childhood came at a time when psychotic illness in the adult was being successfully treated by physical methods and by drugs, and it was obviously very important that efforts should be made to find analogous means of treating psychotic children. It was therefore necessary that clinicians should be able to recognise psychotic illnesses in children, distinguishing them from the neuroses on the one hand and from various other conditions which could lead to severe subnormality on the other. At the same time it was apparent that there were wide differences between various psychotic children, and the question arose how many different psychotic disease processes were included under the term 'childhood psychosis'.

2

Classification

Recently several authors have emphasised the need for some sort of classification of childhood schizophrenia. Delage (11), for example, asks for clarification of the clinical identity of childhood schizophrenia, especially in view of the need to arrive at an accurate prognosis. Classifications which have appeared hitherto have indeed mostly been concerned with 'childhood schizophrenia', but obviously this cannot be the only type of deviation within the group of the 'childhood psychoses'.

The first and most obvious difficulty of course is that we do not have a satisfactory definition of the word 'psychosis' either in children or in adults. Psychosis in adults has been defined as a mental illness involving the whole personality rather than one aspect or function thereof; as being not susceptible to psychotherapy; as being characterised by the presence of delusions or hallucinations; as being endogenous rather than exogenous in causation; or as a condition resulting from a conflict between the ego and the external world; and there have been attempts to define childhood psychosis in the same way. In adults there are so many exceptions and qualifications to these definitions that none of them has won universal acceptance, nor is it agreed where neurosis ends and psychosis begins. In fact there is nowadays decreasing insistence on the importance of consigning psychiatric patients to exclusive diagnostic categories; the tendency is to regard each patient separately, trying to understand his illness in the light of his previous personality and experience, and recognising that more than one morbid process may be going on in the same individual at the same time. This tendency applies to children even more than to adults, and of course in view of the diversity of human personality and environment it would be surprising if children who are mentally sick fitted neatly into clearly defined diagnostic boxes. Indeed if physical illness is any guide, it would be the exception rather than the rule for an individual to suffer from one disease and no other during his whole childhood. The fact that a child has chronic asthma does not mean he will never get measles. Clearly, what has to be done is to recognise the kind of deviation the child is suffering from and to assess the relative importance of the aetiological factors which may be responsible for it; only thus can a satisfactory programme of treatment be planned. Nevertheless it is important that we should know exactly what we mean when we use the term psychosis, what types of illness are embraced by this term, and what are the essential features of these illnesses.

On none of these questions has there so far been general agreement among children's psychiatrists. Some authors, for example, would use 'childhood psychosis' and 'childhood schizophrenia' and 'infantile autism' as apparently interchangeable terms describing a single disease entity whose manifestations differ from case to case though certain features occur frequently throughout the group. Others would regard Kanner's syndrome, childhood schizophrenia, infantile autism, primitive catatonic psychosis of idiocy, the psychosis of phenylketonurea, the symbiotic syndrome of Mahler, and Heller's syndrome as different diseases. Others again have regarded all these syndromes as being related, but have questioned whether there are not also entirely different types of psychotic reaction in childhood —manic-depressive illness, for example, or 'organic psychosis'.

3

'The Schizophrenic Syndrome'

Clinical Picture

The difficulties of classification were emphasised, however, when Creak gathered together a Working Party whose members had much experience of childhood psychosis, with the object among others of defining what was meant by the term (Creak (10)). The Working Party appreciated that the term 'psychosis' was too vague and inclusive, but eventually set out to suggest criteria for what is called the 'schizophrenic syndrome' in childhood, without committing themselves as to the nature of the syndrome, the extent to which it was truly analogous to the adult schizophrenias, or its relationship with other types of childhood psychosis. The nine criteria which they suggested for use in diagnosing the schizophrenic syndrome were as follows:

(1) Gross and sustained impairment of emotional relationships with people. This includes the more usual aloofness and the empty clinging (so-called symbiosis), and also abnormal behaviour towards other people as persons, such as using them, or parts of them, impersonally. Difficulty in mixing and playing with other children is often outstanding and long-lasting.
(2) The child's apparent unawareness of his own personal identity to a degree inappropriate to his age. This may be seen in abnormal behaviour towards himself, such as posturing or exploration and scrutinising of parts of his body. Repeated self-directed aggression, sometimes resulting in actual damage, may be another aspect of his lack of integration (see also point 5), as may also the confusion of personal pronouns (see point 7).
(3) Pathological preoccupation with particular objects or certain characteristics of them, without regard to their accepted functions.
(4) Sustained resistance to change in the environment and a striving to

maintain or restore sameness. In some instances behaviour appears to aim at producing a state of perceptual monotony.

(5) Abnormal perceptual experience (in the absence of discernible organic abnormality), as implied by excessive, diminished or unpredictable response to sensory stimuli—for example, visual and auditory avoidance (see also points 2 and 4), insensitivity to pain and temperature.

(6) Acute, excessive and seemingly illogical anxiety is a frequent phenomenon. This tends to be precipitated by change, whether in material environment or in routine, as well as by temporary interruption of a symbiotic attachment to persons or things (compare points 3 and 4, and also 1 and 2). (Apparently commonplace phenomena or objects seem to become invested with terrifying qualities. On the other hand an appropriate sense of fear in the face of real danger may be lacking.)

(7) Speech may have been lost or never acquired, or may have failed to develop beyond a level appropriate to an earlier stage. There may be confusion of personal pronouns (see point 2), echolalia or other mannerisms of use and diction. Though words or phrases may be uttered, they may convey no sense of ordinary communication.

(8) Distortion in motility patterns—for example (a) excess as in hyperkinesis, (b) immobility as in catatonia, (c) bizarre postures, or ritualistic mannerisms, such as rocking and spinning (himself or objects).

(9) A background of serious retardation, in which islets of normal, near-normal or exceptional intellectual function or skill may appear.

These nine criteria give a fair summary of the clinical picture of the schizophrenic syndrome in childhood, and many psychiatrists would be inclined to include a child in this group if he showed the first and two or three of the other 'points'. Certainly the withdrawal of the schizophrenic child is far and away the most important feature. Sometimes however it would seem more accurate to speak not of withdrawal but of 'non-involvement', because there is a large group of patients who seem never to become properly involved with people, or indeed with reality in general. These are children who used to be described as being 'defective from birth', but it might be more accurate to suggest that they are psychotic (i.e. schizophrenic or autistic) from birth. It is also important to emphasise that in many cases the withdrawal is only partial, that is to say the child remains partly in contact with reality but at a very superficial level. Many of them also are withdrawn for most of the time but may make almost normal contact when under severe emotional excitement, or when they are physically ill. Many children are also selectively withdrawn—that is to say they are withdrawn from certain aspects of reality, certain fields of experience, or they may be withdrawn from everyone but one or two familiar people with whom they have a partial or superficial contact. Probably the most important example of selective withdrawal is that from the field of hearing and communication, the child as a result failing to develop intellectually so that he becomes also mentally defective. Such a child may however have almost normal or at any rate partial contact with people, and if this contact improves under treatment the child may cease to be regarded as psychotic, although still functioning as partially deaf or as grossly retarded or abnormal in the field of communication.

There seems very little evidence that these children are unaware of their own personal identity, as suggested in the Working Party's Point 2. Indeed the total reaction of the child may be looked upon as an attempt to preserve inviolate his own personality, his own inner thoughts and his own body from interference by the outside world. To suggest that posturing or exploration or scrutiny or mutilation of his own body indicates unawareness of his own personal identity seems to be an entirely gratuitous assumption. The work of Norman (37) on which this theory is founded, though of great interest, does not seem to justify this subjective interpretation. The confusion of personal pronouns is better understood as part of the general speech disorder shown by these children, remembering that much of their speech is echolalia or a playing aimlessly with words, just as they play aimlessly with sand or water.

The characteristics mentioned under points 3 and 4 are seen particularly in early cases, and in children who are emerging to some extent from their withdrawal. The anxiety—or panic, or rage—mentioned in point 6 is usually aroused by threatened interference with the sameness of the environment. If the threat is maintained or increased the child usually reacts by a more severe degree of withdrawal. With regard to point 5, it is certainly true that the patients show excessive, diminished or unpredictable response to sensory stimuli. Whether this necessarily implies abnormal perceptual experience seems very doubtful, although abnormal perceptual experiences do seem to occur. It should be emphasised however that formal delusions or hallucinations are rare except in older psychotic children.

Because there are so many causes of intellectual retardation it does not seem very helpful to advance serious retardation as a criterion for diagnosing the schizophrenic syndrome, although undoubtedly most of the children are seriously retarded. On the other hand islets of normal intellectual functioning against a background of serious retardation must be regarded as strongly suggestive of this diagnosis.

In spite of these objections, it appears that the Working Party has made a very useful contribution towards providing a basis for teaching and discussion as well as research into psychotic children, and the decision to use the term 'the schizophrenic syndrome' instead of alternative names was important and far-reaching.

Aetiology

'Organic' or 'Non-organic'? The criteria suggested by Creak's Working Party for the 'schizophrenic syndrome' apply both to cases where there is

clinical or pathological evidence of disease of the central nervous system and to those where there is no such evidence. Some cases, for example, arise in children suffering from epiloia or the lipoidoses or phenylketonuria. In others the disease seems to have been precipitated by environmental stress—although it is a fact that many children subjected to equally severe environmental stress do not show schizophrenic symptoms. Creak (9) in commenting on the nine points says they were framed to include the possibility of the schizophrenic syndrome arising from 'multiple causes, among them organic factors'. She asks whether childhood psychotics are to be regarded as a homogeneous group or whether they include cases arising from varied aetiologies, quoting cases of the syndrome affecting children who prove to be suffering from lipoidosis. She refers to work by Heller (23), Yakolev (50) and Tramer (47) which attributes at least some cases of childhood psychosis to 'deteriorating organically determined illness'. Certainly every pychiatrist who works with psychotic children will encounter cases of the schizophrenic syndrome who turn out to be suffering from deteriorating organic disease of the central nervous system. On the other hand prolonged observation shows that most of these children do not in fact die young, nor do neurological signs usually appear in childhood or young adult life; nor, in the few cases who die of intercurrent disease or accident, is there usually recognisable evidence of brain disease at autopsy. This suggests that if they are suffering from organic disease of the central nervous system it must be an entirely different type of organic disease from any so far described.

Epilepsy and the Schizophrenic Syndrome. The frequency of cerebral dysrhythmia among children suffering from this 'schizophrenic syndrome' has been advanced as favouring an organic aetiology; for some of these patients do have abnormal EEGs, either typically epileptic or showing 'non-specific' abnormalities, and some have epileptic attacks of various kinds. Cerebral dysrhythmia must arise ultimately from a physiological disturbance in the brain, and perhaps this disturbance can be caused not only by 'organic' disease but also by constitutional instability, by emotional upset, or by metabolic disorder. Inherited constitutional instability is well recognised, and it is known that fits may be provoked by emotional stress. Moreover Ounsted (39) has shown that in some cases 'fits' and the abnormal EEG pattern that accompanies them may be aborted by a sharp command or by an effort of will. 'Idiopathic' epilepsy is in fact so called because the physical changes found in the brain at autopsy in these cases seem more likely to be the result than the cause of the epileptic attacks. The work of Hill (24) has suggested not only that epilepsy does not exclude the diagnosis of schizophrenia, but also that in some cases epileptic attacks may be a symptom of schizophrenic disease, at any rate in the adult. At this stage it may be pertinent to enquire whether abnormal electrical activity in the brain necessarily implies 'organic' disease in the usually accepted meaning of the term, and whether the occurrence of fits in psychotic children necessarily means that emotional factors have little importance in the aetiology.

Asynchronous Maturation. Among other theories on aetiology, Bender's views are by now well known and merit close attention. She speaks of a failure of integration and patterning of the central nervous system, and seems to regard childhood schizophrenia as being the outcome of disturbance or delay in the process of neurological maturation. Similar views are held by, among others, Fish (17) and Nouillhat (36). Nouillhat suggests that psychotic children have irregular or 'anarchic' growth patterns. This again is in accordance with clinical experience in this country, the history in many cases indicating that such children have an excessive tendency to mature rapidly at times in some, thought not all, fields of development after a period of stagnation of growth. Simon and Gillies (45) have shown that a proportion of children showing the schizophrenic syndrome have significant retardation of bone age. Other evidence of delayed physical maturation in these children is accumulating—for example it appears that a significant proportion of them are below average in height and weight. Cases have also occurred in children where the jaw and pharynx are not sufficiently well formed at birth to enable them to suck or swallow properly. It is now being suggested that this asynchronous development renders the child vulnerable to emotional stresses and thus more liable to develop a schizophrenic type of disturbance. There is a tendency in some quarters to regard all cases of childhood schizophrenia (and perhaps of adult schizophrenia too) as being due basically to some such abnormality of growth.

Environmental Factors. On the other hand some of those who postulate a basic inherited abnormality in the child also implicate environmental factors. Goldfarb *et al.* (22), for example, have prepared an aetiological schema on the lines shown on page 480. They suggest that the aberrant speech of a schizophrenic child is produced by one or more of the following factors: (1) impairments in physiological equipment for speech at receptor, central, or executive levels; (2) an abnormal speech model (to imitate); (3) a family pattern of inter-personal behaviour which actively blocks or interferes with the learning of speech.

Goldfarb does not really make plain why the child should be 'deviant' in those cases where such deviation is primary; but he is clearly thinking of an organic abnormality in the central nervous system, though he suggests that the organic physical signs are rarely definite. He seems however to assign most importance to emotional and environmental factors, and blames 'parental perplexity' as being important among such factors. This point of view is, of course, that of the analytically oriented, who regard parental disturbances as the main features in aetiology (Kaufmann *et al.* (27)). Klebanoff (28) on the other hand found that the mothers of schizophrenic children show fewer 'pathological attitudes' than the mothers of brain-damaged and retarded children, though more than those of normal children.

Clearly he considers that constitutional rather than environmental factors are of predominating importance in aetiology, regarding the disturbances in parents as secondary to the illness of the children. Further work is being carried out on this problem, but it will always be difficult to be sure whether emotional disturbance in parents of children suffering from psychotic disorders precedes or results from the child's illness.

Parental inadequacy and perplexity, absence of positive reinforcements, stimulus confusion.

Either of these may be primary.

⇃⇂

Deviant child

⇃⇂

Ego deficiency with absence of normal guides for self-directed action and self-regulation, and defect in self-identity, diffusion of boundaries of self and non-self.

⇃⇂

Absence of predictable expectancies, loss of reference and anchoring.

⇃⇂

Catastrophic feelings of strangeness and unfamiliarity.

⇃⇂

Panic (primordial anxiety) with seeking for sameness and constancy.

Bender also seems not to assign primary importance to emotional factors in determining the onset of disease, but she does apparently see the schizophrenic's progress around the time of puberty in terms of his attempts to deal with emotional stresses:

Sometimes they can at puberty reorganise their defences against the disorganising effect of schizophrenia . . . to handle the anxiety so well that it ceases to be overt, and neurotic defences are no longer needed . . . intellectual functioning in tests is increased. But later, up against more difficulties, his defences break down, schizophrenic symptoms begin—either as psychopathic or as severe schizophrenic breakdown, e.g. catatonic.

Bender's views are, of course, well supported by clinical experience. There is no doubt that some of these cases improve (Creak (10)). A few can lead normal lives, some can live limited, sheltered lives at home, and a good proportion end up as dull, inert but high-grade mentally subnormals instead of deteriorating to idiocy. But many do not improve, in spite of all our efforts, and nearly all ultimately have peculiar or psychopathic or inert and ineffectual personalities.

Relationship to Adult Schizophrenia. There is a considerable body of workers who consider childhood schizophrenia to be fundamentally the same as the adult form of the disease (Werkman (49)), and certainly the similarities between the two are striking if allowances are made for the effects of the psychotic process at different ages. It is well known, for example, that the symptoms of schizophrenia vary according to the age at which the disorder develops, paranoid schizophrenia being more common in later life whereas the simple schizophrenias tend to begin in young adult life or even earlier. Lucas *et al.* (33) have pointed out that delusions in schizophrenia occur much more in older than in younger patients, and in the present author's experience formalised delusions and hallucinations are very rare in childhood schizophrenics, just as they are rare in adolescents and uncommon in the simple schizophrenias of young adults. In fact, prolonged observation of young schizophrenics suggests that the symptoms of schizophrenia in adolescence form a continuum merging into those of the young adult patients at one end and into those of childhood schizophrenics at the other. Eisenberg (14) suggests that 'the separation of cases of early infantile autism from other cases of childhood schizophrenia continues to be justified clinically', though he adds that 'the syndrome can be logically classified as one of the schizophrenias'. If childhood schizophrenia is truly analogous to the adult forms of the disorder, it might be anticipated that schizophrenic children would show the same response to tranquillising drugs as adult patients do; whereas in fact the tranquillisers have been extremely disappointing when given to childhood schizophrenics, and in the present author's experience they are only useful when given in enormous doses to relieve violent symptoms in certain severely deteriorated patients. This is not to suggest the tranquillisers have no effect on the less deteriorated children—the effect is nearly always to increase their anxiety, their restlessness and tension and to make them even less responsive. The explanation might lie in metabolic changes around puberty; or it might be that the 'simple' kind of schizophrenia of young adults and adolescents is the disorder to which childhood schizophrenia is truly analogous, the catatonic and paranoid forms which are more responsive to tranquillisers being disorders of a different type.

Genetic Factors. Kallmann and Roth (26), writing about genetic aspects of pre-adolescent schizophrenia, excluded from their sample 'very young children who presented the clinical picture of a psychosis with mental deficiency, perhaps simulating a severe intellectual defect as the result of a very early schizophrenic process'. They were therefore presumably excluding most of the cases of what Kanner and Eisenberg would call 'infantile autism'. We do not know whether they also excluded cases where there were signs of organic disease or of asynchronous maturation, but their criteria were fairly similar to those proposed subsequently by Creak *et al.* (9). They found that the inheritance of these 'schizophrenic' children was strikingly similar to that of adult schizophrenics. They claim that these findings indicate an early effect in childhood schizophrenia of the same genotype (gene-specific deficiency state) assumed to be responsible for the basic symptoms of adult schizophrenia. They also suggest that there is 'an increase in the number of early schizophrenia cases among the co-twins and sibs of early index cases, and there is a definite excess of males over females in the pre-adolescent group. Theories attempting to explain either finding on non-biological grounds lack substantiation.' Impressive as their figures and their arguments undoubtedly were, not all their readers were thereby convinced that what seemed to be a genetic effect could not be accounted for to some extent by post-natal environmental influences, particularly the emotional states of parents.

Biochemical Aspects. The work of Gjessing (20) showing disturbed nitrogen metabolism in periodic catatonia remains the most important contribution in this field, in spite of the immense amount of work which has been carried out since attention was directed towards metabolic aspects of schizophrenia by the success of the tranquillisers. A large number of observations have been made on the levels of various substances in the blood or brain of schizophrenics, but we are a long way from understanding their significance. 'It has to be clearly understood that whilst alterations in the level of substances, such as serotonin and the catecholamines, in the brain are affected by the amine oxydase inhibitors, there is no conclusive evidence that these amines are causally involved' (Quastel (40)). Perhaps the most provocative observation is that of Basowitz *et al.* (4) on abnormalities in the excretion of hippuric acid after benzoic acid administration in persons under emotional stress, as well as in catatonic schizophrenics and subjects under the influence of mescaline (Georgi *et al.* (18)). More recently Hoagland *et al.* (25) have detected a very labile factor in fractions of human globulin which exists in greater quantities in schizophrenics than in normals, and which produces behaviour disturbances in rats. Frequently results and conclusions reached by one group of workers have not been confirmed in other hands. Presumably the ultimate disorder in the brains of schizophrenic children must be a physiological one, and this must be mediated by biochemical changes. At the present time however we are very far from any real knowledge what these changes are.

*   *   *

Thus it seems that one group of authors is thinking of this schizophrenic syndrome in terms of a deteriorating organic disease of the central nervous system, another in terms of a disorder of development as the result of which the child undergoes a schizophrenic reaction to emotional stress, and a third in terms of a metabolic disorder. There is no general agreement whether the childhood schizophrenias form a group truly analagous to or even identical with these disorders in adults. While some authors regard the illness as being determined almost entirely by emotional factors, others produce evidence, which they regard as conclusive, of the preponderating importance of genetic factors.

The 'Pseudo-schizophrenic Syndromes'. Perhaps it is appropriate at this point to consider whether these authors have apparently conflicting opinions because they are not talking about the same disorder. Perhaps there are two or even several diseases or combinations of disease processes, culminating in what some call childhood schizophrenia and some call the schizophrenic syndrome; and if so it is possible that closer observation and more careful investigation may reveal means of differentiating these disease processes both clinically and pathologically. There is, for example, a 'pseudo-schizophrenic' psychosis of twins, in which two apparently severely psychotic children show a remarkable improvement under treatment aimed at persuading them to regard themselves as separate individuals rather than identical halves of the same person. As another example, the present writer has been much impressed by a group of cases in which extreme negativism towards the parents, in particular the mother, is manifested throughout childhood, and appears to be responsible, in part at any rate, for a clinical condition showing many resemblances to the schizophrenic syndrome. These are children who have no friends among their contemporaries, who function as subnormal although from time to time they show glimpses of intelligence at a much higher level, and who are babyish and dependent to an extreme degree. They are always much worse when in the presence of their mothers, whom they plague and punish with their stupidity and babyish idependence but from whom they refuse to be separated. It seems as though they are aware that these symptoms are exceedingly distressing to the mother and therefore use them as a weapon in the oedipal struggle. In a few cases such children have shown the 'functional' deafness or mutism which may be found in some psychotic children, and this again is used as a weapon, the symptom appearing to have value because of the distress it causes to the parent and the relief of responsibility for learning or growing up which it confers. If they remain with their mothers (and the mother is of course so much involved emotionally that she is usually loth to part with her child) they reach young adult life as mentally defective invalids completely dependent on their mothers, whose social and family life is largely ruined as a result. The end state is not unlike an adult form of the symbiotic relationship described by Mahler. Although they have severe difficulty in personal relationships, although they function as severely subnormal and may have difficulties in communication and hearing, although their movements are often peculiar—although, in fact, they would conform with most of the criteria of the schizophrenic syndrome outlined by Creak's Working Party—

they certainly appear to constitute a different group from all the others who show symptoms of the schizophrenic syndrome. They are mentioned here as an example of a pathological process which may in the end lead to a condition very similar to that shown by other patients, suffering from different disease processes, who also may be grouped under the 'schizophrenic syndrome'.

The above group of cases introduces another very difficult problem, namely the relationship between psychotic illness and the neuroses, for example between childhood schizophrenia and hysteria. For there seems to be a strong resemblance between the mutism, or deafness, or visual avoidance, or refusal to make any attempt to learn shown by these patients, and the hysterical aphonia, deafness, blindness or regression shown by some adults under severe stress—for example by soldiers in battle. It is worth recalling that a very large proportion of children showing the schizophrenic syndrome are accused at some time or other of being deaf, and that even more have some difficulties in communication which apparently are not based on organic disease, because often these children will talk, in well formed phrases, when they are alone in their cots at night or under severe emotional excitement. Adult hysterics may of course behave similarly. The suggestion here is that hysterical symptoms may be found in children showing the schizophrenic syndrome. A further example of neurotic symptoms in such children is their obsessive-compulsive mannerisms and rituals. The fact that these neurotic symptoms may be seen in psychotic children may partly explain why the differential diagnosis in some of these cases is so difficult. It also emphasises how unwise it may be to attempt to consign a child irrevocably into a particular diagnostic category. An individual child may be reacting in some ways psychotically and in other ways neurotically.

With all the above considerations in mind it seems justifiable to regard the schizophrenic syndrome in childhood as an end state, a condition which may be produced by several different kinds of disease process, often acting in combination and aggravating one another reciprocally. Few writers on this subject are prepared to deny that emotional factors derived from the environment have at least some importance in aetiology, and some assign the main role to such factors. On the other hand there is impressive evidence that organic factors are present in a great many cases; and some degree of inherited constitutional predisposition towards schizophrenic illness is probably an essential aetiological element in the vast majority.

The main aetiological factors producing the schizophrenic syndrome in childhood can be listed as follows:

A. *ORGANIC DISORDERS*, including

Inherited predisposition to schizophrenic illness;
Infections, including meningitis or encephalitis of various types;

Head injury;

Tumours, including epiloia;

Degenerations, including Schilder's disease, Huntingdon's chorea;

Vascular accidents;

Growth anomalies, including asynchronous or disorganised maturation, mongolism, Klinefelter's syndrome;

Metabolic disorders, including phenylketonurea, the lipoidoses,
foetal or neonatal anoxia;

Poisons, including certain drugs.

B. *EMOTIONAL STRESS*, such as that caused by

Disturbed parental attitudes or relationships;

Sibling rivalry;

Separations;

Feeding difficulties;

Severe physical disease in early life;

Sensory privation—blindness or deafness;

Exposure to sudden shock or terror.

4

Depressive Psychoses

The Reactive Depressions of Childhood

Aetiology. In recent years the work of Bowlby (8) and of Spitz (46) has drawn attention to these disorders, and significant contributions to theories of aetiology have been made by Klein (29a), Scott (44), Despert (12) and Abraham (1). From the writings of these authors it might be deduced that depressions in childhood often result from a persistence of the 'depressive position' which Klein regarded as a normal stage in emotional development. Clinicians whose orientation is not predominantly psychoanalytical point to the more obvious environmental factors as precipitating causes, among which separations from the mother are probably the commonest, though the condition can be precipitated by a variety of emotional traumata including the arrival of a new sibling, loss of some member of the family other than mother, disturbed parental relationships, and of course physical disease in the child or his mother. Depressions may occur in children who are entirely normal before and after the period of the illness, although many of them appear to have a con-stitutional predisposition to develop depressions and their liability to a fresh attack appears to be increased by having had similar troubles in the past. It seems, in fact, that a pattern of depressive reaction may thus be acquired which can persist into later years. In some cases the patient develops a chronically pessimistic attitude towards life rather than further attacks of clinical depression, while in others a child who has become depressed as a reaction to emotional privation or trauma may show chronic insecurity and anxiety in adolescence and adult life.

Clinical Picture. Not every authority would regard these childhood depressions as being truly psychotic, some preferring to classify them with the neuroses and regarding them as analogous to the so called neurotic depressions of adult life (Lewis (32)). Here again the distinction between neurotic and psychotic manifestations is often difficult to make, and certainly many of the symptoms of childhood depression are indistinguishable from those of the neuroses. They include obsessional or repetitive mannerisms, tantrums, and apparently excessive fears. Many patients have psychosomatic symptoms, including constipation, anorexia, vomiting and weakness. Very often there is regression to a more infantile level of behaviour, loss of recently acquired skills, and intellectual backsliding. Control of bowels and bladder are often lost, and severe encopresis, which usually indicates a serious underlying illness, often masks a depression. It usually indicates a strongly aggressive component in the psychopathology, which may also show itself in more openly aggressive behaviour, often directed towards the rival sibling, in contrast to depression in adults, who usually manage to keep their strongly hostile feelings at an unconscious level.

The above symptoms are those most commonly seen in older children with depressive illness. In infants and younger children the common symptoms are an excess of normal grief, with inconsolable weeping or wailing for hours on end, or apparent apathy and inertia with failure to respond or to feed. Indeed many of these children appear for the time being to be genuinely withdrawn in the same way as children suffering from a schizophrenic type of illness, so that it might be suggested that withdrawal can be a symptom of depression in young children, just as it can of schizophrenia. The difference, of course, is that in depressed children the symptoms are recoverable and usually respond to environmental readjustment fairly quickly, though they may relapse if the unfavourable circumstances recur. Moreover depressed children do not as a rule appear to be depressed all the time; they may laugh at times and play actively, only to return to their inert or hypochondriacal state after a little while. The relationships which they make during their better phases are however usually on a superficial level, and difficulty in forming deeper relationships may persist after severe or repeated attacks of depression and become a permanent feature of the individual's personality.

It will be seen that the clinical picture of depression merges on the one hand into that of neurotic illness, and on the other hand into that of the schizophrenic type of disorder. Moreover a child may suffer from more than one kind of deviation at a given time. Thus although most schizophrenic children are apparently unmoved by being separated from their mothers, in a good many cases children admitted for schizophrenic symptoms may also become depressed for a time after coming in to hospital. This seems to emphasise the importance of trying to assess accurately in every case not only the kinds of deviation from which the child is suffering but also the aetiological factors behind his illness, and planning treatment accordingly, rather than consigning him to a diagnostic category and treating the disease rather than the patient.

Manic-depressive Psychoses

The present position seems very little different from that described by Barton Hall (3), who when writing about manic-depressive illness in childhood observed 'It is generally believed that affective disorders of this type do not occur in children and are infrequent in adolescence.' She quoted two large series, one of 1,000 children in whom no case of affective disorder was found under the age of thirteen, and another of 1,200 psychiatric patients in whom no patient suffering from mania or melancholia was discovered under the age of fifteen. Lurie and Lurie (34) stated firmly that manic-depressive psychosis did not occur in childhood. Gillespie (19) thought that manic-depressive illness in childhood was very rare, though in a few cases depression in childhood was described in the previous history of manic-depressive adults. On the other hand Kraeplin (30a) quoted a case of mania in a five-year-old boy, and reported that 0·4% of a series of nine hundred patients appeared to have had a manic-depressive episode by the age of ten years. More recently Anthony and Scott (2) have reviewed the literature of manic-depressive psychosis in childhood, and described a case occurring in a boy aged twelve years and continuing into adult life; these authors concluded that true manic-depressive illness in early childhood *as a clinical phenomenon* has yet to be demonstrated, but that as a psychodynamic entity there is good reason to believe in its existence. They refer to the work of Klein (29a), who contended that the child in his early development goes through a transitory manic-depressive state. Her description of the 'depressive position' in childhood has been echoed by other psychoanalysts, including Abraham (1), Rank *et al.* (41) and Spitz (46). These authors, however, appear to regard the 'depressive position' or something like it as a normal phase of development; indeed Glover (21) did not believe that healthy emotional development could take place without the occurrence of these infantile psychotic phases. But it does not appear from the writing of these authors that the so-called infantile psychotic episodes are necessarily related to the development of manic-depressive illness in later life. There is in non-psychoanalytical circles a good deal of scepticism about this piece of psychopathology, though it would certainly explain some of the depressive and excited phases for which there is no obvious precipitating cause in the environment.

It seems doubtful whether the 'depressive condition' described by the psychoanalysts is related to the manic-depressive or cyclothymic temperament. Although there are comparatively few psychiatrists who would agree that true mania or manic-depressive psychosis occurs before puberty, there are many who would maintain that mood-swings and evidence of cyclothymic temperament may be seen in young children who in later life undergo an exaggeration of such temperamental features and suffer from manic-depressive psychosis. Here again diagnostic difficulties occur, and it is often hard to distinguish the hyperkinetic syndrome in a child from hypomania or mania. In the vast majority of these cases of hyperkinetic psychosis however there is no infectious quality about the hilarity or excitement of the child, who appears to remain largely indifferent to the people in his environment and whose ideas, if there is flight of ideas, seem to be more divorced from reality than those of the manic adult. The present author cannot recall any case in which the hyperkinetic or excited condition exhibited by a psychotic child did not appear to have much more in common with the schizophrenic rather than the manic-depressive psychosis in the adult. In fact the consensus of opinion among psychiatrists with most experience seems to be that true manic-depressive insanity, if it occurs at all, is exceedingly rare before puberty, and almost unknown in earlier childhood. On the other hand, evidence of mood-swings and the cyclothymic temperament as a prelude to the development of manic-depressive psychosis in later life seems to be well recognised.

5

The Organic Psychoses

Aetiology. Sir Charles Symonds, speaking about the effects of head injury, once said that it is not only the kind of injury that matters but also the kind of head; the implication being that the previous personality of the victim, as well as the nature of the injury, was of considerable importance in determining the symptoms. Probably most children's psychiatrists today would endorse this view, though with the addition that the emotional stresses which the patient encounters after his head injury are also of considerable importance. What applies to head injuries probably applies to most other organic affections of the brain. Certainly it is true of, for example, cerebral malaria, for almost any kind of psychotic or neurotic picture may supervene as a sequela to this disease; and also of several other infections and poisons. Some disease processes are particularly liable to attack specific areas of the central nervous system; the best example of these is the virus of epidemic encephalitis, whose effects in chronic cases are most marked in, though not confined to, the brain stem, in particular the substantia nigra and the globus pallidus. Even in these cases however it is the neurological rather than the psychiatric side of the picture which tends to be specific, although some illnesses do produce their own characteristic mental symptoms—for example, the upset of sleep rhythm in the acute phase and the hallucinations in the chronic phase of epidemic encephalitis.

For practical purposes the present tendency is not to speak of specific psychiatric disorders resulting from different organic pathologies, but to group them all together and speak of the 'acute organic syndrome' and the 'chronic organic syndrome', recognising that there may be slight variations in the final clinical picture which will depend partly on what pathology is responsible but to a much greater extent on the pre-morbid personality of the patient and the environmental stresses to which he is subjected after the acute illness.

Clinical Picture. No attempt will be made here to describe in detail the acute organic syndrome, which in non-fatal cases follows, in children as in adults, the reversible sequence of coma, stupor, delirium, cerebral irritability, automatism, recovery of consciousness.

The psychiatrist is more often concerned with the chronic organic syndrome, the leading symptoms of which are headache, irritability, excessive fatigue, increased emotional lability and intolerance of stress, cerebral dysrhythmia with or without epileptic manifestations, and intellectual inertia. Over and above this, symptoms will depend in large measure upon the previous personality of the individual. Thus a child prone to anxiety before the onset of the cerebral pathology will tend to become more anxious and less tolerant of stress than he was previously; a child who previously showed outbursts of rage against a rival sibling may become dangerously aggressive towards him in response to the mildest provocation; a child already liable to depressive episodes may now begin to have them more easily and more frequently; and a child of schizoid personality may show an increased tendency to withdrawal. It is, of course, extremely difficult in some cases to distinguish between a schizophrenic type of withdrawal and the inertia and loss of interest which may supervene in the postconcussional syndrome—especially since in some cases an element of both may be present. The essential difference is that the brain-injured child can and does make deep emotional relationships, except in the most severely affected cases where the child does eventually become incapable of relating to his environment.

It must be pointed out that at this stage most of these children will exhibit several of the characteristics mentioned in the nine points proposed by Creak's Working Party on the Schizophrenic Syndrome; it is for this reason that so many patients in the mental deficiency hospitals will be regarded as suffering from the schizophrenic syndrome if the criteria for diagnosis of that syndrome remain as in Creak's nine points. Probably the relationship between the schizophrenic syndrome and the effects of brain damage in childhood will always remain controversial. The task of the physician, however, is quite clear: he must try and assess the relative importance of the aetiological factors involved in the individual case and base his treatment upon this, not allowing the existence of brain damage to prevent him from treating the psychosis by psychotherapy if this seems indicated. And it must be emphasised that most brain-damaged children will benefit from psychotherapy or environmental or 'relationship' therapy to a considerable extent. Whether or not the child develops features of the schizophrenic syndrome, the intellectual inertia of the brain damaged-child will usually result in his functioning at an intellectual and academic level a good deal below his potential, and in some cases of course the child may undergo severe intellectual deterioration, occasionally to idiot level. These cases follow a melancholy course and have to be cared for ultimately in hospitals for the mentally subnormal.

Social Effects of Brain Damage

With regard to the less severely brain-damaged children, the loss of social sense, of self-control and of intellectual energy which are so often seen even in the mild cases, together with the inability to tolerate stress which may also be a feature, makes these children very liable to fall foul of society in adolescence and young adult life. Time and again cases are brought before the courts in which chronic delinquency, usually minor but often peculiar in its features and occasionally very serious and violent, can be ascribed to the chronic effects of brain damage. It is of extreme importance that children who have had illness or injuries affecting their central nervous system should be kept under surveillance for a long period so that symptoms of brain damage can be recognised and treated, while at the same time any necessary adjustments can be made in their environment to help them steer clear of anti-social behaviour. Referring to Sir Charles Symonds' aphorism once again, it should be pointed out that there is no simple correlation between the severity of the cerebral pathology on the one hand, and the seriousness of the subsequent intellectual and emotional disturbance on the other.

6

A Definition of Childhood Psychosis

With the above descriptions of the various syndromes included under the term 'childhood psychosis' in modern psychiatric practice, it may be permissible at this stage to consider again the question of a definition of what we mean by psychotic illness. The characteristic which seems to be common to all the psychotic syndromes described above is an altered relationship with reality. Thus a child suffering from a schizophrenic type of psychosis is withdrawn from—or perhaps never involved with—the real world of people and their emotional relationships, their aspirations and endeavours. A child who is psychotically depressed sees reality falsely as hostile, rejecting, punishing and unforgiving. A child suffering from an organic psychosis may have an altered relationship with reality as the result of withdrawal or depression, and in addition his inertia of mind shows itself in a lack of interest in the events of the world around him and a growing self-centredness, with a loss of social sense and self-control. Attempts to analyse the essential features of large numbers of cases diagnosed as psychotic by experienced psychiatrists have suggested that the vast majority of them shared this characteristic of an altered relationship with reality. They also showed, without exception, a disturbance or inappropriateness of mood.

Perhaps therefore a definition of childhood psychosis might tentatively be advanced, and in these terms: a psychotic illness in childhood is one in which there is a disturbance and inappropriateness of mood, plus an abnormal relationship with reality.

7

Treatment

An adequate account of methods of treatment of childhood psychosis with an assessment of results is much beyond the scope of this chapter. A brief summary can however be given.

Drugs

The tranquillisers. These have given extremely disappointing results with psychotic children. As mentioned above, their effect is usually to make the child more distressed, tense and restless, with no apparent diminution in withdrawal. Large-scale multi-centred trials are now being planned, and many claims have now been made about the efficacy of different types of tranquilliser, but it is rare indeed for an experienced child psychiatrist to claim that he has had more than isolated successes with these drugs. They are however occasionally useful in controlling symptoms in severely deteriorated children, though they have to be given on an empirical basis, no rationale having been worked out why one drug should succeed better than another in a particular case.

Once puberty is past the tranquillisers appear to have a much greater chance of helping the individual patient, and in these cases tranquillising drugs should be tried, again on an empirical basis, though for older adolescents the indications for using particular drugs approximate to those which apply to adult patients.

Anti-convulsants. These have to be given only occasionally in children suffering from the schizophrenic syndrome. They are, of course, of great importance in the treatment of brain-damaged children.

The mono-amine oxydase inhibitors, so successful in treating depressions in the adult, have not so far been shown to help very much in dealing with depressions in childhood.

Amphetamine has a transient effect on depressed children, but most physicians who have prescribed it for this condition are unwilling to prescribe it a second time. On the other hand amphetamine is of undoubted benefit in a few cases of hyperkinetic syndrome and is often worth a trial, especially when the condition appears to have an 'organic' basis.

Convulsion Therapy

Electro-convulsive therapy also has proved disappointing in the treatment of children suffering from the schizophrenic syndrome, though there is a place for it in the management of particular symptoms such as.

self-mutilation and of severely disturbed phases in children who are usually placid. It can rarely be justifiable to give ECT in the depressions of childhood, since these are usually reactive and convulsion therapy cannot improve an unsatisfactory environment. In adolescent schizophrenics and in very young manic-depressive patients the indications for ECT are similar to those in adults (Sargant and Slater (43)).

Insulin Treatment

Deep insulin therapy seems to be used very rarely on psychotic children at the present time. For ill-thriven patients suffering from the schizophrenic syndrome modified insulin may be of assistance in improving physical states. Its effect on mental symptoms appears slight.

Psychotherapy

Although children suffering from the schizophrenic syndrome are in general exceedingly difficult to treat, so that the prognosis in established cases is often poor, there seems little doubt that some form of psychotherapy offers the best chance of success. Such therapy is more likely to be successful with children in whom there is no evident 'organic' pathology, but even in these cases some response will usually be shown to sustained treatment. Most of the methods are derived from an application of psychoanalytic techniques and no attempt will be made to describe them in detail here, though the reader's attention is directed to the work of Klein (29), Betz (6), Bettelheim (7), Fabian (16), Eckstein (15), Mahler (35), Bender (5), Waal (48) and des Lauriers (31). Nearly all these authors have had their successes, usually only partial and always after an enormous output of the therapist's time and energy. Moreover in most cases the therapist has a feeling that treatment would have been even more successful had it been more intensive. In fact it would seem that each child under treatment needs about one fifth of a therapist's total working time to himself. And of course this is economically impossible.

It seems that success in treatment depends not so much upon the interpretations given to the child as upon the relationship which the therapist is able to establish; for a child's interest in the real world must be based on his interest in people, and our first task must be to persuade the child to form a relationship with one human being. It seems open to doubt whether the psychiatrist or play therapist is necessarily the best person to carry out the individual treatment which these children need. Perhaps ultimately it will be found that in schizophrenics as well as in other disturbed children the main emphasis should be on treating not the child but the mother, or, more accurately, on treating the child through the mother or the mother substitute. It is possible that for practical purposes the best course is to offer in-patient care to those patients whose relationship with other members of the family is so disturbed that it must be broken for a time in order to prevent further deterioration; to continue in-patient care with a mother substitute providing under close medical supervision the intensive relationship which the child needs, while the therapist attempts to readjust the mother's attitudes towards the child as far as possible; and then gradually to reintegrate the child into the family life, the mother spending an increasing amount of time in the hospital during the period of in-patient care, and treatment of both child and mother being carried on after the child's eventual return home. In the less severe cases it may be possible to dispense with the period of in-patient care, though this may be found to apply to only a minority of the patients. Once the child has been returned to live with his family treatment can be carried on as out-patient therapy, with the main emphasis once again on the treatment of the child through the mother. Without such a plan of treatment it might be that only the children of the very rich or some other specially selected group could be given adequate therapy.

In the present state of our knowledge, and in the foreseeable future, the treatment of childhood psychosis will be difficult and generally disappointing, because often irreparable damage has occurred before the child comes for treatment. Indeed it may be that in some cases treatment would have been unsuccessful however early it were undertaken. Nevertheless attempts at treating psychotic children are abundantly worth while, not only because of the occasional brilliant result, but also because in the majority of cases we can produce some improvement, or at least prevent some of the deterioration which would otherwise have occurred. If we can stabilise a child as a high grade imbecile, capable of living at home under sheltered conditions, requiring little or no nursing, and perhaps even working at a simple job, rather than watch him deteriorate to helpless idiocy, we shall have performed a useful function.

REFERENCES

1. ABRAHAM, K., 1949. The infantile prototype of melancholic depression. *Selected Papers of Karl Abraham.* London: Hogarth.
2. ANTHONY, J. and SCOTT, P., 1960. Manic-depressive psychosis in childhood. *J. Child Psychol. and Psychiat.*, 1, No. 1 (January).
3. BARTON HALL, M., 1952. Our present knowledge about manic-depressive states in childhood. *Nerv. Child*, 9.
4. BASOWITZ, H., PERSKY, H., KORCHIN, S. J. and GRINKER, I. G., 1955. *Anxiety and Stress.* Chicago: McGraw-Hill.
5. BENDER, LAURETTA and GUREVITZ, S., 1955. Results of psychotherapy with young schizophrenic children. *Amer. J. Orthopsychiat.*, 25.
6. BETZ, B. J., 1947. A study of tactics for resolving the autistic barrier in the psychotherapy of the schizophrenic personality. *Amer. J. Psychiat.*, 104.
7. BETTELHEIM, B., 1950. *Love is Not Enough.* Glencoe, Ill.: Free Press.

494 THE PSYCHOSES OF CHILDHOOD

8. BOWLBY, J., 1951. *Maternal Care and Mental Health.* Geneva: W.H.O.
9. CREAK, E. M. *et al.*, 1961. The schizophrenic syndrome in childhood. Progress report of a working party. *Brit. Med. J.*, ii: 889-890.
10. CREAK, E. M., 1963. Childhood psychosis. *Brit. J. of Psychiatry*, **109**, No. 458 (January).
11. DELAGE, J., 1960. Critical review of infantile schizophrenia. *Laval Méd.*, **30**: 496-561 (November).
12. DESPERT, J. L., 1952. Suicide and depression in children. *Nerv. Child*, **9**: 378-389.
13. EARLE, C. J. C., 1934. *Brit. J. Med. Psychol.*, **14**: 111, 230.
14. EISENBERG, L., 1956. The course of childhood schizophrenia. *A.M.A. Archs. Neurol. Psychiat.*, **78**: 69-83 (July).
15. EKSTEIN, R. and WRIGHT, D., 1952. The space child. A note on the psychotherapeutic treatment of a 'schizophrenic' child. *Bull. Menninger Clin.*, **16**.
16. FABIAN, A. A. and HOLDEN, M. S., 1951. Treatment of childhood schizophrenia in a child guidance clinic. *Amer. J. Orthopsychiat.*, **21**.
17. FISH, B., 1960. Involvement of the central nervous system in infants with schizophrenia. *A.M.A. Archs. Neurol.*, **2**: 115-121 (February).
18. GEORGI, F., 1946. Indications respectives de l'insulinothérapie de la cardiazol thérapie et de l'ecletrothérapie. *C.R. Congr. Méd. Alién. Neurol.* (July).
19. GILLESPIE, R. D., 1939. *A Survey of Child Psychiatry.* London: Oxford University Press.
20. GJESSING, R., 1938. Disturbance of somatic function in catatonic periodic courses and their compensation. *J. Ment. Sci.*, **84**: 608 (1939). *Arch. Psychiat. Nervenkr.*, **109**: 525.
21. GLOZER, E., 1957. Medico-psychological aspects of normality. *Brit. J. Psychol.*, **23**, 2.
22. GOLDFARB, W., BRAUNSTEIN, P. and SCHOLL, H., 1959. An approach to the investigation of childhood schizophrenia: the speech of schizophrenic children and their mothers. *Amer. J. Orthopsychiat.*, **29**: 481-490 (July).
23. HELLER, T., 1930. Über dementia infantilis. *Ztschr. f. Kinderforsch.*, **73**: 661. Translated by Hulse, C. W. (1954) in *J. Nerv. Mental Dis.*, **119**: 671.
24. HILL, DENNIS, 1948. Relationship between epilepsy and schizophrenia. E.E.G. Studies. *Folia Psychiat. Neurol. Neurochir. Neerland.*, **51**: 95-111.
25. HOAGLAND, H., BERGEN, J. R., KOELLA, W. P. and FREEMAN, H., 1962. *Ann. N.Y. Acad. Sci.*, **96**: 469.
26. KALLMAN, F. J. and ROTH, B., 1956. Genetic aspects of pre-adolescent schizophrenia. *Amer. J. Psychiat.*, **112**, No. 8 (February).
27. KAUFMANN, I., FRANK, T., HEIMS, L., HERRICK, J. and WILLER, L., 1958. Parents of schizophrenic children: Workshop, 1958. 3. Four types of defense in mothers and fathers of schizophrenic children. *Amer. J. Orthopsychiat.*, **29**: 460-472 (July).
28. KLEBANOFF, L. B., 1958. Parents of schizophrenic children: Workshop, 1958. *Amer. J. Orthopsychiat.*, **29**: 445-465 (July).
29. KLEIN, M., 1932. *The Psychoanalysis of Children.* London: Hogarth Press.
29a. 1934. The psychogenesis of manic-depressive states. *Contributions to Psychoanalysis.* London: Hogarth Press.
30. KRAEPLIN, E., 1919. *Dementia Praecox and Paraphrenia.* Edinburgh.
30a. 1921. *Manic-depressive Insanity and Paranoia.* Edinburgh: E. & S. Livingstone.
31. LAURIERS, A. M. DES, 1962. *The Experience of Reality in Childhood Schizophrenia.* London: Tavistock Publications.

32. Lewis, A., 1934. Melancholia: a clinical survey of depressive states. *J. Ment. Sci.*, **10**: 277.

33. Lucas, L., Sainsbury, P. and Collins, J. G., 1962. A social and clinical study of delusions in schizophrenia. *J. Ment. Sci.*, **108**: 747-758 (November).

34. Lurie, L. A. and Lurie, M. L., 1950. Psychosis in children: a review. *J. Pediat.*, **36**: 801-809.

35. Mahler, M. S., 1952. On child psychosis and schizophrenia: autistic and symbiotic psychoses. *The Psychoanalytic Study of the Child*, Vol. 7. New York: Internat. Universities Press.

36. Nouailhat, F., 1960. Schizophrenia in children. Early neurological aspects. *France Méd.*, **23**: 414-415 (Aug.-Sept.).

37. Norman, E., 1955. Affect and withdrawal in schizophrenic children. *Brit. J. Med. Psychol.*, **28**: 1-18.

38. O'Gorman, G., 1954. Psychosis as a cause of mental defect. *J. Ment. Sci.*, **100**, No. 421 (October): 934-943.

39. Ounsted, Christopher, 1961. Personal communication.

40. Quastel, J. H. and Quastel, D. M. J., 1962. *The Chemistry of Brain Metabolism in Health and Disease*. Springfield, Ill.: Thomas.

41. Rank, B., Putnam, M. and Kaplan, S., 1951. A case of primal depression in an infant. In *The Psychoanalytic Study of the Child*, Vol. 6, pp. 38-58.

42. Sanctis, S. de, 1906. *Riv. Speriment. di. Freniat.*, **32**: 141.

43. Sargant, W. and Slater, E., 1963. *An Introduction to Physical Methods of Treatment in Psychiatry*. London: E. & S. Livingstone.

44. Scott, W. C. M., 1948. A psycho-analytic concept of the origin of depression. *Brit. Med. J.*, 538-540.

45. Simon, G. B. and Gillies, S., 1963. Personal communication.

46. Spitz, R., 1946. Anaclitic depression. *Psychoanalytic Study of the Child*, Vol. 2, pp. 313-342. New York: Internat. Univ. Press.

47. Tramer, M., 1935-36. *Zeitsch. f. Kinderpsych.*, **1**: 91.

48. Waal, N., 1955. A special technique of psychotherapy with an autistic child. In *Emotional Problems in Early Childhood*, ed. G. Caplan. New York: Basic Books.

49. Werkman, L. S., 1959. Present trends in schizophrenia research: implications for childhood schizophrenia. *Amer. J. Orthopsychiat.*, **29**: 473-480 (July).

50. Yakolev, P., Weinberger, M. and Chipman, C., 1948. Heller's Syndrome as a pattern of schizophrenic behaviour disturbance in early childhood. *Amer. J. Ment. Def.*, **55** (2): 318.

XXI

THE AETIOLOGY OF

MENTAL SUBNORMALITY

BRIAN KIRMAN

M.D., D.P.M.

Director of Research, Fountain Unit, and Consultant Psychiatrist, Fountain and Carshalton Hospital Group, Surrey
Hon. Associate Consultant Physician, St. George's and Maudsley Hospitals, London

1

Introduction

When a child is mentally backward, we seldom know the precise cause. This applies particularly to mild degrees of retardation, i.e. educational subnormality, with an intelligence quotient on formal tests of 50–70. In 200 consecutive admissions of idiot and imbecile children to the Fountain Hospital (Berg and Kirman (1)), we were able to suggest aetiology in 13·5% and implicate some specific factor in 55·5%, but in 31% no factors could be incriminated. These results were obtained after an exhaustive study of the social, obstetric, paediatric and other aspects of the history plus detailed clinical examination.

It is now generally recognised that, when the curve of distribution of intelligence is followed downwards, evidence of somatic and neurological abnormality increases. In other words an idiot is much more likely to look physically abnormal or to have a motor lesion than a child of normal intelligence. The physical errors of development associated with mental defect were at one time referred to as 'stigmata of degeneration', a vestige of Morel's (64) doctrine which still colours thinking in this field. The presence of these signs has diagnostic value as they sometimes permit classification into syndromes; or they may enable a judgement to be made as to the time of onset of the developmental anomaly, e.g. if a child has markedly low-set ears, epicanthic folds and other physical peculiarities, a diagnosis of birth injury is improbable. Even if somatic errors do not at present permit classification into a syndrome, they may eventually suggest aetiological factors. For example, the syndrome noted by Edwards and others (31), consisting of a peculiar facies, small triangular mouth, head narrow in front and wide at the back, low-set ears and congenital defect of the heart, is now known to be associated with tripling of chromosome 17. No doubt these features had been noted many times before without being assigned to any particular category.

In the study of 200 consecutive cases mentioned above, we considered the physical signs and found that 46 were cases of Down's disease (mongolism), and that of the remainder 68% had either a gross somatic abnormality, eye defect, motor lesion or malformation of the skull. Only 21% were free of gross physical signs. Thus, in the severely subnormal, physical abnormalities can be of great assistance in suggesting the cause of the mental retardation.

Few exhaustive autopsy studies have been done of series of mentally defective children. Cases coming to post-mortem examination are necessarily self-selected, but nevertheless such series add to our knowledge of the relative incidence of different forms of cerebral abnormality and throw light on causation. Crome (25) was able to allot 91 out of a series of 228 brains of mental defectives to recognised syndromes, but of the 191 unclassified brains only 8 showed no morphological change.

2

Relative Importance of Social Factors

Very many studies have shown that mental retardation is commoner if the social and economic environment is unfavourable. This does not imply that the problem of mental defect causes more concern in underdeveloped countries. The reverse is true: the higher the economic level and the better the social and educational services, the more attention is paid to mental retardation. Burt (10) was one of the earlier workers to draw attention to the coincidence of educational retardation and poverty in particular areas. He considered that 20% of the schoolchildren in Lambeth, Hoxton and Poplar were backward, while in the then 'better' neighbourhoods such as Hampstead, Lewisham and Dulwich the backward numbered barely 1%. Attempts have been made in the past to distinguish between scholastic backwardness on the one hand and 'genuine' mental defect on the other. This is always a difficult exercise, and it has lost some of its point since it has become more generally recognised that intelligence as measured by standard tests can also be considerably modified by environmental factors (Clarke and Clarke (13)). These workers found that retarded adolescents from unfavourable homes tended to show a significant increment in intelligence quotient in a stimulating environment. Over a 2-year period the group from homes judged to be unfavourable showed an average increase of 10 points of IQ, compared with an average of 4 points improvement for those from a less adverse environment.

Penrose (69) has demonstrated that a family history investigation which starts with higher-grade cases leads to different results from that which starts with lower-grade cases. He found that, if feebleminded and borderline patients are separated from idiots and imbeciles, in the first group home conditions tended to be subnormal, while in the second they were distributed as in the general population. These findings are similar to those of a number of other workers, but the facts are open to various interpretations. It may be argued that the adverse social conditions of the 'borderline and feebleminded group' are indeed responsible for their mental retardation, whereas factors which are less dependent on the social environment play a major part among the more severely handicapped. This notion is sometimes expressed by referring to the first group, i.e. the milder cases, as having 'sub-cultural defect' and to the second group as having 'pathological defect'. As Penrose emphasises, there is considerable overlap in any such classification. Another consideration which he mentions is that mild cases may transmit their defect since they are fertile, whereas severe cases do not reproduce. Mild defect in the parents of the first group may therefore be to some extent responsible for the poor state of the homes of the milder cases of defect.

It is, however, very difficult to disentangle the relative weight of economic and genetic factors. Brandon (8) reviewed the intellectual and social status of children of mental defectives; 73 mothers were considered who had been certified as mentally defective. The average intelligence quotient of these mothers was 73·5 and they were similar to other groups of institutionalised feebleminded persons. They had an average of 14 years in an institution. They bore 109 live children, of whom 74 were tested: the average IQ was 89·1; 34 more children were assessed on the information available, and this brought the average for the whole group to 91·3 for 108 children. Four children scored below 65 consistently. The 109 children were survivors of a total of 150 children of these mothers, an unduly high death-rate, and it was thought that a number of them had suffered from adverse social factors. None the less these findings, like those of Charles (11), show that the effect of having a mentally defective parent is less overwhelming than was often suggested.

In considering the effect of environment in studies of this kind, allowance should be made for selection of the sample. Some 3% of a given population may be arbitrarily classed as 'mentally defective' on the basis of test results, using a cut-off point of IQ 70 (Wechsler (85)). In a population of some 46 million in England and Wales this would mean a matter of 1,380,000 suffering from a serious impairment of intellectual capacity. But the number for whom it has been found necessary to provide beds in hospitals was 61,245 in 1961, with 5,000 on the waiting lists (1960). In the case of the more severely defective, it is the mental defect as such which is often the chief reason for seeking one of the few hospital beds available. With the feebleminded or subnormal the reverse is the case, only a small minority of this group finding their way into hospital; usually they are accepted by society and form an integral part of it. Admission may be necessary when there are neurotic features, and these in their turn are commonest where there are pressing social problems, commonly lack of an adequate home.

Therefore Penrose's findings mentioned above may simply indicate that socially 'better' households seek to place their severely mentally subnormal children in hospital, while it is the least adequate homes which cannot provide for their subnormal (feebleminded) members. To some extent, then, the inadequacy of the home may not be directly causal in regard to limited intelligence. If however mental retardation is regarded as a failure of social adjustment, then indeed the inadequacy of the home background may well be a prime factor. Such a view might very likely be supported by a more intensive study of children classed as educationally subnormal. These children pose a similar statistical problem to that mentioned above in regard to their relationship to others of a similar level of intelligence. Special schools and classes for the educationally subnormal provide for only a fraction of the total of children who are poor in their performance in intelligence tests. Often the reasons for deciding that a child needs a special school or class are not so much his backwardness as such, as a degree of emotional disturbance resulting in failure to adjust to the group. As a result it is not uncommon for a child with a test performance giving him a formal intelligence quotient above 70 to be classed as educationally subnormal, while a more stable and better adjusted child with an IQ well below that figure may remain in the ordinary class. Intelligence quotient thresholds for ascertainment as educationally subnormal are set at different levels for different social groups (Stein and Susser (78)). In 1959 there were 31,504 children in schools for the educationally subnormal and a further 12,277 judged to be in need of such provision, making a total of 43,781. If this is compared with the figure of nearly 7 million children in the age group 5–14 in England and Wales and subject to compulsory attendance at school, this gives a proportion of approximately 0·63%. In 1961 there were 34,500 places for the ESN.

Gulliford (39) noted that, of ESN school leavers, those with a lower IQ tended to hold their jobs while the more intelligent often failed for personality reasons.

A dichotomy similar to that suggested by Penrose and other workers between the aetiology of severe subnormality on the one hand and subnormality on the other is also emphasised by Stein and Susser (77). They noted that an undue proportion of educationally subnormal children from 'dysmorphic' homes were admitted to hospitals for the mentally subnormal after leaving school. Dysmorphic homes were defined as those in which there was no parent or substitute up to the age of 10 years. A possible interpretation of this finding is that there was simply nobody to assume responsibility for these children when they left school, and therefore the authorities 'played safe' by placing them in hospital. Stein and Susser have revived the view that, if a family with adequate economic and intellectual resources has a mentally defective child, then this is probably due to some pathological change, but that children of inadequate families may suffer from mental subnormality as a natural result of the milieu in which they are reared (Stein and Susser (78)). This dichotomy is similar to that of Lewis (52). The concept is useful, but in practice no such division is clear-cut. In some cases of feeble-mindedness, the home may be quite adequate in regard to the economic and intellectual status of the parents, but it proves impossible to define any precise pathological process in the patient. The converse is also true. An unsatisfactory home environment may operate by producing gross brain lesions. It is now well established that unfavourable socio-economic circumstances tend to produce a low birth weight and that this in its turn favours reduced intelligence and an increased incidence of gross mental defect or cerebral palsy. One example of such a less favoured group is illegitimate births, which carry both a higher infant mortality and a higher rate of premature births. The evidence on this subject has been recently reviewed by Knobloch and Pasamanick (49).

In considering the causation of mental backwardness in any one individual, it will be seen that social and psychological factors are of the utmost importance in all but the most vegetative of idiots. Woodward (87) assessed a group of severely mentally subnormal children for evidence of emotional disturbance. She then quantified her findings, and correlated them with an independent assessment of the adequacy of the home. There was a significant positive correlation of emotional disturbance with domestic inadequacy. This work indicates how much personal relationships influence mental function and social acceptability, even of patients with gross brain lesions.

A similar finding in regard to the level of intellectual function is shown by the work of Tizard and Lyle in the Brooklands experiment (Tizard (82); Lyle (54, 55)). This work demonstrated that if imbecile children were taken out of an unfavourable institutional environment and placed in a smaller unit with more individual attention, they progressed more than a control group remaining in the larger institution. The difference in vocabulary was statistically significant, while many improvements in social behaviour were noted. A similar finding was made by Lyle (56) when he compared imbeciles living at home with an institutional group of the same level by means of performance tests. The home group, as might have been expected, had a better vocabulary level. Apart from proving the point that backward children usually progress better at home, and showing that institutions can be improved, these researches show that the mentally severely subnormal, like normal children, are influenced by their mode of upbringing. An inborn error such as trisomy in Down's disease or an absent enzyme in phenylketonuria may determine that a child will be of imbecile grade, but the precise level of social and intellectual function will vary according to the immediate environment of the child. Within the normal range of intelligence also it may be assumed that cerebral structure and biochemical function prescribe within certain limits the intellectual potential of the individual; but the realisation of these potentialities will depend on circumstances, especially those of early life.

3
Surveys of Hospital Populations

From the above considerations it will be clear that surveys of hospital populations of defectives provide a somewhat biased sample of the total problem of mental retardation. The bias favours severe subnormality, i.e. idiocy and imbecility; it also favours patients with disturbed behaviour or inadequate homes. But there are few adequate clinical reviews of non-institutionalised defectives, and it seems likely that work based on hospital populations will continue to provide the main source of information on the clinical causes of mental backwardness. It appears that at present an increasing proportion of hospital patients are severely subnormal. There were 46,669 (76%) patients in England and Wales in hospital in 1961 classed as severely subnormal and 14,576 (24%) as subnormal. (It should be remembered that different hospitals may use different criteria in making this distinction.)

While, as has been suggested, psychological and social factors are more important in the less severely handicapped group, the majority of whom are retained in the community, gross brain lesions and malfunction are probably very important in this group also. Numerous examples can be quoted of a 'shading off' process, whereby lesions which in severe form may produce idiocy, in their milder manifestations are compatible with feeblemindedness or even normal intellectual capacity.

In the case of tuberous sclerosis (Corlett and Kirman (17)) we studied 13 patients, and found that of these 10 had probably arisen by new mutation since there was no relevant family history. In two cases the mother was affected by the disease but to a minor extent. Both mothers were able to manage their homes; one had worked as a laboratory assistant in a paint factory and the other as canteen hand. Both were judged to be of dull normal intelligence. A number of examples have been recorded of untreated children with phenylketonuria reaching a normal level of intelligence (Cowie and Brandon (19)). Laurence (50) found that a majority of children with arrested hydrocephalus have intelligence within the normal range.

It follows from these considerations that hospital surveys, while focusing attention on gross abnormalities and dealing primarily with the severely mentally subnormal, none the less have considerable significance for the aetiology of feeblemindedness. The classical example, unrivalled in many respects for its thoroughness, is Penrose's Colchester Survey (67) of 1938. This study ably demonstrated the heterogeneity of the material and emphasised the role of multiple specific genetic and environmental factors. Using the title of *The Biology of Mental Defect* (68) for his subsequent text, Penrose was a pioneer in the application to this field of modern biological principles of genetics and ecology. He demonstrated the role of balancing factors in human social adaptation. He also did much to re-educate public opinion, which had been misinformed on the subject by earlier eugenic enthusiasts. Penrose demonstrated the role of environmental factors. He also pointed out the absurdity of the notion, which had been current in 1912 when the Mental Deficiency Act was being prepared, that it was possible in some way to segregate the 'unfit' from the community and thus purge it of abnormality. Penrose (68) stated, '. . . the genes carried by the fertile scholastically retarded may be just as valuable to the human race, in the long run, as those carried by people of high intellectual capacity', and 'Civilised communities must learn to tolerate, to absorb and to employ the scholastically retarded and to pay more attention to their welfare.' The better understanding of the nature and cause of mental defect which we owe to Penrose and similar workers is one of the main factors which led to the change in public attitude clearly reflected in the 1959 Mental Health Act.

The results of the Colchester survey were published 24 years ago. Since that time a number of specific genetic and environmental factors producing mental retardation have been discovered, and a great deal of fresh light has been thrown on previously recognised syndromes. At the same time there has probably been some alteration in the relative frequency of conditions encountered in a representative sample of mental defectives. Examples of newly discovered genetically determined conditions include 'oast house disease' (Smith and Strang (76)) and maple syrup urine disease (Menkes, J. H., Hurst, P. L. and Craig, J. M. (61); Mackenzie and Woolf (57)) among the many rare conditions which occasionally result in impaired brain function. The recognition of the harmful effect of maternal rubella (Gregg (38)) and of toxoplasmosis during pregnancy exemplify the extension of our knowledge of the role of the environment in producing intellectual defect. The discovery of the 47th chromosome in Down's disease (Lejeune *et al.* (51)) is one of the most dramatic advances in the whole field of mental retardation, and indeed of human biology. Some of the more obvious changes in frequency of syndromes are the virtual disappearance of congenital syphilis as a cause of mental defect (Berg and Kirman (2)), and the sudden emergence of a large number of cases of retrolental fibroplasia resulting in blindness and sensory deprivation and complicating mental defect which was perhaps caused by other factors than those producing the retrolental fibroplasia itself (Williams (86)).

Table 1 (Berg and Kirman (3)) shows some of the aetiological factors in 1,900 patients admitted to the Fountain Hospital Group. Seven-eighths of these were idiot or imbecile children. Certain distinct syndromes have been listed, but anatomical abnormalities of mixed aetiology such as hydrocephalus and microcephaly have not been included. The most

TABLE 1

Aetiological Factors and Distinct Syndromes in 1,900 Mental Defectives

FINDING	No. of cases (% incidence in brackets)			Sex distribution	
	Likely or certain	Possible	Total	M	F
Mongolism	249 (13·1)	0	249 (13·1)	135	114
Meningitis	34 (1·8)	6 (0·3)	40 (2·1)	20	20
Phenylketonuria	28 (1·5)	0	28 (1·5)	14	14
Kernicterus	21 (1·1)	0	21 (1·1)	14	7
Tuberous sclerosis (epiloia)	15 (0·8)	0	15 (0·8)	6	9
Encephalitis	6 (0·3)	9 (0·5)	15 (0·8)	7	8
Maternal rubella	8 (0·4)	2 (0·1)	10 (0·5)	6	4
Congenital syphilis	8 (0·4)	0	8 (0·4)	3	5
Cerebral lipoidosis	7 (0·4)	1 (0·1)	8 (0·4)	6	2
Cretinism	2 (0·1)	3 (0·2)	5 (0·3)	2	3
Post-natal head injury	2 (0·1)	3 (0·2)	5 (0·3)	4	1
Sturge-Weber syndrome (naevoid amentia)	4 (0·2)	0	4 (0·2)	1	3
Von Recklinghausen's disease (neurofibromatosis)	4 (0·2)	0	4 (0·2)	1	3
Infantile gastro-enteritis	1 (0.1)	3 (0·2)	4 (0·2)	2	2
X-ray irradiation during pregnancy (child defective)	1 ⎫	0	1 ⎫	0	1
Pertussis immunisation	1 ⎪ (0·2)	0	1 ⎪	1	0
Galactosaemia	1 ⎬	0	1 ⎪	1	0
Hypoglycaemia	1 ⎭	0	1 ⎬ (0·4)	1	0
Thiouracil treatment during pregnancy (child defective)	0	1 ⎫	1 ⎪	1	0
Neonatal septicaemia	0	1 ⎪ (0·2)	1 ⎪	1	0
Sagittal sinus thrombosis	0	1 ⎬	1 ⎭	0	1
Lead poisoning	0	1 ⎭	1	1	0
Totals	393 (20·7)	31 (1·6)	424 (22·3)	227	197

Reproduced from Berg and Kirman (3).

striking finding is that in this series, consisting mainly of severely mentally subnormal patients, it was possible to suggest causation in less than one-fifth of the cases. This fact underlines the extent of our ignorance of the problem. Another feature of this series is that, despite its size, it contains no examples of many conditions known to produce or be associated with mental defect. For example there were no instances of the Laurence-Moon-Biedl syndrome or of Wilson's disease.

4

Classification of Aetiological Factors

The customary division of factors into genetic and environmental is simple and useful. To do this does not commit one on the vexed question of the relative roles of 'nature' and 'nurture'. As has been shown above, both nature and nurture must be considered in understanding the mental development of any individual. Further, many cases of mental defect are doubtless due to the operation of more than one factor. In still other cases there are mitigating factors which reduce the impact of the unfavourable gene or injurious environment.

It should not be assumed that in 'simple' or undiagnosed amentia the cause of the backwardness is necessarily genetic. Until Gregg (38) showed that maternal rubella could cause mental defect, any such cases would have been described as 'simple'. It is likely that many unclassified instances of mental retardation are due primarily to environmental factors. It should also be emphasised that the terms 'genetic' and 'congenital' are by no means synonymous. Thus congenital syphilis is clearly environmental in origin, while the group of conditions referred to as 'Schilder's disease' is equally clearly genetically determined, though the symptoms (including dementia) do not usually manifest themselves until some years after birth. These distinctions are of great importance in advising parents about the risk of another child being affected by mental retardation. In the undifferentiated case the risk is usually not much greater than 3% in the absence of a family history of a similar condition or of parental consanguinity; but in the case of a clearly diagnosed genetic syndrome the risk is likely to be much higher, unless we are dealing with a new mutation or an isolated example of chromosome anomaly.

5

Genetically Determined Conditions

It seems likely that there are hundreds of discrete genetically determined syndromes which produce mental defect by interference with cerebral development or function. Most of these are extremely rare and the majority have not yet been recognised. Understanding of those genetic syndromes which are recognised is at very different levels in different conditions. Garrod's (36) original text did not list any inborn errors of metabolism known to produce intellectual defect. On the other hand, as the extreme delicacy of the balance of biochemical processes in the brain becomes better known, it is surprising that anomalies are not more frequent. The discovery of phenylketonuria by Fölling (33) produced a model for a whole group of conditions interfering with cerebral metabolism. Study of this condition, which occurs in perhaps 1 : 20,000 of the population, has also thrown light on the normal chemistry of brain function, while current studies of prevalence (Harding and Shaddick (40)) illuminate human ecology and will help us to understand the survival of such adverse genetic factors in the population.

It is not possible to assign any precise proportion of defect to genetic causes. This is partly because many cases may be due equally to genetic predisposition and unfavourable environment, partly from lack of precise knowledge. In the series of imbeciles and idiots at the Fountain Hospital mentioned above, it was possible to suggest the role of genetic factors in some 40% of cases. But these results would not necessarily hold good for educationally subnormal children, in whom there is more scope for the action of cultural factors. Even in this series of idiots and imbeciles the proportion of clearly defined genetic conditions amounts to little more than 20% of admissions; and of these cases of Down's disease make up the vast majority.

Multifactorial inheritance is of great importance in mental defect, but the very nature of this concept is such that cases so produced cannot be related to any particular clinical entity. The notion is that a constellation of genetic factors, all of which impinge upon intelligence, are all unfavourable in the given individual. The result is a clinically undifferentiated example of mental retardation. In considering actual cases in order to study genetic causation, therefore, attention is now concentrated on three groups, though others will doubtless emerge with increasing knowledge of how heredity operates.

Recessive and Sex-linked Factors

The majority of mentally backward children presenting with a family history of other examples of the same condition owe their defect to indirectly transmitted factors. In most such cases the syndrome cannot be given a name, though the observer may be struck by the remarkable similarity of the affected individuals and feel that he is in fact faced with a new but unnamed disease. Gradually however the list of known conditions of this nature, most of which conform in their pattern of inheritance to the classical Mendelian recessive concept, is being extended. The best known and commonest of these is phenylketonuria, whose carrier state affects perhaps one in 100 people; others such as galactosaemia are much less frequent. In some of these conditions it is known that a single enzyme is either missing or, more likely, abnormal and functionless. Such enzyme defect may affect a great variety of metabolic systems. There is a group of metabolic disorders characterised by aminoaciduria. In phenylketonuria there is an inability to convert phenylalanine to tyrosine, a process which is essential for normal body chemistry and brain function. In the few cases of maple syrup urine disease so far reported there has been an excessive excretion of valine, leucine and isoleucine and of the corresponding keto-acids (Mackenzie and Woolf (57)). These cases have been associated with a more profound mental defect than is usually found in phenylketonuria, and have succumbed in early life. The disease is an inborn error of metabolism, with a block in the oxidative decarboxylation of the three amino-acids concerned. Another entity with involvement of the brain is oast house disease, in which, as in phenylketonuria, there is excessive excretion in the urine of phenylpyruvic acid, phenylalanine, tyrosine and phenylacetic acid, but in addition there is also alpha-hydroxybutyric acid, which produces the characteristic odour (Smith and Strang (76)). Paine (66) uses the classification shown in Table 2, which depends on whether there is a generalised aminoaciduria, or one in which several amino-acids are excreted but in a definite pattern, or one in which only one amino-acid appears. In fact however these boundaries are not sharp. For example, Ottaway (65) found a greatly increased excretion of tyrosine as well as of phenylalanine in phenylketonuria.

TABLE 2

Classification of Syndromes of Mental Defect and Aminoaciduria according to Patterns of Amino-acids present in the Urine

SINGLE AMINOACIDURIAS
  Phenylketonuria
  Allan-Dent disease (l-arginosuccinic acid)
  Cystathioninuria (Harris)
MULTIPLE BUT PATTERNED AMINOACIDURIAS
  Maple syrup urine disease (Menkes)
  Hartnup disease (Dent)
  Cystinuria (Berry)
  Oast house disease (Smith and Strang)
GENERALISED AMINOACIDURIAS
  Heavy metal poisoning (Pb, Cd, Hg, U)
  Wilson's disease (Cu)

Galactosaemia
Congenital renal tubular acidosis and de Toni-Fanconi syndrome
Buphthalmos and decreased renal ammonia production (Lowe)
Syndromes with muscular wasting (including dystrophy)
? Kernicterus
Sex-linked microcephaly and spastic diplegia
Some cases of hypsarhythmia?
Others

Reproduced from Paine (66).

Disturbances of amino-acid metabolism may well be of direct importance for brain activity. Secondary effects are also important, and in phenylketonuria it is known that there are abnormalities in 5-hydroxytryptamine (serotonin) levels (Kirman and Pare (48)) and adrenaline and melanin metabolism (Cowie and Penrose, 1951 (18)).

In some conditions producing mental defect, aminoaciduria may be a secondary manifestation. This applies to galactosaemia and possibly Wilson's disease (hepatolenticular degeneration), both of which are transmitted in a classical recessive manner. It is still not certain how the brain is damaged in these conditions. One attractive suggestion is that the brain of the infant with galactosaemia is denied an adequate supply of glucose because of 'competition' by galactose, which being present in excess blocks the pathway. This is probably an over-simplification. In hepatolenticular degeneration the loss of mental capacity is probably due to the deposition of copper in the lenticular nucleus and related structures, the fundamental abnormality being a shortage of the ceruloplasmin which normally acts as a vehicle for copper. It may be, however, that this shortage in turn is due to leakage through the kidney.

Errors in metabolism of protein, carbohydrate and fatty substances can all cause inefficient brain function. Some of the amino-acid disturbances have been mentioned. In addition to galactosaemia, the familial type of hypoglycaemia can result in severe defect. It is not certain how frequent hypoglycaemia is in the young, especially in the premature infant, nor how much brain damage is due to this. Certainly hypoglycaemia is rare after the neonatal stage. It may be due to a variety of conditions, but whatever the prime cause it will, if prolonged and severe, inevitably lead to brain damage. One genetic variety seems to be connected with a hypoglycaemic effect of protein, notably leucine and isovaleric acid (Cochrane et al., (14); Woolf (88)).

Some of the large group of disturbances of lipid metabolism are associated with mental defect. Hurler's disease (gargoylism or lipochondrodystrophy) is now included in this group, though the disturbance is characterised by an accumulation of a muco-polysaccharide, chondroitin sulphate. There is also storage of a water-soluble lipid. Lipochondrodystrophy indeed is the commonest member of this group in mental deficiency hospital practice, partly because it is a less obviously progressive disease than most conditions of the cerebro-macular or Niemann-Pick type, so that a few cases may accumulate in a hospital population. With lipochondrodystrophy, as with other such disorders, many cases are probably not diagnosed because the anatomical features which until now have been the basis for recognition are minimal. With phenylketonuria and such abnormalities, in which the chemical basis of the disorder is better understood, marginal cases may be recognised without too much difficulty, even though intelligence may be within the normal range (Cowie and Brandon (19)). In Hurler's syndrome laboratory techniques for recognition during life are only now being evaluated. It is possible to recognise the condition by characteristic inclusions in the lymphocytes (Mittwoch (63)) and by excessive excretion of chondroitin sulphate (Berry and Spinanger (5)). As such techniques become developed and perfected, it will be seen that the proportion of mental defect attributable to metabolic disorders is somewhat greater than appeared at first sight. There are at least two biologically distinct forms of gargoylism (Herndon (44)). One, the commoner, is autosomally transmitted and shows no preference for either sex, while the other is sex-linked and peculiar to boys. There are some clinical differences, the sex-linked form being distinguished by rarity of corneal clouding, infrequent dwarfing and frequent deafness.

Very many metabolic pathways are vital to cerebral activity. In considering recessively transmitted traits some of the forms of cretinism may be mentioned. It seems that genetically determined forms are more important in England than those due to dietary peculiarities. There appear to be quite a number of distinct genetic entities under the general head of 'cretinism' corresponding to a block at different points in the synthesis, storage and activity of thyroxine. A well known example is provided by a much studied family of goitrous tinkers (McGirr and Hutchison (60)). In them, di-iodotyrosine was lost in the urine. The thyroid gland seems unable to bind the iodotyrosyl groups, mono- and di-iodotyrosine being found in the blood. Another error is due to inability to convert inorganic to organic iodine compounds, and yet another involves difficulty in conjugating two molecules of di-iodotyrosine to make thyroxine. A relevant but distinct anomaly was described by Fraser (34), who reported four cases of sporadic goitre and congenital deafness. Despite this, the mental and physical development of the patients was said to be otherwise normal. However it is obvious that such a syndrome could give rise to mental defect, either directly from thyroid inadequacy or indirectly through the deafness. In these cases also the defect appeared to be recessively transmitted.

There are some not uncommon metabolic disorders which have been recognised for many years, but in which so far the nature of the metabolic disturbance remains obscure. This applies to the group of conditions included under the general head of Schilder's disease. Like the lipidoses, these disorders are not so commonly found among groups of severely retarded children because of the tendency to steady progression and removal by death. This group of conditions again appears to comprise a considerable number of distinct genetic entities, though the clinical course is similar. They are usually characterised by an initial period of normality, unlike most cases of idiocy or imbecility, though selective destruction of the white matter may occasionally be seen as a congenital phenomenon (Brandon et al. (9)). One sub-group of leucodystrophy is now categorised as 'metachromatic' because of the peculiarity of staining of myelin with cresyl violet, which Diezel (30) ascribes to a melanin-like catacholamin. This material may also be excreted in the urine. Diezel attempts a rational classification of these disorders based on chemical studies of the brain and other tissues. He puts the various forms of amaurotic family idiocy, Niemann-Pick's disease, Gaucher's disease and gargoylism into the group of storage diseases with an increase in the quantity of sphingolipids, while the demyelinating group of leucodystrophies are characterised by a decrease of sphingolipids. Diezel suggests the possibility that in the storage diseases there is a defect in the 'energetic system of the cell', i.e. the substances stored are normal metabolic substances which accumulate in abnormal quantity because the cell cannot use them. His approach has the merit of putting this type of disorder on the same kind of level as the better known metabolic defects, though it is not yet possible to say precisely what enzymes are involved. Richter (72) points out that a large proportion of the possible 20,000 enzymes in man may be involved in cerebral activity. Further, even in normal physiology these may vary in their availability by a factor of 100. It will be seen from this that there are a tremendous number of possibilities of metabolic error, and it may well be some time before a clearer picture emerges. Advance is at present proceeding on the lines of cerebral chemistry, histo-chemistry, and work on the metabolism of the living patient by more refined techniques and family studies.

A practical contribution to knowledge of the aetiology of mental defect has been made by family studies. Originally these took the form of collection of pedigrees, often incomplete and biased by inclusion of irrelevant material, which tended to imply the attribution of all social ills to a single cause, e.g. Tredgold's (83) chart entitled 'alcoholic, psychopathic and tuberculous ancestry' showing two imbeciles and a third sibling who was 'epileptic and decidedly queer at times'. More sophisticated methods have gradually developed, and in a number of the recognised disease entities it now is possible to identify with fair probability the carriers of recessively inherited conditions. Further development of this work should provide a good basis for family counselling. Increasingly advice is also sought in regard to siblings of affected patients who may be carriers. In galactosaemia, gargoylism, phenylketonuria, pitressin resistant diabetes insipidus and a number of other conditions, there is a prospect of a fairly reliable technique for detection. Methods involve precise chemical measurement of the effect of a dose of a test substance, as in phenylketonuria where a phenylalanine tolerance curve can be obtained, or a search in the potential carrier for histologically recognisable features, e.g. the lymphocytic inclusions found in gargoylism.

Some genetically determined syndromes such as familial microcephaly and lipochondrodystrophy are distinguished by anatomical peculiarities, while others such as phenylketonuria and galactosuria are diagnosable by chemical tests. This made it convenient to describe syndromes as 'anatomical' or 'metabolic'. It is now becoming increasingly possible to achieve a unified view of these two groups of processes. In the lipidoses, for example, the clinical form of the syndrome depends on the extent to which the enzyme abnormality in different diseases affects different tissues. In cerebro-macular degeneration damage is more obvious in the brain, though a careful study of the liver and spleen will also reveal abnormalities. In Niemann-Pick's disease the liver and spleen are very strikingly involved, while in Hurler's disease it is the skeletal alterations which impart much of the recognisable anatomical picture. The duration of the abnormality also determines the degree of anatomical picture. Crome and Pare (24) showed a loss of myelin in long-standing cases of phenylketonuria, while myelination is probably impaired (Crome et al. (28)). In a case of galactosaemia dying at 8 years with idiocy Crome (27) showed a degree of micrencephaly with gliosis and loss of Purkinje cells.

There is still no clue to what biochemical processes are faulty in such a condition as familial microcephaly. It would, however, be reasonable to assume by analogy with other similarly transmitted conditions that each such syndrome is dependent on a single metabolic error. The difference between this and some other conditions is that the effect of the error becomes obvious at a very early stage of development, indeed probably in the first few weeks of intra-uterine life. This applies to most of the forms of mental defect accompanied by obvious malformation or anatomically recognisable syndromes.

A very important practical distinction obtains between those conditions in which the infant is protected by the mother's metabolism during intra-uterine life and those where it is not so. For example, a working hypothesis which is used as a basis for treatment in both phenylketonuria and galactosaemia is that the baby is normal at birth and that effective dietary treatment will prevent damage to the brain. On theoretical grounds this is a reasonable assumption, since in phenylketonuria the placenta should be able to remove the excess of phenylalanine into the maternal circulation for disposal and to supply adequate amounts of tyrosine and other metabolites to the foetus; in galactosaemia no problem arises before birth since no considerable amounts of galactose are supplied to the unborn child. On the other hand, in lipochondrodystrophy the brain is already abnormal at birth. Newborn babies with phenylketonuria do not, as a rule, excrete phenylpyruvic acid, which usually appears at about a three-week stage, and similarly the blood level of phenylalanine slowly rises, suggesting that they start extra-uterine life with normal levels (Gibbs and Woolf (37); Woolf (89)). In the two examples quoted of maladies in which the baby is clinically normal at birth, the fault lies at an early metabolic stage in the elaboration of raw materials. In the lipidoses the block may occur at a much later metabolic stage and concern the ability of the brain cells, among others, to use the more refined metabolites.

Condition Characterised by Direct Transmission

A number of conditions which produce severe mental defect are sub-lethal in their effect. The individual has a very precarious hold on life and is most unlikely to reproduce. Data on the genetic features of some of the rarer gross malformations are for this reason not readily available. With some of the better known syndromes, however, *formes frustes* do occur, and these milder cases may have children. In this way it has become evident that certain syndromes are directly transmissible from parent to child along the classical lines of Mendelian dominance. The best known example of this pattern in mental defect is tuberous sclerosis. The majority of parents of children with this disease are themselves normal. In our series of 13 cases (Corlett and Kirman (17)) we found an affected parent in three, and assumed in the other 10 families with no affected relative that a new mutation had occurred. It is just possible that there may have been examples of irregular dominance among these. As mentioned above, the affected parents, though not of a high order of intelligence, had a mild form of the disorder and were able to look after their affairs and play the role of parent and spouse without difficulty. Very little is known of the cause of 'naturally' occurring mutations, though some agencies which produce an increase in the rate are now recognised. It is presumed that any increase in background ionising radiation would lead to an increase in the number of cases of mental defect produced in this way. An increase in diseases such as tuberous sclerosis would be observed quickly, since the characteristic rash of adenoma sebaceum is obvious at about the age of four years, and a dominant factor would reveal itself in the first generation after the mutation. In the case of recessive factors, however, the effect might only become noticeable after a number of generations, since most persons affected by the mutation would be carriers and not actually suffering from the disease.

Amongst backward children are a few characterised by malformation of both hands and skull. These include cases of acrocephalo-syndactyly (Apert's syndrome). This condition is also transmissible in a dominant manner, but as affected individuals do not make attractive mates, most of the cases are attributed to new mutations. Blank (6) distinguishes between typical cases, which he considers form a genetic entity, and atypical cases. In the former he noted a sharp increase in paternal age. This condition is very rare, being present in only 1 in 160,000 live births, as compared with 1 in 20,000 for phenylketonuria. It is present in perhaps 1 in 2 million of the general population, the difference being accounted for by the high mortality and possibly by under-reporting. This is characteristic of all forms of severe mental defect. As the age scale is ascended, there is a big shift in the nature of the problem of the mentally handicapped away from the extreme forms, as in idiocy, to the milder forms, as in dull normality and the educationally subnormal.

The question of parental age also has relevance to a number of other discrete conditions, some of which, such as Down's disease (mongolism), are very much commoner (1 in 600 of the population at birth) than Apert's syndrome. Maternal age in hydrocephalus has a J-shaped curve, showing that older mothers are much more prone to have affected children. Any decrease in the average age at which mothers have children or decrease in the number born to parents over 40 would reduce the number of defective offspring. Economic measures such as allowances to students, family allowances and housing programmes may therefore be directly relevant to this aspect of the problem. In both Apert's syndrome and mongolism the elderly parent is apparently more prone to mutation of the germ cell, but in the former it is the father in whom the change takes place whereas in mongolism it is usually the mother, though Penrose (70) has pointed out that the unusual form in which two 21 chromosomes are attached to each other is also distinguished by high paternal age. He also suggests that in this condition there may be failure in the case of the aged parent to select against abnormal sperms rather than an increase in the number of abnormal forms.

Some other dominantly transmitted conditions occasionally cause mental defect. Huntington's chorea commonly affects a middle-aged or post-reproductive group, but cases in children do occur. This applies also to the ataxias of the Marie type. Dystrophia myotonica tends to be associated with limited intelligence and is directly transmitted. Also very rare is a central form of neurofibromatosis which is biologically akin to tuberous sclerosis and may cause very severe mental defect (Crome (21, 29)).

Chromosome Anomalies

Until recently studies on the aetiology of Down's disease (mongolism) concentrated on events occurring during the first few weeks of pregnancy, since it was clear that associated anomalies such as heart lesions and faults in the lens suggested an early origin in the organogenetic period. The

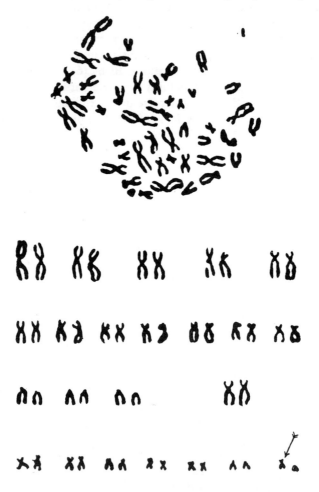

FIG. 1. Chromosomes from a girl with Down's disease (mongolism) showing 21/22 type of translocation (marked with arrow). Larger member of last pair represents in effect 2 chromosomes joined together. Thus 46 chromosomes only can be counted, the normal number, but effect is that of 47 as in 'regular' Down's disease.

(Preparation by Dr. R. G. Chitham.)

discovery of the additional 21st chromosome by Lejeune and his colleagues (51) has definitely enabled Down's disease to be classified as a genetic error. This simply means that the cause of the anomaly must now be sought before conception instead of after it. The recognition of at least three distinct types of chromosome anomaly in Down's disease has greatly stimulated research in this field, particularly in regard to other forms of mental defect. It now seems clear that Down's disease is the only common syndrome in the field of mental retardation which can be ascribed to a gross chromosome anomaly, visible under the microscope.

Several instances have been described of the simultaneous occurrence of Down's disease with an additional 21st chromosome and Klinefelter's syndrome with an additional female (X) chromosome (Harnden et al. (43); Hamerton et al. (42)). The former authors estimate the random risk of such a double event as 1 in 560,000. It seems likely that there is some similarity in the factors predisposing to the two conditions and that the incidence will be more than that expected on a random basis. The Kline-felter syndrome (XXY) itself seems to have an undue incidence in popul-ations of the mentally handicapped (Ferguson-Smith (32)), and the average intelligence of cases so far reported has been below the norm. There is less definite evidence for an association between Turner's syndrome (XO) and mental retardation, though instances have been reported, including a chromatin positive imbecile (XX) in whom one of the female chromosomes was abnormally big, appearing to be an isochromosome of the long arms. It seems that the XXX 'super-female' syndrome is not incompatible with normal intelligence, but in this syndrome also a number of cases have been reported of very low intelligence. In the study by Johnston and others (46), 3 patients were possibly of normal intelligence while 15 were mentally defective (below IQ 70).

Both fine classical mutations involving only one locus, and grosser chromosome anomalies which are microscopically visible, are probably fairly common, though the sex cells involved often fail to produce a zygote which goes to term. Very little is known about the factors favouring these deviations from the normal in man. On general principles, any increase in background radiation is likely to favour such changes. The influence of parental age in the examples mentioned above also suggests the importance of hormonal factors. Some supporting evidence for this was produced by Coppen and Cowie (16), who demonstrated that younger mothers of children with Down's disease tend to be more masculine in body build and to have a hormone output distinguished by excess of dehydroepiandro-sterone (Rundle et al. (73)).

6

Environmental Factors

It should again be stressed that environment plays a very important role in the development of any individual, however backward. This fact is the basis of treatment, education and management of the mentally retarded. As yet we know only a few instances where an environmental factor has produced gross derangement of the developing nervous system, but there are undoubtedly many other cases where we have failed to recognise the external agent. This was true, for example, of babies damaged by maternal rubella before Gregg's discovery. It also applied to the rarer examples of backwardness attributable to toxoplasmosis or cytomegalic inclusion body disease (Crome (26)). In addition to massive single factors of this kind there are doubtless many others which operate in a more subtle fashion, often in combination. Thus, a baby was jaundiced as a result of rhesus incompatibility; it survived but was very feeble and of idiot level. This baby was the product of incest and at autopsy was found to be suffering from cerebral lipidosis. This illustrates multifactorial causation and the interplay of heredity and environment.

Timing of Insult

It is convenient to think of aetiological factors in mental retardation in chronological order. Viewed in this way, some factors are potentially operative before the formation of the zygote. This applies to all genetic factors which depend upon the constitution of the parental sex cells. Conception introduces a 'chance' factor, in that there is a big choice of sperms which may be 'right' or 'wrong' in so far as the intelligence of the new individual is concerned. It seems likely, however, that this is not always 'pure' chance but that some selective factors may operate even at this stage in favour of normality (Hamerton et al. (41)).

Any unfavourable factor impinging on the zygote after conception will be looked upon as 'environmental'. It should be remembered that genetic factors, although by definition implying an abnormal biochemical constitution of the zygote, may not manifest themselves until late in life, an extreme example being Huntington's chorea. In other cases the genetic defect implies an inability to cope with a particular aspect of the environment. Thus the galactosuric child is potentially normal in his mental development if he is not exposed to lactose. In the present state of our knowledge it seems likely that a similar combination of hereditary and environmental factors is necessary to produce infantile schizophrenia, examples of which are found among any considerable group of institutionalised mental defectives.

The environmental factors productive of mental defect can conveniently be divided into those operating before, during and after delivery.

The Intra-uterine Environment

Very little is known about the effect of the mother's state of health on defect of the central nervous system. The age differences mentioned above in relation to such conditions as hydrocephalus and anencephaly emphasise the importance of the foetal environment, as does the fact that these conditions are commoner in less privileged social classes. By analogy with animal work, for example that of Millen and Woollam (62), it seems likely that much congenital defect is produced or made possible by defects in maternal health and diet. It should be emphasised that this type of factor, like all other adverse circumstances, is not absolute. In Millen and Woollam's work they found, in common with other experimenters, that a deficiency in the maternal diet may increase the proportion of deformed offspring, but does not necessarily mean that all the newborn will be deformed. This principle should be remembered in considering pathogenesis at any stage in development. It disposes of the facile argument that, because one individual did not succumb to a given stress to which he was exposed, then the factor under consideration cannot be causal of an abnormality in another individual.

Defects in maternal diet and the influence of toxic substances are interrelated, since poisonous substances may act by interfering with the availability of essential metabolites. A vast number of toxic substances are known to produce foetal anomalies in animals, of which a high proportion are defects in the central nervous system (Warkany (84)). Research on the effects of drugs and poisons in humans has, however, devoted little attention to the effect of these substances on the child if they are given to the pregnant woman. The recent widespread public concern at the large number of congenital malformations produced by the administration of 'thalidomide' during pregnancy may do something to remedy this situation and lead to specially designed research. It is true that most of the 'thalidomide babies' do not appear to have brain defects, but it is also true that brain abnormalities are not always conspicuous at birth in the way that absence of limbs is. The relationship between drugs or other noxious substances and intellectual defect may, therefore, be missed.

Infections during Pregnancy

The role of infectious diseases in regard to congenital abnormality and future development of the exposed foetus is also obscure. It is now well established that maternal rubella during the organogenetic first trimester of pregnancy frequently produces anomalies. In Pitt's series (71) 13 children out of 61 at risk appeared to have been damaged. He estimated that during the first 4 weeks over half the embryos are adversely affected. Mental defect, however, is a rare complication, there being only one case in his series. The British survey (Manson, Logan and Loy (58)) also shows a much lower incidence of gross anomalies than had been suggested by retrospective studies. Jackson and Fisch (45) found 30% of babies deaf after rubella in early pregnancy. Evidence about the role of most other viruses is not very convincing. An exception is the case of cytomegalic inclusion body disease. Very few examples of foetal abnormalities due to this condition have been reported; on the other hand the disease itself is widespread, and it is possible that its role in the production of defect has not been fully recognised owing to its insidious nature. This consideration may well apply to a number of other common diseases.

Influenza is an example of a common condition which is still under suspicion as a cause of foetal abnormality. Coffey and Jessop (15) thought they were able to demonstrate an increase in neonatal defect as a result of a Dublin epidemic of influenza, but the prospective British survey mentioned above (which considered also other viruses than that of rubella in the aetiology of congenital anomalies) did not provide supporting evidence for the role of influenza in this connection.

The part played by most of the maternal infections not due to viruses is also an open question. Maternal syphilis is an exception, and it has long been acknowledged as a cause of mental defect in the offspring, though it seems likely that even in the past, when it was commoner and treatment was less effective, its importance was exaggerated. It is now rare as a cause of mental retardation in children. The increase in the acquired form of the disease during and after the second World War was not paralleled by an increase in the congenital form. We (Berg and Kirman (2)) found a history of maternal syphilis in 12 cases among 1,900 imbeciles and idiots. Among these 12 there were 3 examples of taboparesis, 2 of meningovascular syphilis, and in 3 children we were uncertain whether the defect was due to the maternal disease. In the remaining 4 cases we thought the maternal syphilis coincidental.

McDonald (59) found major defects more common in infants of mothers who during pregnancy had pulmonary tuberculosis, acute febrile infections or were engaged in heavy work. Her study was based on questioning 3,300 women at the time of booking for their confinement.

Perinatal Factors

Little (53) believed that permanent damage to the brain could result from 'the want of a few breathings'. The general view at present is also that oxygen lack is the most important cause of mental defect and cerebral palsy among the factors operating about the time of birth. But there is still no agreement what proportion of all mental retardation is due to damage at birth, nor what part is played by factors other than oxygen shortage. Sylvester (80) described 3 cases of marbling of the basal ganglia, a condition which is often attributed to anoxia. In these three cases there was a history of obstruction of the cord: one was prolapsed, one was knotted and one tightly coiled round the neck. However, there was a history of cord complications in only 7 other cases out of a total of 1,058 admissions to the Fountain Hospital during a 10-year period, an incidence of 1·1%, whereas some degree of coiling of the cord round the neck is common and may occur in as much as 23·3% of all deliveries. A severe degree of neonatal asphyxia, whatever the cause, always suggests the possibility of gross brain damage with subsequent mental defect or cerebral palsy. But there are many recorded instances of normal development following a complicated delivery with asphyxia and difficulty in establishing breathing. Asphyxia in the newborn is not necessarily due to birth difficulty. In cases where the brain is ill-developed the very first sign of malfunction of that organ may be difficulty in establishing breathing. Neonatal death in children with malformed brains is commonly due to impaired respiratory control.

Sylvester (81) found haemorrhage in 44 of 101 brains examined after perinatal deaths. There was 10 times the normal incidence of breech deliveries in this series. There was also a suggestion that smallness of the placenta was related to foetal distress in the mature infants in this series. It is not easy to relate these findings to mental defect, since Crome (personal communication) is of the opinion that the majority of infants with any considerable degree of brain haemorrhage usually succumb. At autopsies of mentally defective children he does not commonly find evidence of old haemorrhage. He has set out some of the evidence on this question (Crome (23)). A number of well documented cases, however, occur with good clinical and radiological evidence of birth injury with haemorrhage followed by severe mental defect, often associated with a motor lesion. In this connection the concept of the 'brain-injured child' (Strauss and Lehtinen (79)) may be mentioned. There is no good evidence that a child damaged during the birth process exhibits a particular behaviour pattern as described by Strauss and his colleagues, neither is there evidence that children with this behaviour pattern were all damaged at birth. So far as the clinical pattern of mental defect goes, there is little to distinguish children whose abnormality derives from a perinatal insult from those whose defect is due to other causes. An important exception to this statement is that somatic and visible anomalies are often associated with cerebral anomalies developing at an early stage in pregnancy. Thus syndromes which include cleft palate, malformed ears, heart abnormality, bifid digits and the like are probably of early origin and are less likely to be due to birth damage. Behaviour patterns and emotional stability seem to be related to the post-natal environment, whatever the cause of the backwardness (Woodward (87)).

Specific Post-natal Factors

As mentioned above, the impact of the social and cultural background on intelligence is undeniable. There is still, however, no agreement about the relative weight of these factors compared with those discussed in the preceding sections, i.e. factors of heredity and disease. The Scottish survey (74) showed the tendency of children from large sibships to do badly on tests, but this finding can be interpreted either as meaning that such children are less favoured because of poorer circumstances, or that intellectually less well endowed parents tend to have more children. The tendency for the first and last children in the family to do better argues in favour of environmental factors. The Clarkes (12) have reviewed some of the more recent work on this subject, notably the study by Skeels and Harms (75) of children placed in foster-homes. The striking thing about such studies is that foster-children from poor homes achieve above-average results in tests as a group when fostered in good homes. One of the complicating factors was that on first assessment of the children no correlation was found between their intelligence and that of their true mothers, but when they were tested at the age of 13 the correlation had risen to 0·44. However, the average intelligence quotient of the mothers was 20 points less than that of the children, and it seems likely that a considerable share of the improvement was due to the much better environment into which the children had been placed.

Specific post-natal adverse factors are easier to define. Hyperbilirubinaemia is now a well recognised hazard. We (Crome, Kirman and Marrs (22)) found 10 cases of kernicterus due to rhesus factor incompatibility among 1,260 admissions. A more recent survey (Tarsh and Kirman, awaiting publication) shows that an appreciable number of cases still occur despite the improvements in treatment. We found, however, that most of the cases had had what must now be judged as inadequate treatment. Kernicterus is occasionally due to other blood-group incompatibilities, Kell or ABO, or to prematurity. A recent survey of premature infants (Freedman et al. (35)) showed that hyperbilirubinaemia, considered separately, i.e. apart from each of the three factors of hypoxia, excessive post-natal weight loss and infection, had an adverse effect on subsequent attainment of the child. The adverse effect of high blood bilirubin was particularly reflected in impaired motor performance. This work confirms the view that hyperbilirubinaemia may have an ill effect in the absence of clinical evidence of gross kernicterus.

Meningitis, encephalitis and occasionally severe gastro-enteritis with dehydration are the infections most likely to produce mental defect in post-natal life. Meningitis must be classed with hyperbilirubinaemia as a factor capable of being combated successfully with adequate early treatment. Late treatment of tuberculous meningitis now accounts for a number of cases of hydrocephalus and severe brain damage (Kirman (47)). In spite of modern antibiotics there were still 11 instances of mental defect due to septic meningitis among 800 admissions (Berg (4)). Ill defined 'encephalitis' is often blamed for brain lesions which declare themselves with fits or fever (Bourne (7)), but, after exclusion of dubious instances, we considered that this group of conditions accounted for at least 6 of our 1,900 cases. The encephalitis may be epidemic, sporadic, post-measles or other viral exanthem. Encephalitis lethargica is now, fortunately, rare, though after the early 1920s it made a considerable contribution to the population of mental deficiency hospitals. In severe gastro-enteritis associated with extreme dehydration and coma there may be irreversible brain damage due to sinus thrombosis (Crome (20)).

The role of early electrolyte disturbance in regard to brain damage has not been fully assessed, and it is possible that this is a contributory factor in impaired cerebral function, particularly in the premature. Similar considerations apply to non-specific and temporary hypoglycaemia.

Some degree of hypoglycaemia is common among the newborn, especially those of low birth-weight. On the other hand the newborn brain may be a little more tolerant of such variations. This problem is the subject of current research.

A vast number of poisons are theoretically capable of producing brain damage with intellectual defect, but fortunately such cases are rare. Lead and carbon monoxide are two of the best known examples, though both are rare. There was only one doubtful case of the former in our series of 1,900; it is possible however, in view of the insidious nature of the symptoms, that some cases were missed. The hazards of carbon monoxide are illustrated by the following case. A.E., born 5.8.60, aged 20 months, was left in a room with her brother, aged 5. An armchair in the room was ignited and smouldered for some time before it was discovered. Both children were by then unconscious. The brother made an apparently complete recovery, but the little girl, previously normal, appeared to have been reduced to idiot level. Two months after the incident she had lost her ability to sit, stand or walk, showed a marked tremor and appeared blind. 7 months after it, when she was 2 years and 3 months, she had made a remarkable degree of recovery, but functioned like a 15-month child. Prognosis must be guarded, but it seems likely that she may function at educationally subnormal level and need special education. There is probably no definite threshold for damage in such cases, and it is possible that the brother, despite an apparently complete recovery, may function at a somewhat lower level than might otherwise have been the case.

★　　★　　★

As yet we are still ignorant of many of the causes of mental defect. With increasing knowledge there is every reason to hope that the possibilities of prevention will increase. In the absence of precise knowledge, all factors which improve the health and cultural level of the community, in particular of mother and child, can be expected to reduce the total incidence. Once defect is established, remedial and palliative measures will help to reduce the burden on the family and society in many cases, irrespective of cause. This very considerable social problem can, however, only be tackled rationally and fundamentally when much more is known about aetiology. This demands a co-ordinated and extensive research programme.

REFERENCES

1. BERG, J. M. and KIRMAN, B. H., 1959a. *Brit. Med. J.*, ii: 848.
2.   1959b. *Brit. Med. J.*, ii: 400.
3.   1959c. *Proc. Roy. Soc. Med.*, **52**: 787.
4. BERG, J. M., 1962. *Proc. London Conference on Scientific Study of Menta Deficiency*, 1960, p. 160. London.
5. BERRY, H. K. and SPINANGER, J., 1960. *J. Lab. Clin. Med.*, **55**: 136.
6. BLANK, C. E., 1960. *Ann. Hum. Genet., Lond.*, **24**: 151.
7. BOURNE, H., 1955. *J. Nerv. Ment. Dis.*, **122**: 288.
8. BRANDON, M. W. G., 1957. *J. Ment. Sci.*, **103**: 710.
9. BRANDON, M. W. G., KIRMAN, B. H. and WILLIAMS, C. E., 1959. *J. Ment. Sci.*, **105**: 721.
10. BURT, C. L., 1937. *The Subnormal Mind*, p. 121. London.
11. CHARLES, D. C., 1953. *Genet. Psychol. Monogr.*, **47**: 3.
12. CLARKE, A. M. and CLARKE, A. D. B., 1958. *Mental Deficiency: the Changing Outlook*, p. 93. London.
13. CLARKE, A. D. B. and CLARKE, A. M., 1959. *Acta Psychol.*, **16**: 137.
14. COCHRANE, W. A., PAYNE, W. W., SIMPKISS, M. J. and WOOLF, L. I., 1956. *J. Clin. Invest.*, **35**: 411.
15. COFFEY, V. and JESSOP, W. J. N., 1959. *Lancet*, ii: 935.
16. COPPEN, A. and COWIE, V., 1960. *Brit. Med. J.*, i: 1843.
17. CORLETT, K. and KIRMAN, B. H., 1957. *Brit. Med. J.*, ii: 1174.
18. COWIE, V. and PENROSE, L. S., 1951. *Ann. Eugen.*, **15**: 297.
19. COWIE, V. and BRANDON, M. W. G., 1958. *J. Ment. Defic. Res.*, **2**: 55.
20. CROME, L., 1952. *Archs. Disease in Childh.*, **27**: 468.
21.   1954. *J. Path. Bact.*, **67**: 407.
22. CROME, L., KIRMAN, B. H. and MARRS, M., 1955. *Brain*, **78**: 514.
23. CROME, L., 1957. *In* Hilliard and Kirman's *Mental Deficiency*, p. 143. London.
24. CROME, L. and PARE, C. M. B., 1960. *J. Ment. Sci.*, **106**: 862.
25. CROME, L., 1960. *Brit. Med. J.*, i: 897.
26.   1961. *Wld. Neurol.*, **2**: 447.
27.   1962a. *Archs. Disease in Childh.*, 37, 415.
28. CROME, L., TYMMS, V. and WOOLF, L. I., 1962. *J. Neurol. Neurosurg. Psychiat.*, **25**: 143.
29. CROME, L., 1962b. *Archs. Disease in Childh.*, **37**: 640.
30. DIEZEL, P. H., 1960. In *Mental Retardation* (ed. Bowman, P. W. and Mautner, H. V.), p. 277. New York and London.
31. EDWARDS, J. H., HARNDEN, D. G., CAMERON, A. H., CROSSE, V. M. and WOLFF, O. H., 1960. *Lancet*, i: 787.
32. FERGUSON-SMITH, M. A., 1959. *Lancet*, i: 219.
33. FÖLLING, A., 1934. *Hoppe-Seylers Z. physiol. Chem.*, **227**: 169.
34. FRASER, G. R., 1959. *Proc. Roy. Soc. Med.*, **52**: 1039.
35. FREEDMAN, A. M. *et al.*, 1961. *The Effect of Hyperbilirubinaemia on Premature Infants. Progress Report.* New York.
36. GARROD, A. E., 1909. *Inborn Errors of Metabolism.* London.
37. GIBBS, N. K. and WOOLF, L. I., 1959. *Brit. Med. J.*, ii: 532.
38. GREGG, N. M., 1941. *Trans. Ophthal. Soc. Aust.*, **3**: 35.
39. GULLIFORD, R., 1960. *Bull. Brit. Psychol. Soc.*, **40**: 53.
40. HARDING, W. G. and SHADDICK, C. W., 1961. *Med. Offr.*, **106**: 51.

41. HAMERTON, J. L., COWIE, V. A., GIANELLI, F., BRIGGS, S. M. and POLANI, P. E., 1961. *Lancet*, ii: 956.
42. HAMERTON, J. L., JAGIELLO, G. M. and KIRMAN, B. H., 1962. *Brit. Med. J.*, i: 220.
43. HARNDEN, D. G., MILLER, O. J. and PENROSE, L. S., 1960. *Ann. Hum. Genet.*, 24: 165.
44. HERNDON, C. N., 1954. *Res. Publ. Ass. Nerv. Ment. Dis.*, 32: 239.
45. JACKSON, A. D. M., and FISCH, L., 1958. *Lancet*, ii: 1241.
46. JOHNSTON, A. W., FERGUSON-SMITH, M. A. and HANDMAKER, S. D., 1961. *Brit. Med. J.*, ii: 1047.
47. KIRMAN, B. H., 1958. *Brit. Med. J.*, ii: 1515.
48. KIRMAN, B. H. and PARE, C. M. B., 1961. *Lancet*, i: 117.
49. KNOBLOCH, H. and PASAMANICK, B., 1962. *New Engl. J. Med.*, 266: 1045, 1092, 1155.
50. LAURENCE, K. M., 1958. *Lancet*, ii: 1152.
51. LEJEUNE, J., GAUTIER, M. and TURPIN, R., 1959. *C.R. Acad. Sci., Paris*, 248: 602.
52. LEWIS, E. O., 1933. *J. Ment. Sci.*, 79: 298.
53. LITTLE, W. J., 1862. *Trans. Obst. Soc. Lond.*, 3: 293.
54. LYLE, J. G., 1960a. *Child Psychol. and Psychiat.*, 1: 121.
55. 1960b. *J. Ment. Defic. Res.*, 4: 14.
56. 1960c. *J. Ment. Defic. Res.*, 4: 1.
57. MACKENZIE, D. Y. and WOOLF, L. I., 1959. *Brit. Med. J.*, i: 90.
58. MANSON, M. N., LOGAN, W. P. D. and LOY, R. M., 1960. Rubella and other Virus Infections during Pregnancy. *Ministry of Health Reports on Public Health and Medical Subjects*, No. 101.
59. McDONALD, A. D., 1958. *New Eng. J. Med.*, 258: 767.
60. McGIRR, E. M. and HUTCHISON, J. H., 1956. *Lancet*, i: 106.
61. MENKES, J. H., HURST, P. L. and CRAIG, J. M., 1954. *Pediatrics*, 14: 462.
62. MILLEN, J. W. and WOOLLAM, D. H. M., 1957. *Brit. Med. J.*, ii: 196.
63. MITTWOCH, U., 1961. *Nature*, 191: 1315.
64. MOREL, B. A., 1857. *Traité des Dégénérescences physiques, intellectuelles et morales de l'Espèce humaine*. Paris.
65. OTTAWAY, J. H., 1957. *Biochem. J.*, 66: 8.
66. PAINE, R. S., 1960. In *Mental Retardation* (ed. Bowman, P. W. and Mautner, H. V.), p. 263. New York. London.
67. PENROSE, L. S., 1938. *A Clinical and Genetic Study of 1,280 Cases of Mental Defect*. London.
68. 1949. *The Biology of Mental Defect*, p. 240. London.
69. 1954. *The Biology of Mental Defect*, p. 54. London.
70. 1962. *Lancet*, i: 101.
71. PITT, D. B., 1961. *Med. J. Austral.*, 1, 881.
72. RICHTER, D., 1959. *Brit. Med. J.*, i: 1255.
73. RUNDLE, A., COPPEN, A. and COWIE, V., 1961. *Lancet*, ii: 846.
74. Scottish Council for Research in Education, 1949. *The Trend of Scottish Intelligence*, p. 101. London.
75. SKEELS, M. and HARMS, I., 1948. *J. Genet. Psychol.*, 72: 283.
76. SMITH, A. J., and STRANG, L. B., 1958. *Archs. Disease in Childh.*, 33: 109.
77. STEIN, Z. and SUSSER, M., 1960a. *Brit. J. prev. soc. Med.*, 14: 83.
78. 1960b. *J. Ment. Sci.*, 106: 1304.
79. STRAUSS, A. A. and LEHTINEN, L. E., 1947. *Psychopathology and Education of the Brain-injured Child*. New York.
80. SYLVESTER, P. E., 1960a. *Acta Paediat. (Uppsala)*, 49: 338.
81. 1960b. *J. Obstet. Gynæc. Brit. Emp.*, 67: 219.

82. TIZARD, J., 1960. *Brit. Med. J.*, i: 1041.
83. TREDGOLD, H. F., 1952. *Mental Deficiency*, p. 43. London.
84. WARKANY, J., 1960. In *Mental Retardation* (ed. Bowman, P. W. and Mautner, H. V.), p. 44. New York and London.
85. WECHSLER, D., 1944. *Measurement of Adult Intelligence*, p. 40. Baltimore.
86. WILLIAMS, C., 1958. *Brit. J. Ophthal.*, 42: 549.
87. WOODWARD, M., 1960. *Brit. J. Med. Psychol.*, 33: 123.
88. WOOLF, L. I., 1960. *Clin. Chim. Acta*, 5: 327.
89.   1961. *Cerebral Palsy Bull.*, 3: 249.

XXII

CHILD THERAPY
A CASE OF ANTI-SOCIAL BEHAVIOUR

D. W. WINNICOTT
M.A., F.R.C.P.

Consulting Physician, Paddington Green Children's Hospital
(St. Mary's Group), London

1

Introductory

In this chapter I propose to illustrate a principle. I shall do this by giving a child psychiatry case, describing a psycho-therapeutic interview that was significant.*

Whereas in psychoanalysis the motto could be: 'How much may I be allowed to do in this case?', in child psychiatry the motto often must be: 'How little need I do?' In very many instances there is a good environmental provision and the persons involved are able and willing to carry the child through to health, provided, however, that someone will first release the child's emotional development which has become hitched up at some point. In the favourable (and common) case the correct procedure is to do the work through the child, in order to arrive at the area of distress in the child's life in relation to which the child's defences became organised. The block to further growth lies in the presence of these organised defences.

It can be wasteful of time in these cases to gather an accurate history from the parents, and on the other hand it is economical to work with the child. It is the child who can take the psychiatrist to the area of distress

---

* Naturally no one case can cover the vast range of child psychiatry; nevertheless it is to be hoped that theas cases that I am engaged in describing at the present time in various books and journals, when added up, and perhaps published in one book, will give a comprehensive picture while illustrating a principle that is not complex.

and *at the same time* give the psychiatrist an opportunity to make a significant contribution. This may be of the nature of a remark or an interpretation, and it may move the block. The parents and perhaps the school can then continue with what amounts to mental nursing, and it is this that completes the process. The psychiatrist may help those who are doing the mental nursing to understand the value of what is being done, and usually the parents are only too pleased to play their part. In this way quite severe child cases can be seen through with economy, with perhaps no more than a few hours of the psychiatrist's work and a few telephone calls. (Nevertheless the training for this work is the psychoanalytic training, in which cases are treated on the other principle: How much may one do?)

If a Psychiatric Social Worker is to be employed in the task of helping the parents to understand what they are doing, then it is economical to have the P.S.W. in the room during the psycho-therapeutic interview. This does no harm to the interview if the psychiatrist is unselfconscious enough, and it avoids the necessity for time-wasting case conferences, except for those required for teaching purposes.

In child psychiatry the accent needs to be on the economic aspect of the work, since it is only in this way that our social services can ever hope to cater for the psychiatric needs of the child population; yet the work must go deep in each case or else it is useless. The only thing is to go as deep as possible at the right moment and as early as possible in those cases in which a setting is 'pre-arranged' because of an environment that is all the time waiting to be helpful. If help cannot be given in the first or the first two or three interviews, then the case automatically changes over into a long-term problem of management or therapy, and the resources of the clinic allow for this development.

The following case is chosen for no special reason except that it can be described relatively briefly.

2

Case of Mark, aet. 12 years

(at the time of the consultation in 1948)

Family:	Girl	16 years
	Patient	12 years
	Boy	8 years
	Boy	7 years

Mark was brought to me at the age of 12 years by his parents. The father was a medical colleague. In this case I first saw the two parents together as they wished to get my help in orientating to the problem (usually I see the child first). Much detail emerged in the usual way of an interview that takes its natural course.

The family was intact. The following significant landmarks in Mark's emotional development were reported:

Mark was breast-fed and *difficult to wean.* 'He resisted weaning very strongly.'

Mark *had never been truthful.* (Later the parents said that this had been a fixed characteristic from 2 years.)

Mark became at 7 (or earlier) a boy who *'if he wants must have'.*

Mark started *to steal at* 8 *years.* (See below for minor correction of this detail.) This happened when he was away staying with friends. At 10 years he was taking money from his mother's bag and telling lies. There was the usual story of refusal to confess. Recently (12 years) serious stealing had taken place. This was associated with his passion for fishing. Stealing was from father's wallet and elder sister's bag, and in amounts of £5 and £10. He swore he had not stolen, and by doing so he incriminated his brother, to whom he was devoted. He confessed only when confronted with a fingerprint investigation. Then he bought a fishing rod and elaborate tackle. He spoke of 'my dealer' and claimed he would be given a special fishing rod on his birthday by this dealer. He had in fact bought two rods and had hidden them. He had taken elaborate precautions against detection.

The family's attitude was reasonable, which was possible since the general relationships in the family were good. If Mark confessed he was never punished, but the parents were especially puzzled by the compulsive lying. Also they marvelled that all these troubles produced no unhappiness in the boy.

At last, after further incidents, the father, who was at a loss to know what to do, put Mark in disgrace; he must have his meals in the kitchen, and fishing was stopped. Mark remained without a sense of guilt, and continued to say his prayers.

The parents went on, in the interview with me, to build up a history of Mark's early life. He was happy. In fact at 2 years he said *'I'm so happy to be alive'*, conscious of a love of living. (There is probably a tie-up here with the parents' philosophy of life, which includes a 'cultivated joy of life'.)

Mark chose to live at home, rather than to continue at his Preparatory Boarding School. School reports said: 'Mark could do better if he tried.' He was good at games and was thought to have average ability. Eventually he went to a Grammar School as a day-boy, and there he made an attempt to 'redeem himself by hard work'. Mark was very fond of nature study and had an incredible knowledge in this speciality, using books intelligently.

When I asked about sleep techniques, the parents reported: *'Mark adopts incredible postures* in his sleep. He is like a log. On going to bed he sleeps immediately, and he has never told his dreams.' Also Mark had had a twitching face recently, including blinking.

Mark had many friends, they said, but no bosom friend; also he was attractive to older people. He had been sensibly informed in regard to sex by his father. When excited Mark would sweat and work his face, and in this way he became thought of as nervous. Mark liked handwork but showed no special artistic ability. He had taste however, and could be moved by beauty. A feature in his life was the brilliance of his older sister. He was well aware of this, and possibly associated with this was a fear of his father, which developed over a phase in which he was doing badly at school.

Mark was courageous physically, swimming being his favourite sport. In fact *Mark's main interests concerned water*. He was set on going into the Navy from 3 years to 8 years, but he temporarily lost this (at 9 and 10 years) when he was told he would have to work to get accepted.

The parents brought out the point that he was affected by the new baby boy, born when Mark was 5. He called him 'our baby', and he had always been especially fond of him. They now said that it was *when he shared a room with this boy that he first stole from his mother*. (Previously the mother had dated the first theft at 8 years.)

The day after the consultation with the parents I had the first of two significant interviews (and two subsidiary interviews) with Mark. Although I knew a good deal about him it would have been valueless to have worked on the basis of this knowledge. What was needed was a new history-taking of a different kind. A great deal happened during this first session, but that which can be reported here centres round the 'squiggle game' which we played together.

The First Interview

In my first personal contact with Mark, I adopted the game in which, in alternating fashion, one makes a squiggle and the other turns the squiggle into something. He was pleased to play this game, a game with no rules.

A1. My squiggle, which he turned into a shoe.
A2. His squiggle, which I turned into a jug.
A3. My squiggle, which he turned into a man with a moustache (rather fantastic).
A4. His squiggle, which I turned into a kind of animal.
A5. My squiggle, which he turned into a face.
A6. His squiggle, which I turned into two worms close to each other. There was a good deal of conversation about this, including a discussion on his part of the function of the 'saddle'. He indicated on the drawing the way in which worms copulate.
A7. My squiggle, which he turned into a curious kind of a man's face. *Here I was already aware of the boy's tendency to undervalue fantasy.*
A8. His squiggle, which I turned into a schoolmaster.
A9. A drawing of his of a man. This resulted from my having used the fantastic part of the drawing to introduce the subject of dreams. He seemed surprised that I should talk about dreams, and the drawing of the man indicated a dream figure which gradually lost definition from the waist down. I spoke about the stealing at this point, using a word that he supplied, which was 'impulse'. I said that

in stealing he was acting out ideas which were in his mind, like dreams. He had spoken about forgotten dreams, and I had said that when dreams become unavailable there may be a need to recapture them through acting on impulse, so that the dream dominates what happens and in this way reappears in the person's own life and conduct.

I now knew of Mark's ability to make use of my approach to the unconscious and to dream material; this approach was somewhat new to him, partly because of his own defence organisation and partly because of the family pattern.

After this first consultation the mother wrote:

After leaving your house with Mark last week, my husband made only casual inquiries, avoiding direct questions. The boy showed no reaction of disturbance or pleasure. Later on in the evening he spoke to me at some length about his visit to you, and quite spontaneously. He was particularly struck by your questions about dreams and their meaning. He seemed puzzled by the importance of dreams and by your insistence in the matter. I hope all this will be of some use. His comment about the toys was that it would be a 'paradise for his young brother'. There were toys which are used by younger patients in the room.)

A fortnight after the first interview with the boy and the day before the second interview, the father rang me up to report. After the first visit to me Mark was not allowed to go fishing. He wanted to take a particular boat to the pond with his brother, and he said to his mother that it was a present for his birthday: could he have £1 to get it? He was so obsessed by the boat that he had only one idea, which was to get this particular one immediately. The mother was firm in refusing. He had already told the brother about the boat. The parents were struck by the way in which eventually he gave in and so was unable to buy the boat. This seemed worth noting by them because of its newness, which they attributed to the fact of the first interview with me. It will be seen that water is again involved in this incident.

The Second Interview

On the second occasion that I saw Mark, he was ready to play the squiggle game again.

B1. My squiggle, which he rather skilfully turned into a human head.

B2. His squiggle, which I made into a tortoise.

B3. He turned his own squiggle into a teacup, appropriately decorated. *Here appeared his wish to take full responsibility for a drawing and for the ideas that lie latent in it. Rather naturally, this was not markedly imaginative.*

B4. My squiggle, which he turned into a man very precariously climbing a rock surface with a pack on his back.

B5. His squiggle, which I turned into the drawing of a girl.

B6. My squiggle, which he turned into a surprising drawing of a pond with bulrushes and reeds, and a water-fowl enjoying the scene and just about to dive its head down for food.

Here was a picture. This showed me Mark's integrative capacity and also his capacity to love. The whole symbolised the persisting love relationship (both instinctual and dependent) with his mother, his fondness for water, and his concern with nature generally and with fertility. It also gave me a glimpse of his special knowledge. The strength of Mark's ego organisation being evident, I knew I had the right to go ahead with interpretation of material presented.

B7. His squiggle, which I turned into a lady's foot and shoe.

B8. My squiggle, which he turned into a most extraordinary and fantastic face.

Here fantasy was appearing again in the form of the fantastic, which is not free dream material. Along with all this there was a good deal of talk, not particularly about anything. Mark could feel however, from what happened, that I was interested equally in fact and in fantasy, whichever should turn up. Also he could understand my appreciation of the picture.

Th Third Interview

At the third interview we again played the squiggle game.

C1. My squiggle, which he turned into a bird with long legs.

C2. His squiggle, which he turned into a bird with a big beak warming itself before a fire.

The game had led Mark to express fantasy without feeling foolish about it. The picture which he had in front of him was entirely his, and the whole idea came unexpectedly to him from his own unconscious. My function here was not to interpret. The main therapeutic was that the boy had found a bridge to the inner world in a way which was quite natural. This drawing was like a dream that has value because it has been dreamed and remembered.

C3. My squiggle, which he turned into the man in the moon. Fantasy continued.

C4. His squiggle, which I turned into a head and shoulders.

C5. My squiggle, which he turned into a bird rather effectively flying upwards. He did this with a minimum of additions and got a good deal of satisfaction from the movement implied.

C6. His squiggle, which I made into a face, and he named it 'Mr. Facing-Both-Ways'. He justified this by a quick drawing of what would be eyebrows from my point of view but what from his point of view was a mouth, the mouth that I had drawn being eyebrows from his point of view. This was all done in a flash.

Here was indicated the dissociation in Mark's personality, relative to stealing. At this point Mark reached a stage at which he was nearly aware of the split. I made no interpretation of this.

C7. My squiggle, which he turned into a most extraordinary being with arms and one leg, a floppy sort of individual, rather bird-like, and certainly humorous.

Here came, among other things, a sense of humour, always a sign of freedom affording elbow room, so to speak, and in this way assisting the therapist.

C8. His squiggle, which I made into a face and which he called an Eskimo.

C9. My squiggle, which he turned into a weird face of a man. At this point it was easy for me to ask him about *dreams*. He said: 'I forget them. In any case they are only ridiculous', and he was obviously afraid of being laughed at if he should remember them. He did however start to draw the next, which was not based on a squiggle.

C10. Here he is kneeling in the road making squiggles in the dust. This was a dream.

This was the significant moment. The drawing led to the subject of depression. He called this 'feeling bored'. 'I only feel it for a few seconds just when I am waking up. I often think it is a strange life; perhaps it *is* a dream.' Here he was a very serious person.

In answer to a question whether he had ever felt really down, he referred to a time when he had stayed away on account of his sister's having measles. *He was perhaps 8.* He said he was homesick, sad and lonely. *Here, as is commonly found in this work, the patient takes the therapist to the date of the period of maximum strain.* At 8 years Mark had had intolerable dreams and a nightmare that indicates a severe depression mood. *The mood indicates ego organisation and maturity and some capacity to cope with the threat of disintegration of the personality.* I referred to *the love of his mother* which was at the back of his sadness at parting from her, remembering the history of difficult weaning. His comment on this was: '*If mother's away things are different.*'

We then talked about fishing. The love of his mother was the thing that he clearly expressed and in a deep way, as it came out of his remembering feeling depressed to the extent of hopelessness, in relation to being parted from her.

C11. As a final drawing I made a squiggle, which he turned into a weird kind of human being.

In this way the consultation did not end with the patient at the depth of a depression mood. He had emerged from the depression that accompanied the report of the dream.

3

General Comment

In this series of three psycho-therapeutic consultations there came about a natural development of a bridge between Mark's conscious and unconscious. If asked about dreams at the beginning he would not have been able to remember any ('He sleeps like a log and never reports dreams.'). By the end of the third interview Mark was able to tell me about his period of maximum strain, which he remembered because of a dream that brought him right into the depression that was reactive to his separation from his mother. This was at the age at which he started stealing (except that he stole once before, from his mother, at the time when he first shared a bedroom with the baby brother).

Naturally, there are precursors to all this. In Mark's case the anti-social tendency indicating a continuing reaction to a deprivation reaches back to the actual weaning from the breast. (No doubt the mother's psychology needs to be taken into consideration here, since it is almost always true that the mother of a baby that is difficult to wean is herself somewhat depressed at the time, or somewhat depressive by nature.)

The anti-social tendency was represented, before the stealing at the time of separation, by: (a) Stealing from the mother (5 years); (b) 'What I want I must have' (from 7 years); (c) Pseudologia fantastica (from 2 years).

4

Discussion

This case illustrates three main themes:

(1) The first interview with the parents gave a clear picture of the case, which however was relatively useless except in so far as it enabled the parents to reorientate to the problem.

(2) The interviews with Mark gave me a new view of the same problem, and gave me opportunity for doing fairly deep psychotherapy. All the essentials were in the material, and in usable form:

> The mother-fixation.
> The significant separation at 8 years.
> The stealing as a reaching across the 'weaning' gap.
> The depression at the time of maximum distress.
> The undervaluation of fantasy.
> The splitting defence, which cleared up as a result of the consultation.
> The sea-fixation, which alternated with a water obsession and which proved to be a satisfactory sublimation of the mother-fixation.

The case also illustrates:

(3) The theory of the anti-social tendency as a reaction to deprivation (not privation), and appearing clinically along with hope in regard to object relationships. In this case the stealing was related to a manic defence against the depression felt as such at 8 years, and was also related to a split in Mark's personality which made him clinically two people, one who had a compulsion to steal and the other who had strong

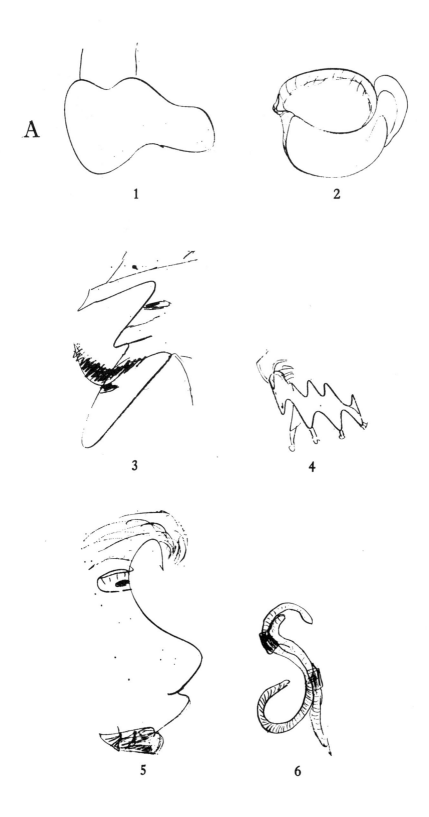

A

1

2

3

4

5

6

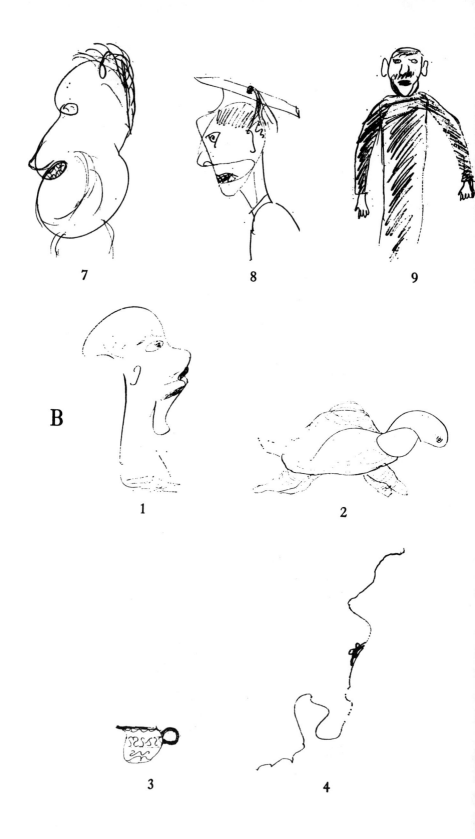

7

8

9

B

1

2

3

4

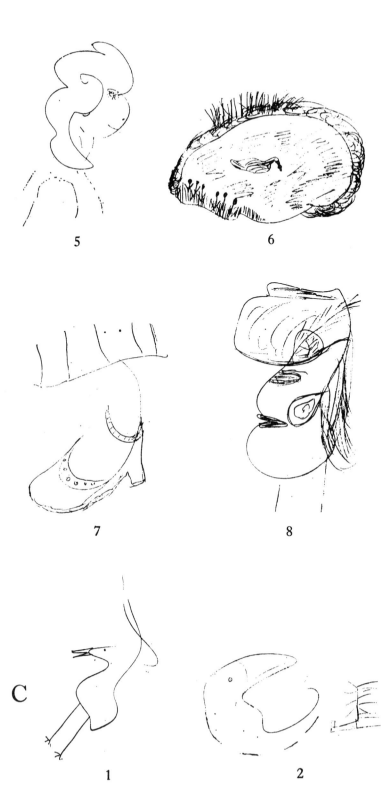

5

6

7

8

C

1

2

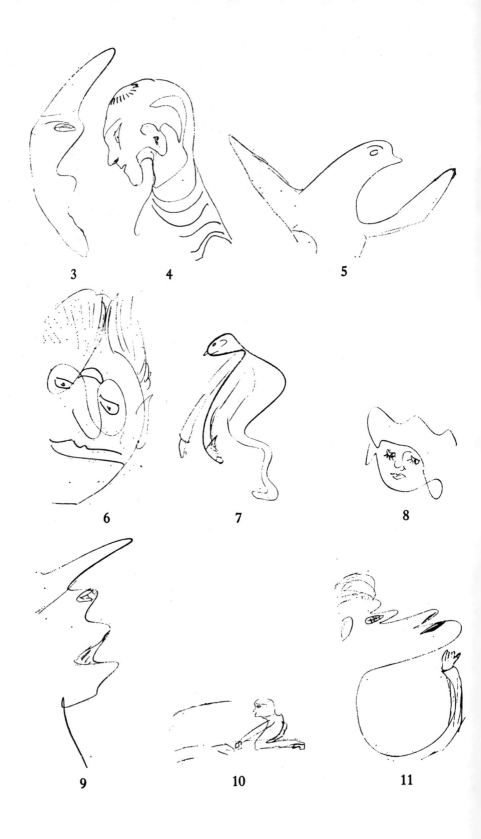

3   4   5

6   7   8

9   10   11

moral principles and a wish to be like his parents and to do well in the world (in Mr. Facing-Both-Ways).

According to the theory on which all this work is based*, the boy in stealing was unconsciously looking for the mother from whom he had the right to steal; in fact from whom he could take because she was his own mother, *the mother that he created out of his own capacity to love.* In other words, he was looking for the mother from whom he had been weaned but from whom he had refused to be weaned. His difficulty in weaning, which indicated at the time his inability to stand *disillusionment*, was turning up again in the present in the form of impatience at frustrations and the need to steal in order to circumvent frustrations. There was a clinical improvement following the first interview, which showed as a new acceptance of reality.

5

Result

After a month the father wrote:

Mark is in very good condition in every way, so far as we can see. In particular, he is far more interested in his work at school than ever before and he is taking it much more seriously, with improved results. He has started to learn a wind instrument, which was his own idea; and he is very keen on it indeed. He formerly learned the piano, but was indifferent to it and had to be pressed to practise, whereas he is eager to practise the wind instrument.

We took him away to . . . for a couple of weeks at Easter to stay with a relative by the sea. He did not ask to fish, which he knows is still forbidden, but was nevertheless exceedingly happy by the seashore. He has transferred his interest in fishing to sailing model boats. He makes these boats quite skilfully, but he shows signs sometimes of becoming obsessed by them, and this makes us a little anxious, as the previous trouble arose (it seemed to us) from an obsession with fishing. He wants to talk incessantly about them and about his expeditions to the pond.

After a further three months the father wrote:

We have been very pleased with Mark's progress this term. He has done very well at school, came out top of his form, and had an excellent report in all respects. He seems stronger morally and appears to derive strength from a habit I have got him to adopt of saying to me each morning that he will put honesty and truthfulness first today.

We are just about to send him off for a long summer holiday at some boys' camps under suitable supervision. He is greatly looking forward to it. After that he will go to stay for a week with an old friend of mine and I have told him that—for the first time—he can resume fishing while he is there if he feels strong enough to be sensible about it. He says he does. We shall see how it works out. He has been very happy again.

* D. W. WINNICOTT. *Collected Papers: Through Paediatrics to Psycho-analysis.* Tavistock Publications, 1958. Chapter xxv, The Anti-social Tendency.

Here the father shows that he has continued his active technique for instilling moral strength, which is part of the family pattern, and which I made no attempt to alter. Also he has played a more vital role in Mark's life, and corresponding with this the boy's mother has stepped somewhat into the background since the time of the first consultation.

The father wrote again in 1956:

Thank you for your letter. I am very glad to give you an account of Mark's progress during the past four or five years.

He has pursued unswervingly his chosen vocation as a sailor, and this very week he has completed his four years' apprenticeship as a midshipman in the . . . Line. He always goes to the Far East and is usually away for several months on a voyage. He has a deep satisfaction in the life at sea, although he found it involved great physical and emotional hardship, especially in the early years. He faced it with great fortitude.

He has of course developed in every way and is much more mature. He has great pride in the line in which he serves and also a sense of duty and of responsibility.

Our home means a great deal to him, and he spends the whole of his leave here. He obviously feels this to be the stable element in his life at present. He appreciates frequent letters from the family more than anything else and he writes to us and to his brother and sister from every port. This is a notable fact considering that he is not a literary type in any way. He is very affectionate in his letters, but appears rather casual outwardly when he is at home. He has one great friend whom he knew at school and they are inseparable when he is at home. The boy in question is at a university.

Mark is much attracted by girls and enjoys going to dances with them when ashore. He talks freely to myself and my wife about his girl friends and brings them to the house. He talks openly about wishing to get married, when he has qualified as an officer, though I don't think he has found a girl he wants to marry.

The timeless quality of life at sea seems to appeal to him. He often writes in his letters about the days slipping past, and of time moving past him in an effortless passage. At sea there is a fixed routine, but no pressure of time, no sense of the day of the week or the date, all of which he finds very irksome on land.

He has become much more sensible about money. He sends me an allotment of his pay every month and I accumulate this for him. He brings home from the East very generous presents and to do this means a great deal to him.

When he is at home, he needs an unplanned life without obligations or engagements, except for dates with girls. His room is always in great disorder, in contrast with the strict neatness imposed on midshipmen in regard to their cabins. But he is very careful about his personal appearance and always wears smart clothes, whereas as a boy he was particularly neglectful of his clothes and appearance.

We are expecting Mark home next month after a very long absence of 10 months and he will then be at home attending a navigation college for about 3 months. It will be interesting to see how he reacts to a very different kind of life to the one he has been leading.

If there is anything else you would like to know, please do not hesitate to mention it. So far as we can see, the lad is getting on satisfactorily. If you have any advice or warnings to give us, we should naturally appreciate your giving them to us.

In a final follow-up, in 1962, the father reported that Mark had continued to follow his calling, and to be successful in it. He was then 26 years old.

6

Conclusion

This is a satisfactory child psychiatry result; the treatment did not overtax the parents' resources, and it put but little strain on the psychiatrist. The parents did the bulk of the work and provided the continuity of management that was essential.

Essential, however, were the three significant psycho-therapeutic interviews which are described, and which centred round the squiggle game.

XXIII

CHILDREN'S IN-PATIENT PSYCHIATRIC UNITS

W. J. Blachford Rogers
M.A., M.B., B.Chir., M.R.C.P., D.P.M.

Physician in Charge, Department of Child Psychiatry, Crichton Royal Hospital, Dumfries

1

Introduction

In-patient psychiatric units for children in Britain are few in number and widely scattered throughout the country. Each one has grown up in response to local needs and as the result of initiative of one or more people in the area they have been designed to serve. Each unit has taken a very distinctive character derived from the situation in which it is placed, the type of building, the relation, if any, to a paediatric or mental hospital, the particular staffing arrangements and the personality of the physician in charge. There are widely varying criteria for the types of children admitted, the area from which they may come, which may include the whole of Britain or of Scotland or may be restricted to a particular region, and they differ in the kind of treatment offered. One of the few features which all units have in common is the enormous pressure on their beds. Many units have a waiting list of two years or more. It is doubtful whether there is any other branch of medicine in which a wait of two to four years for admission for an urgent case would be tolerated. It is impossible to be dogmatic about what the structure, composition and organisation of such a unit should be, and the following account is a very personal one, based on my experiences in the Department of Child Psychiatry of the Crichton Royal Hospital, known as Ladyfield, over the last ten years.

This unit consists of three houses. Two of them were originally medium-sized private houses, each standing in its own grounds outside the grounds of the main hospital, and each accommodates seventeen or eighteen children. These children are of primary school age, of average or above-average intelligence, and suffer from all kinds of psychiatric disorders, psychoses, neurotic disorders, organic brain damage or disease, epilepsy, psychosomatic disturbances, reactive behaviour disorders and the so-called 'personality disorders'. The 'average or above-average' intelligence should be qualified to mean 'potentially average or above-average'. Some children, especially psychotic children, may be functioning at a level well below average on psychometric testing and in their social behaviour, but may still be taken on for long-term treatment. The division between the two houses is mainly by age, one having children of approximately eight to twelve and the other from five to ten. There is a considerable overlap; a very shy or withdrawn child of eleven might well fit in better with the younger age group, at least until he has found his feet. The third house, near the others and also in its own grounds, is a converted drill hall, and is used for the assessment and treatment of twenty-five disturbed children with mental and also in some cases with physical handicaps, It started as a separate entity, but the problems presented for treatment are essentially the same, and it is being integrated more and more closely with the rest of the unit, though it has not so far been possible to extend to it the same intensity of treatment for all the children there as exists in the other two houses.

2

Functions of an In-patient Unit

(1) *Diagnostic.* This is obviously of very great importance. In all young children and in many older children in whom communication by speech is poor, a disorder can only be described in terms of observed behaviour. The limitations of assessing a child's problems by a series of individual interviews and by interviews with parents has long been recognised, and many out-patient clinics now have special facilities for observing children either in groups or individually. Examples of these are play diagnosis sessions which Howells (6) has organised at Ipswich, a very promising small unit attended by parents and P.S.W.s which Haffner has developed at Portsmouth, and a nursery school attached to Anna Freud's clinic at Hampstead (5). A further example is the day hospital facilities developed by Connell (1) at Newcastle. All these represent important contributions to diagnostic facilities, but they cannot take the place of the observation throughout the day which a residential unit can provide. In their extreme form the reactions to dependence on adults, with the frustrations arising from such dependence, are seen most clearly at such times as getting up in the morning, bathing and going to bed at night.

Childhood behaviour disorders, irrespective of the mechanisms involved, may be regarded as forming a continuum: at the one end of the scale is a 'pure' reactive behaviour disorder, i.e. that of a child potentially normal who has reacted to severe and immediate stress by maladapted behaviour, but who, when removed from the situation of stress and placed in a more accepting environment, settles down very quickly and responds appropriately to the demands made on him; at the other end of the scale come severe neurotic disturbances, in which the maladapted behaviour patterns persist even when the stresses which appear to have caused them are no longer operative. The problem of so-called 'personality disorders' in children is a very vexed one. The children who have come to Ladyfield with that label have usually been institutional children or children who have had many changes of foster parents or guardians. After a period of treatment in the unit, these children begin to show phobic or other anxiety symptoms and are then indistinguishable from the children originally referred as neurotic, and their progress continues along the same lines.

At this age children are highly malleable and readily develop new behaviour patterns in response to different stimuli. I think there is a risk that such a diagnosis in young children may be used to evade the intensive and long-term treatment which these children need. There is strong indication for more intensive work on this problem together with very careful follow-up studies. At the present time when facilities for psychiatric treatment of children of any intensity are so few and far between, control groups should be used to attempt to find out which is the best way of handling these problems, and whether there is in fact any justification for such labels as 'personality' or 'character' disorder in children of this age group. Were facilities adequate, control groups of this kind would be hardly justified, but as things are there is a wonderful opportunity for using the diagnostic facilities of an in-patient unit to establish criteria on which adequate comparisons can be made.

Diagnosis in a child may take a period of up to three months of observation, and of treatment, before it can be finally established. All too often the diagnosis is concentrated on the symptoms and signs of disturbance which the child shows. Too little attention is paid to his assets, which should form at least half the diagnostic assessment and formulation. There is yet another important aspect of diagnosis which can only be established over a period of one, two or three months, and that is the child's capacity for change. For assessing the outcome and even the desirability of a particular form of treatment, this may well be the most important aspect.

In addition to diagnosing behaviour disorders, the facilities provided by an in-patient unit can be used very effectively for establishing the diagnosis in cases of epilepsy and other problems of minimal brain damage or brain disease. The advantages of such an organisation in the diagnosis and treatment of epilepsy are obvious. The child is in a setting in which his play with other children can be observed, as also his routine throughout the day. He can be observed minutely in school in the very small groups in which school is organised, and also in occupational therapy sessions and in individual sessions with the therapist. Only in this way can the child's original condition and the response to particular lines of treatment be assessed with any accuracy.

Psychomatic disorders in children are occupying more and more attention. Here again they can often be observed more accurately in this kind of setting than in a hospital ward. Psychiatric units attached to a mental hospital tend to get relatively few of such problems, whereas those units which have been established in connection with paediatric hospitals tend naturally to have a much larger share.

For diagnosis of the very different problems of psychosis in childhood, observation in a residential setting is often essential, and indeed much more careful observation over a long period of time, together with an assessment of the results of treatment, is necessary before a real understanding of the many different disorders now labelled 'psychotic' will be reached; in many cases the solution of these problems will be found only after many years of careful follow-up study.

(2) *Short-term treatment* of disturbed children in whom a particular crisis has led to an especially difficult situation at home. Removal from the environment for a few weeks can allow the child and the parents to settle down, and when the immediate tensions are past, continued treatment on an out-patient basis becomes very much easier. This short-term treatment policy can also give most valuable diagnostic information. This particular aspect of in-patient treatment (8) is very important and is too widely recognised to need further emphasis.

(3) The third function of an in-patient psychiatric unit is to undertake *long-term treatment* (9) of certain childhood disorders. The most important groups of these are:

(a) Severe neurotic disorders, especially where the home situation is so difficult that the child cannot be expected to improve as long as he is living at home (7).

(b) Severe psychotic disorders. By psychotic I mean those which come within the category of the 'schizophrenic syndrome' as defined by Creak (2, 3) and others. This 'syndrome' almost certainly includes a heterogeneous group of cases, of which a few are childhood schizophrenia but many others have some specific handicap or disorder of brain function that makes normal adjustment and normal learning processes in the child extremely difficult; the so-called 'autism' may well be a reaction of the child to these particular handicaps. It is now established that, although a long-term prognosis of many of these children is still uncertain, many respond well to residential treatment.

(c) Brain disease or injury, often with epileptic manifestations, together with the behaviour disorders which often go with these problems. These difficulties again are so well known that they need no more emphasis.

3

Type and Character of the Unit

There are four main settings in which a children's psychiatric unit may develop: (i) attached to a mental hospital; (ii) attached to a paediatric hospital; (iii) attached to a general hospital; and (iv) as a completely separate establishment. Each of these has its own particular advantages and disadvantages. The first big question is whether it should be attached to a hospital or be completely independent. Being completely independent has some advantages in that people approach the problem with no preconceived ideas about what the nursing or treatment should be, and it is often very well accepted by parents. The buildings, grounds, and locus of the unit can be arranged to suit the demand of the population which it serves and to provide the best facilities inside and outside for the children. The disadvantage of a detached unit is that the staff has to be entirely self-contained. The selection of staff for such work is very difficult, and I know no tests or interview techniques which will tell me whether a person is going to be successful in this type of work. Perhaps the most important single factor is that they should be interested enough to want to do it. One difficulty is that some of the people most attracted to this type of work are not the ones most fitted to do it. Where such a unit is attached to a hospital, the hospital forms a pool from which staff can be drawn and given a trial period in the children's unit. If successful they can carry on, but if they do not like it or are obviously out of their depth they can return to the main hospital, having had some useful experience but without having to face the distress of giving up after an obvious failure.

Ladyfield is attached to a mental hospital and staffed by psychiatric nurses, some of the senior nurses having had a general training as well. All nurses, whether their original training is mental, paediatric or general, have to effect a very considerable reorientation when faced with children's problems, and my own view is that the personality of the individual concerned is more important than particular basic training. Units attached to paediatric hospitals have all the advantages of the facilities such hospitals provide, but tend to be rather cramped for space as regards schoolrooms, day rooms and above all grounds. The same applies to units attached to general hospitals. This is the particular stage of development of some units at present, and there is of course no reason why perfectly suitable accommodation with suitable grounds for children should not be built near any hospital where there is space.

The facilities needed for children's units are, first of all, a trained staff, of whom at least some members should be trained nurses. Some units employ house-mothers for the most important part of the day-to-day handling and care of the children. This system has a great advantage in that small groups of children can be arranged with particular house-mothers and an attempt made to build up a kind of family relationship. Very withdrawn children get on the whole more attention and more individual care in such a unit than they do in a unit such as Ladyfield, where there is less opportunity for the nursing staff to develop the very close relationships with shy and withdrawn children.

The services of educational and clinical psychologists are essential for helping with the assessment of the children, with the problems of treatment, of education and also with research projects. Occupational therapists form part of the staff of many units and they are mainly concerned with group therapy. This forms a very important part of the general therapeutic plan. Teachers are essential since these children are all of school age. They may be employed directly by the hospital or by the local education authority. Domestic staff should be very carefully selected, and in my opinion it is an advantage for much of the domestic work to be done by trained staff. The reason for this is that children readily attach themselves to any member of the staff and often like helping to do odd jobs about the place although their capacity for sustained effort may be very limited; they like the attention of an individual they can attach themselves to.

Doctors are usually in charge of these units, and I think it advisable that these should be responsible for the general health of the children. A close link with paediatric departments is essential. Finally, the vexed question of therapists. There are rarely enough doctors to go round to cover individual therapy with children or even the detailed observation which is often necessary, and there is great shortage of trained therapists for individual work with the children. More training schemes for play therapists are an urgent need at present.

Other facilities required for a children's unit include an adequate laboratory for biochemical investigations, ready access to an EEG Department and X-ray facilities. A gymnasium and swimming bath are so helpful as to be almost essential.

4

Therapy and Ward Routine

Introductory

Therapy and ward routine will be described together, as it is difficult to discuss therapy without reference to ward routine. In an in-patient unit the staff must function together as a therapeutic community, with a closely integrated therapeutic plan for each child and with very free communication between the various people involved. The problems can be described under four main headings. Although the staff who carry out the various functions may vary from place to place, the functions must, I think, remain basically the same.

(1) *General Nursing Care.* The basis of the whole plan of treatment is the nursing care of the children. The nursing staff are responsible for the

day-to-day care of the children, getting them up, putting them to bed, clothing them, feeding them, and looking after them at all times when they are not in school or engaged in other activities with therapists. It is their job also to take over a child when he becomes too difficult and disruptive in any group situation, such as school or occupational therapy. These calls are rarely necessary, but when they are they occur at times of crisis, and the fact that a child disrupting a group can be quietly taken from the group and dealt with on his own and given all the attention he needs during the temper tantrum or other period of upset is essential for the smooth working of any group. The nursing care represents the social pressures which are brought to bear on a child, the everyday problems of bringing him up which in his home are the responsibility of his parents.

(2) *School.* Children in in-patient units are normally of school age and the structure of this unit is very much that of a boarding school; as far as possible the day is planned in accordance with a school day. Very disturbed children may be able to participate for only limited times in the organised activities, but gradually as they improve their life corresponds more and more closely to a normal day.

(3) *Group Therapy.* This is normally carried out by the occupational therapists, and forms an essential part of the investigation and treatment of each child. The groups are very small, consisting of two, three or rarely four children. In a way, these group situations represent one of the most natural activities that can be found in such a unit. A child usually works constructively with an adult, learning to share the attention of the adult, tools and activities with other children.

(4) *Individual Therapy.* Each child in the unit has an individual therapist. Where this is impossible owing to shortage of people available to give therapy, the lack of much essential information about the child's thinking and organisation of his ideas means that therapy is carried out on a much more hit-or-miss basis than should ever occur in a well-organised unit.

The particular problems of these four main influences in the children's lives will now be described in more detail.

(1) *General Nursing Care*

In Ladyfield this is performed by nursing staff who are part of the staff of Crichton Royal, but most of the staff who work in the children's unit do so on a long-term basis. There are two important considerations here: firstly the number of nurses required for a particular group of children, and secondly the type of nurse and the training they need. First of all, numbers. In the two houses at Ladyfield which have seventeen or eighteen children in each, the ideal staffing would be eleven nurses. This, with off-duty hours, allows for seven nurses on duty each day. This is not too many when it is considered that the children have to be dealt with in very small groups, and also that in a children's unit much of the domestic work will be done by the nursing staff. While it is obviously important to free nurses from all unnecessary chores, it is nevertheless true that the outsiders of the group and the most withdrawn children who tend to drift away from the group have attached themselves to nurses working around the place. If these people to whom they attach themselves are domestic staff outside the therapy situation, then nothing is known about the child's warmth, confidences and progress, and moreover there is no control over what is said to the child or the way the particular problems are handled. It is therefore essential that as far as possible all people working in the unit should be within the therapeutic situation and part of the therapeutic community.

With nine or ten nurses, which gives five or six on duty at a time, the unit can be run, but with the inevitable sicknesses and holiday periods there will be times when they are very short-handed, and since this type of work is very exacting the strain on the members of the nursing staff on duty is immediately apparent. It must be remembered that the strain is never off them. They are constantly in contact with children, and unlike therapists and teachers get relatively short breaks from the constant demands the children make on them. With eight nurses the ward is often left with only four or five staff on duty. This involves one nurse engaged mainly in administrative work, which is inevitable in coping with the many demands of feeding and clothing and looking after children; one will be working in the kitchen; and this leaves only two nurses to perform all other duties and to be with the children in groups. It can easily be seen that nurses after a day engaged in this way are extremely tired and liable to turn up for duty next day unrefreshed and inclined to be irritable. The very detailed pictures of the numbers and type of staff required is given without any apology, as there is great controversy on this point.

Secondly, composition of staff. This should be: one charge-nurse, one deputy charge-nurse, and two staff nurses, together with seven junior nurses. Ideally the charge-nurse, deputy and staff nurses should have a general and mental nursing training, but several nurses in the unit have been extremely successful who have had the mental training and not a general training. Nurses should have at least a year's experience in a residential unit before being appointed to one of the senior positions, and two years is preferable. The junior nurses should be either assistant nurses or nurses attached to the unit for special training for a period of a year or more. It is undesirable to have probationer nurses under training who come to the unit for periods of three months, as is the practice in the other departments of the hospital. It involves too many changes, which are very unsettling for the children, and the nurses themselves do not have sufficient time to gain confidence in handling the children.

With regard to the distribution of male and female nurses: both are, I think, essential. I think it is relatively unimportant whether the charge-nurse is a man or a woman. I have a slight preference for a matriarchal society in dealing with small children, but in Ladyfield and in several other units the charge-nurses are men because they tend to stay on and eventually achieve promotion. Where children over ten are accommodated, there should be four men on the staff, so that with off-duty times there is never less than one man on duty at a time, and most of the time there will be two. Ideally the remainder of the staff should be women. It is very important that both men and women should be represented among the senior nurses. The nursing staff remain the basis on which any successful therapeutic community must rest. This is equally true if the nursing staff are replaced by 'house-mothers', as in some other units. These have to perform the same functions and I think that the staff/children ratio should be similar.

Another highly controversial point is whether the shift system or a 'long day' system of working is preferable in children's units. In Ladyfield a long day is worked, and I think from the children's point of view this has many advantages. The nurses seem to accept this reasonably happily, although certainly at times the long day, especially when staff is cut by sickness or other unavoidable difficulties, can be very long indeed. I think the disadvantage of the shift system is that a child becomes involved with one lot of people, and particularly that if any severe difficulties arise they cannot be resolved before the end of the day. The hours between bedtimes represent very definite units to children, and it is very important that if a child has intense arguments or quarrels with members of the staff these should be resolved by the time he goes to bed. This often happens, and it is in the heat of emotional disturbances that the really strong relationships with the staff are forged. Many a child has been seen calling a nurse every imaginable name that he has heard, and even being violently aggressive, only to seek out that same nurse to demand a cuddle and bid a very affectionate farewell to him when he goes off duty. There is a danger that if a child falls out with one group of people, largely owing to his own restlessness and irritability, when they go off duty to be replaced by another group for the second half of the day one group will become the good ones and the other the bad ones, and the difficulties will never be properly resolved. The same criticism might be applied to changes-over between the day and night staff, but on the whole this is not found to be such a problem. The day staff are responsible for putting the children to bed at night or at least getting them ready for bed; and it is this time, traditionally a family affair where close relationships are developed, and where the care of the children is exercised in bathing them and dressing them, telling them stories and getting them ready for bed, which is an ideal situation in which tensions can be released and the children go to bed feeling the security and goodwill of the people who are looking after them, which is so essential a part of their treatment.

As for the all-important problem of the actual handling of the children by the nursing staff, I think it difficult to lay down a set of rules; but certain principles can be recognised, and the nursing staff are trained to under-

be illustrated by an example which occurred a little time ago in the unit. This illustrates the day-to-day work of the nurses—not that disturbances as severe as this one are at all common; they do occur, and the principles which are used in dealing with such a problem are applicable to all kinds of disturbances which may upset the smooth working of the groups.

The particular example concerns a boy of eleven who was tough, of superior intelligence, was epileptic and had been excluded from a series of schools throughout his time; finally he had the distinction of being expelled from a school for maladjusted children. He arrived at Ladyfield suspicious, wary and extremely anxious. No place had yet been able to contain him, and it was obvious to him that whenever he left a place it was with enormous relief on the part of a number of people whose hostility he had incurred. For the first two days he fitted in quite well with ward routine, and caused no particular difficulty in discipline or in any other way. At the end of this time his observations told him that the routine seemed to be fairly easy-going, that the relations between the adults and the children were very friendly, and he saw no reason why he should not be able to dominate the situation here as he had done elsewhere. In any case he had, it appeared, a compelling urge to try.

He chose as his first battle-ground tea-time. There was a shortage of staff and the disturbance he was creating would have the largest audience. He began shouting, swearing, became extremely defiant and started throwing food and cutlery about. As usual, when a child is disrupting a group, he is removed from the group. Usually just taking him outside the dining room, waiting till he quietens down and then saying to him, 'All right, if you're feeling better now, you can go back and finish your tea' is quite sufficient. But in this case the shouting and swearing continued and the boy was removed to one of the bedrooms by the charge-nurse. He became extremely frightened and very aggressive, rushing round the room, disturbing the beds, abusing and attacking the nurse. The nurse confined himself to saying quietly to the boy that he would have to stay with him in the room until he settled down, and to preventing him from hurting himself, from hurting the nurse and from doing any actual damage to the room. This extremely aggressive behaviour continued for almost three-quarters of an hour, and all the time the nurse continued to talk quietly to him and to use the minimum of gentle restraint to prevent any damage.

By the end of this time both he and the nurse were rather weary, and each sat down on a disordered bed to talk things over. The boy looked at the nurse thoughtfully and said, 'Well, you're the first man who's managed to control me.' The nurse, who is skilled at putting things in a realistic way to the children at appropriate times, suggested to him that in fact he probably felt safer with grown-ups who could control him; he was not very old and not yet capable of running all his own affairs, and people who could not control him were not much good to him as they would be unable to help him, protect him or look after him as a boy of his age should be looked after. The boy thought this over and agreed that this was so. The conversation continued in this friendly way for a short time and then the boy said, 'I don't suppose you get many as bad as me.' The nurse said reassuringly, 'Well, that was quite an upset, but this is frequent with children when they first come here. They are frightened; all sorts of unpleasant things have happened to them and they wonder what will be the result of defying authority. When they find that we can deal with it and that nothing very dreadful happens to them, they settle down quickly and feel much happier.' The boy said, 'Do you mean to say that was not very bad?' The nurse said, 'Well, it was quite an upset, but not very extraordinary.' The boy said angrily, 'Huh! You haven't seen anything yet', and away he went with a temper tantrum which lasted another half-hour.

At the end of this time he found that he was still getting nowhere. There are no sanctions imposed for this extremely disturbed behaviour in the early stages, which is a mixture of extreme fear and violent aggression. When he had settled down, he washed his hands again, combed his hair and went back down to tea, which had been saved for him. After this, he had a few more mild temper tantrums and remained very demanding of staff attention, but after quite a short time he settled well to the ward routine, made friends with the other children, and after a few months had learned to accept the ordinary frustrations and the ordinary discipline which could be expected from a child of his age. Many children have episodes like this, not quite so violent in most cases, during which they defy the authority of the staff, but they soon settle down with similar skilful handling.

In dealing with very withdrawn children, the method is very different from that described above, but not altogether. In these cases the problem is not to control the child in this way but gradually to gain his confidence, and without pushing him too far at any stage to encourage him to take part in the activities of the other children, and above all to seek the help of the staff whenever he is in trouble. Such children when they begin to gain confidence often go through a mild or even fairly severe aggressive stage, but when they have learned to control their aggression, of which they are very frightened, both in themselves and other people, they settle down well and are able to lead a much more normal and active life.

One boy, who was so withdrawn and with behaviour so bizarre and manner-istic that he was off school for a year before admission with a diagnosis of possible psychosis, was obviously terrified of other children. He was observed frequently at the end of the garden engaged in violent fights against phantom opponents. He was induced to take it out of pillows and even large sheets of paper represent-ing his chief tormentors among the children, which he did with startling violence. The next step was quite violent attacks on members of the male staff whom he really trusted. The next step is holding his own with the other children. There is no danger of this child turning into a bully, but if he can gain enough confidence to establish normal relationships with adults, and to hold his own with other children, a whole new life opens up for him. The importance of this process can-not be overestimated.

Various drugs have been tried out at different times to try to help children get over these difficult phases more quickly and more smoothly, but the results of such treatment have so far been very disappointing. Chlorpromazine has a certain use in the treatment of these children, but only to tide them over crises when they are so restless and so disturbed they can accept no authority whatever and are liable to run away, possibly taking other children with them. Two or three children are far more likely to indulge in wild or destructive anti-social behaviour than any one child on his own, and careful watch has to be kept on any groups which may be formed during a very disturbed phase of a particular child. Chlorpromazine given in sufficiently large doses, sometimes up to 75 mg. three times a day, will definitely slow down the children and inhibit their motor activity, but in my experience it very rarely makes them more accessible and it is not a short cut to getting closer to them or gaining their confidence; it is only useful when a child is so disturbed that he cannot accept even the least frustration and is liable to run off or indulge in some wild or destructive activity at any moment. Librium and other tranquillisers have also been tried, but with even less effect than Chlorpromazine.

It would be very helpful indeed if some tranquilliser could be found which would both settle the children down and make them more accessible to the influence of adults. Barbiturates have even less use in the treatment of such children. On one or two occasions I have given them in fairly large doses, and this has produced a state of confusion with violent abreactions which I have occasionally thought useful, but these abreactions are even more difficult to control than the disturbed behaviour of the children normally is. The staff find them more disquieting and they feel that they are even less able to get close to the children and give them the reassurance they need. Barbiturates, of course, have their use in cases of cerebral dysrhythmia of an epileptic kind, but in other children they tend to produce a great deal of fast activity in the EEG and an irritable rather than a settled state in the child.

A great deal of space has been occupied in describing the handling of children by the nursing staff, but the reason is that this is the particularly difficult part of in-patient treatment, i.e. the day-to-day handling of the children. Both group therapy and individual therapy and also the work with the parents present their own special problems, but in general the lines follow much more closely those familiar to all who treat children in an out-patient setting. The work of day-to-day handling of the children is unique; it presents the greatest problem and is also the most difficult from the point of view of training of staff. Much of the training of new members of staff must be done by precept and example, and a skilled charge-nurse or senior nurse will help the other nurses to cope with the difficult behaviour of the children by quietly and unobtrusively taking over when the child is becoming too much for a junior nurse, but allowing them to carry on when they have gained confidence themselves. There is no short cut to gaining confidence by the nursing staff, and we find that it takes about a year before a nurse is fully competent to deal with all situations. For this reason it is extremely important that as few changes as possible should take place in the nursing staff, and particularly that the night nurses should be drawn from the regular staff of the unit as their turn comes round. We had a very striking example of that recently when one of the regular staff had to be off duty unexpectedly and a nurse entirely new to the unit took over. Although he did his best, a state of chaos resulted, which is never seen when the regular staff are on duty.

Another very important aspect of the nurses' training is training in accurate observation and reporting. So much of childhood disorder is, in the present state of our knowledge, described in terms of 'overt behaviour' that all nurses must know how to describe and report accurately the behaviour of the children. This is equally important for junior nurses, as with them often the most difficult behaviour of the children is seen. Children will try things on with a less experienced nurse which they would not attempt with senior nurses. It is also very important that the nurses should be able to describe accurately such specific phenomena as epileptic fits in all their various manifestations. An exact record of the time and an exact description of the course and progress of the fits enables anticonvulsant therapy to be given in an in-patient unit with great accuracy, and in fact when the children are under constant observation in this way much more accurate control can be achieved than is possible in an ordinary hospital ward.

In some units the duties described as being carried out here by the nursing staff are performed by house-mothers, who have each a small group of children whom they look after, with whom they have meals and whom they get up in the morning and put to bed at night. There are advantages and disadvantages in each way of working. There is certainly a place for a psychiatric in-patient unit attached to a hospital where the care of the children is in the hands of trained nursing staff. Such a unit can undertake the investigation and treatment of all kinds of problems such as children with epilepsy, children with organic brain damage, and various psycho-somatic complaints which would worry and be beyond the skills of lay house-mothers. On the other hand, with certain types of children, particularly perhaps a group of autistic and psychotic children, the system of house-mothers, in which each child becomes attached to one or two particular people, has I think very distinct advantages. One thing is certain, whichever way the staff of a children's unit is recruited and trained: they need a great deal of support during the whole of the time they are working with the children, and direct contact and frequent consultation with the physician responsible for integrating the whole plan of treatment for the children. Without this, and without very free and frequent communication with other members of the staff, teachers, occupational therapists and the people doing individual therapy, no co-ordinated plan is possible and treatment becomes a very haphazard business dependent entirely on the whims of a number of individuals. This may sound too obvious to be stated, but in fact the difficulty in communication at all levels in such a unit and the appreciation of their particular roles by different members of the staff presents one of the greatest problems which has to be faced. On the successful outcome of this depends in large measure both the success of treatment and the morale of those concerned with it.

All these observations produce a vast amount of data—valuable, but in it it is not always easy to see the wood for the trees. In order to bring it into some kind of order and to see the trends of development, often only clear in retrospect, summaries of the daily and weekly notes are made at the end of each school term. These are read out at a staff meeting, recorded on tape, and typed copies included in the case records. The nurses' notes are included in their own section, along with those of the doctors, occupational therapists, psychologists, psychiatric social workers and teachers.

(2) *School*

School plays a very important part in the lives of all children up to the age of fifteen, and as far as possible, even with very disturbed children, their day is organised in terms of an ordinary school day. Teachers in this unit are appointed by the local education authority, from whom we have always had the greatest co-operation, and are paid by this authority. The equipment and desks are also provided by the local education authority. The actual classrooms are within the building in which the children live. Teachers work normal school hours and have the same holidays as teachers in the local schools. During the holidays most of the children go home, and as far as possible they go for the full school holiday.

With very disturbed children, teaching has to be organised in very small groups. On the whole five or six is as large a group as is convenient to take, although for certain school activities, such as watching films or film strips and certain other classes, two or three groups may be joined together; it is useful for the children to feel that they are doing some things in a large group. The problems of schooling are considerable; it is rather like a very small village school, with age-ranges in one house from five to twelve, in the other from eight to twelve, but with the children almost all with some degree of retardation and with IQs varying from seventy to one hundred and forty or more. A number of the children have been excluded from school for difficult behaviour before they arrive. In spite of this, school is generally very well accepted by the children. The general plan is that children are taken in these groups in the morning and then individually or in twos or threes in the afternoon, when most of the important new steps in learning are undertaken. At first, many of the children have to get used to the idea of being at school again after a period of absence. This is usually accomplished fairly quickly. As far as possible the more hectic disturbances are kept outside the school situation, and, as always in this plan of treatment, if a child is disrupting the group severely he is removed, the nurse taking over. Children on the whole do not like being away from their group, and except in times of very great anxiety dodging school is surprisingly rare. The teachers take a part in all the staff meetings and have to know the stages through which each individual child is going. In the early stages when a child is very anxious, no pressure is put on him in school, but later on when he is settled and secure, but considerably behind in some subjects, the teacher may well say to him, 'You are now almost ready to go home, but you will find it difficult when you get to your ordinary school if you cannot do a little better than this. We can give you a good deal more individual attention than you will get in your ordinary school, and it is your difficulties here which are now holding you up and stopping you from going home.' Children respond to this very well when they are settled, but it is useless to expect much in the way of concentration or sustained effort from a child who is only just learning to cope with his aggression and who is still extremely anxious about his home situation. There is a tendency sometimes for teachers to become very interested in the problems of therapy and to carry these into the school situation. In a unit like this every situation is in a sense a therapeutic situation, but as far as school is concerned the nearer it gets to ordinary schooling and the more regular are the hours which the children keep, the better progress they make. They get satisfaction from the constructive activities in school, and school is, after all, one of the closest links for them with everyday life as they have known it. The special problems of teaching autistic children, some of whom have only just begun the difficult business of communication, cannot be dealt with here, but as far as the general organisation of school is concerned, these children have their own groups and their own school times which they can look forward to.

(3) Group Therapy

Group therapy in this unit is carried out by the occupational therapists, of whom at present there are two on the staff. It is the aim in treatment to provide all children with group therapy as part of their régime. The groups are very small, usually two children, sometimes three and occasionally four. On the whole, the work the children do is constructive. A limited amount of actual craft work is undertaken since the children have very limited powers of concentration and application, although their ability may be quite good; but as they become more settled during their stay in the unit they may do quite good work, such as making baskets or other long-term projects, occupying several sessions. In the early stages they usually wish to make toys, swords, guns, holsters etc., and they are usually willing to undertake only those tasks which can be finished at the end of the session, three-quarters of an hour to an hour, so that they can take what they have made away with them. These sessions provide one of the most natural and relaxed settings for work with the children in the unit, one adult working with two or three children; they do things which they enjoy doing and they learn to share tools with each other, to share the attention of the adult and to co-operate in their various activities. Occasionally, when children are going through a very disturbed phase, little or no constructive work may be done, and these sessions may involve messy play with water, sand or clay, but these phases usually last for a short time only and then constructive work is resumed.

In these group sessions, more relaxed and intimate than school, where some pressure however slight to get on with some work is always present, and should be, important scraps of information are often gleaned. One boy, whose mother was separated from her husband and was unable to control the boy, had been ejected in quick succession from no less than seven children's homes and other institutions before coming to Ladyfield. Just before one holiday he demanded to be taken for a walk in his occupational therapy session to collect 'conkers'—otherwise 'You'll have me in Borstal.' He explained that if he had conkers he would be able to keep his friend and his brother amused, instead of going off on wild expeditions. He came back from the holiday triumphant, saying to his therapist, 'I never hit my mother. I lit no fires. And I never stole.' At this time in his individual therapy he was going through a regressive phase, even enjoying a feeding bottle, and was not talking about home.

In other cases particular groupings can be very helpful. One boy, of superior intelligence but completely lacking in confidence, worked with an older boy, very stable, in for treatment of *petit mal*. The younger boy's confidence improved, and he produced the best work of any kind he had done in the unit.

Two other boys, one the ugly duckling of the family, went through a very hectic phase, one going so far as to urinate in the corner before settling down to work well. At this time the second boy, though not so disturbed, was quite unable to work in school, but his work in his occupational therapy sessions was of such a standard that it astonished his parents, and was one of the things that caused them to begin to think better of him.

It is interesting to note that some children, though they may be very disturbed in their play with the main group of children and unable to settle at school, yet in the sheltered group situation may for the first time show concentration, ability to co-operate and work with others, and a fair degree of constructive activity. On the other hand—and this applies especially to rather shy children—in this protected group session they may for the first time begin to show some aggression or defiance, and they may gain confidence to test out grown-ups or other children in a way which they would find quite impossible to do in the larger groups. It is only when all these various activities can be observed at the same time, that is, their reaction to the group as a whole, school, group therapy and individual therapy, that the particular contrapuntal development of the child's different relationships with people can be observed. In some cases occupational therapy can be used specifically for observation on a particular child, for example to test the concentration of a child who is suffering, or suspected to be suffering, from *petit mal* attacks. In other cases, where children with minimal degrees of brain damage are being treated, both their motor skills can be tested and they can be given help in developing them. Group therapy should, I think, never be used as a substitute for any of the other methods of treatment of a child, but in my opinion it plays a vital part in the treatment of all children.

There are other forms of group therapy which can be used for children, such as discussion groups, and these can be of great value. In this unit such discussions usually take place informally with the nursing staff and in school, but I think there is a real place for more formal groups of this kind in the treatment of children, although in the age group with which we normally work, i.e. children of primary school age, it has a more limited application than with adolescents.

(4) *Individual Therapy*

The problem of individual therapy is one of the most controversial in any discussion of the treatment of children, whether in a residential or an out-patient setting. My own view is that without individual therapy the treatment of the child is very much on a 'hit-or-miss' basis. I think that the aim of individual therapy is above all to attempt to make sense of the world to the child. A setting in which a child has a grown-up to himself, whom he sees at regular intervals which he can depend on, who is not responsible for the ordinary everyday discipline, for putting him to bed, making him do things etc. or for applying any of the sanctions which necessarily follow his less acceptable behaviour, forms an ideal situation in which the child's confidence can be gained. During the first few sessions the therapist plays a very passive role, finding out the child's interests, which may be settling down to talk or more often playing with the sand tray or painting, either of which may form a useful means of communication. The therapist who listens patiently soon begins to see the world through the child's eyes, and at first it is wise to make very few comments. Any child in residential care lives in three worlds: the world of his immediate environment, in this case Ladyfield; the world of fantasy, often terrifying, but offering compensations by providing situations which can be manipulated, and where the child can give expression to his wishes for omnipotence; and the world of home.

A great deal of information can be gained about the child's view of Ladyfield from his talk and from his play, and this can be checked against the information which is constantly available from members of the nursing staff, teachers and group therapists, so that the discrepancy between the child's view of reality and reality as seen by other people is readily appreciated. It is this aspect which is, I think, absolutely essential in the diagnostic assessment of the child and without which treatment can only be guesswork. Otherwise you would depend entirely on observations of his behaviour, and important though this is, you have only to read any psychological or psychopathological work on children to see how many different interpretations can be placed on any one particular aspect of the behaviour of a child. Few people would attempt to make a diagnostic assessment of an adult patient without a very careful examination of his mental state and of his thinking processes, and the same is true of children. Without these individual interviews, I think it is impossible to obtain this information. Psychological tests and projective tests of various kinds may help, but cannot, I think, take the place of regular individual interviews carried on over months during the course of a child's treatment.

An example of the course of the early stages of therapy is that of a boy from a problem family, excluded from school. The first goal in individual therapy, both from the diagnostic and the therapeutic angle, is to gain the child's confidence. Children usually come readily to interviews, and it is not difficult to keep their interest, so that the therapist can at first adopt a very passive role. The importance of this was illustrated by this boy, whose first few interviews were entirely silent, though his play with the toys was varied and highly imaginative. After a few sessions he began to talk; every other word was a swearword—f . . . ing this, etc. The therapist made no comment for a few more sessions, and then suggested mildly that this was not a very nice word. The boy asked, 'What would you suggest instead?' She suggested 'flipping' as being a little more acceptable. He thought this over, then said, 'F . . . ing square word, isn't it.' But from this time on he continued to talk freely, but he rarely swore. He described his father coming home drunk, a very different picture from the idealised pattern of family life represented in his earlier play. The points illustrated by this are numerous and clear. All that needs emphasising is that I know no short cut to the goals so far achieved, nor to the further goals to which they lead.

The second important world of a child's thoughts is the world of fantasy, often far more terrifying than reality is or is ever likely to be. This is readily seen even in the very early stages of the children, when they hear perhaps of the illness of one of their parents. Even if reassured that mother or father has only a slight cold, they will often tell other children or their therapist that they are afraid their parent is dead. This sort of remark is of course open to various forms of interpretation, but the observed behaviour of the child confirms that these ideas are accompanied by a great deal of anxiety. The world of fantasy is often explored along with the slow process of getting to know the child's view of the world and his immediate environment, and it is often very difficult to sort out fantasy from reality as it appears to the child; but when the child's confidence has been gained, first of all he can be helped to understand much more clearly the reality of Ladyfield and his various relationships with people there, and secondly many of his fears in fantasy can be helped by reassurance and by their being brought into relation to reality by someone whom the child has learned to trust.

An example of a very persistent type of fantasy, which appeared only in therapy sessions, was shown by a boy of superior intelligence who had been excluded from two schools for aggressive behaviour before he came to the unit. His play in the sand-tray always started, 'It was a dark and stormy night.' He once turned to his surprised therapist and remarked, 'You may wonder why the stories always start, "It was a dark and stormy night." Well, that was how it was.' There followed scenes of violence, anti-aircraft guns, bandits (he was always one) against the police, and so on. His family had lived in one room during the first five years of his life, and during this time his mother, terrified of childbirth, had had a baby. His father was a quiet intelligent man. There are, of course, many different ways of interpreting this material. What was certain was that the child's extreme tension and anxiety were centred in the home (he regressed markedly after his first few holidays, even to smearing of faeces), and that there were no obvious stresses operating currently there sufficient to cause anything like this degree of tension.

The third important world of the child is the world of home. Here the child may at once talk freely about his life at home, but much more often this comes only after quite a long period of time. Here again the child's known reactions to frustration and other stress situations in Ladyfield can be used to discuss with him his difficulties at home with parents, siblings and other people, and by gaining insight into his own and other people's reactions he can be helped to deal with them more appropriately. It is remarkable how quite young children can appreciate grown-ups' difficulties with extraordinary insight, and sometimes the child is ready to make allowances for the grown-ups and to tolerate their difficulties more readily than the grown-up is willing to make adjustments and tolerate the child's problems.

The following is an example of the kind of information about the home which can in most cases only be obtained by someone who is alone with the child and who has his complete confidence:

A child, son of professional people, whose parents both died during his stay in the unit, was admitted with a diagnosis of psychosis. His speech was odd and babyish. He had all kinds of bizarre manneristic movements, and showed the rigid behaviour patterns associated with psychotic children. In his therapy sessions at first he was very distractable; later he played games such as 'shops', and then went through a phase during which he attacked the therapist, using physical violence viciously and all the time upbraiding her in the tones of an exasperated old woman bitterly taking it out of a child whose oddities are beyond her comprehension. So bitter was this attack that the therapist, although she was a girl of quite outstanding skill and with good experience, found it very hard to cope with, but it gave a startling insight into the treatment the child had had from his grandmother, about which we had had no previous hints. Later this same child, when he was anxious about the holidays and wondering where he would stay, would draw up a chair and sit down to discuss his problems with his therapist. He never unburdened himself so freely outside the therapy situation, and in no other situation did he appear so obviously aware of his problems, or so coherent about them. The very important information about the child's attitude to home and his anxieties was not obtainable in any other way, and the terrifying episodes about the grandmother were unknown to anyone but the child, the grandmother being then dead. The child's communication, except with someone he knew very well indeed, was fragmentary and often bizarre.

This principle of making sense of the world to the child applies equally strongly if the discussions involve helping the child to understand why he has come to the unit, what people there are trying to do to help him, and what is likely to happen to him when he returns again to the outside world. For example some children from broken homes suffer a series of rejections very hard to accept. One boy, whose mother had deserted the family, was for a time well treated by his stepfather. He then refused to have any more to do with the boy (he had met another woman). After a further stay in Ladyfield fostering was tried, with careful preparations. All went well for five months; then the foster-parents, who had seemed stable and warm, threw him out on his birthday. The boy's main support throughout this came from Ladyfield, and later also from his children's officer and the house-mother and house-father of a children's home. Throughout the time, through the good contact made with him initially, it was possible to talk to him about these and other changes in his life and to help him to accept them. Without this support over many years it is certain he would have developed an entirely anti-social attitude, trusting no one, the attitude reinforced by many clashes with the law.

The therapy may take a different line and involve discussion of his psycho-sexual development in Freudian terms or in those of any other psychological theory to which the therapist is himself an adherent. The course of the therapy and the form it takes will depend mainly, of course, on what are thought to be the child's needs, and also on the experience and inclinations of the individual therapist. All therapy is under the immediate direction of the physician in charge, and very regular sessions with the therapist are held, whenever possible at least once a week, so that the interviews, normally three a week, are discussed and the programme for the next sessions formulated. This is very time-consuming, but it is essential if therapy for all the children is to be undertaken. Therapy is not confined to the doctors but is also undertaken here by psychologists and by the occupational therapists. As their experience to begin with is often very limited (and this applies to the doctors as well as to other members of the staff), this very close supervision of therapy is essential. This insistence on individual therapy by such relatively inexperienced therapists may be criticised on many grounds, but I think it works well in practice, and certainly as a matter of practical politics there is no alternative if the diagnostic and therapeutic needs of the children are to be met.

The problem of the therapy of psychotic children is too complex and specialised to be dealt with here. My own view is that individual therapy forms an essential part of the treatment of all such children. It is often very difficult to see exactly what is happening at any particular time, and observation of sessions, through a one-way screen by the doctor supervising the therapy and cinematograph recordings of the child's behaviour and progress, are of great value.

Another form of therapy which offers great possibilities for the future is behaviour therapy (4). Conditioning techniques have long been used with success for treating enuresis, and more recently success has been reported with cases of encopresis. The treatment of such symptoms, where the results can clearly be seen (and smelt), is less difficult than the treatment of less well defined anxieties of children. It is claimed that with adults most neuroses can be reduced by careful anamnesis to a specific phobia, and a hierarchy of tension-provoking situations can be constructed to form the basis for the deconditioning process. This is obviously much more difficult with children, and in any case all too often they are reacting, not by inappropriate responses to stress, but by real anxiety to real stress with which they cannot cope. Nevertheless learning processes form such a large part of the life of a child that the scientific investigation of such processes offers great opportunities for an increase in our knowledge of child development and of the development of neurotic illnesses, even though for the time being we still have to rely on our patiently-acquired empirical skills for much of the treatment of disturbed children. I think there will always be a need for such skills, though advances in understanding may put them on a more scientific basis. Clearly in-patient units should be used for such research projects, and this may well come to be one of their most important functions.

5

Work with Families

During a child's stay in Ladyfield, intensive casework is undertaken with the family. There are no fixed visiting hours and children can see their parents at any time. Normally of course parents visit during the week-ends, and wherever possible if a child's home is near the hospital he goes home and spends each week-end with the family. Psychiatric social workers deal with the family problems and see the families wherever possible, either when they come to fetch the child or when they visit him or when they bring him back. As far as possible the children have full school holidays at home. In the early stages when the children are very disturbed, or the family are not yet ready to cope with them, the holiday may be cut down to a week or even to a long week-end, but these periods are extended gradually until the child can cope with the full holiday at home. When I first started to work in the unit I considered these long holiday periods were a waste of therapeutic time, but I am quite certain that this is not so, and in fact the children make very much better real progress where there is the closest possible interaction with the family during their stay in the unit. In spite of the obvious problems, it should never be too difficult to settle even very disturbed children in a unit where everything is run for the children and where a large and skilled staff are available. This is, of course, an over-simplification; but it is true that a child may become very well adjusted in this protected environment and yet make no further progress in coping with the outside world unless very close contact with the outside world is maintained.

In some cases the families do not visit regularly; when they live distances of up to two hundred miles away this is of course extremely difficult. Wherever possible the children are visited weekly by their parents. Fortnightly visits form a very fair working basis for treatment, but occasionally visits as infrequent as monthly have to be accepted. In some cases the parents do not visit, and one of the most difficult experiences the children have to cope with is parents who constantly promise and then let them down, sometimes without even letting them know that they are not coming. There are few experiences more distressing for the children than when they get ready for the visit and then are disappointed for no apparent reason. In all cases, wherever possible, visits to the home are made by the staff at some stage during the treatment, and in some cases when the parents are uncooperative many such visits have to be made.

There are a number of special problems which arise in the handling of family relationships when a child has come to a residential unit. At first the parents, often near the end of their tether, are very relieved that some-one can take over and cope with the problem and accept both the child and them. Later, as the child begins to improve, the unit and the people working in it become a threat to their security. They feel that the obvious improvement the child has made in other people's care reflects very much on their own handling. The child's improvement is felt as an indictment of themselves. This stage is accompanied by great anxiety on the part of the parents, and often by threats to take the child away from the unit. Parents need a great deal of reassurance at this stage; they need to feel that all people with whom they come in contact are trying to help them with this problem and are sympathetic about their own difficulties. It is always a good idea when dealing with parents to tell them a great deal of what goes on, and it is often very reassuring to parents to hear that we have found a child difficult, and to have us, without over-emphasising the difficulties, making quite clear that we share the parents' own problems.

Some children come to the unit while in the care of children's departments. In some cases they are living with relatives, foster-parents or even with their own families, but some come from children's homes or other institutions. In these cases we make the same demands on the children's officer as we do on the parent. Actually it is extremely difficult for children's officers to visit as often as do parents, but it is of the greatest importance that when such children come to a unit of this kind they should receive a great deal of support from the people looking after them. Normally they go home to their foster-parents or to the institution they come from for holidays, just as do the other children. We encourage all the people who have been looking after them to write them letters and postcards and send them parcels, and we try to persuade them to visit as often as possible. However much children may appear to be settled in an institution, and however little they ask about their own families, as soon as they come in contact with a group of other children whose parents visit regularly and take them out they at once demand the same things for themselves, and it is extremely important that they should not feel different from the other children, or at least that the difference should be minimised as far as possible. Most children's departments are very understanding and co-operative with this work, but in some cases there is a tendency to feel that once the child has been placed in a suitable treatment centre their responsibility ends; it is sometimes a difficult task to disillusion them.

These children, especially those from institutions, are some of the ones who particularly need help in explaining their situation to them. This is best done in their individual therapy sessions, although other members of the staff must be kept informed of the way things have been explained to the child, so that when he asks them they can say the same things. Children need very constant reassurance, especially when there has been a good deal of insecurity and change in their lives; therapists must be prepared to go over the same ground time and time again with deprived children before they really can accept reassurance. It is also of the utmost importance that any arrangements made for them should be carefully thought out and that the child should never be let down. We attach such importance to the communication with the outside world, both with children in care and those within their own families, that an exact record of the number of letters and parcels, as well as of the number of visits the child has had, is kept in each case.

There are many other aspects of social work done by the psychiatric social workers which could be discussed, but only those particular points in which residential care presents special problems have been touched upon. In all instances, the whole family wherever possible, or in the case of children in care as many of the people involved with the child as can manage it, are brought into the situation and encouraged to visit the child in Ladyfield. Visits are encouraged not only from fathers and mothers but also from siblings and friends and relatives. In some cases it is necessary to do a good deal of intensive work with, say, grandparents in order that a settled plan of campaign may be agreed upon in the family, particularly when a child has become expert at playing off one grown-up against another. With the very disturbed children admitted to an in-patient unit, intensive work has to be done with the child himself in the various fields already described, but in the great majority of cases this goes for nothing if a very real modification has not been possible in the environment and in the attitude to the child of people looking after him. The work with the families may be said to represent at least half the battle.

6

Conclusion

So far the description of children's residential psychiatric units has been in terms of children of primary school age, and it is true that the majority of psychiatric in-patient units at present cater for this age group. The problems of adolescents are no less important, but the provision of psychiatric in-patient units for this group is even more inadequate than that for younger children. The Mental Health Sub-Committee in Scotland in a recent report (*Medical Services for Child Guidance*, 1962) has recommended that there should be no split in medical care at the age of twelve. With this I would certainly agree, but at present such few adolescent units as exist are not usually in the same hospital as children's units. The needs of adolescents are very similar. They require school, and here the problem providing secondary education with all the additional equipment and wider range of subjects presents a much greater problem and is considerably more expensive than for primary school children, especially for the small numbers which would be present in each unit. Group therapy and individual therapy are equally important, and the handling of adolescents requires at least as much skill and understanding as that of younger children. Acting-out is often even more difficult to cope with, and the methods used by adolescents in showing their disapproval of society are often more enterprising and more difficult to cope with than those of the younger children. The same high standard of care is required; real therapeutic communities must be established, with all members of the staff working closely together, understanding what each one is doing and what their own role in the therapy of the child must be. Warren (10), in a recent follow-up at Bethlem Hospital, has shown clearly the close link between child psychiatry and adult psychiatry, indicating that many problems presenting as behaviour disorder in adolescents all too often progress to crippling psychiatric illness in early adult life.

There is great need for integration of in-patient units with other services for children. Some children and adolescents are ready after treatment to return home and to attend their ordinary schools. Others require residential schooling in schools for maladjusted children. It would certainly be a great advantage if such schools were situated within reasonable distance of children's units, so that a close link between the staff of the children's unit and the residential school to which the children progressed could be maintained, and if necessary a further spell of treatment in the children's unit be undertaken should this become necessary. There should also be close links with children's homes, reception centres and approved schools. At present criteria for assessment of disturbed children are extremely arbitrary, and the long waiting lists for children's units also makes selection procedures arbitrary. If our knowledge of the problems of disturbed children is to extend, it is necessary that a survey of the whole range of children's problems be made. Whether they are taken into care by children's committees, sent to residential schools, psychiatric units or approved schools, their assessment should be undertaken by people using the same criteria. This should be linked with a very careful long-term follow-up to determine both the immediate effects of various methods of dealing with the children and also the long-term effects. This could very well be undertaken in a country such as Scotland, where there is a small population; a legal system of its own—and services which are at present totally inadequate to deal with the problems presented. If such a comprehensive survey is not made in the near future, there is danger that the development of services for children will continue to be inadequate to meet their needs, and even that the wrong type of services will be developed to the neglect of some more essential needs.

The other age group which has not so far been dealt with is the preschool child. Here the problem of residential treatment is very much more difficult; indeed in many cases it is undesirable to remove the child from the care of his parent. There is a strong case here for establishing units to which the mother and child can be admitted. Attention is being focused more and more on this age group, in which the seeds of many of the more severe disturbances of later life probably develop.

A recent development in children's services is that of day hospital facilities. These are developed in some cases, as in Newcastle, in connection with an out-patient unit, but some in-patient units take a small number of children as day patients. There is a very strong case for the extension of day hospitals for children, particularly in large population areas. In Ladyfield there are, at present, eight day patients attending regularly. They come on each of the normal school days and take part in all the activities of the children, including school, returning home in the evening. This is a particularly promising experiment in the treatment of cases such as school phobia, and a number of other problems have been treated successfully in this way. It is too early yet to assess fully the results of this treatment, but at present it seems to be a very promising adjunct and in some cases a very useful substitute for residential treatment.

Wherever children are taken from their home and treated in a residential unit of any kind, very careful follow-up studies should be undertaken. As the numbers of such children in any one unit are small, there is a very strong case for a much closer liaison between the different units so that similar problems and results of different forms of treatment of these problems can be studied. Until this is done, much of the work which is undertaken must be empirical, the selection of cases for treatment remain arbitrary and the prognosis and ultimate fate of the children a matter of guesswork.

REFERENCES

1. CONNELL, P., 1961. The day hospital approach in child psychiatry. *J. Ment. Sci.*, **107**: 969.
2. CREAK, M., 1938. Psychoses in children. *Proc. Roy. Soc. Med.*, **31**: 519.
3. —— 1951. Psychoses in childhood. *J. Ment. Sci.*, **97**: 545.
4. EYSENCK, H. J. and RACHMAN, S., 1964. The application of learning theory to child psychiatry. In *Modern Perspectives in Child Psychiatry* (ed. J. G. Howells). Edinburgh: Oliver & Boyd.
5. HELLMAN, I., 1960. *Research in a Child Guidance Clinic*. Paper presented at the W.H.O. Seminar in Child Guidance, Brussels.
6. HOWELLS, J. G., 1963a. *Family Psychiatry*. Edinburgh: Oliver & Boyd.
7. —— 1963b. Child-parent separation as a therapeutic procedure. *Amer. J. Psychiat.*, **119**: 922.
8. Royal Medico-Psychological Association, 1956. *In-patient Accommodation for Child and Adolescent Psychiatric Patients*.
9. —— 1960. *Units for the Long-term Medical Care of Emotionally Disturbed Children and Adolescents*.
10. WARREN and STEIN. Unpublished paper.

XXIV

THE CONTRIBUTION OF PSYCHOLOGICAL TESTS TO CHILD PSYCHIATRY

JOHN R. LICKORISH

B.A.

Senior Clinical Psychologist, Department of Family Psychiatry, Ipswich and East Suffolk Hospital

1

Introduction

Aim of the Chapter

This chapter describes the contribution of diagnostic psychological testing to clinical practice in Child Psychiatry. It is not a survey of all the psychodiagnostic procedures in current use; still less is it a disguised manual of instruction in the use of psychological tests. It describes the broad features of the most useful tests currently available, and indicates how they assist in the investigation of psychiatric disorders in children. The limitations of the tests are indicated and emphasis is laid upon the value of using a battery of tests whenever possible. The results of the tests should be evaluated not only in the light of each other but also in the light of all the available information about the particular case.

It is quite fallacious to suppose that a test is valueless because it does not provide 'objective' information with a high degree of statistical reliability. Many tests of low reliability are clinically valuable, because they enable the psychologist to gain information by structuring an interview, especially when working with young children.

This discussion assumes that the tests will be administered by a fully trained psychologist, who will decide what tests to employ when consulted about a particular problem. It is also assumed that the results of the tests administered will be discussed by those handling the case, so that the results may be integrated into the general diagnostic appraisal of the situation. The broad principles outlined in this chapter provide a background against which the detailed discussion and interpretation of individual test results may take place.

Psychological Measurement

Psychological tests are frequently said to 'measure' various aspects of personality and to give 'objective' assessments of personal traits. Some psychologists lay great emphasis upon the need for 'objective measures' of personality, and much research has been devoted to the compilation and testing of objective measures. The results of this quest for 'objectivity' in psychological 'measurement' are not impressive, and it is doubtful whether 'objective' measurements are, strictly speaking, possible in Psychology. It is certain that 'measurements' in the ordinary physical meaning of that word are not applicable to *psychological* investigations. The reason for this is very simple. Physical measurements as used in the natural sciences are expressed in appropriate units, like centimetres, grams and seconds; once we have defined these units, we can measure weight, volume, duration, acceleration and other physical attributes in terms of these fundamental units. But there are no similar fundamental units in which to express 'psychological measures', with the exception of units of time. Measurement in psychology consists in assigning a *number* to certain data and not in evaluating the data in terms of fundamental units. Thus when we 'measure' a child's intelligence we place him in a certain position on a scale relative to other children who have taken the same test. His 'IQ' is a number, which denotes his position on this scale. Alternatively, his intelligence is expressed as a *ratio* between two numbers, one being his chronological age and the other being the score (expressed in terms of his 'mental age') that he gains on a given test. It is clear that the unit of time or duration enters into psychological assessments, but this is the only such unit and it indicates change in a psychological feature, and is not itself a direct psychological measure.

It is advisable to avoid the term 'measure' in psychological statements, owing to its ambiguity and its traditional association with physics. On almost every occasion another and more suitable word can be employed, such as assess, estimate, ascertain or evaluate. These words do not suggest the use of c.g.s. units and imply nothing more than the process of counting.

Objectivity

The word 'objective' occurs frequently in psychological discussion, but it is very difficult both to define and to use correctly. In Psychology it has two quite different implications. Its fundamental psychological meaning as defined by English and English (12) is 'not dependent upon the judgment or accuracy of the individual observer; free from personal and emotional bias; hence, open to observation by any competent observer'.

A sixth definition by the same authority reads 'localised by the observer outside his own body'. It may be argued that no psychological test is 'objective' in the sense of the first of the above definitions, since some personal bias is inevitable at some stage of the compilation, administration or scoring of the test. Various devices are employed to eliminate bias as far as possible, and they are highly successful in many tests of intelligence. The term 'objective' is also applied to that *method* of scoring a test in which the judgement of the examiner is not required. An 'objective' *test* on the other hand is one in which the examiner's influence is reduced to an absolute minimum. This type of test may or may not be objectively scored. Provided these definitions are kept in mind, the term 'objective' may be properly used in discussing psychological tests. Yet it still remains true that the presence of the examiner in the test situation will influence the test procedure and probably the test results also. A coldly 'scientific' attitude on the part of the examiner will tend to discourage the patient and depress his score, whilst a warm, sympathetic, understanding attitude will put him at ease and encourage him to make the maximum effort of which he is capable. Strictly speaking neither of these attitudes is 'objective', but the latter is the correct approach to the patient in clinical psychological work.

Current Trends in Testing

There is an increasing tendency for the assessment of children's disorders to be 'family-centred'. Less attention is being paid to the 'child-in-isolation' and more attention is being given to the 'child-within-the-family'. This influences test procedures in two ways. First, there is a tendency to assess the other members of the family and hence to test adults even in a children's clinic. Secondly, the test results will be viewed in relation to the social, economic and cultural characteristics of the family and not regarded as simple 'measures' of an isolated individual's abilities.

A further important trend is to regard the objective, or quantitative, test as the source of valuable qualitative information. This means that the manner in which a child responds to the various items presented during the test is almost as important, clinically, as the numerical result of the test.

Another trend, made possible by the work of Gesell (14), is the increased interest in the testing of pre-school children and of those referred to the paediatrician. This frequently enables an early diagnosis of intellectual defect to be made and also assists in differentiating between those who are simply retarded and those who are mentally subnormal.

These trends have taken the Psychologist away from the view that a single test of intellectual ability, applied objectively to an isolated individual, would give an invariable IQ. This view was probably a by-product of nineteenth-century determinism, which entered psychological thinking via Freud and the Behaviourists. It is now realised that the IQ is not invariable, although it probably has a maximum possible value for any given individual. However measured, the IQ is essentially an indication of the individual's ability to perform a series of specified tasks. These tasks usually, but not always, sample a wide range of knowledge and abilities.

Types of Tests Available

There are literally hundreds of tests available for use by the Psychologist, and others are frequently being devised. Many of them are intended for research use only, but scores of standardised tests are listed in the catalogues of firms who supply psychological equipment. Although most of these tests will be used by a Psychologist at one time or another there are a relatively small number which are in daily use, and it is these which are described in this chapter. While special investigations naturally require the use of specialised tests, it is good clinical practice to extract the maximum amount of information from a few tests rather than to use many tests and gain little data from each. Familiarity with a few well known tests is of more value to the Psychiatrist than a passing acquaintance with a large number of psychological techniques which require specialised knowledge for their application.

The tests to be discussed are classified under five headings, as follows: I, Tests of Intelligence; II, Projection Tests; III, Tests of Educational Attainments; IV, Vocational Guidance Tests; V, Tests of Organic Involvement.

2

Tests of Intelligence

Intelligence tests may be divided into verbal and non-verbal types, and further subdivided into the age-range for which they are suitable. Verbal tests, as the name implies, are 'question and answer' tests, in which the question and the reply may be either oral or written. Non-verbal tests require material to be manipulated in response to oral, or written, instructions. The non-verbal tests are especially useful for testing children with poor speech or low educational attainments. These tests are less dependent upon cultural and social factors than verbal tests and are frequently valuable in assessing the abilities of handicapped children.

Both verbal and non-verbal tests are designed for specified age-ranges, as follows: (i) under 5 years or pre-school; (ii) 5 to 15 years inclusive; (iii) 16 years and upwards. Some tests are applicable to age-ranges lying within or overlapping these groupings.

TESTS FOR PRE-SCHOOL CHILDREN

There are three very useful tests for children below the age of 5 years, namely the Gesell Schedules, the Griffiths Mental Development Scale and the Merrill-Palmer Scale. Generally speaking below the age of five, the younger the child, the more the tests tend to depend upon physical activities rather than upon psychological abilities. During the first twelve months of life a psychological test will add very little to the assessment of development made by a paediatrician. But by the second year a psychological assessment may usefully be undertaken, in addition to a physical examination. By the age of three it is often possible to estimate the psychological ability of a child who is physically defective, or who has been deprived emotionally or socially and so gives the impression of being mentally retarded.

The Gesell Developmental Schedules. These schedules were devised by the late Dr. Arnold Gesell and his colleagues and are described in detail in Gesell and Amatruda, *Developmental Diagnosis* (15). The schedules are used to assess four areas of development, namely Motor Development, Language Ability, Adaptive Behaviour and Personal-Social Development. Each area is assessed and 'scored' separately and a Developmental Quotient (DQ) is calculated for each developmental area. It is important to remember that this 'DQ' is *not* related to the 'IQ', although for normally developed children the numerical values of the two may be quite close together. The schedules are based on the general principle that at a certain age a child is normally able to perform certain actions, either on request or after they have been demonstrated to him. Thus a two-year-old is normally able to run; to kick a ball (without being shown how to do it); to imitate the shapes O and V; to give his name and to use simple phrases or sentences. Similarly at other ages he is normally able to perform a well defined series of actions. Up to the age of twelve months the child's abilities are assessed at four-week intervals, from the age of 56 weeks to 24 months the intervals are 3 months, and thereafter assessments are made at 6-month intervals. Scoring consists of counting the items passed at the various age-levels in each of the four developmental areas. The age-level at which items are successfully completed is the child's Developmental Age. The Developmental Quotient or DQ is given by the following formula:

$$DQ = \frac{\text{Developmental Age}}{\text{Chronological Age}} \times 100.$$

Each of the four developmental areas provides its own DQ, so that *four* quotients, not one, are required for the overall assessment.

Normally these four values of the DQ are quite close to each other, but in assessing emotionally disturbed children it is frequently found that there is a wide divergence between the values. This divergence obviously indicates that the child is backward in one or more areas of development. This backwardness may, or may not, be due to his emotional disorder; the schedules may indicate that he is backward, but they cannot indicate the reason for it.

The schedules may be employed for assessing all pre-school children. Mentally subnormal children may attempt them at almost any age.

The Griffiths Mental Development Scale. This scale is described in detail by Griffiths (17), and is similar to the Gesell Schedules but more elaborate. It covers the period from birth to 24 months only. The child's ability is assessed by using the following five sub-scales: Locomotor; Personal-Social; Hearing and Speech; Eye and Hand; Performance. Each sub-scale consists of 52 items arranged in order of difficulty. One, two, or three items are provided for each month of developmental age. The test items may be taken in any order, but they are continued in each sub-scale until the child has failed six successive items. The scores for each of the five sub-scales are totalled and converted to a Mental Age (MA). A General Intelligence Quotient (GQ) is derived from the formula

$$GQ = \frac{MA}{CA} \times 100$$

where CA is the child's Chronological Age. A quotient may be obtained for each sub-scale and a 'profile' of GQs or of raw scores may be drawn.

In clinical work the profile is the most illuminating method of recording the results, and wide differences between the five scores or sub-quotients may be expected.

For children under two years of age this test may be used in conjunction with the Gesell Schedules. Each may act as a re-test for the other, or used together they may corroborate each other.

The Merrill-Palmer Scale. This scale, described in detail by Stutsman (39), covers the age-range 18 to 71 months. There are 93 items in the scale, but these are not all different, since extra credit is given for some items if they are completed within specified time limits. These items predominate in the scale and include picture puzzles, matching and buttoning exercises and the Seguin Formboard. The verbal items included in the scale consist of simple directions, repetition of words and phrases, questions and the meanings of words.

The scoring is arranged so that if the child refuses to attempt an item or 'spoils' an attempt, allowance may be made for this in the total score. It is also possible to omit the verbal items and obtain an estimate of the child's ability based upon the performance items only. The total score may be expressed in terms of Mental Age, Percentiles, or Standard Deviations from the Mean. An *approximate* value for the IQ may be found from the formula

$$IQ = \frac{MA}{CA} \times 100,$$

but the IQ derived in this way is only approximate and is not strictly comparable with IQs obtained by other tests at other age-levels. Nor is it strictly comparable with the DQ or the GQ. Scores obtained on one test are frequently related to scores obtained on another, and the correlation between specific tests is given in the manuals which describe them. The clinician must beware of comparing the quotients obtained in different tests unless he knows the correlation between them. A *general* comparison of the results of different tests is permissible even if their inter-correlations are unknown, but this should be made on an item basis, when the discrepancies between the tests will be clinically more illuminating than their agreements.

When testing pre-school children for clinical purposes it is usually sufficient to place them within one of the following categories: mentally subnormal; borderline; dull; below average; about average; above average; superior. The precise value of the quotient obtained is of secondary importance.

TESTS FOR CHILDREN OF SCHOOL AGE

Wechsler Intelligence Scale for Children. The most useful intelligence test for clinical purposes, for the age-range 5-15 years, is the Wechsler Intelligence Scale for Children. This is described by Wechsler (44), and although American in origin it has been modified for use with English children. Commonly known as the W.I.S.C. ('wisk'), it consists of a Verbal Scale and a Performance Scale with six sub-tests in each.

The *Verbal Scale* comprises:—(1) *General Information*, which consists of 30 questions, like a wide-ranging general knowledge 'quiz'. (2) *General Comprehension*, which tests the child's understanding of social life. (3) *Arithmetic*, a graded series of problems ranging from simple counting to a complex calculation. (4) *Similarities*. This sub-test is divided into two parts: the first part consists of four sentence completion items and the second part of the names of twelve pairs of objects, the subject being required to say how each member of the pair is similar to the other. (5) *Vocabulary*. A list of 40 words of graded difficulty are presented for definition. (6) *Digit Span* consists of a series of numbers for repetition both forwards and backwards.

The *Performance Scale* consists of:—(1) *Picture Completion*, a set of 20 pictures with one significant detail omitted in each. (2) *Picture Arrangement* is similar to a 'strip cartoon': a series of pictures is presented in random order and the subject is required to arrange them in a logical sequence. (3) *Block Design* consists of making patterns with red and white blocks in accordance with specified designs. (4) *Object Assembly*, as its name implies, consists in putting together a Mannikin, a Horse, a Face and a Motor Car. (5) *Coding* requires geometrical shapes to be matched with numbers in a specified manner. (6) *Mazes* requires the tracing of paths through a graded series of mazes.

Each sub-test is administered and scored independently. There are time limits for most items and additional credit is also given for the speedy completion of most performance items. Three estimates of the subject's IQ are obtained, one from each scale and one from the combined scales. The IQ is not based upon the concept of mental age, but is derived from the statistical distribution of the scores at each age-level. The IQ values for different ages are strictly comparable.

The W.I.S.C. possesses a number of features which make it especially useful in clinical work. It employs a wide variety of material which stimulates the child's interest. A wide range of knowledge and ability is tested, and several sub-tests are largely free from educational influences. Children who have difficulty in talking, or deaf children, may be tested by the Performance Scale only. The interest of apathetic children is often aroused by the items in the Performance Scale and it is then possible to present the Verbal Scale; if only verbal items were available, no result would probably be obtained from such children. It is not essential to present all twelve sub-tests; a selection may be made from them if time prevents the administration of both Scales. If for any reason a sub-test is 'spoiled' or interrupted, its score may be discarded and the total score pro-rated to give an IQ. The omission of one or two sub-tests does not usually appreciably influence the final result. There are several 'short forms' of the test which may be used when the time for the test is severely restricted. These short forms show a fairly high correlation with the complete test, but they should never be used if there is time to administer the whole test. Much useful clinical information may often be gained from the *manner in which* the child attempts to answer the items presented.

The scores for the sub-tests considered separately, or in combination with each other, are often useful 'diagnostic pointers'. Suppose the following scores are obtained from a boy of 11 years of age:

Verbal Scale	Scaled Score	*Performance Scale*	Scaled Score
General Information	5	Picture Completion	14
General Comprehension	12	Picture Arrangement	13
Arithmetic	6	Block Design	16
Similarities	12	Object Assembly	10
Vocabulary	8	Coding	7
Digit Span	4	Mazes	9
Sum	47	Sum	69
IQ	96	IQ	127

The low scores of 5, 6 and 8 would suggest poor school attainments since the corresponding sub-tests are greatly influenced by school work. The score of 4 for Digit Span suggests inability to concentrate and a poor memory. These facts are congruent with poor educational progress. The two high scores of 12 indicate an above-average basic ability, since success in these two sub-tests depends more upon the ability to reason and to observe than upon formal education.

The lower scores in the Performance Scale are indicative of anxiety. The higher scores indicate a basically good ability. The Block Design score of 16 indicates facility in handling material (manual dexterity) and good perceptual ability.

The overall assessment of these results indicates that the boy is basically of above average ability and that the Performance IQ of 127 is probably a better estimate of his ability than the Verbal IQ of 96. He is making poor progress at school, he lacks concentration and is anxious. He can reason well, is observant and is socially well informed.

These scores and the deductions made from them illustrate how the results of the W.I.S.C. may be used in making a clinical assessment of a child. Many variations in the pattern of the scores are possible. Relatively *low* scores for Block Design, Object Assembly and Picture Arrangement might indicate perceptual difficulties, which might be due to organic brain damage. *High* scores for General Information, General Comprehension and Vocabulary might be gained by a child from a culturally good home. No combination of scores by itself is an adequate basis for a diagnosis of psychological disorder; but the clinician should look for these 'patterns' in the scores and regard them either as corroborating other evidence or as indicating the need for further investigation.

Progressive Matrices. This test, devised by Raven (32), may be used to obtain quickly an estimate of a child's intellectual ability. It can be completed in 20 minutes or half an hour, compared with at least one hour required for administration of the W.I.S.C. It is also scored in a much shorter time. The Matrices do not sample such a wide range of ability as the W.I.S.C. since they require a rather special reasoning ability and perceptual discrimination. The full test consists of five series, lettered A to E, of twelve items each. Each item is of the 'completion' variety, and consists of a large rectangle containing either an 'overall pattern' or a series of geometrical figures. There is also a blank space in the rectangle which may be filled by just *one* of several figures or patterns which are printed beneath it; the test consists of choosing the appropriate pattern or figure which will complete the large rectangle. The test is suitable for an age range of 6–13½ yrs. The final score does not provide an IQ but is expressed in terms of percentiles. Owing to its rather specialised nature it does not appear to correlate very closely with tests like the W.I.S.C.

Stanford-Binet Intelligence Scale. This is still the most widely used of all tests of mental ability. It is described in detail by Terman and Merrill (42), and has recently been issued in a third revised form (43). This test was developed from the intelligence scales devised by Binet and Simon, which were first published in 1905 and subsequently modified in 1908 and 1911. In 1916 the Stanford Revision of the Binet-Simon intelligence scale was published; this was revised in 1937 and in 1960.

The S-B Scale tests a range of ability extending from a normal two-year-old to a superior adult. There are two forms, L and M, which enable re-tests to be carried out effectively. The scale is heavily loaded with verbal items and so depends largely upon linguistic ability for its completion. It is also educationally loaded and does not separate verbal from performance items as the W.I.S.C. does. It is a useful scale for assessing mental ability within an educational context, but it is inferior to the W.I.S.C. for clinical purposes.

Wechsler Adult Intelligence Scale (W.A.I.S.). Since the upper limit of the W.I.S.C. is 15 years 11 months it is necessary to use the W.A.I.S. (45) when assessing the mental ability of the older adolescent. This adult version of the W.I.S.C. covers an age-range of 16–75 years. It is very similar to the W.I.S.C. in administration and construction and has the same clinical usefulness; it is not necessary therefore to discuss it in detail. The handbook (46) gives a full account of the test.

The Diagnostic Use of Intelligence Tests

The use of the W.I.S.C. as an aid in diagnosing educational retardation or perceptual difficulties has already been mentioned. The test may also be used, within the appropriate age-range, for differentiating between lack of basic ability and remediable retardation due to adverse family, emotional or personal influences. Thus a child may appear apathetic and make little educational progress and therefore be regarded as mentally backward or educationally subnormal (E.S.N.), but in an encouraging environment, together with the stimulus of intrinsically interesting test material, his test score may make it quite clear that his basic ability is much greater than it appears to be.

This concept of 'basic' or 'potential' mental ability is very important in clinical work. It is now known that the IQ as measured by an intelligence test does not have an invariable value, but is influenced by many factors, including error due to the test procedure and practice effects. If a subject undergoes a series of intelligence tests at regular intervals, his IQ may show a successive increase on each test, up to a maximum or limiting value. This maximum value represents his 'potential' or 'basic' ability. If the subject were 'emotionally disturbed' he would obtain an IQ which misrepresented his real ability. A consideration of the pattern of the scores in the W.I.S.C. often enables the examiner to tell whether or not the IQ is indicative of the subject's basic ability.

In assessing the reliability of the final result of an intelligence test, it is necessary to consider the behaviour of the subject in the test situation. It is almost as important to assess correctly the manner in which the subject attempts the test as it is to score the test correctly. An occasional high score combined with restlessness, lack of concentration and impulsive behaviour would indicate that the child's basic ability is greater than the IQ suggests. It is being increasingly recognised that the subject's general reaction to the test procedure is as clinically important as the test results. The test may therefore be regarded as a highly structured interview rather than as a mechanical 'psychometric' procedure.

There are some ages at which the diagnostic use of an intelligence test is especially valuable. It is sometimes possible to tell whether pre-school children are basically of low intelligence or simply retarded. Occasionally it is possible to reassure parents that their child is not mentally subnormal on the basis of his test performance. If a child is 'emotionally disturbed' and performs at a subnormal level, it is not possible to say that he *is* subnormal. If he *appears* to be sub-normal but performs at a 'near-average' level of ability, then it is safe to say that the child is *not* subnormal.

Neurotic breakdown may occur in school children because they are under pressure to attempt work which is too difficult for them. The W.I.S.C. results show whether or not they are capable of mastering the work they are attempting.

The results of an intelligence test may also help to prepare parents for their child's possible failure in the 'eleven plus' or the G.C.E. exams, or alternatively they may help to explain the unexpected failure which has already occurred. The W.I.S.C., by differentiating between basic ability and educational achievement, may show that although the child has made good educational progress through hard work he does not possess the basic ability to enable him to meet successfully the demands of higher education.

When assessing a child's ability to pass a given examination, it should be remembered that he is likely to gain a higher score on an individually administered intelligence test than on a corresponding group test or in an examination.

INTELLIGENCE TESTS FOR PHYSICALLY HANDICAPPED CHILDREN

The testing of physically handicapped children may be undertaken either by a test devised specially for them or by a modified form of the test appropriate to normal children. Skill in improvising a test procedure is frequently demanded from the Examiner, and often he must *estimate* the level at which the child succeeds with an item rather than measure it accurately. Sometimes it is possible to use a selection of items from two or more comparable tests. A high correlation between the results of these partial tests encourages confidence in the resulting assessment of the child.

Deaf or Partially Deaf Children. Provided that the deaf child under-stands what the Examiner wishes him to do, either by gesture or sign language, the performance items only from one of the standard tests may be administered. Alternatively the Drever-Collins (9) or the Alexander Passalong Test (1) may be presented.

Partially Sighted Children. The verbal items or the verbal scale from a standard test may be employed to test children whose sight is so poor that they cannot use the performance material. The Williams Intelligence

Test for Children with Defective Vision (47) uses many items from, or similar to, the Terman Merrill Test (42), together with some specially designed material for use with very young children.

Children with Impaired Motor Ability. Children who are unable to use their limbs efficiently cannot usually complete performance items satisfactorily. They may be able to complete performance items which are *not* timed, while timed items may be attempted on a pass-or-fail basis. If these items are taken from a standard test, only an approximate score can be obtained. The Examiner may, however, assess the *quality* of the child's performance and make some allowance for this in the final assessment. Provided there are no defects of speech or hearing, verbal items only may be used to assess the ability of these children. The Progressive Matrices devised by Raven (32) may also be used provided the child can point accurately to the solution chosen.

Brain-damaged Children. The nature and extent of damage to the brain will determine the test to be used. Aphasic patients may be able to indicate their choice if alternative solutions are presented. A test employing this technique has been devised by Kogan and Crager (24) for pre-school children. The tests currently available for this class of children have been listed and discussed by Graham and Berman (16).

Validity of the Results. The scores obtained by brain-damaged and physically handicapped children in the tests already mentioned must be treated with caution. Only a few tests have been standardised on handicapped populations, and even their validity is not beyond dispute. It cannot be assumed that the average scores of normal children will correspond exactly to the mean scores of handicapped children, even when the same test is applied to both groups. In assessing the intelligence of handicapped children the Examiner must rely to some extent upon his wisdom and experience. He may be able to assign approximate scores to some items and to estimate the degree of success attained in others. This method of 'estimating' the child's success is not entirely satisfactory, but it is sometimes all that the Examiner can do. Although it will not provide an *accurate* estimate of the child's intelligence, it may often enable the Psychologist to say that the child is 'at least of average ability' or that 'he is certainly not mentally subnormal'. If a small battery of 'part-tests' is administered, the results may confirm each other and so give added weight to the estimate of the child's intelligence.

Factors Influencing Test Results and their Interpretation

It is generally agreed that the raw scores in an intelligence test do not differ, fundamentally, from the scores gained in a scholastic test or examination. The intelligence test differs from other types of test in being more carefully constructed, more precisely marked and more closely related to the level of performance of a representative group of children of a given age. But so far as the child is concerned, it is one test amongst others and the 'marks' (i.e. raw scores) he receives for it are related to the level of his performance just like the marks he receives for his work at school. It follows that the results of the intelligence test are influenced by the factors which influence his school performance. In addition to basic ability, these factors include cultural background, degree of neuroticism and anxiety, parental influence and personality traits.

Cultural influences, or socio-economic factors, are important because they determine the amount of stimulation that a child receives from home and the range of experience that is open to him. Stimulation may be either personal or material. 'Personal stimulation' by his parents encourages the child to experiment with new ideas and activities and rewards successful achievement. It also sets a good example of effort and conduct, and provides a cultural milieu of good conversation and ideas in which the child may develop. 'Material stimulation' is provided by an adequate supply of play material and expressive media during the pre-school stage, and books and equipment for crafts, hobbies and games during later school life. Curry (8) claims that 'as the intellectual ability decreases from high to low, the effect of social and economic conditions on scholastic achievement increases greatly.' While favourable socio-economic factors cannot, as far as we know, improve the child's basic ability, they provide the optimal conditions under which his ability may develop. A child from a cultured home is therefore likely to score rather higher, especially on the culturally and educationally loaded tests, than a child with the same basic ability who comes from a home of a lower socio-economic level. It may be that the socio-economic status of the family has a differential effect upon the child's ability according to his basic intellectual level.

The child's degree of anxiety, or 'emotional disturbance', also affects his test scores. Hoch and Zubin (20) have summarised some of the results of anxiety upon test performance. In a clinical psychological setting anxiety may diminish concentration, interfere with recall, produce 'thoughtless' answers and decrease the span of attention. Young children may be so over-active and lacking in concentration that they may be untestable.

Some degree of neuroticism or anxiety may, however, be beneficial to test performance, since Lynn and Gordon (26) suggest that 'the optimum level of neuroticism for academic performance appears to be in the region of half a standard deviation above the national average.'

Parental pressure upon a child may 'drive' him to work very hard, and so his educational attainments may be appreciably greater than his basic intellectual ability would indicate. This state of affairs is sometimes disclosed by a high score on Vocabulary, Information and Comprehension and a relatively low score on most of the Performance sub-tests. Occasionally some 'parental pressure' may be advisable. If it is excessive it may produce a breakdown, because the child is being driven to try to achieve a standard of academic success of which he is not capable.

Personality traits also influence test performance. Other factors being constant, traits like persistence, independence and interest are, according to Astington (3), favourable to high scoring—whereas irritability, indifference or sullenness probably depress test scores.

It is perhaps advisable to mention two 'cautions' which should be observed in making a preliminary assessment of a child's ability. The well-dressed child who has a highly cultured home may have acquired pleasing manners and good speech. A good initial impression may therefore be created and the Examiner may associate this with high intelligence, whereas the child may be intellectually dull, as the W.I.S.C. results will make clear. Conversely, the unkempt child from a problem family may be of average or even above-average ability.

The other 'caution' refers to school reports. Very occasionally it happens that a child of more than average ability has sunk to the bottom of his class and has remained there, or has even been transferred to a special class. The school reports on such a child are unfavourable and so he acquires almost a reputation for failure.

Because the factors just mentioned may have important effects upon test performance, it is important to review the test results in the light of all the information that is available about the child.

3

Projective Techniques

Nature and Definition

There are a large number of projective techniques for use with children, which are reviewed in detail by Rabin and Haworth (30). A projective technique is defined by English and English (12) as 'a procedure for discovering a person's characteristic modes of behaviour (his attitudes, motivations or dynamic traits) by observing his behaviour in response to a situation that does not elicit or compel a particular response'. The administration of a projective technique may be divided into: the situation, the stimulus, and the response.

The *situation* in which the test is administered may determine the success or failure of the procedure. It is essential for the maximum possible rapport to be established between the Subject and the Examiner. The child must be made to feel that the Examiner is positively friendly towards him and that within this relationship it is 'safe' for him to disclose his personal thoughts and feelings. It follows that it is frequently impossible to establish an adequate degree of rapport during the first interview with the child, so that the administration of a projective technique may have to be delayed until the child's second or his third interview. The initial interviews may be utilised for administering more formal tests, or they may be devoted to playing with the child and gaining his confidence.

The *stimulus* consists of the material used to evoke the child's response. It may consist of pictures; words or phrases; material for manipulation and arrangement; or 'expressive' material, including drawing and dramatic materials. Examples of these different types of stimuli are described in the next section.

The *responses* that the child makes to the stimulus material are determined by: (a) his own past experience, (b) his imagination, and occasionally (c) recent events which have impressed or interested him. Most responses will reflect his own experience, since he will usually rely upon this to provide him with a meaning for an ambiguous stimulus. Sometimes he will respond by describing what he would like his experience to be, rather than by describing it as it actually is. Occasionally accounts of recent incidents which have impressed the child may be included in his responses. It is therefore not always possible to distinguish clearly between these sources (a), (b) and (c). Hence it is unwise to *interpret* the results of a projective technique in isolation from the other information which is available concerning the subject. It is however advisable to *score* the test results without this addionatil knowledge.

Because elements of phantasy and wishful thinking may influence the responses, projective techniques are frequently unreliable and poorly validated from a statistical point of view. They have therefore been strongly criticised by Eysenck (13) and others. But in spite of this statistical objection they are very useful clinically, when used in conjunction with other methods of investigation.

Classification of Projective Techniques

Projective techniques may be classified according to the type of response which they elicit. This classification is favoured by Rabin and Haworth (30), who enumerate the following kinds of responses: association; construction; completion; choice; expression. A modified form of this classification is used in the present discussion.

' Association' Techniques

Under this heading are included three picture techniques which require the child to 'associate' the figures in the pictures with the members of his family and his friends. He is asked to describe what is taking place in the pictures, or else to eompose a story about them. The pictures are introduced quite informally and the child's responses are recorded verbatim.

Symonds Picture Story Test. This consists of twenty pictures showing adult and adolescent figures, singly or in groups. Seven cards include parental figures and five portray sibling figures; the other eight cards show solitary figures. The cards are intended to be used by adolescents and should enable them to disclose their conflicts, phantasies, latent wishes, impulses and anxieties. Several of the cards also encourage the subject to describe his relationships with his family. It is presented as a test of 'creative imagination', and should be interpreted in the light of all the available case material. An extensive discussion of the test is provided by

PLATE 1

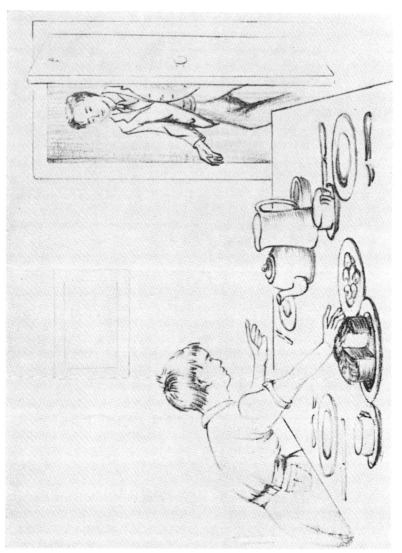

Specimen card from the Family-relations Indicator.

Symonds (40), who considers in some detail the picture method of studying personality.

A Test of Family Attitudes. This was devised by Jackson (23), and comprises eight pictures showing family scenes. The figures in the pictures have blurred outlines as if drawn in charcoal, and several of the scenes are highly structured. A set of questions is provided for use with each picture, in case the child's spontaneous responses are inadequate. The author claims that there are significant differences between the types of responses given to the pictures by normal, neurotic and delinquent groups of children. Although there is a psychoanalytic background to the test, it may be used effectively by those who subscribe to other psychological theories.

The Family Relations Indicator. This projective technique, developed by Howells and Lickorish (22), is specifically intended to disclose the relationships that exist between the child and the members of his family. It consists of 33 cards measuring 8 in. × 6 in., which were drawn to specifications laid down by the authors. Each card shows one of more members of a family in a domestic or an out-of-doors setting. They are so arranged that the following sequence is repeated three times: family group, father and child, mother and child, child alone, sibling group, and child and baby. The figures are clearly drawn but show a minimum of emotional expression. There are separate cards for use with boys and girls. The test has been given a clinical trial over a period of four years. No special procedure is required for its administration beyond good rapport. It is scored simply by inspecting the responses and grouping similar items.

The validation study was based on a detailed knowledge of the case histories of 50 families. On a simple 'agree-disagree' basis, the mother-child relationships given by the Indicator were shown to be correct in 80% of the cases and the father-child relationships in 70% of the cases. Other valuable clinical information is often provided by the Indicator. It is not based on any particular psychological theory and does not need to be 'interpreted', but provides factual information about family relationships. The picture in Plate 1 is an example of the type of card used in this Indicator.

The Children's Apperception Test. This test by Bellak (4) is especially suitable for young children. Instead of human figures, the pictures portray animal figures acting like humans. The test is based upon psychoanalytical theory and also upon the view that children respond more readily to pictures of animals than to pictures of human beings. Some doubt has been thrown upon this view by Biersdorf and Marcuse (7), but it has not been disproved. It is possible that these animal pictures may be used successfully by non-analysts to gain an understanding of the child's personal traits and personal relationships.

'Constructive' Techniques

These projective methods form a link between the more formal diagnostic procedures and the type of investigation used in play therapy;

they are also akin to the expressive methods mentioned below. A widely used formal test requiring constructive ability is the Make-A-Picture-Story Test (M.A.P.S.) devised by Shneidman (38). This test consists of a number of background pictures showing scenes of home, school and the outside world, together with a large number of assorted 'cut-out' figures. The child is presented with a background picture and asked to chose cut-out figures and arrange them upon it. As the child 'makes the picture' he is also encouraged to tell a story about it.

There are several methods of interpreting the 'picture-story' and the Examiner adopts the method which is consistent with his general psychological outlook. This type of test allows the child to become 'absorbed' in the manipulative aspect of the test and so be less 'self-conscious' in expressing himself verbally.

'Completion' Techniques

The most useful completion techniques are story completion, sentence completion and the Rosenzweig Picture-Frustration Test.

Story completions are usually based upon psychoanalytical concepts, but even those who do not accept the tenets of psychoanalysis may find these stories useful. They may help to establish rapport between the child and the Examiner, ir, as Rabin and Haworth (30) point out, they may 'lead children to express some of their difficulties . . . in an indirect way . . . with a minimum of discomfort' (p. 195). The stories cannot be scored 'objectively' but are interpreted according to the theoretical framework favoured by the Examiner. Story-completion techniques have been devised by Thomas (28) and Raven (31). These procedures should be regarded as 'structured interviews' rather than as formal tests.

The *sentence completion technique* of Rotter (35) is not suited to primary school children, but it may be presented to secondary school children of average or above-average ability. It is most suitable for adolescents, especially those who are well able to express themselves in writing. Each item consists of the initial word or phrase of a sentence and the subject is asked to complete the sentence. The completed items may be formally assessed, or evaluated simply by inspection.

The *Rosenzweig Picture Frustration Test* (34) consists of twenty-four cartoons showing children, with or without adults, in domestic, school and out-of-doors settings. In each cartoon one of the figures has spoken and the subject is required to insert a suitable reply in the space provided. A formal method of scoring the responses is provided.

'Forced Choice' Techniques

This method is usually more suitable for adults than for children, and is employed extensively in the construction of Questionnaires. Two examples of this technique which may be used with children and adolescents are the Family Relations Test and the Mooney Problem Check List.

The *Family Relations Test* was devised by Anthony and Bene (2). It consists of a number of cardboard figures from which the child chooses those he would like to represent the members of his family. He is next given a number of small cards on which are printed statements which could apply to various members of his family. The child is asked to 'post' these cards, one at a time, in the little boxes attached to the family figures. If any statement does not apply to a member of the family it is given to a figure called Nobody. The results are scored in terms of 'ingoing' and 'outgoing'; 'positive' and 'negative' feelings; degree of involvement, over-protection and over-indulgence.

The *Mooney Problem Check List* (29) consists of 330 statements (College Form) of personal, domestic and other problems. The subject is asked to underline those statements which describe his present worries and problems. A wide range of problems may be quickly surveyed in the initial interview, with a consequent saving of time.

'Expressive' Techniques

There are a large number of techniques which allow the child to express himself in various media and so encourage him to disclose some of his problems and difficulties. None of these techniques can be regarded as a formal test, but they provide means for establishing rapport, and also provide the *occasion* for the child to exhibit or even to discuss his difficulties. These techniques are frequently very dependent upon the interpretation given by the Examiner, and some of them require appreciable verbalisation by the child.

The need for verbalisation and interpretation is greatest when the child is presented with a 'squiggle', and asked to make it into some sort of drawing and then to talk about.

A more formal procedure is to request the drawing of specified objects, like the House-Tree-Person (H-T-P) Drawing Test devised by Hammer (18.)

The child may be requested to draw 'a person', followed by a drawing of one of the opposite sex. A formal enquiry may be carried out with regard to each figure along the lines suggested by Machover (27).

A method by which the child may indicate his preferences for certain members of his family was described by Szyrynski (41) in a paper read before the Western Regional Meeting of the Royal College of Physicians and Surgeons of Canada in 1961. It is called the Two-Houses Technique. The child enumerates all the members of his family and these are recorded on a sheet of paper. Two houses are drawn on the sheet and the child is invited to divide up the family, including himself, between the two houses. The subject is next asked to invite anyone from the *other* house into his *own* house. Later the families are again divided between the two houses as at first, and the subject is invited to *send away* one or more persons from his house to the other. In this way the child's order of preference for the members of his family may be investigated. The technique is still being developed and a manual describing it is in preparation.

Other 'expressive' methods may be used in investigating personality traits and inter-personal relationships. But the more expressive methods require more interpretation by the Examiner and require to be corroborated by information derived from other clinical sources. The use of Doll Play has been well reviewed by Levin and Wardwell (25), while drawing, painting and puppetry are other expressive techniques which may be used diagnostically. Generally, the expressive techniques form a link between formal diagnostic tests and therapeutic procedures: the one merges into the other, and any well conducted psychological interview probably has some therapeutic value.

A number of projective procedures have been described, because the application of projection techniques must be varied according to the nature of the patient as well as according to the problem being investigated. Some children will write their answers rather than verbalise them; others will attempt to draw, when they cannot write and are unable to verbalise, while many are more inclined to talk if they have material to manipulate. Projective procedures have a much lower statistical validity than tests of intelligence; it is therefore advisable to present at least two projective tests whenever possible, while the use of a small 'battery' of them is better still.

The 'projective' value of the standard intelligence tests themselves should not be underestimated. Considerable information about the child's personality may be gleaned by a careful observation of his behaviour in the test situation. The importance of relating the scores in an intelligence test to the child's behaviour during the test has already been pointed out. It is now emphasised that the behaviour itself is a useful source of information about the child's personality, although this is more formally investigated by projective techniques. It is therefore clinically worth while to devote considerable time and attention to observing and recording the child's behaviour during every test situation, irrespective of the formal test which is being presented.

4

Tests of Educational Attainment

The application of these tests is the concern of the Educational Psychologist rather than the Clinical Worker. However, psychiatric problems are sometimes intertwined with educational difficulties, so that it is advisable for the Clinical Psychologist to be familiar with at least the more usual tests of educational attainments.

The scores on certain sub-tests in the W.I.S.C. or W.A.I.S. are very valuable indicators of educational progress, as already mentioned. A more formal estimate of the child's attainments may be obtained by using the tests for reading, comprehension, spelling, word recognition and arithmetic devised by Schonell (36). The task of elucidating the causes of backwardness in any specific ability may be complex, requiring neurological, psychological and educational investigations. It should also be remembered that the child may have 'learned to fail' if he has had repeated lack of educational success over a period of years. In such circumstances it will be necessary for him to learn to gain confidence in himself as well as to learn the necessary reading or arithmetical processes.

Children are sometimes encouraged, or even forced, to attempt to learn to read before they are really able to do so. Hildreth and Griffiths (19) have devised a method of assessing whether or not the child is ready to begin to learn to read. An analysis of the difficulties encountered in reading may be made by using the scheme arranged by Durrell (10). The possibility of perceptual or neurological disorders must be considered in cases of read ng disability, since these disorders may occasionally be present. Similar diagnostic investigations may be required for analysing disabilities in writing and arithmetic. The effects of inappropriate teaching methods (consequent upon the special perceptual needs of the patient), absences from school at critical periods in the teaching program, and frequent changes of school, must all be considered when investigating educational backwardness. In addition sensory defects, and poor personal relationships within the family or within the school, may retard the child's educational progress. The diagnostic procedures mentioned are by no means exhaustive, but they may assist in distinguishing between the purely educational and the 'emotional' causes of backwardness.

5

Vocational Guidance

In clinical work, the psychologist will be called upon to give vocational guidance mainly to those young people who have either failed to obtain employment through the usual channels or are unable to remain in employment for any appreciable length of time. Those who frequently change their employment may be repeatedly discharged by their employers because they are incompetent, or else may leave their work because of their own personal problems or inter-personal difficulties. In such cases vocational guidance is concerned not only with assessing the aptitudes and abilities of the subject, but also with trying to ensure that the work recommended shall be consistent with his personal traits and shall not exacerbate his personal difficulties. There is no single test, or even any battery of tests, which will certainly determine what work the disturbed adolescent should do. Many of the tests already mentioned must be used to assess the subject's intelligence, his educational attainments, his personal traits and inter-personal relationships. The results of the test must be supplemented by his personal and family history, school record, and work record if any. In addition, one or more 'job preference' lists may be presented to the subject, in which he is asked to indicate which of the activities listed he would like to do. One or more informal interviews are necessary to gain information about his likes and dislikes, hobbies and other interests. An analysis of the information thus gained should enable the psychologist to assess the kind of work suited to the subject, and also the type of person (manager, foreman or employer) with whom he would be most likely to establish a good personal relationship. It will presumably be the duty of the Social Worker to discover the employment which most closely satisfies the recommendations. It should be clear that vocational guidance in a clinical setting is a very complex procedure and that there are no short, clear-cut methods of discovering the employment which any given young person should undertake. It may also be added that some form of psychotherapy is frequently an essential adjunct to the type of vocational guidance just described. The therapeutic measures, whether 'intra-' or 'extra-clinical', group or individual, should be aimed at assisting the adolescent to make the necessary adjustment to his new job, since it is unlikely that there will be complete accord between the ideal recommendations and the actual work available.

6

Tests of Organic Involvement

The phrase 'organic involvement' denotes that psychological skill or ability is impaired because of some identifiable physical defect in the child. Usually such a defect lies in the brain or C.N.S. or in the special senses, and is discovered as a result of a physical or neurological examination. Psychological tests cannot by themselves identify organic defects, but they may suggest the existence of defects and indicate the need for further investigation.

Colour vision may be tested by asking the young child to match and select the coloured blocks of the W.I.S.C., or even the coloured discs of the Merrill-Palmer Scale. Older children may attempt the Ishihara test of colour vision. Simple hearing tests may also be carried out along the lines suggested by Sheridan (37).

Less specific organic defects may be indicated by the use of the Visual Motor Gestalt Test by Bender (5). This test consists in copying a number of line drawings of a geometrical kind. The accuracy of the reproductions naturally increases with the age of the child. Levels of accuracy corresponding to ages from 4 to 11 years have been established, so that any serious deviation from these standards might indicate the possibility of organic disorder. Other indications of organic involvement are marked difficulty in arranging Block Designs, and inability to complete satisfactorily those items which require an appreciable degree of conceptualisation or 'abstract' thinking.

The younger the child, the less is the likelihood of obtaining useful results from these tests. Much depends upon the child's general ability and the degree of co-operation established between the child and the Examiner. Older children may attempt the Visual Retention Test by Benton (6), or Tests for Aphasia and Related Disturbances by Eisenson (11).

Older adolescents whose behaviour appears to be deteriorating may show this defect in their Wechsler scores, especially when these are evaluated by means of the deterioration formula (46). It must however be emphasised that the results of any of these tests, with the possible exception of Eisenson's, must be treated with extreme caution. Psychological deficiencies which may at first sight seem to be due to organic involvement may on careful investigation prove to be the result of under-stimulation, emotional disorder, or general retardation. The results of tests for organic involvement must be carefully correlated with other test results and with all other information available about the child.

7

Conclusion

The value of any psychological test is enhanced when it is seen in relation to the total amount of information about the child. This includes not only what is known about the child's personal behaviour, but also information about his whole environment, especially his family and school relationships. If the Psychologist is to interpret correctly the results of his tests, he must relate them to the rest of the information available. This may be accomplished by having adequate interviews with the child and his parents, and by presenting a small battery of tests rather than a single test. Pressure of time may often preclude the administration of more than one test, but this should be undertaken in a leisurely manner. It is much more valuable to administer, say, only half the W.I.S.C. under conditions of leisurely co-operation than to attempt to complete the whole test in a hurry. Adequate observation of the child in the test situation requires an unhurried approach in the test interview, and it is false economy of time and effort to speed up the procedure.

The use of a battery of tests whenever possible has been urged, but this implies that adequate time must be available for their presentation. One test, thoroughly and carefully administered, is of far more value than several which have been hastily completed. It is often not possible to present more than one test during the child's first attendance at the clinic, and occasionally the first interview must be used to establish rapport with the child and accustom him to his new surroundings. The establishment of good rapport is an essential prerequisite for psychological testing, and if necessary much time should be spent initially in making a good relationship with the child.

The assessment of the test results and the writing of the psychological report may require as much time, or more, than the actual administration of the test. The process of psychological testing is therefore a time-consuming procedure. To economise in time, a request for a psychological assessment should be as specific as possible. A vague request for 'personality tests' or 'assessment of ability' is inadequate, nor is it usually sufficient to ask for a specific test to be administered to the child. The Psychologist should be asked a specific question or questions, or alternatively be asked to investigate a specific problem. He will then be able to decide which tests and procedures should be used in the investigation. In order to interpret his results correctly the psychologist will also need further information about the child, its parents and its background. This may be obtained either from interviews or from other clinical sources.

When the psychologist is a member of a clinical team and does not take full responsibility for the case, there should be the fullest possible discussion between him and the clinical workers concerned. This will enable each member of the team to understand and appreciate the contribution made by each of the others. It will also prevent them from seeing the child simply as a 'problem'. For by sharing each other's insights and knowledge, they may appreciate that the child *has* a 'problem', which is due to distorted relationships and an unfavourable environment. By pooling their techniques and experience the clinical team may attack the problem from several angles, with better hope of success than an unidimensional approach would provide.

REFERENCES

1. ALEXANDER, W. P., 1946. *A Performance Scale for the Measurement of Practical Ability*. London: Nelson.
2. ANTHONY, E. J. and BENE, E., 1957. A technique for the objective assessment of the child's family relationships. *J. Ment. Sci.*, **103**: 541-555.
3. ASTINGTON, E., 1960. Personality assessments and academic performance in a Boys' Grammar School. *Brit. J. Educ. Psychol.*, **30**: 225-236.
4. BELLAK, L., 1954. *The T.A.T. and C.A.T. in Clinical Use*. New York: Grune & Stratton.
5. BENDER, L., 1938. A visual motor gestalt test and its clinical use. *Res. Monogr. Amer. Orthopsychiat. Ass.*, No. 3.
6. BENTON, A. L., 1955. *The Revised Visual Retention Test*. New York: Psychological Corporation.
7. BIERSDORF, K. R. and MARCUSE, F. L., 1953. Responses of children to human and animal pictures. *J. Proj. Tech.*, **17**: 455-459.
8. CURRY, R. L., 1962. The effect of socio-economic status on the scholastic achievement of Sixth Grade children. *Brit. J. Educ. Psychol.*, **32**: 46-49.
9. DREVER, J. and COLLINS, M., 1944. *Performance Tests of Intelligence* (3rd ed.). Edinburgh: Oliver & Boyd.
10. DURRELL, D. D., 1955. *Durrell Analysis of Reading Difficulty*. New York: World Book Co.
11. EISENSON, J., 1946. *Examining for Aphasia*. New York: Psychological Corporation.

12. ENGLISH, H. B. and A. C., 1958. *A Comprehensive Dictionary of Psychological and Psychoanalytical Terms.* New York: Longmans Green.
13. EYSENCK, H. J., 1959. Learning Theory and Behaviour Therapy. *J. Ment. Sci.,* 105: 61-75.
14. GESELL, A. *et al.,* 1940. *The First Five Years of Life.* New York: Harper Bros.
15. GESELL, A. and AMATRUDA, C. S., 1947. *Developmental Diagnosis* (2nd ed.). New York: P. B. Hoeber.
16. GRAHAM, F. K. and BERMAN, P. W., 1961. Current status of behaviour tests for brain damage in infants and pre-school children. *Amer. J. Orthopsychiat.,* 31: 713-727.
17. GRIFFITHS, R., 1954. *The Abilities of Babies.* Univ. of London Press.
18. HAMMER, E. F., 1955. *The H—T—P Clinical Research Manual.* Western Psychological Services, U.S.A.
19. HILDRETH, G. H. and GRIFFITHS, N. L., 1949. *Metropolitan Readiness Tests.* New York: World Book Co.
20. HOCH, P. H. and ZUBIN, J., 1952. *Relation of Psychological Tests to Psychiatry.* New York: Grune & Stratton.
21. HOWELLS, J. G. and LICKORISH, J. R., 1962. *The Family Relations Indicator.* National Foundation for Educational Research in England and Wales, 79 Wimpole Street, London, W.1.
22. 1963. The Family Relations Indicator: a projective technique for investigating intra-family relationships designed for use with emotionally disturbed children. *Brit. J. Educ. Psychol.,* 33: 286-296.
23. JACKSON, L., 1952. *A Test of Family Attitudes.* London: Methuen.
24. KOGAN, K. L. and CRAGER, R. L., 1959. A Standardisation of the Children's Picture Information Test. *J. Clin. Psychol.,* 15: 405-411.
25. LEVIN, H. and WARDWELL, E., 1962. The research uses of doll play. *Psychol. Bull.,* 59: 27-56.
26. LYNN, R. and GORDON, I. E., 1961. The relation of neuroticism and extraversion to intelligence and educational attainment. *Brit. J. Educ. Psychol.,* 31: 194-203.
27. MACHOVER, K., 1949. *Personality Projection in the Drawing of the Human Figure.* Springfield, Ill.: Thomas.
28. MILLS, E. S., 1953. The Madeleine Thomas Completion Stories Test. *J. Consult. Psychol.,* 17: 139-141.
29. MOONEY, R. L. and GORDON, L. V., 1950. *Mooney Problem Check List* (revised ed.). New York: Psychological Corporation.
30. RABIN, A. I. and HAWORTH, M. R., 1960. *Projective Techniques with Children.* New York: Grune & Stratton.
31. RAVEN, J. C., 1951. *Controlled Projection for Children* (2nd ed.). London: H. K. Lewis.
32. 1956. *Guide to the Standard Progressive Matrices* (revised ed.). London: H. K. Lewis.
33. 1958. *Guide to Using the Mill Hill Vocabulary Scale with the Progressive Matrices* (revised ed.). London: H. K. Lewis.
34. ROSENZWEIG, S., FLEMING, E. E. and ROSENZWEIG, L., 1948. The Children's Form of the Rosenzweig Picture-Frustration Study. *J. Psychol.,* 26: 141-191.
35. ROTTER, J. B. and RAFFERTY, J. E., 1950. *The Rotter Incomplete Sentences Blank.* New York: Psychological Corporation.
36. SCHONELL, F. J. and F. E., 1960. *Diagnostic and Attainment Testing* (4th ed.). Edinburgh: Oliver & Boyd.
37. SHERIDAN, M. D., 1958. Simple clinical hearing-tests for very young or mentally retarded children. *Brit. Med. J.,* ii, 999-1004.

38. SHNEIDMAN, E. S., 1949. *The Make a Picture Story Test*. New York: Psychological Corporation.
39. STUTSMAN, R., 1949. *Guide for Administering the Merrill-Palmer Scale of Mental Tests*. New York: World Book Co.
40. SYMONDS, P. M., 1949. Adolescent Phantasy. New York: Columbia Univ. Press.
41. SZYRYNSKI, V., 1963. A New Technique to Investigate Family Dynamics in Child Psychiatry. *Canadian Psychiat. Ass. J.*, 8: 94-103.
42. TERMAN, L. M. and MERRILL, M. A., 1937. *Measuring Intelligence*. London: Harrap.
43.   1960. *Stanford-Binet Intelligence Scale. Third Revision. Form L-M*. London Harrap.
44. WECHSLER, D., 1949. *Wechsler Intelligence Scale for Children*. New York: Psychological Corporation.
45.   1955. *Wechsler Adult Intelligence Scale*. New York: Psychological Corporation.
46.   1958. *The Measurement and Appraisal of Adult Intelligence* (4th ed.). The Williams and Wilkins Co., U.S.A.
47. WILLIAMS, M., 1956. *Williams Intelligence Test for Children with Defective Vision*. University of Birmingham, England.

AUTHOR INDEX

SUBJECT INDEX

DATE DUE

MAY 3 0 1982		
MAY 3 4 1983		
GAYLORD		PRINTED IN U.S.A.